BSAVA Manual of Abdominal Surgery
second edition

Editors:

John M. Williams
MA VetMB LLB CertVR DipECVS FRCVS
Northwest Surgeons, Delamere House,
Ashville Point, Sutton Weaver,
Cheshire WA7 3FW

Jacqui D. Niles
BVetMed CertSAS DipACVS
Metropolitan Veterinary Associates,
2626 Van Buren Avenue,
Norristown, PA 19403, USA

Published by:

British Small Animal Veterinary Association
Woodrow House, 1 Telford Way,
Waterwells Business Park, Quedgeley,
Gloucester GL2 2AB

A Company Limited by Guarantee in England
Registered Company No. 2837793
Registered as a Charity

The drawings in Operative Techniques 5.1, 5.2, 5.3, 5.4, 5.5, 5.6, 5.7, 5.8, 6.1, 6.2, 6.3, 8.1, 8.2, 8.3, 8.5, 8.6, 8.7, 8.8, 8.9, 8.10, 8.11, 9.1, 9.2, 9.3, 9.4, 9.5, 11.1, 12.1, 13.1, 14.1, 14.2, 14.4, 15.1, 15.2, 15.3, 15.4, 15.6, 16.3, 17.1, 17.3 and 17.6 and Figures 3.16, 4.3, 4.4, 4.5, 4.6, 4.14, 4.21, 5.1, 5.7, 5.12, 6.1, 6.15, 7.1, 7.8, 7.9, 7.14, 7.16, 8.1, 8.11, 8.12, 8.18, 8.21, 8.22, 9.1, 9.8, 9.9, 9.13, 9.14, 9.15, 10.2, 10.3, 11.1, 11.2, 12.3, 13.1, 14.17, 15.1, 15.2, 15.5, 15.11, 16.2, 17.1 and 17.2 were drawn by S.J. Elmhurst BA Hons (www.livingart.org.uk) and are printed with her permission.

A catalogue record for this book is available from the British Library.

ISBN 978 1 905319 62 6

The publishers, editors and contributors cannot take responsibility for information provided on dosages and methods of application of drugs mentioned or referred to in this publication. Details of this kind must be verified in each case by individual users from up to date literature published by the manufacturers or suppliers of those drugs. Veterinary surgeons are reminded that in each case they must follow all appropriate national legislation and regulations (for example, in the United Kingdom, the prescribing cascade) from time to time in force.

Printed in the UK by Severn, Gloucester GL2 5EU – a carbon neutral printer
Printed on ECF paper made from sustainable forests

Titles in the BSAVA Manuals series

For further information on these and all BSAVA publications, please visit our website: **www.bsava.com**

Contents

Contributors

Davina M. Anderson
MA VetMB PhD DSAS (ST) DipECVS MRCVS
Anderson Moores Veterinary Specialists,
The Granary, Bunstead Barns,
Poles Lane, Hursley,
Winchester, Hampshire SO21 2LL

Floryne O. Buishand
DVM
Department of Clinical Sciences of Companion Animals,
Faculty of Veterinary Medicine,
Utrecht University, Yalelaan 108,
3584 CM, Utrecht, The Netherlands

Gary W. Ellison
DVM MS DipACVS
Small Animal Surgery Department,
Small Animal Clinical Sciences,
College of Veterinary Medicine, University of Florida,
PO Box 100126, Health Science Center,
Gainsville, FL 32610-0126, USA

Alasdair Hotston Moore
MA VetMB CertSAC CertVR CertSAS MRCVS
Bath Veterinary Referrals,
Rosemary Lodge, Wellsway, Bath BA2 5RL

Geraldine B. Hunt
BCSc MVetClinStud PhD FACVSc
Department of Surgical and Radiological Sciences,
School of Veterinary Medicine,
University of California-Davis,
Shields Avenue, Davis, CA 95618, USA

Jolle Kirpensteijn
DVM PhD DipACVS DipECVS
Hills Pet Nutrition,
4010 SW 8th Avenue, Topeko, KS 66603, USA

Jane Ladlow
MA VetMB CertSAS CertVR DipECVS MRCVS
Department of Veterinary Medicine,
University of Cambridge, Madingley Road,
Cambridge CB3 0ES

Lori Ludwig
VMD MS DipACVS
Veterinary Speciality Care,
985 Johnnie Dodds Blvd,
Mount Pleasant, SC 29464, USA

Philipp D. Mayhew
BVM&S DipACVS MRCVS
Department of Surgical and Radiological Sciences,
School of Veterinary Medicine,
University of California-Davis,
Shields Avenue, Davis, CA 95618, USA

Mary A. McLoughlin
DVM MS DipACVS
Department of Veterinary Clinical Sciences,
The Ohio State University Veterinary Medical Center,
601 Vernon Tharp Street,
Columbus, OH 43210, USA

Alison Moores
BVSc(Hons) CertSAS DipECVS MRCVS
Anderson Moores Veterinary Specialists,
The Granary, Bunstead Barns,
Poles Lane, Hursley, Winchester,
Hampshire SO21 2LL

Prue Neath
BSc(Hons) BVetMed DipACVS DipECVS MRCVS
Oakwood Veterinary Referrals,
267 Chester Road,
Hartford, Cheshire CW8 1LP

Jacqui D. Niles
BVetMed CertSAS DipACVS
Metropolitan Veterinary Associates,
2626 Van Buren Avenue,
Norristown, PA 19403, USA

Brian A. Scansen
DVM MS DipACVIM (Cardiology)
Department of Veterinary Clinical Sciences,
The Ohio State University Veterinary Medical Center,
601 Vernon Tharp Street,
Columbus, OH 43210, USA

Catherine Sturgeon
BVetMed (Hons) CertSAS DipECVS MRCVS
Visiting Vet Specialists,
Chester

Elizabeth Welsh
BVMS PhD CertVA CertSAS MRCVS
Vets-Now Referrals,
123–145 North Street,
Glasgow, G3 7DA

Richard A.S. White
BVetMed PhD DVR DSAS (ST) DipACVS DipECVS MRCVS
Dick White Referrals,
Veterinary Specialist Centre, Station Farm,
London Road, Six Mile Bottom,
Suffolk CB8 0HU

John M. Williams
MA VetMB LLB CertVR DipECVS FRCVS
Northwest Surgeons,
Delamere House, Ashville Point,
Sutton Weaver,
Cheshire WA7 3FW

Foreword

In the 10 years since the publication of the first edition of the *BSAVA Manual of Canine and Feline Abdominal Surgery* there have been significant advances in the field of soft tissue surgery. From the materials used, to the procedures performed, this second edition of the Manual has been extensively revised and updated to take account of these new developments.

Abdominal surgery is an essential component of general small animal practice and as such I am proud to be President of the organization that has produced this excellent guide to the many procedures that many clinicians may be called upon to perform on a daily basis. *The BSAVA Manual of Canine and Feline Abdominal Surgery* provides a valuable resource dedicated to helping veterinary surgeons explore and evaluate abdominal surgical options in an easy to follow and practical way. I am particularly proud of the photographs and illustrations in this Manual which greatly facilitate its use.

Although open surgery remains the mainstay of small animal practice, laparoscopic procedures are gaining in popularity as clinicians become more familiar with the equipment and techniques. This increase in the use of minimally invasive techniques is reflected by the inclusion of a chapter dedicated to laparoscopic instrumentation and the fundamentals of laparoscopic surgery.

I extend my congratulations to the contributors to this Manual, who are all experts in their field, and to the editors, John Williams and Jacqui Niles, in putting together a new edition that will be sure to find a place on every practice shelf.

Patricia Colville BVMS MRCVS
BSAVA President 2015–16

Preface

'The incision must be as long as necessary'
Theodor Kocher (1841–1917)

The *BSAVA Manual of Canine and Feline Abdominal Surgery, 2nd edition* is a welcome update on the first edition and aims to provide the veterinary practitioner with an up-to-date reference which is easy to read and follow.

The style of the book is faithful to the BSAVA Surgical Manual series featuring a combination of detailed text together with a series of Operative Techniques, which makes this a truly practical manual. The book not only allows the busy practitioner to read in-depth about the indications and perioperative management of a procedure, but also provides a step-by-step illustrated guide to the surgical procedures themselves.

The Manual has been structured with introductory chapters on surgical principles and equipment, before going on to consider in-depth approaches to the various organ systems within the abdominal cavity. The Manual provides a comprehensive review of current techniques in abdominal surgery. A new chapter on laparoscopic surgery has been included, along with a chapter dedicated to urinary incontinence. Emphasis is placed throughout the Manual on the important adage that surgery does not begin and end in the operating theatre – it is essential that appropriate preoperative and postoperative management is available for all surgical cases.

The *BSAVA Manual of Canine and Feline Abdominal Surgery* is aimed at clinical veterinary students, general practitioners and those seeking to improve their surgical knowledge and ability through further postgraduate qualifications. With this in mind, the procedures described in the book range from those that most veterinary surgeons in general practice will be familiar with, to those which should only be approached by the more experienced surgeon.

We have chosen contributors who are recognized both nationally and internationally to ensure that this Manual is comprehensive in its make-up and we are indebted to all the authors for their hard work. We are grateful to Samantha Elmhurst for her excellent artwork and would also like to thank the Publishing Team at the BSAVA.

John Williams
Jacqui Niles
October 2015

Chapter 1

Principles of abdominal surgery

Liz Welsh

Coeliotomy	Surgical incision into the abdominal cavity
Laparotomy	Surgical incision through the flank Used as a synonym for coeliotomy

Abdominal surgery is a commonplace procedure in modern veterinary practice and one that most veterinary surgeons (veterinarians) feel confident in their ability to perform. This confidence stems from the familiarity with the procedure that arises from almost daily exposure to the technique when neutering animals. This familiarity can tempt the unwary to perform abdominal surgery unnecessarily or inappropriately, to the potential detriment of the patient.

There are currently no controlled veterinary studies that quantify the risk:benefit ratio of abdominal surgery in companion animals (Osborne and Lulich, 2000), and cats and dogs may still be operated on needlessly, albeit in good faith. Consequently it behoves the responsible veterinary surgeon to:

- Evaluate the patient and make an informed decision on the need for surgery
- Communicate with the owner promptly and clearly regarding the planned procedure(s) and provide regular updates on their pet's progress
- Prepare and stabilize the patient prior to surgery
- Provide competent anaesthesia and analgesia for the procedure to be performed
- Be familiar with the surgical principles and techniques required for abdominal surgery, to minimize perioperative morbidity and mortality in the patient
- Provide appropriate postoperative care for the patient
- Recognize the limitations of personal ability and experience, the available equipment and facilities and the procedure.

Indications for abdominal surgery

Animals may present to the veterinary surgeon for abdominal surgery without the need for medical investigation (e.g. neutering or prophylactic procedures), but many cats and dogs will require initial investigations before the decision for surgery is made. Advances in diagnostic imaging (e.g. flexible endoscopy, ultrasonography, computed tomography (CT), magnetic resonance imaging (MRI)) and minimally invasive surgical techniques (e.g. laparoscopy, laparoscopic assisted surgery, cystoscopy) provide veterinary surgeons with increased opportunities to reach a diagnosis and provide treatment without the need for open cavity surgery. However, for a number of reasons, open abdominal surgery still forms a large part of the daily operating list (Figure 1.1).

On occasions, abdominal surgery will be undertaken on an emergency basis. In these cases it is important where possible to collect samples (e.g. blood, urine and other fluids, and material for bacterial culture and cytology) before administering diagnostic, therapeutic or anaesthetic agents to the patient. These samples may provide valuable baseline or historical data as the case progresses.

Diagnostic purposes	A diagnosis may only be made by inspection or palpation of abdominal organs or tissues A diagnosis depends on cytological, histopathological or microbiological examination of tissues, fluids or other biological samples collected at surgery
Assessment of prognosis	Prognosis may be established after diagnosis is achieved (see above) The extent of a disease process may only be established by gross inspection of organs or tissues The feasibility of surgical correction of a disease process may only be assessed by gross evaluation of affected tissues and organs
Therapeutic purposes	Abdominal trauma Internal or external abdominal wall hernias Treatment of abnormal discharges from abdominal organs, abdominal wall sinuses or fistulae Control of ongoing haemorrhage Correction of a source of contamination Investigation and elimination of the source of abdominal pain Investigation of pneumoperitoneum Removal of mass lesions within the peritoneal cavity, from abdominal organs and from the abdominal wall Removal of the cause of visceral obstruction, including visceral torsion Removal of abnormal accumulations of fluids Treatment of congenital abnormalities such as portosystemic shunt or ectopic ureter Surgical treatment of dystocia
Prophylactic procedure	Gastropexy
Neutering	Neutering bitches or queens Neutering cryptorchid dogs or cats

1.1 Indications for abdominal surgery.

Patient evaluation, preparation and stabilization

> For every mistake that is made for not knowing, a hundred are made for not looking. Anon

Preoperative patient evaluation, preparation and stabilization are the most efficient and overlooked ways to improve patient outcomes and reduce client costs associated with abdominal surgery. It is the responsibility of any veterinary surgeon operating on an animal to assess not only the patient but also any relevant information available for the case and to discuss the proposed procedure and attendant risks with the owner. The goals of preoperative evaluation are to identify physiological, pathological and drug-related factors that may complicate the anaesthetic or surgical management of the patient. This allows the veterinary surgeon to:

- *Reduce morbidity and mortality associated with anaesthesia and surgery.* Despite increasing patient baseline risk, perioperative mortality has declined significantly in human surgery in the last 50 years (Bainbridge *et al.*, 2012). However, there is an enduring relationship between the American Society of Anesthesiologists (ASA) Physical Status score and adverse perioperative outcomes for both anaesthesia and surgery (Saubermann and Lagasse, 2012). There are no similar perioperative data for veterinary patients. However, current data for anaesthetized or sedated cats and dogs suggest that approximately 0.1–0.2% of healthy (ASA 1–2) and 0.5–2% of sick (ASA 3–5) cats and dogs suffer an anaesthetic-related death (Brodbelt, 2009). There is clearly room for improvement, with these figures substantially higher than those reported in human anaesthesia
- *Increase the quality of perioperative care.* Prior knowledge of all pre-existing medical or coexisting surgical conditions ensures appropriate therapeutic and supportive care
- *Decrease the cost of perioperative care.* A complete patient history and thorough physical examination allow targeted laboratory testing and patient stabilization prior to surgery and may reduce postoperative morbidity
- *Restore the patient quickly to preoperative function or better.*

Requirements for preoperative patient evaluation vary considerably with the patient and proposed procedure; however, an accurate patient history and physical examination are essential. On the basis of this information, further diagnostic tests may be recommended and the perioperative management tailored to the individual's needs. If patient assessment has been performed before the day of surgery, the assessment should be repeated prior to surgery to ensure that nothing has been overlooked or changed.

Patient history

A standard approach to recording a medical history is essential to ensure that important factors are not missed. The most important aspects are outlined below.

Patient identity and proposed procedure(s): Identity includes species, breed and reproductive status.

- In intact females consider the possibility of oestrus or pregnancy and the effects that a gravid uterus may have on cardiovascular and respiratory function. Additionally, it is important to consider the effect of anaesthesia and surgery on the fetus (e.g. teratogenicity, abortion).
- Consider disease susceptibility in specific breeds (e.g. von Willebrand's disease in the Dobermann).

Confirm patient age: Both very young and geriatric (age ≥75–80% of expected breed lifespan) patients may have increased perioperative risk.

Current health and habits: Careful physical examination is particularly important where the owner reports clinical signs that may be indicative of underlying endocrine, cardio-respiratory, gastrointestinal or urogenital disorders (e.g. weight loss, inappetence, exercise intolerance, coughing, vomiting, diarrhoea or polydipsia). The owner should be questioned about possible exposure of their pet to toxins.

Prior medical and surgical history: It should be established whether the patient has a history of perioperative complications. It is important to know whether the patient has had previous blood transfusions.

Prior adverse reactions to drugs or anaesthetic agents (side effects or allergies): It should be established whether the patient has any known drug allergies. Any anaesthetic records available for the patient should be reviewed.

Recent and current drug therapy: It is important that drugs such as insulin, cardiac medications, anticonvulsants, corticosteroids, mineralocorticoids and immunosuppressants are continued prior to surgery and that the consequences of ongoing drug therapy are considered. For example, diuretics might have significant effects on fluid balance and electrolyte concentrations, while long-term glucocorticoid treatment can impair the ability of the patient to mount an appropriate stress response. The administration of aminoglycoside antibiotics can affect the action of non-depolarizing muscle relaxants. Other drugs that may affect the course or outcome of anaesthesia and surgery include insulin, digoxin, phenobarbital, cimetidine and other H2 blockers, beta-blockers, insecticides, calcium channel blockers, angiotensin converting enzyme (ACE) inhibitors, bronchodilators and non-steroidal anti-inflammatory drugs (NSAIDs).

Physical examination

A complete physical examination incorporating all body systems should be performed. The veterinary surgeon should avoid concentrating solely on the complaint necessitating surgery. The general assessment should consider the following:

- *Obesity* compromises the cardiovascular system and necessitates an increased respiratory effort. Obese patients should receive drug dosages calculated on the basis of ideal body weight
- *Cachexic patients* are physiologically stressed and have little metabolic or homeostatic reserve. They may have a reduced ability to metabolize perioperative drugs because of impaired hepatic function.

System-specific examination should include:

- *Cardiovascular system*: heart rate and rhythm, pulse rate and quality, murmurs, mucous membrane colour, capillary refill time, temperature of extremities and jugular vein examination
- *Respiratory system*: respiratory rate, respiration character, pulmonary auscultation and percussion
- *Central nervous system*: cranial nerve examination and evaluation of conscious proprioception
- *Alimentary system*: careful oral examination to establish the presence of masses, foreign material, ulceration and petechiation. In patients with acute abdominal pain the abdomen should be examined using visual inspection, auscultation, percussion, ballottement, superficial and deep palpation, and a digital rectal examination. A careful body wall inspection is mandatory, to search for deformity or swelling and evidence of bruising or penetrating wounds. Red discoloration at the umbilicus may be indicative of intra-abdominal haemorrhage
- *Urogenital system*: a rectal examination
- *Lymphatic system*: palpation of peripheral lymph nodes
- *Musculoskeletal system*
- *Special senses*
- *Cutaneous system*: particular attention should be paid to the area of the proposed surgical incision.

Following the examination, the patient may be assigned an ASA Physical Status score (Figure 1.2).

Physical status score	Definition
1	A normal healthy patient
2	A patient with mild systemic disease
3	A patient with severe systemic disease
4	A patient with severe systemic disease that is a constant threat to life
5	A moribund patient who is not expected to survive without the operation

1.2 American Society of Anesthesiologists (ASA) Physical Status classifications (available at: http://www.asahq.org).

Laboratory investigations

In many cases further laboratory or diagnostic tests will be required in the pursuit of a diagnosis or to manage comorbidities. Routine preoperative blood testing has been shown to be of little clinical relevance in dogs if no potential problems are identified in the history or on physical examination (Alef *et al.*, 2008). However, it still may be appropriate to obtain baseline data prior to procedures where there is a risk of significant operative or postoperative complications. It is important, when preoperative testing is performed, that any abnormalities detected are noted and/or investigated further as appropriate to the patient. Where routine preoperative testing is performed a reasonable approach would be to perform a minimum pre-anaesthetic database for patients with an ASA Physical Status score of 1–2 (i.e. packed cell volume (PCV), total solids (TS), urea, creatinine, glucose, electrolytes and urinalysis), and a complete pre-anaesthetic database for those patients with an ASA Physical Status score of 3–5 (i.e. complete haematology, blood biochemistry and urinalysis) (Figure 1.3).

Further investigations

Further clinical investigations or interventions may be warranted in individual patients prior to anaesthesia and surgery (Figure 1.4). These may include the following:

- *Cardiovascular system*: coagulation profile (Figure 1.5), electrocardiography, radiography, echocardiography and pericardiocentesis
- *Respiratory system*: blood gas analysis, direct laryngoscopy, radiography (Figure 1.6), fluoroscopy, advanced imaging, tracheoscopy, bronchoscopy, tracheal wash, bronchoalveolar lavage, ultrasonography and thoracocentesis (Figure 1.7)
- *Alimentary system*: radiography, ultrasonography, canine/feline pancreatic lipase immunoreactivity, trypsin-like immunoreactivity (TLI), endoscopic examination and biopsy, faecal examination, folate, cobalamin, bile acid stimulation test, abdominocentesis (Figure 1.8) and diagnostic peritoneal lavage
- *Urogenital system*: protein:creatinine ratio, radiography, ultrasonography, advanced imaging, cystoscopy, biopsy and stone analysis.

Preoperative management of systemic disease

It is beyond the scope of this chapter to describe in detail the management of systemic diseases in patients undergoing abdominal surgery. However, it is important to recognize that, except for emergency procedures, patients with unstable cardiovascular, respiratory, endocrine, renal, hepatic or central nervous system disease have a higher surgical risk than those animals whose disease is well controlled prior to surgery.

Perioperative nutrition

- *Simple starvation* occurs as a consequence of lack of calories and protein in an otherwise healthy animal that is unwilling or unable to eat. Fat becomes the primary energy source, though amino acids are used preferentially for gluconeogenesis. With access to food, metabolism returns to normal within a day and amino acid mobilization decreases.
- In *stress starvation* the shortfall in nutrition is complicated and exacerbated by systemic inflammation or physiological stress. Glycogen stores are depleted rapidly and, again, fat becomes the primary energy source. Protein catabolism increases to fuel gluconeogenesis, but the animal is unable to use glucose efficiently. The protein-sparing adaptations that occur in simple starvation are overridden and a hypermetabolic state exists, resulting in protein–energy malnutrition. Unfortunately, following a return to normal enteral nutrition, the stressed patient's metabolism will not return to normal function within a day, and negative nitrogen balance, accelerated gluconeogenesis and insulin resistance may persist.

A complete patient history and physical examination are critical for the assessment of the nutritional status of the preoperative patient. Many patients undergoing abdominal surgery are initially healthy, but factors affecting preoperative nutritional status include:

- Anorexia (1–2 days in young and 3–5 days in adult animals)

Test	Reason for inclusion	Common abnormalities
Packed cell volume (PCV) or haemoglobin (Hb)	Indicator of: • O₂ carrying capacity of blood • Hydration status • Chronic hypoxia	↑ PCV may indicate dehydration or splenic contraction ↓ PCV may indicate haemodilution, increased red cell destruction or decreased red cell production, or chronic blood loss
Visual appraisal of serum/plasma	Check for changes which could reflect systemic disease, i.e. lipaemia, haemolysis, icterus	
Total solids (TS)	Indicator of: • Hydration status • Inflammatory disease • Hypoproteinaemia	↑ TS may indicate dehydration, increased globulin production ↓ TS may indicate increased protein loss (e.g. third spacing, gastrointestinal, renal), decreased protein production, overhydration or blood loss
Albumin	Indicator of: Hydration status Hypoalbuminaemia	↑ Albumin may indicate dehydration ↓ Albumin may indicate hepatic, renal or gastrointestinal disease. It may also indicate malnutrition or sequestration into body cavity effusions (exudates)
Urea and creatinine	Used as indicators of glomerular function, but can be affected by other processes	↑ Urea level is an indicator of: • Hydration status • Cardiac disease • Recent high protein meal • Intestinal haemorrhage • Post-renal obstruction ↓ Urea may indicate reduced dietary protein intake, diffuse hepatic disease or portosystemic shunting of blood ↑ Creatinine indicates decreased glomerular filtration
Glucose	Hypo- and hyperglycaemia create metabolic disturbances that interfere with anaesthetic management and risk neurological damage	↑ Glucose may indicate stress, diabetes mellitus, glucocorticoid administration ↓ Glucose may indicate sepsis, neoplasia, insulin overdose, neonatal hypoglycaemia, artefact, toy breed hypoglycaemia
Electrolytes	Sodium, potassium, chloride and calcium are the commonly measured electrolytes. Where possible abnormalities should be rectified prior to anaesthesia and surgery	
Urine specific gravity (USG)	Azotaemia with USG <1.030 in dogs and <1.035 in cats	Consider renal disease or other diseases that impair tubular function and produce urine that is not maximally concentrated (e.g. hypercalcaemia, hypoadrenocorticism)
	Azotaemia with USG ≥1.030 in dogs and >1.035 in cats	Consider prerenal causes (e.g. dehydration, cardiac disease)

1.3 Tests included in a minimum pre-anaesthetic blood profile.

Clinical abnormalities noted or reported	Possible causes	Further tests often required to reach a diagnosis
Exercise intolerance	Cardiac disease Respiratory disease Systemic disease including anaemia Neurological disease Musculoskeletal disease	Radiography or advanced imaging Blood gas analysis Electrocardiography Ultrasonography or echocardiography Haematology and biochemistry screen Specific laboratory testing (e.g. acetylcholine receptor antibodies, endocrine testing)
Respiratory embarrassment	Pleural effusion Thoracic wall disease Pulmonary disease Large airway disease Upper airway disease	Blood gas analysis Thoracocentesis Bronchoscopy Radiography or advanced imaging Fluoroscopy Laryngoscopy
Coughing	Cardiac disease Respiratory disease	Thoracic radiography or advanced imaging Bronchoscopy Tracheal wash Therapeutic trials (e.g. diuretic therapy)
Episodic collapse	Cardiac disease Pulmonary disease Neurological disease Hypoglycaemia	Biochemistry profile Blood gas analysis Radiography or advanced imaging Electrocardiography Ultrasonography or echocardiography

1.4 Common causes of physical abnormalities that might be noted, or reported, during a preoperative assessment, and the tests often used to investigate these clinical presentations. Anorexia may be associated with many systemic diseases and is not listed here. (continues) ▶

(Modified from Duncan, 2009)

Clinical abnormalities noted or reported	Possible causes	Further tests often required to reach a diagnosis
Vomiting	Gastric disease Intestinal disease Pancreatic disease Pyometra Renal disease Liver disease Feline hyperthyroidism Diabetes mellitus Hypoadrenocorticism	Radiography including contrast studies Ultrasonography Biochemistry profile including electrolytes For pancreatitis: amylase, lipase and canine/feline pancreatic lipase immunoreactivity, trypsin-like immunoreactivity (TLI) Endoscopy Biopsy
Diarrhoea	Intestinal disease Feline hyperthyroidism Liver disease Hypoadrenocorticism	Radiography including contrast studies Faecal examination Endoscopy Biochemistry profile including electrolytes TLI, folate, cobalamin Feline thyroxine (T4) Breath hydrogen test Biopsy (intestinal or hepatic)
Polydipsia	Renal disease Liver disease Pyometra Feline hyperthyroidism Diabetes mellitus Hyperadrenocorticism Hypercalcaemia Hypoadrenocorticism Diabetes insipidus Psychogenic polydipsia	Radiography including contrast studies Urinalysis, haematology and biochemistry profile including calcium and electrolytes Thyroid-stimulating hormone, T4 Bile acid stimulation test (hepatic function) Low dose dexamethasone suppression test or adrenocorticotropic hormone stimulation test (for hyperadrenocorticism) Biopsy
Petechiation/bruising	Thrombocytopenia Coagulation defects Trauma Vasculitis	Haematology profile with film examination Coagulation profile (e.g. activated clotting time (ACT), prothrombin time (PT), activated partial thromboplastin time (aPTT)) Fibrinogen degradation products, D-dimer analysis, proteins induced by vitamin K antagonism or absence (PIVKA)
Lymphadenopathy	Reactive lymphoid hyperplasia Lymphoma Metastatic neoplasia Lymphadenitis	Examination of drainage region of enlarged nodes Ultrasonography Cytological examination of fine-needle aspirate Histological examination of biopsy sample
Neurological signs/behavioural changes	Primary neurological disease Hepatic encephalopathy (e.g. congenital portosystemic shunt) Hypoglycaemia Hypocalcaemia	Biochemistry profile Diagnostic imaging Cerebrospinal fluid analysis Serology Bile acid stimulation test

1.4 (continued) Common causes of physical abnormalities that might be noted, or reported, during a preoperative assessment, and the tests often used to investigate these clinical presentations. Anorexia may be associated with many systemic diseases and is not listed here. (Modified from Duncan, 2009)

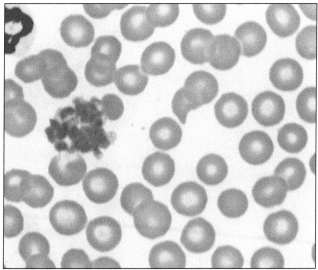

1.5 Manual platelet counts (shown with platelet clumping), activated clotting time (ACT), activated partial thromboplastin time (aPTT), prothrombin time (PT) and buccal mucosal bleeding time, in addition to specific factor estimation, all provide valuable information about a patient's haemostatic ability.
(© Alison Ridyard)

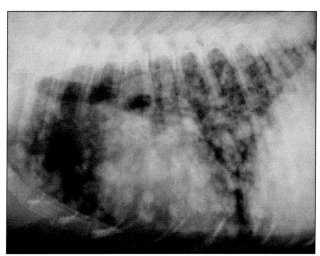

1.6 Patient evaluation for the presence of pulmonary metastatic disease is important prior to abdominal surgery in the treatment of neoplastic diseases.

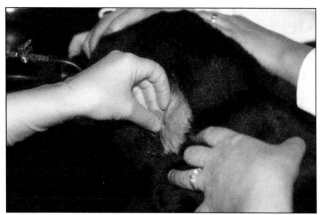

1.7 Thoracocentesis to remove pleural effusion prior to general anaesthesia and abdominal surgery in a dog with a chronic traumatic diaphragmatic rupture.

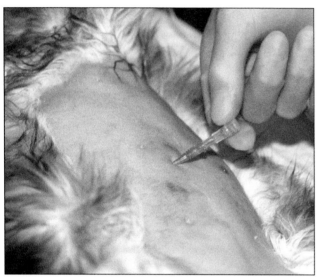

1.8 Abdominocentesis prior to abdominal surgery aided in the diagnosis of uroperitoneum in this patient.

- Weight loss (>5% in young and >10% in adult animals)
- Fever
- Recent trauma, surgery or sepsis with anorexia
- Physical impairments to prehension, mastication and deglutition
- Vomiting and diarrhoea
- Oedema, ascites, open or draining wounds
- Catabolic medications (e.g. glucocorticoids).

In the perioperative period the body increases its energy requirements but its nutritional intake decreases. Initially glycogen stores are depleted and insulin resistance and glucose intolerance develop. This is designed to preserve the function of vital organs and is of short duration (12–24 hours). Subsequently, stress hormones are released (e.g. adrenaline (epinephrine), cortisol and glucagons) that stimulate the breakdown of protein and fat. There are also diminished insulin levels, leading to hyperglycaemia. Finally, the sympathetic response abates and the levels of stress hormones decrease; there is resolution of hyperglycaemia and reduced protein catabolism. Thus energy requirements in healthy patients undergoing elective procedures can increase transiently by 10%, but metabolic processes rapidly return to normal.

Malnourished animals undergoing surgery will not only be suffering the general systemic effects of stress starvation prior to the procedure but will also be at increased risk (during and after surgery) of reduced wound tensile strength, increased wound infection, increased wound dehiscence, decreased immunocompetence and increased perioperative morbidity and mortality (all leading to poor wound healing) and prolonged hospitalization.

> **PRACTICAL TIP**
>
> Nutritional support of malnourished patients, before surgery when possible and certainly following surgical intervention, will lead not only to an improved nutritional status but also to an improved clinical outcome following surgery

Intestinal permeability normally increases transiently after surgery. Increased intestinal permeability is indicative of failure of the gut mucosal barrier to exclude intestinal bacteria and toxins from the systemic circulation. Such agents are proposed as aetiological in the systemic inflammatory response syndrome, sepsis and multiple organ failure. Enteral nutrition helps to minimize gastrointestinal mucosal atrophy and increased intestinal permeability by ensuring production of secretory immunoglobulin (Ig)A, and should be used in the perioperative period whenever possible (Figures 1.9 and 1.10). In the absence of specific contraindications, enteral nutritional support should start in the early postoperative period. This includes patients that have undergone gastrointestinal surgery, because a rapid return to enteral nutrition has not been shown to prolong postoperative ileus or increase the risk of dehiscence of gastrointestinal wounds. For further information see the *BSAVA Manual of Canine and Feline Surgical Principles*.

Enteral nutrition	Increased oral intake or change of diet to high-palatability energy-dense diet Assisted oral feeding Chemical stimulation of appetite Tube feeding: naso-oesophageal, oesophagostomy, gastrostomy and enterostomy tubes Microenteral nutrition (Devey and Crowe, 2000)
Parenteral nutrition	Total parenteral nutrition: all essential nutrients are administered parenterally Partial parenteral nutrition: nutrients are administered parenterally to support enteral feeding

1.9 Methods of providing peri- and postoperative nutritional support.

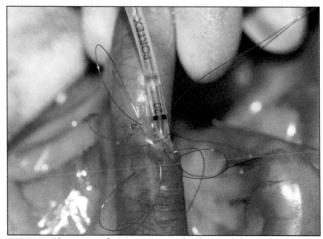

1.10 Placement of a jejunostomy tube during abdominal surgery, allowing enteral nutritional support in the postoperative period in a patient with a pancreatic abscess.

Surgical risk and prognosis

Risk assessment is the critical appraisal of what is potentially harmful, an assessment of its significance, and an evaluation of the measures available to eliminate or reduce that risk. There are several known factors that affect perioperative risk in companion animals, including:

- Pre-existing medical disease
- Age
- Emergency procedures
- Anaesthetic management
- Surgical procedure performed
- Duration of the procedure
- Haemodynamic stability
- Experience of the veterinary surgeon
- Availability of adequate postoperative monitoring
- Inadequate analgesia.

However, there are no universal data to quantify the degree of risk that each of these factors represents. Osborne and Lulich (2000) proposed probable patient risk/benefit outcomes associated with management of some abdominal diseases by exploratory coeliotomy in companion animals (Figure 1.11).

The level of experience of the veterinary surgeon operating on the patient affects surgical outcome in many procedures. It is hoped that each surgeon's outcome improves with further experience of performing individual procedures (Figure 1.12), but assessment of this improvement or of continued success requires that each individual critically evaluates their outcome for each procedure against current published data. As part of this evaluation process, veterinary practices should carry out monthly mortality and morbidity rounds. These have proved to be a powerful tool for reflection and learning in human surgery (Orlander et al., 2002). Evidence of surgical outcomes persistently below those accepted by the profession as a whole requires appropriate remedial action. Although it may be a fault with surgical technique, it is important that the standards for preoperative evaluation, preparation and stabilization are considered, in addition to the level of anaesthetic and postoperative care.

Risks/benefits	Diseases
Benefits probably outweigh risks	Penetrating abdominal trauma Haemoperitoneum in haemodynamically unstable patient Septic peritonitis Evisceration Intestinal obstruction Bile peritonitis Obstructive uropathy of ureter or renal pelvis Uroperitoneum
Risk/benefit ratio requires further study	Intra-abdominal malignancy Haemoperitoneum in haemodynamically stable patient
Risks likely to outweigh benefits	Persistent or intermittent vomiting that has not been localized with non-surgical diagnostic methods Uncomplicated feline lower urinary tract disease (FLUTD) Nephroliths or ureteroliths not obstructing urinary outflow Persistent intermittent diarrhoea that has not been localized with non-surgical diagnostic methods Ascites that has not been localized with non-surgical diagnostic methods

1.11 Risks/benefits of exploratory coeliotomy in patients with abdominal diseases.

Risk or prognosis	When given
Excellent	Minimal potential for negative consequences of the procedure and high probability that surgery will resolve problem
Good	Low potential for complications resulting from surgery and high probability of successful surgical outcome
Fair	Serious complications possible but uncommon; recovery may be prolonged or animal may not return to its presurgical function
Guarded or poor	Recovery expected to be prolonged, high likelihood of death during or after the procedure, or animal unlikely to return to its presurgical form

1.12 Summary of surgical risk.

Client communication

Client communication is extremely important in preoperative planning. Clients should be informed of all clinical problems that have been identified in their pet. This is particularly important if conditions that may affect perianaesthetic morbidity and mortality are identified. Non-surgical as well as surgical treatments for the main condition should be highlighted, with their respective merits, complications and the attendant inpatient, outpatient and home care anticipated. The overall surgical risk to the patient, as it is perceived at the time by the veterinary surgeon, should be discussed. The owner should be advised of the importance of neutering patients with hereditary conditions.

The owner must be given an estimate of the costs involved in the treatment of their pet, and updated as costs rise, especially if they are above those anticipated. It is reasonable for the owner to request a detailed invoice of the costs incurred. The owner should sign their consent for the agreed treatment and the document must be retained as part of the medical record. If verbal consent is obtained, it should be noted in the medical record.

> **PRACTICAL TIP**
>
> Referral of cases should be considered when the procedure required is beyond the experience of the referring veterinary surgeon or where the appropriate level of perioperative care is not available

Preoperative fasting

Except in emergency situations, animals undergoing abdominal surgery should be fasted prior to induction of anaesthesia. The purpose of preoperative fasting is to minimize the volume of the gastric contents, while avoiding unnecessary dehydration. Minimizing the volume of gastric contents is important in reducing the risk of regurgitation, vomiting and gastro-oesophageal reflux (GOR) either at induction of anaesthesia or during the surgical procedure. GOR can cause oesophagitis and in severe cases may lead to oesophageal stricture. Regurgitation and vomiting may cause laryngospasm. Potential complications of aspiration include the development of hypoxia, interstitial oedema, alveolar haemorrhage, atelectasis, airway obstruction, chemical pneumonitis, bronchospasm, postoperative aspiration pneumonia and death. The volume, pH and amount of particulate matter in the material will affect the pulmonary outcome.

There are a number of risk factors for regurgitation, vomiting, aspiration and GOR, including:

- Recent ingestion of food
- Pregnancy and obesity
- Hiatal or diaphragmatic hernia
- Laryngeal paralysis
- Megaoesophagus or oesophageal motility disorders
- Oesophageal, gastric or intestinal surgery
- Anaesthetic drugs that reduce lower oesophageal sphincter pressure
- Opioids delaying gastric emptying
- Vomiting
- Abdominal masses or gross ascites
- Gastric or bowel obstruction
- Recumbency or mental depression
- Head-down surgical position.

The length of time for which patients should be fasted before surgery is controversial. Current recommendations include withholding solid food and water preoperatively for 6 to 8 hours and 2 to 4 hours, respectively. It is important that inpatients scheduled for surgery are clearly identified, to ensure an appropriate period of fasting. However, it is also important to ensure that animals with increased fluid requirements (e.g. renal insufficiency, pyrexia) are identified and appropriately supported with intravenous fluids during preoperative fasting.

Dogs and cats considered at increased risk of regurgitation, vomiting and GOR should be anaesthetized using a rapid intravenous induction technique. This allows prompt tracheal intubation with the patient in a sternal, head-up position using a lubricated cuffed endotracheal tube. Facilities for oropharyngeal suction should be available. Some authors recommend pre-treatment of at-risk patients with prokinetic agents, such as metoclopramide, H2 antagonists or proton pump inhibitors, to increase lower oesophageal sphincter pressure and reduce gastric acid production.

Preoperative bowel preparation

The principle behind mechanical bowel preparation (MBP) is that it reduces the risk of surgical site infections and anastomotic leakage following surgery of the large bowel. Although preoperative enemas decrease faecal bulk they do not decrease the bacterial load in the remaining faeces. In humans, there is no evidence that patients benefit from MBP before elective colorectal surgery (Güenaga et al., 2011). In cats and dogs there is no indication for MBP, and in fact the use of preoperative enemas can cause greater surgical contamination because of the presence of liquefied faecal material within the bowel at the time of surgery (Williams, 2012). Similarly, there is no need or justification for preoperative administration of prophylactic oral antimicrobials before colonic surgery, there being no scientific evidence for this practice.

Preoperative hair removal

Animals that are not scheduled for emergency surgery that have grossly contaminated hair coats may be washed the day before surgery, both to decrease the amount of foreign material on the coat and to reduce the skin's microbial colony count. Products containing chlorhexidine gluconate can be used, but repeated shampooing would be required to obtain the maximum benefit. Currently, routine preoperative shampooing has not been shown to reduce the risk of surgical site infections.

PRACTICAL TIP

The hair coat should ideally be clipped with a 10–15 cm border around the site of the proposed surgical incision

---

WARNING

Clipping the hair coat from the surgical site is performed at the time of surgery, as clipping or shaving of hair before this time increases the risk of surgical site infections. This is believed to be caused by microscopic cuts in the skin acting as foci for bacterial multiplication

---

Anaesthesia, analgesia and fluid therapy

All cats and dogs undergoing abdominal surgery require cardiovascular support in the form of intravenous fluid therapy and must be provided with an appropriate level of anaesthesia and analgesia. These techniques are discussed in detail in the *BSAVA Manual of Canine and Feline Anaesthesia and Analgesia* and the *BSAVA Manual of Canine and Feline Surgical Principles*.

Analgesia

It is the veterinary surgeon's duty to relieve the suffering of animals in their care and therefore they must strive to minimize pain in the perioperative period. Pain may be detrimental to animals undergoing abdominal surgery for a number of reasons, because it:

- Enhances fear, anxiety and stress response, leading to a catabolic state
- Delays wound healing
- Predisposes to intestinal ileus
- Reduces food intake
- Leads to wound interference and self-trauma
- Prolongs anaesthetic recovery, leading to increased morbidity
- Reduces cardiovascular function.

A variety of drugs are available for the provision of analgesia and their use is described in detail in the *BSAVA Manual of Canine and Feline Anaesthesia and Analgesia* and the *BSAVA Manual of Canine and Feline Surgical Principles*. They are listed here with notes relating to their use in patients with abdominal disease.

Opioids

Within the gastrointestinal tract, smooth muscle tone and sphincter tone tend to increase with opioid drugs but peristalsis is decreased, reducing propulsive activity. While most opioid drugs induce nausea and vomiting. In humans, this is much less common in animals and is most frequently seen with morphine. Hyporexia may be observed following prolonged or inappropriate use of opioids in the postoperative period. Pethidine has a spasmolytic action on the gut, due to its anticholinergic activity, but its short duration of action limits its practical use in the postoperative period.

Much emphasis has been placed in the past on the most suitable opioid for use in patients with pancreatitis. It is known that all opioids increase biliary pressure. In humans the bile duct and pancreatic duct are conjoined at the entrance to the duodenum at the level of the sphincter of Oddi. Consequently, it was believed that the administration of opioids, and in particular morphine, could increase the pressure not only within the biliary tree but also within the pancreatic duct, leading to further damage to that organ in patients with pancreatitis. Around 80% of cats have conjoined ducts, while in dogs the bile duct and pancreatic duct enter the duodenum separately in the vast majority of animals. However, as in humans, there is little scientific evidence supporting the deleterious effects of opioid use on the clinical course of pancreatitis in cats or dogs.

Non-steroidal anti-inflammatory drugs

The therapeutic effects of most NSAIDs are due to inhibition of the enzyme cyclo-oxygenase (COX), which converts arachidonic acid into prostaglandins and thromboxane A2. COX exists as two main isoenzymes, COX-1 and COX-2, and NSAIDs are classified according to their activity against these isoenzymes. This classification is useful in understanding the risk of toxic side effects and the individual drugs can be described as COX-1 or -2 sparing, preferential or selective.

The most frequently encountered toxic side effects of NSAIDs are gastrointestinal irritation or ulceration, nephrotoxicity and hepatopathy. Despite the known risk of gastrointestinal side effects there is no clear evidence to support withholding NSAIDs in patients undergoing uncomplicated gastrointestinal surgery, although many surgeons prefer not to use them in this situation. The potential for nephrotoxicity is of concern in the anaesthetized patient, where hypotension may reduce renal blood flow. The administration of an NSAID will inhibit the production of prostaglandins within the kidney that are responsible for maintaining renal perfusion in the face of decreased renal blood flow. This is of particular concern in patients with impairment of renal function that is not clinically apparent prior to anaesthesia and surgery. Appropriate patient monitoring in the perioperative period will alert the surgeon to any fall in arterial blood pressure that could reduce renal perfusion and consequently put the patient at risk of nephrotoxicity. All NSAIDs have the potential to increase bleeding at surgical sites by inhibition of thromboxane A2. However, this is uncommon with therapeutic doses – with the exception of aspirin, a COX-1 selective drug, which binds irreversibly to COX inside platelets, inhibiting thromboxane A2 for the life of the platelet.

There are an increasing number of NSAIDs available with a veterinary authorization for the management of inflammation and pain associated with soft tissue surgery in dogs and also cats. These drugs are not suitable as the sole analgesic in patients requiring abdominal surgery but form an important part of a balanced analgesic protocol. It is important to ensure that the NSAID used is prescribed at the correct dose rate and interval for the species treated.

WARNING

NSAIDs should only be administered to critically ill animals following fluid resuscitation and once the patient is haemodynamically stable

---

Drugs such as dexmedetomidine and medetomidine are potent analgesics and are increasingly used at low doses for continuous rate infusions in multimodal analgesic therapy without dramatic alterations in cardiac output and blood pressure. Ketamine, at subanaesthetic doses, and low-dose lidocaine are also used as adjunctive analgesics via continuous-rate intravenous infusions.

Surgical site infection

Surgical site infections (SSIs) are associated with increased perioperative morbidity and mortality and increased treatment costs in companion animals. The overall risk of developing an SSI in companion animals is approximately 5%. The term encompasses all infections local and regional to the surgical wound, including superficial (skin and subcutaneous tissues) and deep (fascial and muscle layers) incisional SSIs and organ or visceral space infections (Figure 1.13; Nelson, 2011; Shales, 2012). The bacteria most frequently isolated from SSIs in companion animals are endogenous skin flora and include *Staphylococcus* spp. (e.g. *S. pseudintermedius* and *S. aureus*), *Escherichia coli*, *Pasteurella* spp. and *Bacteroides* spp. The flora encountered in organ or visceral space infections may also include *Enterobacter* spp., *Enterococcus* spp. and *Clostridium* spp.

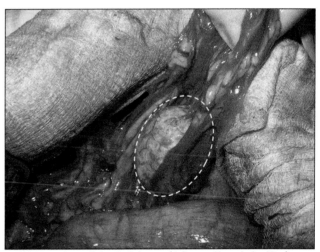

1.13 An intra-abdominal abscess (delineated by a dashed line) following splenectomy in a German Shepherd Dog. The abscess developed at the site of ligation of the splenic artery and vein. The dog had a 3-week history of lethargy, inappetence and diarrhoea following the initial surgery. *Clostridium* was cultured from the abscess.

A wound classification system originally developed by the National Research Council has been used to predict the likelihood of an SSI (Figure 1.14). Many factors are thought to contribute to the susceptibility to and incidence of SSIs and they are usually classified as host, operative and microorganism factors.

Host factors

Systemic host factors that may influence the development of an SSI include ASA Physical Status score ≥3, age, severe malnutrition, neoplasia, pre-existing illness such as endocrinopathies, immunosuppression and distant sources of infection. Local host risk factors are also important, in particular haematoma, seroma and the presence of foreign material and devitalized tissue.

Wound category	Infection rate (Cimino Brown, 2012)	Description	Examples
Clean	2.0–4.8%	Non-traumatic, non-inflamed, elective procedure No entry into the gastrointestinal, genitourinary or respiratory tracts No break in aseptic technique	Ovariohysterectomy, ovariectomy, incisional gastropexy
Clean–contaminated	3.5–5%	Operative wounds in which a hollow viscus (including the gastrointestinal, genitourinary and respiratory tracts) is opened	Routine gastrotomy, enterotomy, enterectomy, colposuspension, cystotomy, cholecystectomy, elective Caesarean section
Contaminated	4.6–12%	Fresh, open accidental wounds Major break in aseptic technique (e.g. gross spillage from the gastrointestinal tract) Surgery in which acute non-purulent inflammation is encountered	Traumatic abdominal hernia, penetrating abdominal wound
Dirty or infected	6.7–18.1%	Old traumatic wounds with devitalized tissue Surgery in the presence of clinical infection or perforated viscera	Septic peritonitis, intraperitoneal abscess, visceral perforation

1.14 Wound classification system.

Operative factors

Surgical time has been identified as a risk factor for the development of SSIs. In humans an operative time of >2 hours is the second greatest independent predictor of risk for an SSI, wound contamination being the greatest. In animals the risk of an SSI in patients that undergo a 90-minute procedure is double that with a 60-minute procedure. The precise aetiology is undetermined but increased wound contamination, tissue desiccation and trauma, cauterized tissue, suture materials, and decreased host resistance due to blood loss and hypothermia may be important. Other important operative factors are wound classification (see Figure 1.14), patient and surgeon preparation, surgical technique, emergency procedures, preoperative hair removal, method of incision, use of biomaterials and surgical implants, previous local radio-therapy and the length of hospitalization.

Specific anaesthetic risk factors for SSIs have been identified, including the duration of anaesthesia independent of the duration of the surgical procedure, and use of the intravenous anaesthetic agent propofol. This does not preclude the use of propofol, but highlights the importance of following the manufacturer's recommendations for storage and using aseptic technique when handling this drug.

Microorganism factors

The infective dose of obligate or facultative aerobic bacteria has been determined to be 10^5 bacteria per gram of tissue. However, this is a relative figure. A smaller inoculum of a virulent microorganism may result in infection, and adverse operative or host factors will increase the chance of infection with a bacterial dose of $<10^5$ bacteria per gram of tissue. Further detailed information can be found in the *BSAVA Manual of Canine and Feline Surgical Principles*.

Reducing surgical site infections

Few of the possible preventative measures that can be taken to reduce the incidence of SSIs in veterinary medicine have been validated (Nelson, 2011). However, the following are important:

- Adequate preoperative assessment of the patient to identify, treat or stabilize host factors that may

influence the development of SSIs prior to surgery (e.g. treatment of sites of distant infection, providing nutritional support)
- Careful monitoring and support of the patient under anaesthesia prior to and during surgery (e.g. maintaining blood pressure, limiting the development of hypothermia)
- Appropriate preparation of the surgical site
- Suitable preparation of the surgical team
- Maintaining asepsis in the surgical theatre
- Adhering to Halsted's principles of surgery (see below)
- Limiting the use of implanted foreign material within the surgical wound (e.g. suture, mesh, drains)
- Providing ongoing care in the postoperative period.

Antibacterial prophylaxis, when appropriate, may reduce the incidence of SSIs, but should never be considered as a substitute for aseptic technique.

Principles of antibacterial prophylaxis

Antibacterial prophylaxis involves the administration of antibiotics in the absence of infection, with the aim of preventing it. The most common reason for the prophylactic use of antibacterials in cats and dogs is for the prevention of infection in the perioperative period. A recent survey of the use of antibacterial prophylaxis in cats and dogs in the UK showed that in general such antibiotics are over-prescribed and that there needs to be improvement with respect to the timing, duration, choice of antibiotic used and selection of surgical cases requiring prophylaxis (Knights *et al.*, 2012).

PRACTICAL TIP

In abdominal surgery, routine antibacterial prophylaxis is not required for short-duration clean procedures performed in healthy tissue unless there are other risk factors to consider (e.g. systemic host factors). The benefit of routine antimicrobial prophylaxis in clean–contaminated procedures is unclear, and the decision should be based on the surgeon's judgement of the potential risk *versus* benefit of their use. Antibacterial prophylaxis is warranted for all contaminated procedures

---

The antibiotics used for prophylaxis should have a narrow spectrum of activity, but be effective against major anticipated contaminating bacterial species; they should be safe, non-toxic, bactericidal and suitable for intravenous administration. They should be present in the serum and target tissues at an adequate concentration at the time of first incision and therapeutic levels maintained throughout surgery.

> **PRACTICAL TIP**
>
> The optimum time for parenteral administration of prophylactic antibiotics is 30–60 minutes before surgical incision

The choice of prophylactic antibiotic will be empirical. So that an informed choice may be made, the normal flora, opportunistic bacteria and likely pathogens at the surgical site in question should be known.

Until recently the first-generation cephalosporin cefazolin was used frequently for antimicrobial prophylaxis prior to abdominal surgery. It has now been withdrawn from the market in the UK (though it is still available in the USA). Now amoxicillin and clavulanate (co-amoxiclav; 20 mg/kg) or cefuroxime (20–50 mg/kg), a second-generation cephalosporin, are common choices. Amoxicillin has a broad spectrum of bactericidal activity against many Gram-positive and Gram-negative microorganisms, but is susceptible to degradation by β-lactamases. Clavulanate inactivates a wide range of β-lactamase enzymes found in microorganisms resistant to amoxicillin, and so it effectively extends the antibiotic spectrum of amoxicillin. Amoxicillin with clavulanate is useful in the treatment of Gram-positive bacilli and cocci, as well as Gram-negative bacilli including *Escherichia coli*. It also has an anaerobic spectrum that includes *Bacteroides* and *Fusobacterium* species and so is adequate for surgery of the colon, where Gram-negative aerobic and anaerobic bacteria predominate. Cefuroxime has activity against Gram-positive and Gram-negative organisms, with some activity against anaerobes, but has a narrower spectrum of activity than the first-generation cephalosporins. However, it is more effective against *Enterobacter* spp., some *Proteus* spp., *Escherichia coli* and *Klebsiella* spp. Clindamycin and metronidazole are suitable for antimicrobial prophylaxis where contamination or infection with anaerobes is anticipated.

There is no evidence to support the prolonged administration of prophylactic antibiotics. They should be continued until the fibrin seal has formed postoperatively, a matter of 4–6 hours (Shales, 2012), but should not be extended beyond 24 hours postoperatively unless assessment of the patient indicates that continued therapy is required.

> **PRACTICAL TIPS**
>
> * The antibiotic administered should cover the pathogens most commonly isolated from SSIs that occur following the surgical procedure being performed
> * Repeat intravenous administration of the antibiotic during the procedure is recommended at intervals of two half-lives of the drug at the same dose (e.g. every 2 hours for amoxicillin and clavulanate, every 3–4 hours for cefuroxime)

Exploratory coeliotomy

Abdominal surgery should be regarded as an opportunity to examine the entire abdominal cavity, and surgeons should avoid the temptation to treat only the obvious lesion prior to closure of the abdomen. Frequently no further abnormalities will be detected, but other significant pathology may be identified and either influence the anticipated surgical procedure or warrant tissue sampling. Limited abdominal incisions are only indicated with organ-specific surgical procedures such as ovariohysterectomy. However, even in these circumstances the veterinary surgeon should examine local organs and tissues and should not hesitate to extend the length of the initial incision to improve surgical exposure if abnormalities are identified. In the cranial abdomen this may necessitate extending the incision into the thorax via a caudal median sternotomy or caudally into the pelvic cavity using pelvic osteotomy procedures.

The abdominal cavity may be divided into five regions for the purposes of exploration; this ensures that all organs and tissues are examined (Figure 1.15):

* Cranial abdomen
* Gastrointestinal tract
* Right paravertebral region
* Left paravertebral region
* Caudal abdomen.

Abdominal region or organ	Organ or tissue assessed	Specific manoeuvres to aid examination
Greater peritoneal cavity	Peritoneal fluid	Excision of falciform ligament Examination of right and left paravertebral 'gutters'
Cranial abdomen	Liver	Tilting surgical table and transection of the triangular ligaments will facilitate examination of diaphragmatic surface of liver. Palpate parenchyma
	Gallbladder and bile ducts	Caudal retraction of the stomach
	Hepatic hilus (portal vein, hepatic artery, caudal vena cava) Epiploic foramen	} Duodenal manoeuvre
	Spleen	Exteriorization
Gastrointestinal tract	Stomach Intestinal tract Pancreas	Exteriorization Exteriorization of spleen facilitates examination of left limb of pancreas. Right limb of pancreas may be examined when assessing descending duodenum. Palpate parenchyma
	Regional lymph nodes	

1.15 Exploration of the abdominal cavity. (continues) ▶

Abdominal region or organ	Organ or tissue assessed	Specific manoeuvres to aid examination	
Right paravertebral region	Hepatic portal vein Caudal vena cava Coeliac artery Hepatic lymph nodes Right adrenal gland Right kidney and proximal ureter Right ovary and uterine horn	Duodenal manoeuvre	
Left paravertebral region	Aorta Left adrenal gland Left kidney and proximal ureter Left ovary and uterine horn	Colonic manoeuvre	
Caudal abdomen	Bladder and distal ureters Proximal urethra Prostate gland and ductus deferens Uterine body and proximal vagina Regional lymph nodes	Cranial traction of the small intestine	Caudal reflection of bladder Cranial traction on bladder Cranial traction on bladder or traction on ductus deferens in neutered males Caudal reflection of bladder
Abdominal wall, peritoneal surface and mesenteries	Diaphragm Oesophageal hiatus Aortic and caval hiatus Greater and lesser omentum Internal inguinal rings	Tilting surgical table and caudal retraction of liver lobes will facilitate examination of the visceral surface of the diaphragm Caudal retraction of the stomach Caudal retraction of liver lobes and sectioning the triangular ligaments Caudal retraction of the stomach (lesser omentum) and exteriorization (greater omentum)	

1.15 (continued) Exploration of the abdominal cavity.

In addition, the abdominal wall, peritoneal surface and mesenteries should be evaluated. Abnormalities in location, shape, size, texture and colour of organs and tissues should be noted, and appropriate tissue or fluid samples taken.

Principles of abdominal surgery

Halsted's principles:
- Asepsis and aseptic surgical technique
- Sharp anatomical dissection
- Atraumatic tissue handling and surgical technique
- Removal of devitalized tissue from the surgical wound
- Precise haemostasis with preservation of blood supply to tissues
- Accurate tissue apposition, minimizing tissue dead space but without excessive tension on tissues

---

These surgical principles, laid down by the surgeon William Halsted (1852–1922), are hard to improve upon and are still of paramount importance in surgery. The principles are designed to improve surgical morbidity and mortality, minimize patient discomfort, promote rapid wound healing, reduce surgical site infection and increase client satisfaction.

Asepsis and aseptic surgical technique

Asepsis and aseptic surgical technique involve appropriate preparation of the patient, surgeon, instruments and operating theatre. In addition, the surgeon and theatre staff must remain aware of the aseptic surgical field throughout the surgical procedure undertaken. Further details can be found in the *BSAVA Manual of Canine and Feline Surgical Principles*.

Patient preparation

1. The patient should be provided with an opportunity to urinate and defecate prior to anaesthesia. It may be necessary to catheterize the urinary bladder or manually evacuate faeces.
2. Following induction of anaesthesia, the hair should be clipped from the ventral abdominal cavity; the clip should extend 10–15 cm beyond the anticipated incision on each side (Figure 1.16).
3. Loose hair is removed from the patient and an antiseptic detergent, e.g. chlorhexidine, or an iodine-based agent, is used to clean the surgical site, working from the site of the proposed incision outwards to the edge of the clipped area in a circular motion. The swab is replaced and the procedure repeated until no further dirt is removed.
4. The prepuce (or vagina if necessary) should be flushed with a non-detergent antiseptic solution (Neihaus *et al.*, 2011).
5. The patient may then be moved to the operating theatre and the procedure repeated.
6. The surgical site is sprayed or wiped with a non-detergent solution of chlorhexidine, 10% povidone–iodine or ethyl or isopropyl alcohol to remove the detergent solution from the site of surgical incision. Sterile saline may also be used for this purpose and is particularly indicated in the presence of open wounds.

Abdominal surgery generally necessitates dorsal recumbency and the patient is stabilized using sandbags, rolled towels (Figure 1.16a), troughs and leg ties. If there is any break in aseptic technique during patient positioning or placement of anaesthetic monitoring devices, skin preparation must be repeated.

The prepuce of male dogs may be clamped to one side of the ventral midline with a sterile Backhaus or cross-action towel clamp. Sterile surgical drapes are used to create a sterile surgical field around the aseptically prepared surgical site and are positioned by a properly prepared surgeon (see below). Four field drapes are

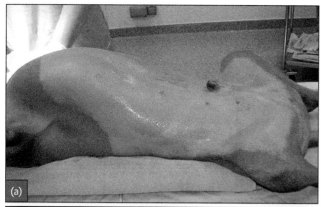

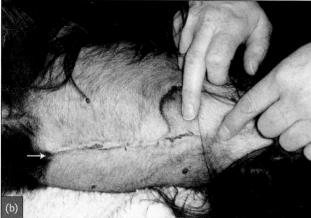

1.16 (a) A wide surgical clip has been performed prior to exploratory abdominal surgery in a dog. (b) An inadequate surgical clip was performed in this dog. Note that the cranial part of the abdominal incision stops within the hair coat (arrowed).

placed initially and secured to the patient with towel clamps, sutures or skin staples. Securing the field drapes with sutures may be advantageous when intraoperative radiography is required. A plain or fenestrated coeliotomy or sheet drape covers the field drapes and is attached to them by either non-penetrating forceps (e.g. Allis tissue forceps) or a plain or impregnated incise (adherent) drape. The sheet drape provides an additional layer of coverage around the surgical site, covers any remaining exposed areas of the patient and provides a continuous sterile field from the area of interest to the surgical table.

Surgeon preparation

The surgeon and theatre staff are a significant source of surgical contamination and therefore the people in the operating theatre should be limited to essential staff. Theatre staff must not wear outdoor clothing in theatre and ideally should wear clean scrub suits. Shoe covers or designated surgical shoes, surgical hoods and masks complete normal surgical attire.

The surgeon and any assistants must perform an adequate surgical scrub using an antimicrobial scrub preparation prior to donning a sterile sleeved operating gown and surgical gloves. Contaminated or perforated gloves must be replaced during the surgical procedure.

Instruments

Theatre staff will be familiar with the instrumentation required for routine abdominal surgery but the veterinary surgeon must inform the relevant staff of any specific requirements for the anticipated procedure (see Chapter

2). The instruments must be sterilized in preparation for surgery. Instruments that become contaminated during the surgical procedure should be discarded and replaced with sterile equipment.

Operating theatre

The operating theatre must not be used for patient or surgeon preparation and is not an appropriate area for storing surgical or other equipment and consumables. At the start and end of each operating day the theatre, table, lights and walls are damp-dusted or wiped down with disinfectant. Any floor spills need to be dealt with promptly, not only from a health and safety point of view but also to minimize ongoing theatre contamination. The surgical table must be disinfected between surgical patients to limit cross-contamination.

Sharp anatomical dissection

A ventral midline incision is most frequently used for abdominal surgery and may extend from the xiphoid process, through the umbilicus to the pubic symphysis. Although the incision can be created using electrosurgery, ultrasonic scalpel or laser, sharp surgical incision with a scalpel is usually employed. The scalpel blade is held perpendicular to the skin to avoid bevelling the skin edge (Figure 1.17). Applying equal lateral tension on either side of the proposed incision facilitates separation of the wound margins and identification of the underlying tissues. Scalpel blades rapidly become dull and may need to be replaced before further sharp dissection is performed.

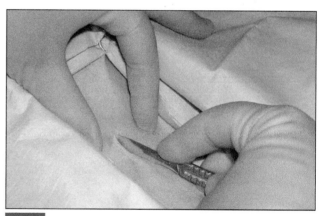

1.17 The scalpel blade should be held perpendicular to the skin.

The following principles of good dissection are used within the abdominal cavity.

* *Dissection of anatomical tissue planes is best performed by blunt dissection.* Blunt dissection incorrectly used significantly increases tissue trauma. The veterinary surgeon's gloved finger, sterile gauze surgical swabs (sponges), pledget Lahey or peanut swabs, sterile cotton buds or surgical instruments such as Metzenbaum scissors, Lahey bile duct forceps or Halsted mosquito forceps may be used for blunt dissection. Recently the use of ultrasonic scalpels has been described for dissection (Figure 1.18). The variety of techniques that are used includes: splitting of muscle, aponeuroses and connective tissue; peeling, wiping, pinching and tearing of adhesions, connective tissue and fibrous tissue; and finger fracture of friable parenchymatous organs.

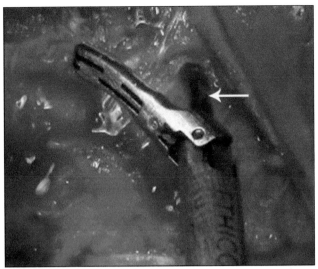

1.18 A Harmonic® scalpel being used to dissect the skin away from a mandible. The active blade (arrowed) vibrates at 55,000 cycles per second.

- *Dissection of scar tissue or in non-anatomical tissue planes is best performed by sharp dissection.* Both scissors and scalpels may be used for sharp dissection. Scissor dissection lacks the control of the scalpel and can crush tissues. This can be minimized by using sharp, well maintained scissors and ensuring that the scissor blades remain in contact with each other when cutting. Sharp incision and dissection make tissue realignment on anastomosis and closure easier and reduce the opportunity for development of tissue dead space.
- *The application of traction and counter-traction facilitates identification of tissue planes.* Applying traction and counter-traction is particularly important during scalpel dissection. It stretches and thins tissue to be dissected and may allow important structures to be identified. In addition, it helps to fix tissues about to be cut so that they do not move away from the scalpel or scissor blade. However, it should be remembered that traction and tension can distort the normal relationship between tissues, obtund arterial pulsations and flatten veins. Consequently, the tissues should be relaxed intermittently and tension reapplied.
- *Dissect from known to unknown in the presence of scarring or abnormal anatomy.* Pathological processes can change the appearance, location and texture of normally familiar tissues and it is advisable to work towards the affected area from normal tissue.

Atraumatic tissue handling

> **WARNING**
>
> Inadequate length of incision or an inappropriately positioned incision increases tissue trauma by decreasing surgical exposure, leading to excessive tissue traction

Tissue trauma can occur easily throughout the surgical procedure:

- The veterinary surgeon should be familiar with the normal anatomical features and organs of the abdominal cavity. This will help to prevent misdiagnosis and inappropriate surgery and thus trauma
- Transection of peritoneal reflections and ligaments can increase surgical access and exposure (e.g. transection of the triangular ligaments of the liver)
- Sharp surgical incision and dissection cause less tissue trauma than blunt dissection and should be used where appropriate
- Tissue desiccation must be prevented by keeping exposed tissues moist with sterile saline or laying moist abdominal swabs over the surface of the exposed tissues (Figure 1.19)
- During abdominal surgery the correct instrument must be used on the correct tissue in the proper way. Common errors include stabilizing and handling visceral and parenchymatous tissue with Allis tissue forceps, plain forceps or rat-toothed forceps (see Chapter 2)
- All surgical instruments should be properly maintained to ensure optimal function
- Stay sutures are atraumatic and facilitate surgical exposure and procedures
- Meticulous haemostasis, lavage and control of surgical fluids by use of an appropriate suction tip (see Chapter 2) will help to maintain a clear surgical field of vision
- Lavage and suction to remove minor haemorrhage are less traumatic than repeated swabbing of organs such as the bladder
- It should be remembered that sacrificing atraumatic technique for surgical speed will increase surgical morbidity.

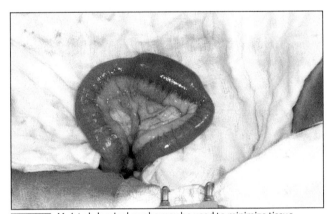

1.19 Moist abdominal swabs may be used to minimize tissue dehydration when operating on isolated tissues, such as this section of jejunum.

Removal of devitalized tissue and lavage

All devitalized tissue and contaminants should be removed as far as possible. In some situations (e.g. septic peritonitis) it may be necessary to provide ongoing drainage. 'Packing off' or isolating tissues and organs with moist sterile surgical or abdominal swabs can help to limit contamination of the abdominal cavity during procedures (see Figure 1.19). When this is done it is essential to record the number and size of swabs used in this way. The contaminated swabs are subsequently discarded. In the presence of gross contamination, surgical gloves and instruments should be changed before proceeding. Finally, the abdomen must be thoroughly lavaged using warmed sterile isotonic saline and the lavage fluid removed as far as possible by suction prior to abdominal closure. The volume of lavage fluid is not clearly defined but volumes of up to 200–300 ml/kg have been recommended in cases of septic peritonitis (Seim, 1995).

Haemostasis

Control of haemorrhage during abdominal surgery is important to prevent significant blood loss, maintain good surgical exposure, minimize strikethrough and prevent the development of haematomas that may compromise wound healing and predispose to SSIs. If significant haemorrhage occurs, it must be dealt with as a priority. Packing the affected area with a moist or dry swab may control haemorrhage temporarily. This provides time for the veterinary surgeon to extend the surgical incision if required or to ask for surgical assistance. All of the standard methods of haemostasis may be used. Further details can be found in the *BSAVA Manual of Canine and Feline Surgical Principles*.

Accurate tissue apposition

Correct closure of the abdominal cavity and anastomosis and apposition of the viscera and abdominal organs are discussed in the relevant chapters.

Complications of abdominal surgery

Appropriate surgical training and guidance, in addition to up to date knowledge of anatomy, pathophysiology and surgical methods, with close adherence to Halsted's surgical principles, will all contribute to a successful surgical outcome. However, complications – secondary conditions that develop during treatment of a primary disease – may still occur following abdominal surgery (Figure 1.20). Rates of perioperative complications following elective procedures (Figure 1.21) in cats and dogs are variably reported as between 10% and 20%, though the incidence of severe complications is lower (1–5%). Exploratory coeliotomy in cats and dogs, for reasons other than elective procedures, has a 25–30% perioperative complication rate (Boothe *et al.*, 1992; Lester *et al.*, 2004). Anaesthetic morbidity and mortality in these animals is similar to that found in elective procedures, with the majority of complications related to the underlying disease process rather than the surgical procedure itself (7–9%).

In addition to surgical complications, human error can occur in both human (McIntyre *et al.*, 2010) and veterinary surgery (Forster *et al.*, 2011) and may cause harm to the patient. The recent introduction of the World Health Organization guidelines for safe surgery (WHO, 2009) has successfully focused efforts worldwide on reducing avoidable errors in the theatre suite to decrease surgical morbidity and mortality (Haynes *et al.*, 2009, 2011). The use of similar checklist-based surgical safety interventions is starting to gain favour in veterinary medicine.

WARNING

One possible error is failure to remove all surgical swabs or instruments from the abdominal cavity (Figure 1.22). Such retained surgical items may cause problems as diverse as abdominal wall sinus formation, septic peritonitis, gastrointestinal perforation and obstruction

---

Simple procedures must be adopted to minimize the incidence of such errors, for example: using surgical swabs with radiopaque markers; counting all surgical swabs used during open cavity surgery, once at the start

Anaesthetic complications

- Perivascular injection of irritant drugs
- Dysphoria on recovery
- Prolonged anaesthetic recovery (e.g. hypothermia, hypotension)
- Inadequate analgesia
- Allergic reaction to anaesthetic agents
- Re-expansion pulmonary oedema (e.g. following repair of chronic diaphragmatic hernia)
- Silent regurgitation and aspiration
- Reflux oesophagitis/oesophageal stricture
- Organ dysfunction or failure (e.g. renal)
- Anaesthetic death (e.g. respiratory arrest)

Abdominal wall complications

- Haemorrhage
- Wound infection/cellulitis
- Seroma
- Ischaemia
- Haematoma/contusion
- Oedema
- Suture sinus
- Wound dehiscence
- Evisceration
- Patient interference
- Incisional hernia

Abdominal cavity complications

- Shock
- Haemorrhage
- Inadequate resection of tissues (e.g. neoplasia)
- Inappropriate resection of tissues
- Inappropriate euthanasia (e.g. visual rather than histopathological diagnosis of neoplasia)
- Suture line leakage or dehiscence (e.g. gastrointestinal dehiscence)
- Localized or generalized peritonitis (e.g. abscess, septic peritonitis, uroperitoneum)
- Organ-specific complications (e.g. gastric stasis following gastric derotation)
- Disease-specific complications (e.g. poor glycaemic control following resection of insulinoma)
- Procedure-specific complications (e.g. thromboembolism following adrenal gland surgery)
- Organ malposition (e.g. small intestinal volvulus)
- Portal hypertension
- Iatrogenic diaphragmatic rupture and pneumothorax
- Adhesions
- Retained surgical swab or instrument

1.20 Complications following abdominal surgery in companion animals.

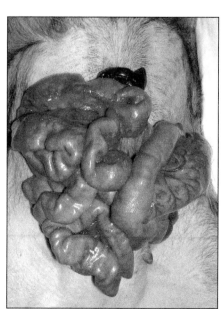

1.21 Evisceration following ovariohysterectomy.

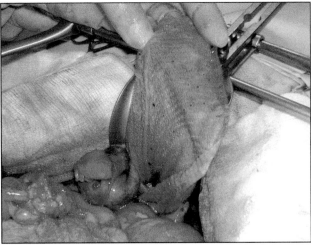

1.22 A surgical swab retained following exploratory abdominal surgery.

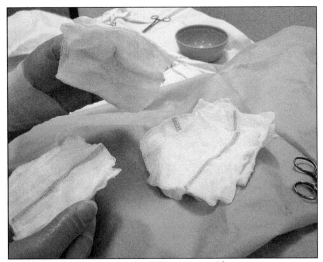

1.23 All surgical swabs should be accounted for prior to abdominal closure. Note the presence of the radiopaque marker in the swabs.

of the procedure and twice at the end (Figure 1.23); recording all surgical swabs packed into the abdomen during a procedure, and checking they are removed; and intraoperative or immediate postoperative radiography of patients following incomplete swab counts. In addition, veterinary surgeons should be aware that such errors occur more readily when surgical procedures are performed on an emergency basis, or when there are unexpected changes in the operation performed.

Routine perioperative monitoring

The importance of continuing patient monitoring into the postoperative period cannot be underestimated. The level of monitoring required is dictated by the patient, the procedure performed (see relevant chapters) and the monitoring equipment and personnel available. The most critical monitoring is frequent personal observation and assessment by the clinician or a suitably trained and qualified veterinary nurse or technician. It should be remembered that trends often provide the best information.

The speed of recovery from general anaesthesia and surgery depends on many factors, including:

- Duration of the procedure
- Breed
- Systemic illness
- Temperature
- Anaesthetic drugs administered and route of administration.

It is important to be vigilant for animals taking an unexpected period of time to become fully conscious. The minimum monitoring provided for every patient recovering from an abdominal surgical procedure should be as follows:

- *Temperature.* Hypothermia is very common during surgery and can be exacerbated by prolonged anaesthesia and surgery, excessive anaesthetic depth, small body size, paediatric or geriatric patients, open body cavities (abdomen), low ambient room temperature, cold intravenous and lavage fluids and an unheated operating table. Hypothermia that is not addressed can lead to prolonged anaesthetic recovery
- *Pulse rate and quality.* Monitoring the pulse rate and quality is the least invasive way to assess the cardiovascular system. More advanced monitoring may be achieved using an electrocardiogram, invasive or non-invasive blood pressure monitoring and sequential central venous pressure measurements
- *Respiratory rate and quality.* Respiratory arrest leading to cardiac arrest is more common in companion animals than cardiac arrest alone. Oxygen supplementation may be required in patients recovering from abdominal surgery and may be provided by a variety of means, including flow-by, mask, nasal oxygen tubes or prongs. More advanced monitoring may be achieved using pulse oximetry or blood gas analysis. Pulse oximetry is widely available, but it is important to remember that arterial oxygen haemoglobin saturation (S_aO_2) does not have a linear relationship with arterial oxygen concentration (P_aO_2)
- *Mucous membrane colour and capillary refill time (CRT).* Mucous membrane colour and CRT taken together give a crude indication of both ventilation and perfusion
- *Mentation and level of analgesia*
- *Position of the patient.* If a patient has not moved voluntarily for 30 minutes, they should be turned over to minimize the risk of hypostatic congestion developing in the dependent lung
- *Wound management.* The surgical wound should be carefully observed for any excessive swelling or discharge in the postoperative period. It is good practice to cover the surgical wound with a light absorptive semi-occlusive adhesive dressing in the immediate postoperative period to protect it from contamination
- *Drug therapy.* Prescribed medications must be given at the appropriate times.

Other easily measured parameters during this time are as follows:

- *Urine production.* The most accurate measurement of urine output is obtained by means of an indwelling urinary catheter and closed drainage system, with frequent measurement of output. Normal urine production (1–2 ml/kg/h) signifies adequate renal perfusion. Causes of oliguria (i.e. <0.5 ml/kg/h) should be investigated

- *Packed cell volume (PCV) and total solids (TS).* These must be monitored in patients with ongoing or suspected haemorrhage. In acute haemorrhage, the fall in PCV and haemoglobin concentration is delayed until plasma volume re-expands. The fall is accelerated by administration of intravenous fluids. Ultrasound examination of the abdomen to detect free fluid, and paracentesis, may be warranted in the interim
- *Blood glucose, electrolytes and other blood biochemistry.* Routine postoperative evaluation of specific electrolytes is dictated by coexisting disease processes, anaesthetic and operative procedures and complications, delayed anaesthetic recovery and clinical findings during postoperative monitoring.

Conclusion

The principles of abdominal surgery vary little from those applied during any operative procedure undertaken in veterinary practice. The value of careful preoperative evaluation of the patient and the importance of operative planning cannot be overestimated. Continued evaluation following surgery is paramount in limiting perioperative morbidity.

References and further reading

Alef M, Von Praun F and Oechtering G (2008) Is routine pre-anaesthetic haematological and biochemical screening justified in dogs? *Veterinary Anaesthesia and Analgesia* **35**, 132–140

Bainbridge D, Martin J, Arango M and Cheng D (2012) Perioperative and anaesthetic-related mortality in developed and developing countries: a systematic review and meta-analysis. *Lancet* **380**, 1075–1081

Boothe HW, Slater MR, Hobson HP, Fossum TW and Jung C (1992) Exploratory coeliotomy in 200 non-traumatized dogs and cats. *Veterinary Surgery* **21**, 452–457

Brodbelt D (2009) Perioperative mortality in small animal anaesthesia. *The Veterinary Journal* **182**, 152–161

Cimino Brown D (2012) Wound infections and antimicrobial use. In: *Veterinary Surgery: Small Animal*, ed. KM Tobias and SA Johnston, pp.135–139. Saunders Elsevier, St Louis

Devey JJ and Crowe DT (2000) Microenteral nutrition. In: *Current Veterinary Therapy XIII*, ed. JD Bonagura, pp.136–140. WB Saunders, London

Duncan J (2009) Preoperative assessment and patient preparation. In: *Anaesthesia for Veterinary Nurses, 2nd edn*, ed. E Welsh, pp.39–60. Wiley-Blackwell, Oxford

Forster K, Anderson D, Yool DA, Wright C and Burrow R (2011) Retained surgical swabs in 13 dogs. *Veterinary Record* **24**, 337

Güenaga KF, Matos D and Wille-Jørgensen P (2011) Mechanical bowel preparation for elective colorectal surgery. *Cochrane Database of Systematic Reviews* **9**, CD001544

Haynes AB, Weiser TG, Berry WR *et al.* (2009) A surgical safety checklist to reduce morbidity and mortality in a global population. *New England Journal of Medicine* **360**, 491–499

Haynes AB, Weiser TG, Berry WR *et al.* (2011) Changes in safety attitude and relationship to decreased postoperative morbidity and mortality following implementation of a checklist-based surgical safety intervention. *British Medical Journal of Quality and Safety* **20**, 102–107

Knights CB, Mateus A and Baines SJ (2012) Current British veterinary attitudes to the use of perioperative antimicrobials in small animal surgery. *Veterinary Record* **170**, 646

Lester S, Welsh E and Pratschke K (2004) Complications of exploratory coeliotomy in 70 cats. *Journal of Feline Medicine and Surgery* **45**, 351–356

McIntyre LK, Jurkovich GJ, Gunn MD and Maier RV (2010) Gossypiboma: tales of lost sponges and lessons learned. *Archives of Surgery* **145**, 770–775

Neihaus SA, Hathcock TL, Boothe DM and Goring RL (2011) Presurgical antiseptic efficacy of chlorhexidine diacetate and providone-iodine in the canine preputial cavity. *Journal of the American Animal Hospital Association* **47**, 406–412

Nelson LL (2011) Surgical site infections in small animal surgery. *Veterinary Clinics of North America: Small Animal Practice* **41**, 1041–1056

Orlander JD, Barber TW and Fincke BG (2002) The morbidity and mortality conference: the delicate nature of learning from error. *Academic Medicine: Journal of the Association of American Medical Colleges* **77(10)**, 1001–1006

Osborne CA and Lulich JP (2000) Alternatives to exploratory celiotomies; first do no harm. In: *Current Veterinary Therapy XIII*, ed. JD Bonagura, pp.17–21. WB Saunders, London

Saubermann AJ and Lagasse RS (2012) Prediction of rate and severity of adverse perioperative outcomes: 'Normal accidents' revisited. *Mount Sinai Journal of Medicine* **79**, 46–55

Seim HB (1995) Management of peritonitis. In: *Kirk's Current Veterinary Therapy XII*, ed. JD Bonagura, pp.764–770. WB Saunders, Philadelphia

Seymour C and Duke-Novakovski T (2007) *BSAVA Manual of Canine and Feline Anaesthesia and Analgesia, 2nd edn.* BSAVA Publications, Gloucester

Shales C (2012) Surgical wound infection and antimicrobial prophylaxis. In: *BSAVA Manual of Canine and Feline Surgical Principles*, ed. S Baines, V Lipscomb and T Hutchinson, pp.220–230. BSAVA Publications, Gloucester

Williams JM (2012) Colon. In: *Veterinary Surgery: Small Animal*, ed. KM Tobias and SA Johnston, pp.1542–1563. Saunders Elsevier, St Louis

World Health Organization (WHO) (2009) WHO guidelines for safe surgery: safe surgery saves lives. http://www.who.int/patientsafety/safesurgery/tools_resources/9789241598552/en/

Chapter 2

Equipment and surgical instrumentation

Prue Neath

This chapter considers the surgical biomaterials, instruments and equipment that aid veterinary surgeons (veterinarians) in performing abdominal surgical procedures to the best of their ability.

Surgical biomaterials

Surgical biomaterials are substances of natural or synthetic origin that are implanted within the body to treat, augment or replace tissue or function of the body.

Suture material

The range of available suture materials has greatly increased since the 1980s. This has assisted the veterinary surgeon in selecting a suture material that is appropriate for each wound, taking into account the typical healing rate of the tissue concerned and any local conditions or systemic factors that might influence healing.

Each suture material is classified according to a variety of properties: flexibility, capillarity, relative knot security, tissue reaction, loss of strength over time, ability to be absorbed, and time to complete absorption.

> **PRACTICAL TIP**
>
> Selection of suture size is guided by the strength of the tissue being repaired. Use of an excessively large suture should be avoided, since this leads to increased trauma to the tissues as the suture passes through, changes to tissue architecture, and an increase in foreign material within the wound

Figure 2.1 lists the wide range of suture materials available, and further details are discussed below. Figure 2.2 compares suture sizes in metric (Ph. Eur.) and United States Pharmacopeia (USP) systems.

Absorbable – rapid loss of strength

Polyglytone 6211: This synthetic monofilament suture material has excellent handling characteristics, good knot security and minimal tissue reactivity. In common with all the synthetic absorbable suture materials, it is broken down by hydrolysis. It loses 50% of its tensile strength by 5 days, 80% by 10 days, and is fully absorbed by 56 days.

Poliglecaprone 25: This synthetic monofilament suture material has good handling characteristics, good knot security and minimal tissue reactivity. The high initial strength of this material indicates that a smaller size than usual may be used. The dyed version loses tensile strength more slowly than the undyed version; strength reduction by 7 days is 40% *versus* 50%, and by 14 days is 70% *versus* 80%, respectively. The suture material is fully absorbed by 90–120 days.

Surgical gut (catgut): Catgut is a natural absorbable suture material created from the submucosa of sheep intestine or the serosa of bovine intestine. Machine-grinding and polishing of the multifilament thread produces a relatively smooth surface.

- Since catgut is composed mainly of collagen, it causes a marked inflammatory reaction and is removed by phagocytosis.
- Catgut is a rapidly absorbed material, losing 33% of its tensile strength by 7 days and 67% by 28 days, with complete absorption by 90 days. Absorption occurs more quickly in the presence of infection, increased vascularity or gastric secretions.
- The 'tanning' process produces chromic catgut, which makes it less inflammatory and more resistant to breakdown.
- Although the handling characteristics of catgut are good, knot security is variable and knots may become loose once the suture is wet.

Lactomer 9–1, polyglactin 910 and polyglycolic acid: These synthetic braided multifilament materials have excellent handling characteristics, good knot security and cause only mild tissue reaction, but do have marked tissue drag. They are removed from the tissues by hydrolysis. These suture materials lose 20–25% of their strength by 14 days, 50–70% by 21 days and are fully absorbed by 56–90 days. Polyglycolic acid may be broken down more quickly when exposed to urine, so its use in bladder closure is not recommended. Irradiated polyglactin 910 is more rapidly absorbed than standard polyglactin 910; it will retain only 50% of its tensile strength at 5 days, and will be completely absorbed by 42 days.

Absorbable – slow loss of strength

Glycomer 631, polyglyconate and polydioxanone: These synthetic monofilament suture materials have good

Generic name	Trade name	Manufacturer	Absorbable or non-absorbable	Multifilament or monofilament	Strength reduction	Complete absorption	Handling	Knot security	Tissue reaction
Irradiated polyglactin 910	Vicryl Rapide	Ethicon	Absorbable	Multifilament	50% at 5 days 100% at 14 days	42 days	+++	+++	++
Polyglytone 6211	Caprosyn	Covidien	Absorbable	Monofilament	50% at 5 days 80% at 10 days	56 days	++++	++	++
Poliglecaprone 25	Monocryl	Ethicon	Absorbable	Monofilament	50% at 7 days 80% at 14 days	90–120 days	++++	++	++
Chromic catgut	n/a	Multiple	Absorbable	Multifilament	33% at 7 days 67% at 28 days	90 days	++	+	++++
Lactomer 9–1	Polysorb	Covidien	Absorbable	Multifilament	20% at 14 days 70% at 21 days	56–70 days	+++	+++	++
Polyglactin 910	Vicryl	Ethicon	Absorbable	Multifilament	25% at 14 days 50% at 21 days	56–70 days	+++	+++	++
Polyglycolic acid	Dexon-S	Covidien	Absorbable	Multifilament	25% at 14 days 50% at 28 days	60–90 days	+++	+++	++
Glycomer 631	Biosyn	Covidien	Absorbable	Monofilament	25% at 14 days 60% at 21 days	90–110 days	+++	++	++
Glycomer 631	V-Loc 90	Covidien	Absorbable	Monofilament	25% at 14 days 60% at 21 days	90–110 days	+++	Knotless, barbed	++
Polyglyconate	Maxon	Covidien	Absorbable	Monofilament	25% at 14 days 75% at 42 days	180 days	++	++	++
Polydioxanone	PDS II	Ethicon	Absorbable	Monofilament	20% at 14 days 40% at 42 days	182–238 days	++	++	++
Silk	Perma-hand Silk	Ethicon Covidien	Non-absorbable	Multifilament	30% at 14 days 50% at 1 year	2 years	++++	+	++++
Polypropylene	Prolene Surgipro	Ethicon Covidien	Non-absorbable	Monofilament	n/a	n/a	++	++++	+
Nylon	Ethilon Monosof Dacron Surgilon	Ethicon Covidien Covidien Covidien	Non-absorbable	Monofilament Multifilament	30% at 2 years 75% at 180 days	n/a n/a	++ ++	++ +++	++ ++
Polymerized caprolactam	Supramid	S. Jackson Inc. B. Braun	Non-absorbable	Multifilament	n/a	n/a	+++	++++	+++
Polyester + Dacron	Ethibond Mersilene	Ethicon Ethicon	Non-absorbable	Multifilament	n/a	n/a	+++	+++	+++
Polyethylene	TiCron Surgidac	Covidien	Non-absorbable	Multifilament	n/a	n/a	+++	+++	+++
Polybutester	Novafil	Covidien	Non-absorbable	Monofilament	n/a	n/a	+++	++	++
Stainless steel	Steel	Ethicon Covidien	Non-absorbable	Monofilament	n/a	n/a	+	++++	+

2.1 Characteristics of selected suture materials. n/a = not applicable.

Metric (Ph. Eur.)	USP
0.5	7/0
0.7	6/0
1	5/0
1.5	4/0
2	3/0
3	2/0
3.5	0
4	1
5	2
6	3

2.2 Equivalent suture sizes.

handling properties, good knot security and minimal tissue reactivity. They vary mostly with regard to their duration of tensile strength retention. Glycomer 631 is absorbed more quickly, with 25% loss of tensile strength by 14 days, 60% loss by 21 days and full absorption by 90–110 days. Polyglyconate loses 25% by 14 days, 35% by 21 days, 50% by 28 days, 75% by 42 days and is fully absorbed by 180 days. Polydioxanone loses 20% by 14 days, 40% by 42 days and is completely absorbed by 180–240 days. The rate of loss of tensile strength is faster with 1.5 metric (4/0 USP) than with 2 metric (3/0 USP) polydioxanone.

Antibacterial

The antiseptic triclosan has been incorporated into three absorbable suture materials: poliglecaprone 25, polyglactin

910 and polydioxanone. There have been varying reports and opinions as to whether this modification has a statistically significant effect on surgical site infections, and a recent veterinary study reported little benefit from their use (Etter *et al.*, 2013). However, a systematic review and meta-analysis of the human literature (Wang *et al.*, 2013) revealed a 30% decrease in surgical site infections when the triclosan-embedded suture material was used. Experimentally, doxycycline-coated suture material has been shown to improve the mechanical strength of intestinal anastomoses (Pasternak *et al.*, 2008). Further development of antibacterial coatings for suture materials is ongoing, and further products are likely to become available.

Non-absorbable

Silk: This is an organic braided multifilament suture material created from the fibres produced by a special type of silkworm. The natural capillarity of the material is decreased by coating with oil, wax or silicone. Silk has excellent handling properties, but poor knot security and marked tissue reactivity. It should never be used to repair the gastrointestinal tract or bladder, nor should it be used in contaminated wounds, where it potentiates the development of infection. Silk is slowly broken down, losing all significant tensile strength by 6 months after implantation, and is eventually absorbed over 2 years.

Polypropylene: This synthetic monofilament suture material is derived from propane gas and is classified as a polyolefin plastic material. It is awkward to handle and tie but the knot security is excellent, owing to a locking action created by flattening of the strands where they cross each other. Polypropylene is highly flexible and has a low thrombogenicity; it is therefore an excellent choice for cardiovascular repairs. It causes minimal tissue reaction, retains its strength in tissues and is the least likely of the suture materials to potentiate infection in contaminated wounds.

Nylon: This synthetic suture material is a polyamide. It is available in a multifilament form but is most commonly used as a monofilament suture material. Nylon is awkward to handle and has poor knot security. It causes minimal tissue reaction, though buried cut ends may cause irritation. Monofilament nylon loses 30% of its tensile strength within 2 years of implantation, whereas the multifilament form loses 75% within 6 months.

Polymerized caprolactam: This synthetic twisted multifilament suture material also belongs to the polyamide group. It has excellent handling properties and tensile strength. Although it is coated with a proteinaceous sheath to decrease tissue drag, any damage to the sheath leads to a marked tissue reaction and this material is therefore not recommended for implantation beneath the skin.

Polyester and polyethylene: The uncoated forms of these braided multifilament suture materials have good knot security but excessive tissue drag. Coating improves handling and decreases tissue drag, but the knot security decreases and a five-throw knot is recommended. Polyester will cause a significant tissue reaction, especially if the coating is damaged, and tissue implantation is not recommended.

Polybutester: This specially modified form of monofilament polyester has improved handling qualities, good knot security and excellent flexibility.

Stainless steel: This is available as a monofilament suture material and although it is very strong, with excellent knot security, it has poor handling qualities. It is an inert material with minimal tissue reaction, but cut ends beneath the skin will cause irritation and may traumatize tissue.

Selection of suture material

The general objective of suture placement is to hold together tissues that have been separated until healing has occurred. It is therefore important to select the suture material for each tissue based on the expected healing rate of that tissue, whilst also taking into account the detrimental effects that the suture material may have on the healing process. General guidelines are summarized below.

Skin

Synthetic monofilament suture material is recommended (e.g. nylon, polypropylene). Some surgeons prefer the superior handling qualities of polymerized caprolactam, but significant skin irritation is often seen.

Subcutaneous tissue

Most skin sutures are removed by 14 days, although skin regains only 20% of its strength by 21 days postoperatively. The subdermal or immediate subcutaneous sutures therefore need to provide support beyond this time. Absorbable suture material is recommended and the synthetic materials have less tissue reactivity (e.g. glycomer 631, polyglactin 910 or polydioxanone). Recently an absorbable (glycomer 631) unidirectional barbed suture (wound closure device) has been introduced to spread tension more evenly when closing a wound, with the added advantage of avoiding bulky knots at either end (Figure 2.3).

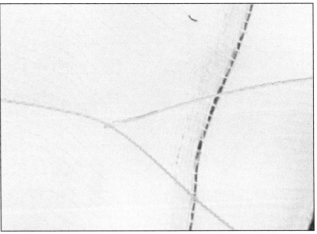

2.3 Barbed absorbable suture being passed through the loop at the distal end of the suture.

Linea alba and fascia

Fascia heals relatively slowly and its tensile strength is only 20% at 20 days postoperatively. A long-acting suture material is therefore recommended. The majority of surgeons recommend a synthetic absorbable suture material that loses its tensile strength relatively slowly (e.g. polydioxanone), but non-absorbable material may be indicated when delayed healing is anticipated.

Hollow viscus organs

Synthetic absorbable suture material is recommended for closure of organs such as the intestine and bladder. Although absorbable multifilament suture material will cause increased tissue drag and potentiate infection, it is used as frequently as absorbable monofilament material for this purpose, with no significant complications reported to date. The barbed version of glycomer 631 has recently been reported to provide a higher leakage pressure compared with the non-barbed version when used for enterotomy closure. Non-absorbable monofilament suture material may be used to repair the gastrointestinal tract when delayed healing is anticipated.

Parenchymal organs

Absorbable monofilament suture material is recommended for repair of organs such as the liver and kidney. Synthetic materials are preferred, owing to less tissue reactivity. Since multifilament suture material may tear through tissue and may potentiate infection, monofilament material is recommended.

Blood vessels

Absorbable suture material is recommended for ligation of the majority of blood vessels within the abdomen. Large blood vessels may be ligated with a non-absorbable suture material such as silk or polypropylene. Repair of large blood vessels should be performed with fine-gauge polypropylene.

Surgical needles

Needles are selected according to the tissue characteristics and the site of the wound. Most surgical needles are made from surgical-grade stainless steel. Needles are classified as eyed or swaged. Eyed needles require threading; they will cause more trauma to the tissues and are less efficient, but they are cheap and reusable.

Editors' note:

Eyed needles should never be used to suture a hollow viscus

Swaged needles form a continuous unit with the suture thread; they cause less tissue trauma, are reliably sharp and easier to use, but are more expensive and can only be used once.

The body of the needle may be straight, or it may be curved as $^5/_8$, $^1/_2$, $^3/_8$ or $^1/_4$ of a circle. Straight needles are used in superficial wounds, as are $^3/_8$ and $^1/_4$ circle needles. Deeper structures may be more easily sutured with a $^5/_8$ or $^1/_2$ circle needle.

The point of the needle is selected according to the type of tissue requiring repair:

- *Cutting needles* are used for tough tissue such as skin. The reverse cutting needle is used more commonly than the standard cutting needle because its design is associated with less tissue cut-out
- *Taper-cut needles* have a rounded body with a cutting point and are best used for dense tissue such as tendon
- *Taper-point needles* have a rounded body with a sharp point and are best used for more delicate tissues such as intestine and fascia

- *Blunt-pointed needles* have a rounded body with a blunt point and are best used for friable structures such as liver or spleen.

Stapling devices and ligating clips

Stapling devices have gradually become more widely used in the veterinary field. They have the advantages of being more consistent in their application, time-saving, and generally provide more reliable haemostasis than suture ligation if used correctly.

Skin staples

These have been used not only for closing skin wounds, but also experimentally for intestinal closure (Coolman *et al.*, 2000). They are single rectangular staples that are supplied in a pre-loaded fixed-head staple gun. Successful application requires that the skin be held in apposition whilst the staple is applied, that the operator ensures that both skin edges are perforated, and that the staple points meet in the midline to prevent rotation.

GIA and EEA staplers

Gastrointestinal anastomosis (GIA) and end-to-end anastomosis (EEA) staplers have been described for use in the dog and cat. Both devices apply a double layer of staples with concurrent resection of intestinal tissue to create a new stoma (see Chapter 7).

TA staplers

Thoracoabdominal (TA) stapling devices can be useful for resection of gastric or hepatic tissue, and can be used for intestinal anastomosis in combination with a GIA or EEA stapler. Three sizes of TA stapler are available (Figure 2.4), producing staple lines of 30, 55 or 90 mm in length. Each staple bends to form a B shape, compressing the tissue within the staple. Each length of cartridge is available in one of two staple depths: the 3.5 mm staple (blue cartridge), which compresses to 1.5 mm; or the 4.8 mm staple (green cartridge), which compresses to 2 mm tissue depth. All three cartridge lengths fire two rows of staples, but the smallest cartridge is also available with three rows of staples (V3). The V3 cartridge is especially useful for ligating tissue that contains large blood vessels. Details of stapling techniques are covered in Chapters 5, 7, 8 and 9.

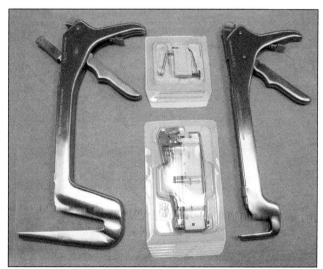

2.4 Thoracoabdominal staplers (left to right): TA90; TA90 and V3 cartridges; TA30.

Ligating clips

These small V-shaped clips can be applied to blood vessels up to 11 mm in diameter in place of suture ligation. Metallic clips (stainless steel, tantalum, titanium) are used most commonly, but absorbable clips are also available. The blood vessel should be dissected free from the surrounding tissue and the clip applied at a level that leaves 2–3 mm of tissue distal to the clip. Ligating clips are useful when multiple small blood vessels require ligation, or when the blood vessels are difficult to access. Use in adrenalectomy, neutering, mastectomy and amputation has been reported. Disadvantages include the expense of the clips and applicator, and insecurity of the clip if incorrectly applied.

LDS™ staplers

The ligate-and-divide stapler (LDS™; Figure 2.5) applies a metallic clip on either side of a pedicle and then cuts the tissue between the clips. It is extremely efficient. Although expensive, it is particularly useful for procedures such as splenectomy or resection of omental adhesions.

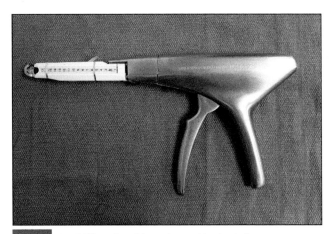

2.5 An LDS™ stapler with staple cartridge loaded.

Mesh and porcine small intestine submucosa

Surgical mesh

The most commonly used surgical mesh is created from polypropylene, but mesh composed of polyester or synthetic absorbable suture materials is also available. Mesh is useful for repairing defects in the body wall, whether the defect is created by trauma or by surgical excision of a tumour (see Chapter 3). If the site is contaminated, non-absorbable mesh should only be used as a temporary measure but absorbable mesh can be left in place. Since mesh is not flexible, it must be used with caution in growing animals. Mesh provides a scaffold for fibrous tissue to cross the defect. Although polypropylene mesh is associated with a granulomatous foreign body response in rats and humans, significant clinical complications are rarely reported in dogs and cats.

Porcine SIS

Porcine small intestine submucosa (SIS) has been developed as a tissue graft as part of the ongoing search for an ideal prosthesis for repair of body wall and hollow viscus defects in humans. Experimental studies in dogs

have shown porcine SIS to be an excellent scaffold for repair of defects of the bladder, body wall, dura, biliary tract and large arteries. The graft initially acts as a scaffold for migration of cells but, as activity by the native fibroblasts and blood vessels leads to collagen production, the porcine SIS material gradually disappears. New tissue specific to the repaired organ has also been found during histological examination of the repair sites, including smooth muscle fibres in bladder repair and biliary mucosa in bile duct repair. Defects repaired with porcine SIS demonstrate a well organized tissue structure with good incorporation into the surrounding normal tissue, in marked contrast to the disorganized repair found with non-biological graft material such as polypropylene mesh. A recent comparison of porcine SIS, fascia lata and polypropylene mesh concluded that fascia lata performed similarly to polypropylene mesh with regards to suture pullout, tensile testing and push-through tension. Porcine SIS was found to perform poorly in high-strain environments (Arnold et al., 2009).

Haemostatic agents

A wide variety of haemostatic products are available on the human and veterinary markets. Figure 2.6 lists a selection of the products in current use. Four categories of haemostatic agents are in general use: cellulose, collagen, gelatin and polysaccharide beads. More advanced products involving application of fibrin sealant or thrombin are used in the human medical field but are not widely used in the veterinary field, owing to their expense and special preparation requirements.

Cellulose

Cellulose is available as oxidized regenerated cellulose that has been knitted into a soft fabric (Figure 2.7) or carded into a textured cottony sheet. A piece is cut from the fabric and gently applied to the site of bleeding. The

Type of haemostatic agent	Material	Trade name	Manufacturer
Oxidized regenerated cellulose	Loose knitted fabric	Surgicel	Johnson & Johnson
	Textured sheet	Surgicel fibrillar	Johnson & Johnson
Calcium carboxycellulose	Plug, gauze, powder, spray	Traumastem	Millpledge
Gelatin	Sponge	Gelfoam	Pfizer
		Surgifoam	Johnson & Johnson
	Powder	Surgifoam	Johnson & Johnson
Collagen	Sponge	INSTAT	Johnson & Johnson
		Lyostypt	B Braun (Europe)
		Ultrafoam	CR Bard Inc. (USA)
	Microfibrillar	INSTAT MCH	Johnson & Johnson
		Avitene MCH	CR Bard Inc. (USA)
Polysaccharide	Microporous beads	HemaBlock	Hemablock LLC

2.6 Guide to various haemostatic agents available commercially.

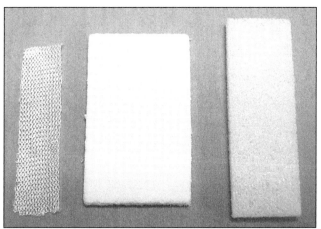

2.7 Haemostatic agents (left to right): cellulose fabric; collagen sponge; gelatin sponge.

woven fabric becomes gelatinous and acts as a matrix for platelet adhesion, thereby encouraging clot formation. Haemostasis occurs within 2–8 minutes. Although the material is absorbable over 1–2 weeks, there are differing opinions as to whether the product may precipitate infection. Some authors recommend that the product should be gently removed once haemostasis has been achieved. The product is only activated by whole blood and will not be effective in halting serous effusion from a tissue surface.

Cellulose is also available as a product made of calcium carboxycellulose. This is available as a sheet, powder, plug and spray. It works on the same principles as described above.

Collagen

Collagen products are created from bovine or porcine collagen and may be supplied as a small sheet of sponge (see Figure 2.7), powder or web. An appropriate amount of the product is applied to the bleeding area. Aggregation of platelets on the collagen activates the clotting cascade. Haemostasis may take 1–5 minutes. The collagen is slowly absorbed over 8–12 weeks.

Gelatin

Gelatin is available in both sponge (see Figure 2.7) and powder formulations. It is created from a purified gelatin solution. An appropriate amount is applied to the wound. It assists haemostasis by applying pressure to the wound as it swells with absorbed blood. The product is slowly absorbed over 4–6 weeks, but gentle removal once haemostasis has been achieved is recommended if the site is infected.

Microporous polysaccharide beads

These are synthesized from a plant-based polysaccharide source. When the particles come into contact with blood they act as a sieve and concentrate blood solids, such as platelets, red blood cells and clotting proteins, thereby accelerating natural haemostasis. The product is supplied in 0.5 g tubes with a tapering applicator. The site of bleeding should be blotted before the product is applied. Gentle pressure is then applied over the product until no re-bleeding is seen. Haemostasis usually occurs within several minutes, and excess powder can be flushed away with saline.

Surgical instruments

This section provides a general classification of instruments commonly used in abdominal surgery, illustrations of many of the examples described, and some brief notes on good handling techniques. The minimum instruments required in a general soft tissue surgical pack are shown in Figure 2.8. For additional instrumentation required for a specific procedure, see the instrument section for each Operative Technique in relevant chapters.

> **PRACTICAL TIP**
>
> It is worth investing in good quality instruments, as their extended lifespan will easily compensate for the initial extra outlay

Scissors

Scissors are available in many different varieties, depending on the use for which they are designed (Figure 2.9). They may have sharp or blunt points, plain or serrated cutting edges, and blades of different shapes. They may be designed with long or short bodies and may be light or heavyweight.

Instrument	Number
Scalpel handles (No. 3)	1–2
Scalpel blades (Nos. 10, 15 and/or 11)	1 of each
Metzenbaum scissors	2 (1 curved and 1 straight)
Mayo scissors	1
Brown Adson thumb forceps	1–2
DeBakey thumb forceps (150 mm/6 in)	1
DeBakey needle holder (6 or 7 in) or Mayo–Hegar needle holder	1
Allis tissue forceps	2
Halsted mosquito forceps (curved 5 in)	6–8
Backhaus towel clamps	8
Surgical swabs (small)[a]	5–10
Surgical swabs (large)[a]	5
Large kidney dish	1

[a] All surgical swabs should contain a radio-detectable marker

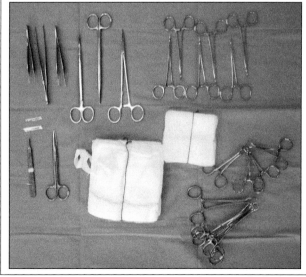

2.8 Minimum instrument requirements for a general soft tissue surgical pack.

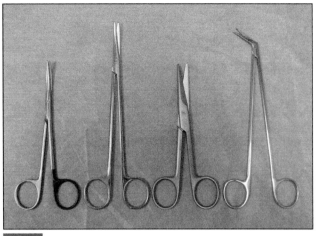

2.9 Scissors (left to right): suture; Metzenbaum; Mayo; Potts.

Metzenbaum scissors

These delicate scissors are the most commonly used dissecting scissors and are available in different lengths, with either curved or straight blunt-tipped blades. The curved blade is preferred by most surgeons, since it acts as an extension of the slightly bent index finger guiding the scissor. This tends to provide a more accurate line of incision than a straight blade. Metzenbaum scissors are particularly useful for controlled dissection through fine or delicate tissues. They should never be used for cutting heavy tissue or sutures, because this will lead to blunting, loosening and separating of the blades.

Mayo scissors

These heavier and sturdier scissors are also used for dissecting but tend to be reserved for heavier tissues such as fascia or cartilage. They may also be used for cutting suture material, though this will lead to blunting of the blades. They are available in a variety of lengths, with either curved or straight blades.

Suture removal scissors

Sutures may be cut during surgery using special scissors with serrated edges or simply a designated pair of Mayo or general-purpose scissors. Suture removal scissors, which are not generally used in the operating theatre, have a concavity on one blade that minimizes pull on the skin as the suture is cut.

Potts scissors

These delicate instruments are designed with a long body that ends in straight blades with pointed tips. The blades are available at varying angles to suit different situations. The scissors are designed specifically for blood vessel surgery and should not be used for general dissection.

Efficient use of scissors

Scissors are used most efficiently if they are held correctly. The wide-based tripod grip is recommended:

- The thumb is inserted into the upper ring and the third finger is inserted into the lower ring (Figure 2.10a)
- The first finger is placed on the shaft near the fulcrum, while the second finger is wrapped around the shaft at the junction with the lower ring.

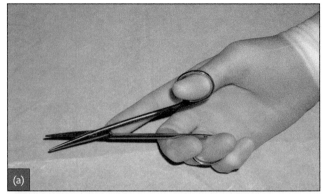

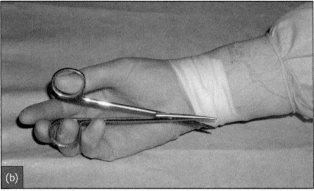

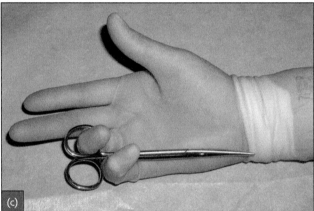

2.10 Scissor grips: (a) wide-based tripod; (b) backhand thumb–third finger; (c) 'palmed', leaving thumb and two fingers free.

This grip improves stability and increases the shearing force and torque of the blades. When the surgeon needs to cut in a reverse direction, towards their body, the scissors can be reversed to a backhand grip, which provides better control of the scissor tips (Figure 2.10b). Some surgeons use the thumb and first finger for this backhand grip, but the author finds the thumb and third finger grip more stable. When scissors are not in use, they can be rotated around the third finger to be 'palmed', leaving the thumb, first and second fingers free to perform another action (Figure 2.10c). The fourth finger holds the scissors in place.

Most scissors are designed for use by right-handed surgeons. Left-handed surgeons will need to use scissors designed for left-hand use or they can practise using right-handed scissors.

Tissue forceps

Tissue forceps are used to grasp or clamp tissue and can be divided into 'thumb' or dissecting forceps, and ratcheted tissue forceps.

Thumb forceps

These pincer-like instruments of varying lengths have either grooves or teeth at their tips. They are designed to retract or stabilize tissue in a non-traumatic way, enabling dissection or suturing to proceed. Thumb forceps should be held in a pencil grip by the non-dominant hand, balancing the blades between the thumb and first finger. When not in use, the forceps can be rotated into a 'palmed' position with the third and fourth fingers holding the forceps against the palm (Figure 2.11). This leaves the thumb, first and second fingers free for another task.

- Thumb forceps with *smooth* grooves or ridges at their tips include dressing forceps and Emmett forceps (Figure 2.12). These may be used simply for manipulating dressings, but the lighter versions can also be used for gentle handling of viscera and serosal surfaces.
- '*Atraumatic*' thumb forceps have interlocking longitudinal rows of tiny teeth and were designed for minimizing damage during vascular surgery, though they may be used for handling many delicate tissues safely. The most commonly used variations are the DeBakey (Figure 2.12) and Cooley forceps. They are available in a variety of lengths suitable for different depths of surgical field. Note that the delicate teeth of these expensive forceps should never be used to grasp needles during suturing.

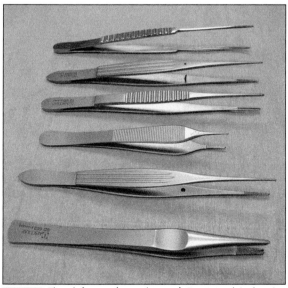

2.11 Thumb forceps grip: 'palmed', leaving thumb and two fingers free to use another instrument.

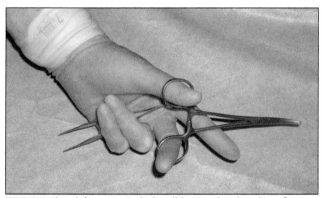

2.12 Thumb forceps (top to bottom): Emmett; plain dressing; DeBakey; Adson; Gillies; Lane's.

Toothed forceps

Toothed forceps are available in three different weights, with variations in the number of teeth depending on the width of the tip.

- The *small fine-toothed* forceps allow a delicate grip of fine tissues with greater security than the non-toothed forceps. They may be used for thin skin but are not strong enough to hold thicker skin or fascia. The Adson forceps are the most commonly used of this group and have a 1 × 2 teeth tip (1 tooth on one tip and 2 teeth on the opposite tip; Figure 2.12).
- The *medium-toothed* forceps are heavier and longer, but still have a narrow tip with only 1 × 2 teeth. They can be used for thicker skin and fascia than the small forceps; the Gillies (Figure 2.12) and Treves forceps are typical examples.
- *Heavy-toothed* forceps are occasionally required for handling of thick fascia or skin in large dogs, and the Lane's forceps are an example of these (Figure 2.12).

Most toothed forceps have a cross-hatched area below the tips that can be used for grasping needles during suturing.

Ratcheted tissue forceps

Ratcheted forceps of various sizes and lengths are available, with tips that are toothed or smooth (Figure 2.13).

- *Toothed* ratcheted forceps have a crushing action when applied to tissue and are therefore only applied to heavy tissue, such as fascia or connective tissue. They should not be used on skin or on any abdominal organs. The Allis tissue forceps are a light version of this category with multiple teeth, whereas the Lane's forceps are heavier forceps with 1 × 2 teeth.
- *Non-toothed* ratcheted forceps are less traumatic to tissues, with more flexible shafts and *atraumatic* tips. They can be used for grasping hollow viscus organs to retract or stabilize them. The Babcock forceps have a

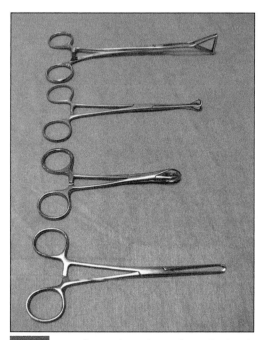

2.13 Tissue forceps (top to bottom): Duval; Babcock; Lane's; Allis.

similar appearance to Allis forceps but they have a wide fenestrated tip with a grooved surface. The Duval forceps have a longer, straighter shaft with a wide fenestrated triangular tip lined with tiny teeth or grooves.

Bowel clamps

Bowel clamps are specialized types of tissue forceps, available in non-crushing and crushing designs (Figure 2.14).

* Doyen intestinal clamps have long flexible bowed jaws with *atraumatic* gripping surfaces. They are designed so that the tips begin to meet as the first ratchet is closed. The pressure applied to the intestine gradually increases along the length of the jaws as the ratchet closes further. This allows occlusion of the lumen without disruption of the blood supply. Doyen clamps are available with straight or curved jaws, and the gripping surfaces are usually covered with longitudinal grooves.
* *Crushing* bowel clamps are ratcheted traumatic instruments with long grooved jaws. They are applied to areas of hollow viscus organs, such as the intestine, stomach or uterus, that are to be resected. The tissue is crushed between the jaws, occluding the lumen before the tissue is transected along the edge of the jaws. The Parker–Kerr and Lang–Stevenson clamps are typical examples of this category.

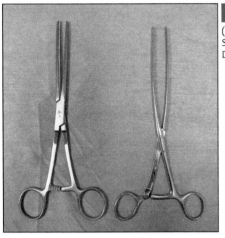

2.14 Bowel clamps: (left) Lang–Stevenson; (right) Doyen.

Haemostatic forceps

These instruments are crushing forceps used primarily to grip blood vessels, though they may also be used for tissue dissection, securing stay sutures and tissue handling. Haemostatic forceps are available in various sizes (Figure 2.15), with either straight or curved tips.

* Halsted mosquito forceps are *small fine-tipped* forceps with transverse serrations along the length of the jaws.
* *Medium-sized* haemostatic forceps include Spencer–Wells, Kelly and Crile forceps. These are able to crush slightly larger amounts of tissue. Jaw serrations vary among these forceps, with transverse serrations extending along only half the length of the Kelly jaws but along the entire length of the Spencer–Wells and Crile jaws.
* The *largest* and heaviest haemostatic forceps can be used for clamping large tissue bundles and include Roberts, Kocher and Rochester–Carmalt forceps. Jaw

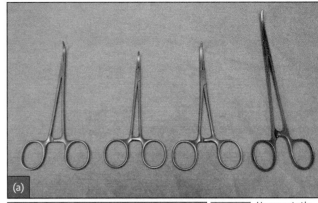

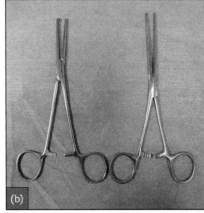

2.15 Haemostatic forceps: (a) (left to right) Mixter; Halsted mosquito; Spencer–Wells; Crile; (b) (left) Kocher; (right) Rochester–Carmalt.

serrations vary among styles and range from transverse serrations extending along the Roberts jaws, to longitudinal serrations along the Rochester–Carmalt jaws with cross-hatching at the tips to help prevent tissue slippage, to the large teeth at the end of the transversely serrated Kocher jaws to help ensure a secure grip.

Haemostatic forceps work most effectively if the blood vessel is not surrounded by excessive tissue. Small low-pressure blood vessels will be sealed by simply applying the crushing haemostat and leaving it in place, but some surgeons recommend twisting the forceps before removal. When applying curved forceps to these small vessels, the tip is pointed down towards the wound during application. This allows the forceps to fall to the side of the incision with the curved surface facing downwards. If the vessel is larger and requires ligation, the curved forceps should be applied with the tips facing upwards to facilitate suture placement below the instrument. The forceps are placed at a level that will leave sufficient vessel wall above the ligature to prevent slippage. Once the first throw of the ligature is in place, the forceps should be released as the ligature is tightened to ensure sufficient crushing of the tissue. A square knot is recommended with at least three or four throws. If excessive tissue is included in the pedicle, the ligature will tighten only on the outer tissue, allowing the enclosed blood vessel to retract and bleed once the pedicle is released. Large pedicles may be secured by division into smaller sections that can each be ligated individually.

Right-angled forceps are ratcheted crushing forceps that are used mainly for tissue dissection and for passing sutures around deep structures, but they can also be used for clamping blood vessels in deep locations. They are designed with the jaws forming a 90-degree bend along their length. They are available in fine and heavy versions and come in varying sizes. The fine version is used most commonly and its tips tend to be tapered to a narrow blunt point, assisting careful dissection of delicate tissues. The Mixter forceps are the most commonly used fine version (Figure 2.15a). The Lahey forceps are an example of the heavier right-angled forceps.

Vascular clamps

Non-crushing vascular clamps are useful for temporary occlusion of large blood vessels during surgery. These clamps are specially designed to minimize trauma to the blood vessel wall and reduce the chances of intravascular thrombus formation. They are available in different lengths and weights with a variety of jaw lengths and shapes. The jaws are lined by atraumatic serrations that allow gentle occlusion. Commonly used vascular clamps include the DeBakey angled and Satinsky vascular clamps, as well as various bulldog vascular clamps (Figure 2.16).

Needle holders

Needle holders are used to grasp needles and push them through tissue. They are available in a variety of lengths and weights. The length of the instrument is selected so that the hands do not obstruct the surgical field. The jaws must hold a needle firmly, and they are usually short when compared with the long shafts. The weight of the instrument and size of the jaws are selected according to the size of the needle. Too large a needle can damage the needle holder; too large a needle holder will distort the needle. The tips are usually cross-hatched to enable a strong grip. Good quality needle holders have either a diamond surface coating of the tips or tungsten carbide inserts that can be replaced once worn. Needle holders can be broadly divided into ratcheted and non-ratcheted designs (Figure 2.17).

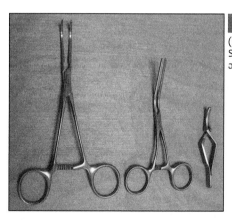

2.16 Vascular clamps (left to right): Satinsky; DeBakey angled; bulldog.

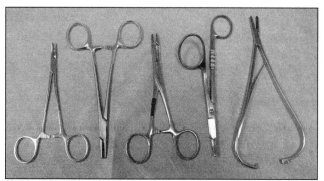

2.17 Needle holders (left to right): Ryder; Mayo–Hegar; Olsen–Hegar; Gillies; MacPhail.

Ratcheted needle holders

The most common ratcheted designs are shaped in a scissor pattern with a ratchet lock near the finger rings.

* The most widely used is the Mayo–Hegar needle holder. It is available in a variety of sizes that are suitable for medium to large needles.
* The Olsen–Hegar needle holder has a very similar design, but scissors are incorporated just above the gripping tips. The ability to allow cutting and suturing with the same instrument is very useful for surgeons working on their own, though some skill must be developed to avoid cutting the suture during tying.
* The Ryder needle holder is designed for delicate work, with narrow jaws that are ideal for small needles.

These ratcheted needle holders may be held in a wide-based tripod grip (as described for scissors above) for precise suturing, or in a palmed thenar eminence grip, which provides greater strength of needle passage and quicker needle release but less precision and greater chance of tissue trauma.

Ratcheted needle holders are also available in a design with the ratchet lock at the end of long arms and no finger rings. The MacPhail and Mathieu needle holders are typical examples of this design. These needle holders are held in a palmed thenar eminence grip and are very strong. They are only required for suturing very thick tissue and are not commonly used in the small animal field.

Non-ratcheted needle holders

Non-ratcheted needle holders require constant pressure to be applied in order to maintain the needle in the jaws. The most commonly used example is the Gillies needle holder. This instrument has the upper shaft shorter than the lower shaft, as well as an offset thumb ring, and this design allows a more comfortable grasp of the instrument with easy needle release. Scissors are incorporated into the blades above the cross-hatched tips, which is useful for the surgeon working alone. The perceived advantages of this design are outweighed by the need to apply constant pressure to the blades during needle handling.

Retractors

Retractors are of great use in soft tissue surgery, especially when working in the abdominal cavity and particularly if no surgical assistant is available. They may be held by hand to expose deeper tissues, or may be self-retaining. Hand-held retractors require the presence of an assistant, who must be instructed in how to use the instrument safely.

Passive retraction is rarely dangerous to the patient, but active retraction often places pressure on the tissues beneath the retractor blade and care must be taken to avoid tissue trauma. It is recommended that tissues are protected with saline-moistened laparotomy swabs if retraction is likely to be required for a prolonged period; for example, moistened laparotomy swabs should be placed along the edges of the abdominal incision prior to placing a self-retaining retractor.

Hand-held retractors

These are made in a variety of shapes and sizes (Figure 2.18), but the majority involve a 'blade' at approximately a right angle to the longer handle.

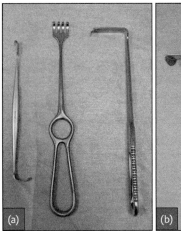
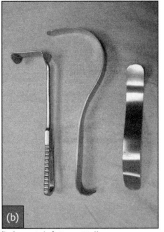

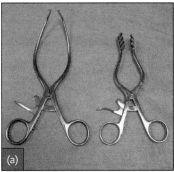

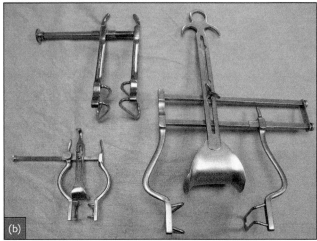

2.19 Self-retaining retractors: (a) (left) Gelpi; (right) West; (b) (left to right) baby Balfour; Gosset; Balfour.

2.18 Hand-held retractors: (a) (left to right) Senn; Volkmann; Langenbeck; (b) (left to right) Morris; Deaver; malleable.

- *Toothed small hand-held retractors* include the Senn (UK/USA), Volkmann (UK) and Meyerding finger (USA) retractors. These grip well, owing to their curved pointed teeth, and are useful for retracting skin and superficial muscle layers. Some varieties can have up to six teeth.
- *Non-toothed small hand-held retractors* include the Langenbeck (UK), Czerny (UK), Parker (USA) and Army–Navy retractors. These have deeper blades, and the Langenbeck and Parker retractors have a small lip at the end. The Langenbeck is available in several sizes. These instruments are useful as general retractors in abdominal surgery for retracting fat and smaller organs.
- *Large hand-held retractors* include the Morris (UK), Deaver (UK), Kelly (UK) and Meyerding (USA) retractors. These have larger wider blades and are useful for retracting large organs and large fat pads. Applying a damp laparotomy swab to the tissues before placing the retractor can help to decrease slippage or trauma.
- *Malleable retractors* are available in varying lengths and widths and are made of soft malleable metal. They can be bent in any combination of angles required, which makes them especially useful for deep abdominal surgery. They may be more effective if combined with a large damp laparotomy swab to retract slippery organs over long periods.

Self-retaining retractors

Self-retaining retractors are able to remain in a fixed position using a locking mechanism such as a ratchet, screws or simply friction. They are available in varying sizes with different lengths and shapes of blades (Figure 2.19).

- *Ratcheted retractors* include the Gelpi (UK/USA), Weitlaner (UK/USA), West (UK), Travers (UK) and Cone (UK) retractors. Gelpi retractors have single sharp outwardly pointed ends, but a blunt-ended version is available in the UK and ball tops placed over the pointed ends are used in the USA. The Weitlaner, West and Travers retractors have several teeth on each blade, with variations in whether the teeth are pointed or blunt, curved or straight, and in the number of teeth on each blade. The Cone retractor is an example of a hinged-arm ratcheted retractor.

- *Friction retractors* include the Balfour and Gosset self-retaining retractors. The Balfour has fenestrated side blades on curved arms supported by a double rail system. An optional short central blade may be attached to the rails to pull at 90 degrees to the side blades. Although some Balfour retractors have a screw to secure the side blades in place, most versions rely on friction to maintain the retraction. The spread of the standard Balfour retractor is 18–25 cm, whilst the smaller paediatric or baby Balfour has a spread of 10 cm. The Gosset retractor has fenestrated side blades on straight arms supported by a single rail. Two different sizes are available with a retraction spread of 10–15 cm. No central blade is available for this retractor.

> **PRACTICAL TIP**
>
> Balfour retractors are an invaluable piece of surgical equipment and should be used routinely in every abdominal exploratory surgery

Additional surgical equipment

Drapes

The goal of draping is to cover the patient and surrounding areas with a sterile barrier that will maintain a sterile field. The ideal draping material would be impervious to blood and fluid, since wet drapes allow migration of microorganisms. The material should ideally be resistant to tearing or puncture, lint free to reduce shedding into the surgical site, and easily drapable to fit around the patient and surgical equipment.

Woven textile drapes

These should be made from cotton with a 270-thread count. This provides a tightly woven finish that may inhibit microorganism migration. Further treatment of the fabric to repel fluids is ideal. Treated cotton drapes will become moisture permeable after 75 washes, whereas untreated cotton drapes become permeable after 30 washes. Holes and tears should be repaired before the next sterilization cycle. Adequate steam sterilization (with a vacuum cycle) requires that each drape pack should be no larger than 30 × 30 × 50 cm and weigh no more than 6 kg, and should be placed in the autoclave with the layers oriented vertically.

Non-woven fabric disposable drapes

These are made from compressed layers of synthetic fibres such as rayon or polyester combined with cellulose. They have the advantages of being moisture repellent, lint free and lightweight but relatively tear resistant. They are pre-packaged and already sterilized, which saves time and labour. The main disadvantage of these disposable drapes is their cost.

Self-adhering disposable drapes

These may be supplied as an 'incise' drape with an adhesive backing over the entire drape, or as a 'towel' drape that has a band of adhesive along only one edge. They may be applied quickly without the need for towel clamp attachment. This is especially useful in cases where imaging may be performed intraoperatively (e.g. portovenogram) because there are no towel clamps to obscure the image. The drapes are waterproof and microorganisms cannot penetrate the material. Previous concerns that microorganisms might multiply rapidly beneath the drape have been disproved. The main disadvantages of these drapes are the high cost and their inconsistent adherence to canine and feline skin.

Swabs (sponges)

Surgical swabs have traditionally been made of cotton gauze, but improved products are more widely used in the human medical field. The commonly used small swabs are composed of single layers of gauze, each folded into 4-ply squares measuring 7.5 × 7.5 cm or 10 × 10 cm. They are generally packed in batches of five (5–10 in the USA) for sterilization and supply.

> **WARNING**
>
> It is essential to use swabs with a radiopaque marker when working in the abdominal cavity

Large laparotomy swabs are composed of several layers of gauze stitched together at the periphery. Radiopaque markers are incorporated into the swab by the manufacturer. The 12-ply 30 × 30 cm laparotomy swab is useful for general tissue protection and retraction, in addition to fluid absorption. The thicker 24-ply 30 × 30 cm laparotomy swabs are especially useful for fluid absorption. Various other sizes are available.

Delicate dissection can be assisted by the use of cotton buds (Q-tips®). Standard cotton buds may be sterilized on site for intraoperative use, but surgical cotton buds with both tapered and round ends are available commercially in pre-sterilized packs (Figure 2.20).

> **PRACTICAL TIP**
>
> Large laparotomy swabs are essential for major abdominal surgery. Organs cannot be effectively packed off from the rest of the abdomen with regular-sized surgical swabs

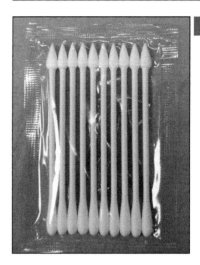

2.20 Surgical cotton buds (Q-tips®).

Suction

Portable suction units are available, but hospitals with multiple operating theatres may have a pipeline vacuum system instead. A unit that provides a vacuum of 80–120 mmHg is ideal to avoid tissue trauma, but an adjustable range of 0–200 mmHg is useful. Suction tubes are available with a simple suction tip or as a sump suction device (Figure 2.21).

- The *Frazier* suction tube has a narrow angled shaft with a single-hole tip and a decompression hole near its handle. It is usually supplied with a stylet which allows any tissue obstruction to be cleared as required. This suction tube is useful for focal suction of fluid.
- The *Yankauer* suction tube also has an angled shaft but it is larger than the Frazier, with no decompression hole. The round end of the shaft has four small holes. This suction tube is useful for removal of large quantities of fluid from the abdominal cavity.
- The *Poole* suction tube is a sump suction device with a fenestrated sheath covering a central tube ending in a single-hole tip. The fenestrated sheath allows suction of large volumes of fluid while preventing pieces of tissue or blood clots from obstructing the central tube. The sheath can be removed or retracted to allow the central tube to be used for focal suction as required.

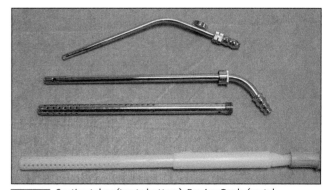

2.21 Suction tubes (top to bottom): Frazier; Poole (metal, unassembled); Poole (disposable, assembled).

Electrosurgery

Electrocoagulation is a very useful method of haemostasis for arteries up to 1 mm and veins up to 2 mm in diameter. An electrosurgical unit provides a highly dampened radio-frequency current that heats the tissue as it passes through it, leading to tissue coagulation. Two different types of electrosurgery can be used, each using a different type of handpiece (Figure 2.22).

Monopolar electrosurgery

Use of monopolar coagulation requires that a groundplate is applied to the patient's body, using conduction gel to ensure maximal contact. The handpiece can then be applied to the tissue requiring coagulation, and the current is turned on by using a hand switch (some units use a foot switch instead). For successful coagulation, the tissue site must be dry at the time of current application. It is recommended that the current is applied by touching the handpiece to a haemostat or thumb forceps in contact with the tissue, rather than by direct application. This allows more precise and effective coagulation of the site. Thermal burns can occur if there is insufficient contact between the groundplate and the patient. Modern machines have a safety system that sounds an alarm and prevents further current application if there is insufficient groundplate contact. The monopolar handpiece can also be used to cut through tissue, but this is used less frequently than coagulation in the veterinary field.

Bipolar electrosurgery

Bipolar coagulation is a more precise method of coagulation that involves the passage of current between the tips of a forceps handpiece, operated by a foot switch. The tips are placed either side of the tissue to be coagulated, leaving at least 1 mm between them. If the tips are touching, the current will short-circuit without coagulation occurring. Coagulation will occur even if the field is wet

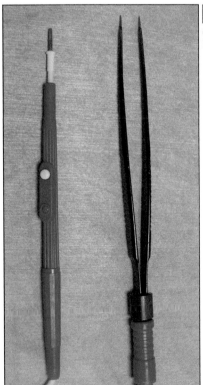

2.22 Electrocautery handpieces: (left) monopolar; (right) bipolar.

at the time of current application. There is no need for a groundplate and there is minimal chance of damage to adjacent structures with this controlled method of application. Less surgical smoke is produced by bipolar electrocautery, which is an advantage for the surgical staff.

Advanced electromagnetic energy coagulation and cutting devices

LigaSure™ and Enseal® vessel sealing systems

These systems were developed as an advanced bipolar system for sealing large vessels (up to 7 mm), but they are also used for grasping, sealing and cutting soft tissues. The energy output of the system alters in response to tissue impedance, and the heating cycle stops when protein coagulation is achieved. The tissue between the seals is then cut with a blade. The main disadvantage of the system is the blunt tip of the device, which makes dissection challenging. There have been reports of the device adhering to tissue and disrupting the seal as the jaws are released. The high cost of these single-use devices has slowed spread of their use in veterinary clinics. Though designed for single use they are frequently reused in veterinary practice, following sterilization with ethylene oxide; this does make them more cost-effective. Their use (together with Harmonic® devices) is particularly valuable in minimally invasive surgery (see Chapter 3).

Harmonic® system

The Harmonic® system (see Figure 1.18) uses a generator to transmit electromagnetic energy to piezoelectric crystals within a transducer in the handpiece. High-frequency ultrasonic mechanical energy is produced and transmitted to a blade or shears attached to the handpiece, which vibrates at 55,000 Hz (cycles per second). The longitudinal vibrations of the blade cause frictional heating, and tissue proteins are denatured by the mechanical energy. Compression encourages bonding of proteins to create a blood vessel seal. Tissue cutting is performed by a combination of mechanical vibration of the sharp blade and cavitational fragmentation at the tip of the blade. Coagulation is best achieved using a low power setting on the generator with low tissue tension, whereas cutting requires a high power setting and increased tissue tension. The blade attachments are best for dissection, but can seal vessels up to 2 mm in diameter. Shear attachments allow sealing of arteries up to 5 mm and veins up to 7 mm in diameter, as well as dissection and cutting. The main disadvantages of the Harmonic® system are the high cost and the risk of accidental damage to adjacent structures through coupling or blade overheating.

References and further reading

Arnold GA, Mathews KG, Roe S, Mente P and Seaboch T (2009) Biomechanical comparison of four soft tissue replacement materials: an in vitro evaluation of single and multilaminate porcine small intestinal submucosa, canine fascia lata, and polypropylene mesh. *Veterinary Surgery* **38**, 834–844

Boothe HW (1998) Selecting suture materials for small animal surgery. *Compendium on Continuing Education for the Practicing Veterinarian* **20**, 155–163

Bowman KLT, Birchard SJ and Bright RM (1998) Complications associated with implantation of polypropylene mesh in dogs and cats: a retrospective study of 21 cases (1984–1996). *Journal of the American Animal Hospital Association* **34**, 225–233

Coolman BR, Ehrhart N, Pijanowski G, Ehrhart EJ and Coolman SL (2000) Comparison of skin staples with sutures for anastomosis of the small intestine in dogs. *Veterinary Surgery* **29**, 293–302

Dubiel B, Shires PK, Korvick D and Chekan EG (2010) Electromagnetic energy sources in surgery. *Veterinary Surgery* **39**, 909–924

Etter SW, Ragetly GR, Bennett RA and Schaeffer DJ (2013) Effect of using triclosan-impregnated suture for incisional closure on surgical site infection and inflammation following tibial plateau leveling osteotomy in dogs. *Journal of the American Veterinary Medical Association* **242(3)**, 355–358

Hansen LA and Monnet EL (2012) Evaluation of a novel suture material for closure of intestinal anastomoses in canine cadavers. *American Journal of Veterinary Research* **73**, 1819–1823

Nieves MA and Wagner SD (2003) Surgical instruments. In: *Textbook of Small Animal Surgery, 3rd edn*, ed. D Slatter, pp.185–198. WB Saunders, Philadelphia

Pasternak B, Rehn M, Andersen L *et al.* (2008) Doxycycline-coated sutures improve mechanical strength of intestinal anastomoses. *International Journal of Colorectal Disease* **23**, 271–276

Skinner I (2000) *Basic Surgical Skills Manual*. McGraw-Hill Book Co. Australia, Roseville

Soiderer EE, Lantz GC, Kazacos EA, Hodde JP and Wiegand RE (2004) Morphological study of three collagen materials for body wall repair. *Journal of Surgical Research* **118**, 161–175

Toombs JP and Clarke KM (2003) Basic operative techniques. In: *Textbook of Small Animal Surgery, 3rd edn*, ed. D Slatter, pp.199–222. WB Saunders, Philadelphia

Wang ZX, Ziang CP, Cao Y *et al.* (2013) Systematic review and meta-analysis of triclosan-coated sutures for the prevention of surgical site infection. *British Journal of Surgery* **100(1)**, 465–473

Chapter 3

Laparoscopic instrumentation and fundamentals of laparoscopic surgery

Philipp Mayhew

Minimally invasive surgery (MIS) is a rapidly developing area of small animal surgery that can offer many advantages over traditional open surgery. Comparative studies in veterinary patients have documented a reduction in postoperative pain, more rapid return to normal activity and a possible reduction in wound healing complications when an MIS approach is used, compared to an open surgical incision (Devitt *et al.*, 2005; Culp *et al.*, 2009; Mayhew *et al.*, 2012).

A large number of totally laparoscopic as well as laparoscopic-assisted procedures have now been described in veterinary patients and new procedures are constantly being reported. Early reports in the veterinary literature documented simple 'assisted' procedures where laparoscopic equipment was used to elevate an organ out of the peritoneal cavity through a small incision. Traditional surgical instrumentation was then used to perform the procedure in an extraperitoneal location. Some of these techniques, such as laparoscopic-assisted gastropexy and gastrointestinal biopsy, have persisted and offer many of the advantages of an MIS approach combined with technical ease and a limited requirement for specialized instrumentation. In some cases both laparoscopic-assisted and totally laparoscopic versions of certain procedures have been described. In other cases, modifications of previously reported techniques have been described. Following the general trend in human medicine, this steady refinement in MIS has also led to a reduction in the number of operative portals used in veterinary medicine, and the use of single-port devices is increasing.

Equipment

High quality instrumentation is paramount to successful performance of laparoscopic surgery. Essential components that are usually housed on a mobile cart or endoscopic 'tower' include a medical grade monitor, endoscopic camera, light source unit and mechanical insufflator (Figure 3.1). A data recording device is preferred, to enable recording of images and videos, but is not essential to the performance of procedures. Telescopes transmit the image from the body cavity to the camera. Cannula and trocar assemblies provide safe and efficient access to the peritoneal cavity, allow for easy instrument exchanges during the procedure and play an essential role in maintenance of the pneumoperitoneum. Laparoscopic instrumentation is

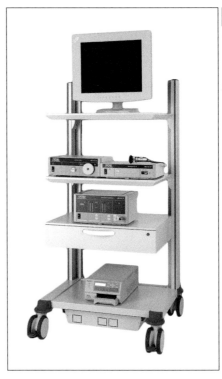

3.1 All the essential components for laparoscopic surgery are usually housed on an endoscopic tower. (Courtesy of Karl Storz Veterinary Endoscopy)

required to perform the surgical procedure. The variety of laparoscopic instrumentation used will depend on the complexity of the procedure being performed.

Camera

The endoscopic camera (Figure 3.2) is the device that turns the images transmitted through the telescope into viewable images on the monitor. The camera attaches to the head of the telescope and has a cord that feeds into the camera control box housed on the tower. Various types of camera exist and quality and cost can vary widely. One-chip cameras use a single computer chip to process colours, whereas in a three-chip camera each chip processes a separate primary colour, namely red, green or blue. One-chip cameras are adequate for most applications whereas three-chip cameras have superior optical clarity and colour reproduction. More recently high definition technology has provided another substantial improvement in the image quality produced by endoscopic cameras.

BSAVA Manual of Canine and Feline Abdominal Surgery, second edition. Edited by John M. Williams and Jacqui D. Niles. ©BSAVA 2015

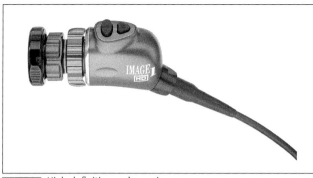

3.2 High-definition endoscopic camera.
(Courtesy of Karl Storz Veterinary Endoscopy)

Light source

The quality of light within the peritoneal cavity is dictated by the quality of the light source, the light cable and the gauge of the telescope being used. Modern light sources are powered by xenon, which reproduces the colour of natural light most closely. Different light cables transmit different light intensities, depending on their gauge, with larger cables being capable of transmitting more light.

> **PRACTICAL TIP**
>
> As telescope diameter decreases, the quality of light will also diminish. Telescopes smaller than 3 mm in diameter will provide poorer illumination within the abdominal cavity of larger patients

Mechanical insufflator

The insufflator is an essential piece of equipment for laparoscopy, allowing safe and regulated insufflation of gas into the peritoneal space. Mechanical insufflators sense intra-abdominal pressure (IAP) and provide regulation of the amount of gas to be insufflated. The IAP as well as flow rate (in litres/minute) and total gas volume infused are usually provided on the unit's visual display (Figure 3.3). Maximal IAP can be preset by the surgeon. In most cases, pressures of 8–12 mmHg are sufficient to perform most laparoscopic procedures in dogs and 4–8 mmHg is usually adequate in cats. Carbon dioxide (CO_2) is the most frequently used gas for insufflation during laparoscopy in small animals because it is inexpensive, colourless, does not support combustion and is rapidly excreted.

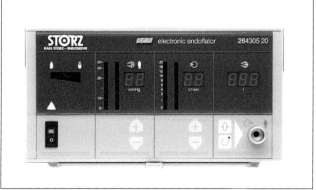

3.3 Mechanical insufflator.
(Courtesy of Karl Storz Veterinary Endoscopy)

Monitor

The ability to visualize the monitor clearly is a prerequisite for successful laparoscopic surgery. High quality medical grade cathode ray tube or flat panel monitors are preferred. Commercial television screens can be used but are usually inferior in quality. There is now a movement towards the use of high definition (HD) monitors in human and veterinary medicine. It is preferable to locate the viewing monitor on the contralateral side of the table from the surgeon, in a way that maintains a straight line from the surgeon to the lesion/organ being operated upon to the monitor. Arrangement of the operating theatre equipment in this fashion tends to augment the surgeon's hand–eye coordination substantially.

Data recording devices

Recording devices vary in complexity from simple printers to more expensive digital capture devices that incorporate their own hard drives from which both still images and video segments can be downloaded.

Telescopes

A variety of telescopes are available to the small animal laparoscopist. Variables include the diameter of the telescope and the angulation of the tip of the laparoscope. The 5 mm laparoscope provides a nice balance of durability, light conductance and image quality and can be passed down relatively narrow-gauge 5.5 or 6 mm cannulae. Telescopes 10 mm in diameter are often available from human hospitals and provide excellent image quality but are unnecessarily large. Smaller (3 mm) telescopes are helpful for very small patients and are the smallest sized telescopes that can be used without a sheath (when used unsheathed smaller telescopes are more easily damaged). Commonly used telescopes either do not incorporate an angulation of the tip (0 degrees) or are angled at 30 degrees (Figure 3.4). The 0-degree telescope is easy to use and provides an image of the organs lying directly in front of the telescope. With 30-degree telescopes the camera is providing an image that is deflected by 30 degrees (Figure 3.5). Rotation of the light cable (and therefore the telescope) allows a much wider viewing angle to be obtained as well as the ability to deflect the image around anatomical structures, allowing some degree of visualization over and around tissues.

> **WARNING**
>
> Inexperienced endoscopic surgeons may find 30-degree telescopes more difficult to use due to the deflected nature of the image

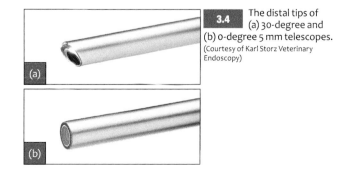

3.4 The distal tips of (a) 30-degree and (b) 0-degree 5 mm telescopes.
(Courtesy of Karl Storz Veterinary Endoscopy)

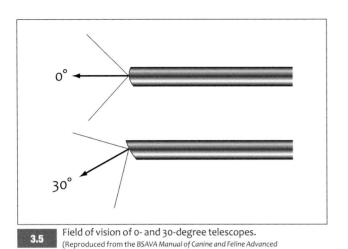

3.5 Field of vision of 0- and 30-degree telescopes.
(Reproduced from the *BSAVA Manual of Canine and Feline Advanced Veterinary Nursing*)

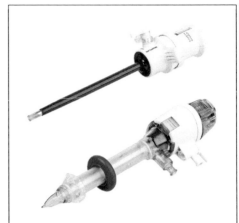

3.7 Disposable trocar–cannula assemblies come in a plethora of different sizes and designs.

Trocar–cannula assemblies

Use of cannulae in laparoscopic surgery is essential for two principal reasons:

- To minimize the leakage of CO_2 from the peritoneal cavity with subsequent loss of working space
- To ensure simple and safe instrument exchanges during surgery.

A multitude of sizes and designs of trocar–cannula assemblies exist on the market. They are generally subdivided into non-disposable (resterilizable) and disposable single-use devices that are principally designed for surgery in humans. Non-disposable cannulae are generally cheaper in the long term and are simpler in design, but may be heavier and more cumbersome. Threaded shaft designs can minimize dislodgement when using heavier cannulae (Figure 3.6). Disposable cannulae often have adjustable diaphragms that can accommodate variably sized instruments, whereas non-disposable types usually require the placement of differently sized reducer caps to allow different-sized instruments to be used. Disposable cannulae also sometimes incorporate helpful features such as radially expanding blades at the trocar tip or shielded trocar tips designed to reduce the chance of iatrogenic tissue damage (Figure 3.7).

The most common cannula sizes are used to accommodate 5 or 10 mm instruments and are generally 5.5–6 mm or 10.5–12 mm in diameter, respectively. Smaller (3.5 mm) graphite cannulae (Figure 3.8) are available for use in small dogs and cats and even smaller cannulae are available for exotic species. Most cannulae are designed for use with the appropriately sized trocar to facilitate placement. Trocars can be sharp or blunt tipped. If the

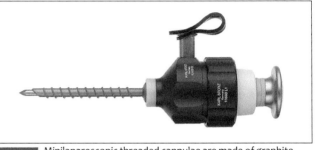

3.8 Minilaparoscopic threaded cannulae are made of graphite. They are very lightweight and ideal for small patients.
(Courtesy of Karl Storz Veterinary Endoscopy)

Hasson technique is being used for initial entry (see Laparoscopic access techniques below), a blunt-tipped trocar should always be used to avoid iatrogenic damage to the underlying organs. During placement of a camera portal after creation of a pneumoperitoneum with a Veress needle, a sharp-tipped trocar can be used because a pneumoperitoneum has been established and there is space between the abdominal organs and the body wall that should protect against iatrogenic damage. Trocarless cannulae (e.g. EndoTIP® cannula, Karl Storz) also exist and have a small protruberance on the end that can be used to 'corkscrew' the end of the cannula through the tissues (Figure 3.9). These cannulae are designed to spread the muscle fibres that they penetrate, rather than creating a hole. They also have the advantage that they can be used with a telescope in place during insertion, to allow direct visualization of the tissues that are being penetrated during entry.

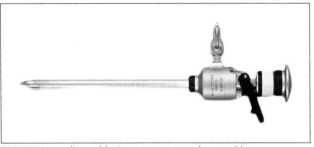

3.6 Non-disposable 6 mm trocar–cannula assembly.
(Courtesy of Karl Storz Veterinary Endoscopy)

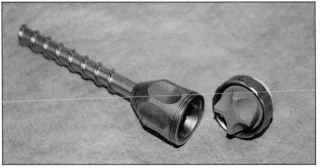

3.9 EndoTIP® cannulae are trocarless threaded cannulae that are designed to 'corkscrew' through the tissue, causing tissue separation.
(Courtesy of Karl Storz Veterinary Endoscopy)

Single-port devices

With the increased interest in MIS in human medicine has come a desire to refine techniques in order to minimize postoperative discomfort and scar formation through a reduction in port numbers. A rapid development in single-port procedures and devices has occurred. These devices are designed in most cases to be used in the umbilical area of human patients, thereby creating no visible scarring. In some cases they have been adapted for use in small animals in an effort to minimize port numbers in such patients. Most incorporate three to five ports within a single device, allowing the passage of the telescope along with multiple instruments (Runge, 2012). Examples include, the SILS™ port (Covidien Inc.), the TriPort™ (Olympus America Inc.), the GelPort® (Applied Medical Inc.) and the EndoCone® (Karl Storz Endoscopy). The SILS™ port can be used for a variety of procedures in small animals, including ovariectomy, cryptorchidectomy and gastropexy (Figure 3.10).

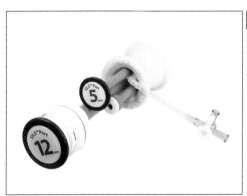

3.10 Single incision laparoscopic surgery device (SILS™, Covidien Inc.).

Laparoscopic instrumentation

The majority of instruments available for open surgery are now available for laparoscopic surgery (Figure 3.11). There are non-disposable as well as disposable instruments but non-disposable instruments are more common in veterinary medicine, mainly owing to their cost. The handles are generally interchangeable and therefore a smaller number of handles are required when compared with the number of instruments that are being used. Many instruments incorporate a monopolar pin that will allow the use of monopolar energy through the device tip.

A basic set of laparoscopic instrumentation should include a blunt probe, Kelly forceps, Babcock forceps, Metzenbaum scissors, suture-cutting scissors and cup

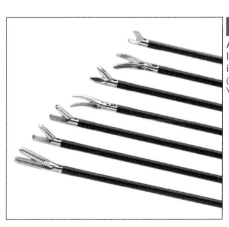

3.11 A selection of 5 mm laparoscopic instrumentation.
(Courtesy of Karl Storz Veterinary Endoscopy)

and/or punch biopsy forceps. Other useful additions to the basic set include right-angle dissection forceps, a knot pusher (if extracorporeal knot-tying is anticipated) and fan or other types of retractors. Most commonly in small animals, 5 mm instruments are used, although 3 mm and 10 mm instrumentation is also available. Instrumentation 1 or 2 mm in size can also be used, and this is sometimes termed minilaparoscopic or needlescopic instrumentation in the human literature. Suction–irrigation wands are available in disposable and non-disposable forms. Suction devices that allow fine control of suction and irrigation functions are ideal. The author uses a suction device that incorporates a trumpet valve to provide fine control of suction (Figure 3.12).

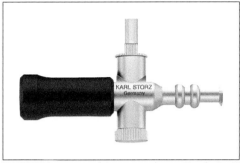

3.12 Laparoscopic trumpet valve suction device. The shaft and tip of the suction wand are not shown.
(Courtesy of Karl Storz Veterinary Endoscopy)

PRACTICAL TIP

Careful use of suction pressure is mandatory in laparoscopic surgery to avoid the rapid loss of the pneumoperitoneum and working space

Specimen retrieval bags (Figure 3.13) are necessary to minimize the risk of port site metastasis when tissue samples that could be neoplastic or infected are withdrawn through small portal incisions. They also allow large tissue samples to be withdrawn through relatively small port incisions. A variety of types and sizes are available for this purpose. For small samples, specimen retrieval bags can be fashioned out of the inverted thumbs of large surgical gloves and placed into the abdominal cavity through 10 or 12 mm cannulae. Specimen retrieval bags are available either loaded on an applicator or come without an applicator. The former are superior as the applicator (Figure 3.13) allows resected organs or tissue specimens to be 'scooped' into the opening of the bag which springs open after deployment. However, they are generally more expensive. Commercially available bags without applicators are more cumbersome to use as instruments are often required to hold the bag open as well as manipulate the tissue into the bag.

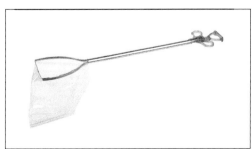

3.13 Specimen retrieval bag.

Laparoscopic access techniques

Safe and efficient abdominal access is the first important step in any laparoscopic procedure. In a number of cases, morbidity associated with laparoscopic surgery in humans has been attributed to complications occurring during peritoneal cavity access, and so a significant effort has been made to design devices and procedures to minimize these risks. Common to all techniques is the requirement to penetrate the abdominal wall to allow access for gas insufflation without causing iatrogenic organ trauma. A number of access techniques exist and can be used in small patients. **The choice between these techniques is largely based on personal preference; there is currently no clear evidence of one being safer than the other.**

Veress needle technique

This specialized device designed specifically for laparoscopic access consists of a sharp-tipped needle which houses within it a blunt-tipped obturator loaded on a spring mechanism (Figures 3.14 and 3.15). For placement, a small skin incision (2–3 mm) is made through which the needle is passed. Upon meeting resistance from the abdominal wall, the blunt-tipped spring-loaded obturator retreats into the shaft of the needle, allowing tissue penetration. Upon penetration of the body wall, however, resistance is lost, allowing the blunt-tipped obturator to spring forward, shielding the abdominal viscera from injury (Figure 3.16). During placement, it is important to drive the needle in while holding on to the shaft of the needle rather than the tip so as not to interfere with the spring mechanism.

Both disposable and non-disposable Veress needles are available. Once the needle has been placed it is essential to confirm correct positioning inside the peritoneal cavity as incorrect placement occurs commonly, especially during the early learning phase. Aspiration of the needle with an attached syringe is performed to ensure that penetration of a vascular structure has not occurred. Subsequently, a 'hanging drop test' can be performed to

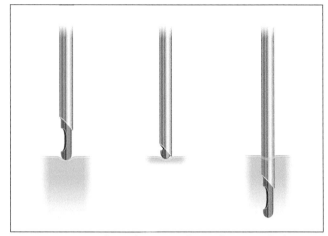

3.16 Veress needle mechanism. As the needle tip is pushed against the tissue, the inner blunt obturator retracts into the shaft, allowing the sharp needle tip to penetrate tissue planes. Upon entry into the peritoneal cavity and with the loss of resistance, the blunt obturator jumps forward, limiting potential iatrogenic damage to tissue.

confirm the position of the Veress needle within the peritoneal cavity. A drop of saline is placed on the hub of the needle. If the needle is within the peritoneal cavity the saline will generally pass down the needle. If the needle is in the subcutaneous space or has penetrated an organ no pressure difference will exist and the saline will remain on the hub. Once entry into the abdominal cavity has been confirmed, the hub of the needle is attached to the gas insufflator to create a pneumoperitoneum.

Modified Hasson technique

The modified Hasson technique involves the creation of a minilaparotomy, usually 1 cm caudal to the umbilicus. After an initial skin incision is made, blunt dissection is used to expose the linea alba, which is then grasped with rat-toothed forceps. A small incision is made using a No. 11 or 15 blade through the linea alba into the peritoneal cavity. Peritoneal cavity penetration is usually confirmed by visualization of the falciform fat (Figure 3.17). Once the surgeon is convinced that the peritoneal cavity has been penetrated a blunt-tipped trocar–cannula assembly can be inserted.

Insufflation

Regardless of which technique is used for abdominal access, the next step in the process of any laparoscopic procedure is the generation of a pneumoperitoneum. To

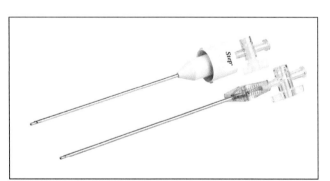

3.14 A variety of designs of disposable Veress needles (shown here) are available, as well as non-disposable types.

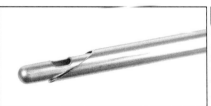

3.15 The tip of the Veress needle is shown, demonstrating the sharp-tipped outer needle that penetrates tissue as well as the spring-loaded inner blunt obturator.

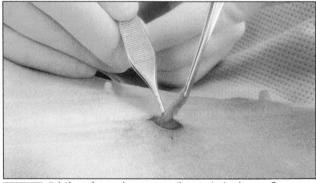

3.17 Falciform fat can be temporarily exteriorized to confirm peritoneal cavity entry when using the Hasson method of laparoscopic access.

achieve this, the insufflator line is attached to the side-port of the cannula or Veress needle and the abdomen is insufflated with CO_2. Other insufflation gases have been used (e.g. nitrous oxide, helium) but none is as rapidly absorbed, inert and inexpensive as CO_2.

> **WARNING**
>
> Air should never be used as an insufflation gas owing to the significant risk of air embolism

Once the gas flow is turned on, the abdomen should begin to become tympanic in the space of a few seconds to a few minutes, depending on the size of the patient and the gas flow rate (usually set at 1–2 l/min). Improper placement of the Veress needle or cannula can result in inadvertent insufflation of the subcutaneous space, resulting in subcutaneous emphysema. Further evidence of improper placement can usually be detected by observation of the insufflator pressure readings: if initial IAP is high (>6 mmHg) and flow of CO_2 is low, it suggests that the end of the trocar might not be positioned within the peritoneal cavity because resistance to flow of gas is being met (Figure 3.18b).

Correct positioning is usually indicated by an initially low IAP (<2 mmHg), which rapidly increases to the preset desired IAP in conjunction with a free and unimpeded flow of insufflation gas (Figure 3.18ac). For completion of most laparoscopic procedures in dogs, an IAP in the range 8–12 mmHg is sufficient. In cats, a lower IAP (4–8 mmHg) is often adequate for performance of many procedures, probably as a consequence of the greater compliance of the feline peritoneal wall.

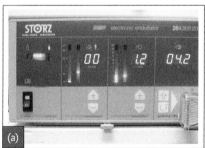

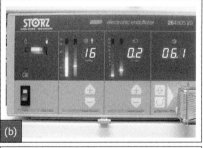

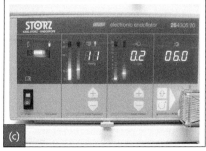

3.18 (a) If the cannula tip is positioned correctly within the peritoneal cavity, initial insufflator readings should indicate a low IAP (left-hand number) and good flow rate (1.2 l/min). (b) If initial readings suggest a high IAP with low flow rate (0.2 l/min), consider a possible occlusion in the line, cannula tip positioning not within the peritoneal cavity or the cannula tip being up against an organ or within the falciform fat. (c) With correct cannula positioning the pressure will rise to the preselected IAP and the flow rate will drop back down (0.2 l/min).
(Courtesy of Karl Storz Veterinary Endoscopy)

Port position

The selection of port locations for laparoscopic surgery is somewhat opinion-based and many procedures may be performed from variable port positions. In the author's practice the majority of laparoscopic procedures are performed using a camera portal located 1 cm caudal to the umbilicus (subumbilical). The subumbilical location is further caudal than the majority of the falciform fat in most dogs and cats and is a central location within the abdomen from where cranially and caudally located organs can easily be visualized. The exception to this rule is when certain dorsally located organs need to be accessed; procedures performed by the author in lateral (or sternal) recumbency using a paramedian camera portal include adrenalectomy, ureteronephrectomy and medial iliac lymph node resection.

Once pneumoperitoneum and camera portal placement have been established, instrument ports can be placed under direct laparoscopic visualization using either sharp-tipped or trocarless cannulae. Most procedures require one to three instrument ports for placement of instruments, and the location of these ports is dependent on the procedure or group of procedures that will be performed. Recommended instrument port locations are described below for each procedure discussed.

Laparoscopic procedures

Ovariectomy and ovariohysterectomy

Case selection

Any dog or cat requiring elective surgical sterilization. Dogs and cats under 2 kg may be more challenging.

Laparoscopic instrumentation

Two or three trocar–cannula assemblies, palpation probe, grasping forceps, vessel-sealing device or laparoscopic clips.

Patient positioning and preparation

The patient is placed in dorsal recumbency and the ventral abdomen is clipped (from the xiphoid to the pubis). When employing the transabdominal suture technique, a particularly wide clip needs to be performed to maintain sterility in the area where the suture is passed through the body wall. After port placement, it is important that the patient be tilted (15–25 degrees) to the left and right to facilitate visualization of the respective ovaries (Figure 3.19). This can be achieved either manually or with a mechanical tilt table. Expression of the urinary bladder prior to surgery aids in visualization. The endoscopic tower is usually positioned at the tail end of the patient.

Surgical technique

A significant number of modifications to the originally described surgical techniques for laparoscopic ovariectomy and ovariohysterectomy have been published. These include laparoscopic *versus* laparoscopic-assisted techniques, variations in port numbers (one-, two- or three-port techniques), as well as a variety of ovarian pedicle ligation techniques. Three-port laparoscopic-assisted ovariohysterectomy and two-port laparoscopic ovariectomy are described below but are not the only available options.

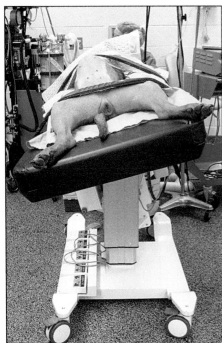

Patients should be tilted laterally on a mechanical tilt table during laparoscopic ovariectomy or ovariohysterectomy to facilitate visualization of the ovaries.

At this point the pneumoperitoneum is evacuated to decrease tension as the uterus and ovaries are exteriorized. The caudal incision is extended as required to exteriorize the right ovary and uterine horn (usually no more than 2 cm is required). After exteriorization of one ovary/ uterine horn further traction will allow exteriorization of the contralateral uterine horn and finally the ovary (Figure 3.21). Care should be taken not to place excessive traction on the tissues, as this can lead to tearing. Once the ovaries and uterus are exteriorized, ligation of the uterine arteries and transection of the uterine body are performed routinely.

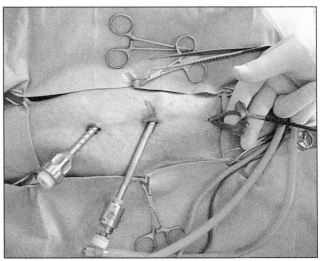

3.21 Exteriorization of both right and left uterine horns from the caudal incision during laparoscopic-assisted ovariohysterectomy.

Laparoscopic-assisted ovariohysterectomy (three-port technique): Following introduction of the laparoscope in routine fashion at the subumbilical site, two 6 mm instrument cannulae (if using a 5 mm laparoscope) are established 3–5 cm cranial to the umbilicus and 3–5 cm cranial to the pubis on the ventral midline (Figure 3.20).

To visualize the left ovary, the patient needs to be tilted to the right and a probe or laparoscopic instrument used to retract organs medially that are obscuring access to the ovary and proper ligament, most commonly the spleen, colon and small intestines with associated mesentery. Laparoscopic Kelly or Babcock forceps are used to grasp the proper ligament and elevate the ovary from the abdominal viscera. A bipolar cautery or vessel-sealing device or laparoscopic clip applier is inserted through the cranial trocar and used to section the ovarian pedicle and cranial aspect of the broad ligament. The surgeon and assistant then move to the opposite side of the animal and the patient is tilted to the left to visualize the right ovary. The procedure is repeated for the right ovary, which is normally covered by small intestine. After sectioning the right ovarian pedicle, the laparoscopic Kelly forceps are used to withdraw the ovary into the caudal cannula.

Laparoscopic ovariectomy (two-port technique): A camera portal is established in a subumbilical location. A single instrument port is established 3–5 cm cranial or caudal to the subumbilical port. The exact location of this port is not particularly important because it will be used simply for pedicle sectioning and not exteriorization of any anatomically fixed structures. The ovary is located in a similar fashion to that described above. Once it has been elevated away from the abdominal viscera, a transabdominal suspension suture is utilized to suspend the ovary from the abdominal wall. A length of 2–3 metric (3/0–2/0 USP) suture material on a large curved needle is introduced percutaneously in a location adjacent to where the ovary is being held up against the body wall (Figure 3.22). Digital pressure on the body wall can aid in identification of a good location to pass the transabdominal suture so that it emerges adjacent to the proper ligament. The suture is passed through the body wall, directed through the proper ligament under direct laparoscopic guidance, and then passed back out through the body wall. Grasping the free ends of the suture next to the body wall with a haemostat serves to suspend the ovary away from the abdominal viscera. The laparoscopic Kelly haemostats are then released and removed from the instrument portal and a bipolar vessel sealing device or clip applier is introduced. The proper ligament, mesovarium, and the ovarian artery and vein are ligated and subsequently transected.

In some cases it can be challenging to transect the proper ligament, in which case transection of the distal uterine horn close to the ovary is acceptable. The procedure is repeated on the contralateral side (Figure 3.23).

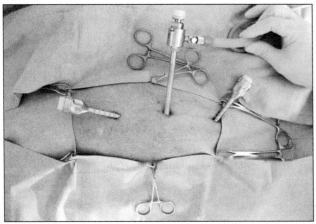

3.20 Three-port laparoscopic-assisted approach for ovariectomy or ovariohysterectomy.

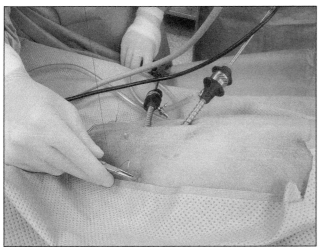

3.22 A transabdominal suspension suture is being passed through the body wall to suspend the ovarian pedicle.

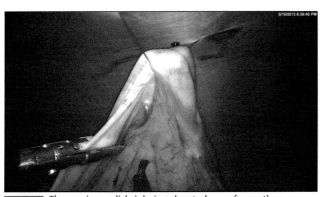

3.23 The ovarian pedicle is being elevated away from other structures and the vessel-sealing device is in position to seal and divide the distal uterine horn during laparoscopic ovariectomy.

Once free, each ovary can be recovered through the instrument port incision or both ovaries can be left attached to their respective suspension sutures until the procedure is complete, facilitating their removal at the end of the procedure. To remove the ovaries, the suspension suture is released after laparoscopic Kelly haemostats have grasped the ovary. If it is very small, the ovary may pass through the instrument cannula, but it is more likely that the instrument cannula will have to be removed with the forceps still attached to the ovary as a unit. Sometimes slight enlargement of the port incision may be necessary to accomplish this. After inspecting the ovarian pedicles for haemorrhage, the port sites are closed routinely. The transabdominal suspension suture technique can also be used to reduce the laparoscopic-assisted ovariohysterectomy technique to a two-port technique.

Orchidectomy

Case selection

Any elective intra-abdominal cryptorchid castration. This may be an appropriate technique for cryptorchid castrations in dogs with modestly sized neoplastic testicles.

Laparoscopic instrumentation

Two or three trocar–cannula assemblies, blunt probe, Kelly or Babcock forceps and a vessel-sealing device or laparoscopic clips.

Patient positioning and preparation

The patient is positioned in dorsal recumbency on the operating room table. Thorough palpation of the inguinal area should be performed in order to rule out an inguinally located testicle. A 20–30 degree 'head down' (Trendelenburg) position can be used to improve visualization of the caudal abdomen but is not always necessary.

Surgical technique

Both laparoscopic-assisted and totally laparoscopic techniques are possible for cryptorchidectomy. Exploration of the caudal abdomen usually reveals the cryptorchid testicle(s) lying adjacent to the bladder or sometimes hidden dorsal to it. If doubt exists as to the location of the testicle, the internal inguinal ring should be visualized. In cryptorchid testicles only the gubernaculum will be seen exiting from the inguinal ring. Traction on this structure should allow localization of the testicle.

Laparoscopic-assisted cryptorchidectomy: A subumbilical telescope port is established and the caudal abdomen is visualized. A 5 or 10 mm trocar–cannula assembly can be established under direct visualization in a paramedian location (lateral to the prepuce in dogs, in the left or right caudal quadrant of the abdomen in cats) on the right or left side, depending on which testicle is cryptorchid. In bilaterally cryptorchid animals, the contralateral testicle can be pulled up to the instrument portal. If too much tension exists, a second instrument portal is placed on the side ipsilateral to that testicle. Laparoscopic Kelly or Babcock forceps can be placed through the instrument port to grasp the testicle.

The pneumoperitoneum is evacuated to decrease tension and elevate the testicle to the end of the cannula. The cannula is then removed over the forceps and the port incision is enlarged as necessary to exteriorize the testicle. At this point routine ligation of the testicular pedicle can be performed. After ligation, the pedicle is returned to the abdomen, making sure that it does not become entrapped in the port incision as it passes back into the abdomen. In bilateral cases this process is repeated with the contralateral testicle, either through the same port or a second port established on the contralateral side.

Totally laparoscopic cryptorchidectomy: A technique can also be used in which the vascular supply and spermatic cord are ligated within the peritoneal cavity, followed by removal of the testicle(s) from the abdomen. This can be done using a three-port technique with two instruments located in paramedian locations on either side of the prepuce or using a single-port device on the ventral midline. With this technique a vessel-sealing device, laparoscopic clips or intra- or extracorporeal suturing will be necessary to ligate the vascular pedicle and spermatic cord. The testicle is elevated with forceps and the ligation is performed intracorporeally. Vessel sealing is a very rapid and safe way of sealing and dividing all the testicular pedicles (Figure 3.24).

Once the testicle is free it can be withdrawn through one of the instrument portals as described previously for the laparoscopic-assisted technique. If a single-port device is used, the device can be exteriorized with the instrument and testicle still in place. The single-port device is then replaced and the contralateral testicle ligated, in cases of bilateral disease. This technique lends itself very well to a single-port approach and obviates the need for any parapreputial port sites.

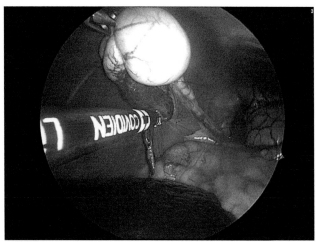

3.24 The vessel-sealing device can be seen in place, sealing and dividing the testicular pedicle.

Liver biopsy
Case selection
Ideal cases are those with diffuse hepatopathies. Great care should be taken when substantial focal hepatic masses are present because these can bleed profusely when biopsied using laparoscopic cup or punch biopsy forceps.

Laparoscopic instrumentation
Two or three trocar–cannula assemblies, blunt probe, cup biopsy forceps and optional use of loop ligature (e.g. ENDOLOOP™, Ethicon Endosurgery Inc.).

Patient positioning
Patients are usually positioned in dorsal recumbency.

Surgical technique
A subumbilical camera port is established. A single instrument port is sufficient for most cases, although a second instrument port can be helpful for placement of a blunt probe for manipulation of the liver lobes or if a loop ligature is to be placed on the tip of a liver lobe prior to biopsy. In cases where a single instrument portal is placed under direct visualization, a paramedian position is chosen in either the right or left cranial abdominal quadrant. A 6 mm trocar–cannula assembly can be placed to accommodate 5 mm cup biopsy forceps.

The simplest way to biopsy the liver is by using 5 mm laparoscopic cup biopsy forceps to harvest pieces of liver from the edge of a lobe. The tissue is grasped and gently twisted until it separates from the rest of the lobe. This technique has been shown to cause minimal bleeding in healthy dogs and to yield good quality tissue samples. It is also possible to coagulate the periphery of the biopsy site with a vessel-sealing device, and this may help to reduce haemorrhage (Vasanjee et al., 2006). Several biopsy specimens should be taken from multiple lobes.

A pre-tied loop ligature or an extracorporeally assembled loop ligature can also be used to ligate the tip of a liver lobe prior to collection of biopsy samples with cup biopsy forceps. This can help to minimize haemorrhage. If significant haemorrhage is seen, gelatin foam or oxidized regenerated cellulose can be placed over biopsy sites to aid in clot formation.

Kidney biopsy
Case selection
Cats and dogs with diffuse nephropathies are suitable patients. Focal renal mass lesions should be biopsied with care owing to the risk of profuse bleeding.

Laparoscopic instrumentation
Two trocar–cannula assemblies, blunt probe and a Tru-cut type biopsy needle.

Patient positioning
Patients are usually positioned in dorsal recumbency.

Surgical technique
A subumbilical camera port is established. An instrument port can be placed 3–5 cm caudal or cranial to the camera port on the ventral midline to allow passage of a blunt probe. The probe is useful for any manipulations that might be required to move the kidney into an optimal position prior to biopsy. Additionally, the probe can be used to tamponade the bleeding that occurs after withdrawal of the biopsy needle. Automatic spring-activated biopsy needles (e.g. BioPince®, Angiotech Inc.) are ideal as they allow harvesting of the sample with minimal movement and aid in procuring good quality samples. Some models allow presetting of the length of sample to be taken, which is very advantageous given the great variation in size of veterinary patients.

Under direct visualization, the core biopsy needle is guided into the parenchyma and directed to pass across the renal cortex in order to maximize the number of glomeruli recovered. The biopsy is performed by activating the biopsy needle, which is subsequently withdrawn from the peritoneal cavity. Usually one to two samples are taken from one or both kidneys, depending on the nature of the pathology suspected. If the needle is placed too deeply into the medulla, fewer glomeruli might be recovered and there is a greater risk of haemorrhage from arcuate vessels. Generally 14–16 G needles are used for larger dogs and 18 G needles are used for small dogs and cats. After the biopsy has been performed, pressure can be put on the small entry hole in the kidney capsule for as long as is required for a clot to form and for haemorrhage to cease.

Pancreatic biopsy
Case selection
Dogs and cats with diffuse pancreatic diseases are suitable patients.

Laparoscopic instrumentation
Two or three trocar–cannula assemblies, blunt probe and punch (or cup) biopsy forceps.

Patient preparation and positioning
Patients are usually positioned in dorsal recumbency.

Surgical technique
For the laparoscopic technique, one instrument port can be used for pancreatic biopsy if a punch technique is used, although a second port will be necessary if use of a vessel-sealing device or ligature is desired. A second

instrument port may also be necessary if significant manipulation of the surrounding organs is needed to obtain an unobstructed view of the pancreas. A pancreatic biopsy is usually performed in addition to sampling of other organs, so access is usually from instrument ports that have been positioned for the biopsy of other organs. The tip of the right (duodenal) limb of the pancreas is usually the simplest to access. Cup or punch biopsy forceps can be used carefully to remove a small piece of pancreas from the periphery of the lobe. Care should be taken to avoid biopsying the body of the pancreas (to avoid damaging larger pancreatic ducts) as well as the area where the caudal pancreaticoduodenal vessels enter the tip of the right pancreatic limb.

To reduce haemorrhage several other techniques can be used. A pre-tied loop ligature can be placed around a piece of pancreas to be biopsied or haemostatic clips can be placed in a V-shape around the tissue segment to be excised. A vessel-sealing device can also be used to harvest the specimen. A recent study compared use of the Harmonic® scalpel device to the placement of haemostatic clips when performing laparoscopic pancreatic biopsy (Barnes et al., 2006). Use of the Harmonic® scalpel led to a reduction in haemorrhage but resulted in significantly greater inflammation.

Splenectomy
Case selection
Dogs and cats with diffuse splenic disease, and those where splenectomy is being performed as an adjunctive therapy for immune-mediated disease, are the best candidates. Those with haemoabdomen or medium- to large-sized splenic masses are not currently recommended as good candidates for this technique by the author.

Laparoscopic instrumentation
Three or four trocar–cannula assemblies, blunt probe, fan retractor, vessel-sealing device, specimen retrieval bag and a morcellator (optional).

Patient positioning
Patients are usually positioned in dorsal recumbency initially and then rotated into right lateral recumbency for final dissection of the head of the spleen.

Surgical technique
A camera portal is established in a subumbilical location on the ventral midline. Two further instrument ports are placed under direct visualization on the ventral midline 3–8 cm (depending on patient size) cranial and 3–8 cm caudal to the subumbilical camera portal. Alternatively, a port can be placed in a paramedian location just caudal to the last rib in the left cranial quadrant, to allow for triangulation around the anticipated location of the splenic hilus. A blunt probe or fan retractor is then placed into one of the instrument portals (usually one of the more cranial ports) and a vessel-sealing device is placed into the other instrument portal. The spleen is manipulated with the blunt probe or retractor so that the hilar vessels become visible (Figure 3.25). Care needs to be taken to ensure that, during splenic manipulation, no perforation of the splenic capsule occurs.

Moving from the tail towards the head of the spleen, the vessels and associated fat are cauterized at the level of the hilus using the vessel-sealer. The most challenging

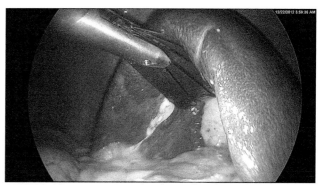

3.25 A fan retractor is used to elevate the spleen away from underlying organs and expose the hilus so that a vessel-sealer can be used to seal and divide the hilar vessels.

aspect of the dissection is sectioning the hilus and short gastric vessels at the splenic head, owing to their less mobile attachment to the greater curvature of the stomach. In cats there is a close association between the splenic head and the left limb of the pancreas, and iatrogenic damage to the pancreas needs to be avoided. In most patients, as dissection of the splenic head is approached, it is usually made much less challenging if the patient is rotated into a more lateral position with its left side facing up. This allows the head of the spleen to become more accessible and reduces the amount of tension that is required to elevate this area of the spleen during attempted dissection with the patient in dorsal recumbency. This can often help to reduce the likelihood of iatrogenic haemorrhage from the splenic capsule during the final dissection. Once dissected free, the spleen should be placed into a specimen retrieval bag (Figure 3.26) or exteriorized through a protected wound retractor. Enlargement of a portal incision will be necessary, proportional to the size of the spleen/lesion to be removed. If available a tissue morcellator can be used to reduce the size of the spleen prior to extraction, possibly reducing the size of the incision required to retrieve the organ.

A laparoscopic-assisted technique, which involves removal of the spleen through a wound retraction device, has also been described in cats and could be used in small dogs (O'Donnell et al., 2013). The success of this technique may vary by species and be affected by other variables that may increase or decrease the degree of splenic mobility, such as relative obesity of the patient. In some cases the mobility of the spleen maybe insufficient to allow a laparoscopic-assisted approach.

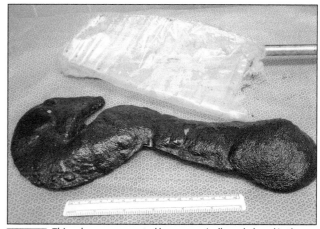

3.26 This spleen was resected laparoscopically and placed in the specimen retrieval device shown before withdrawal from the body cavity.

Laparoscopic-assisted techniques

Cystotomy

Case selection

Most dogs and cats with urinary calculi can be treated via laparoscopic-assisted cystotomy. Those with stones that are too large to be removed by urohydropulsion will be good candidates, as well as those where medical dissolution is unlikely to be successful. Resection of inflammatory polyps has also been described using this technique.

Laparoscopic instrumentation

Two trocar–cannula assemblies, grasping forceps and basket catheters (optional).

Patient positioning

Patients are usually positioned in dorsal recumbency.

Surgical technique

A number of variations of laparoscopic-assisted cystotomy have been described. A camera portal is established in a subumbilical location. The caudal abdomen is inspected and a second instrumental portal is established on the ventral midline in a location directly adjacent to the apex of the bladder. This usually lies approximately halfway between the camera portal and the brim of the pubis. In male dogs it often falls adjacent to the cranial margin of the prepuce. In these cases a small skin incision can be made in a parapreputial location, followed by undermining of the tissue dorsal to the prepuce, allowing an incision to be made in the linea alba to access the bladder apex (Figure 3.27).

Once port placement has been achieved, the next step is exteriorization of a small area of the apex of the bladder. Babcock forceps are placed into the instrument portal and used to grasp the apex of the bladder. The location at which the bladder is grasped is of importance, because if the incision is made into an area of the bladder near the trigone full exploration of the entire bladder is more challenging. As the apex is brought up towards the cannula, the instrument port incision is

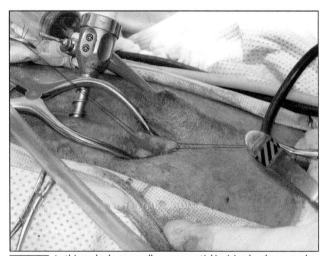

3.27 In this male dog a small parapreputial incision has been made for access to the apex of the bladder, which has been exteriorized by traction on two stay sutures.

enlarged to approximately 2–4 cm (allowing the pneumoperitoneum to be purged and tension to decrease), depending on the size of the animal and the calculi. The cannula is then withdrawn along with the forceps, which are still grasping the bladder. As soon as the bladder is visible, stay sutures of 3 metric (2/0 USP) or 2 metric (3/0 USP) polydioxanone should be placed into the bladder wall to ensure that it does not slip back into the abdomen. While maintaining upward traction on the stay sutures to create a seal with the abdominal wall, a small cystotomy incision is made.

At this time the edges of the cystotomy incision can be temporarily sutured in a simple continuous fashion to the border of the skin to allow temporary marsupialization of the bladder. A 2.7 mm 30-degree cystoscope is then placed into the cystotomy incision within a cystoscopic sheath (Rawlings et al., 2003). Sterile saline is run through one of the ports on the cystoscope sheath to create constant bladder lavage. This is essential to maintain good visualization of the bladder during retrieval of the calculi. Alternatively, if a cystoscope is unavailable, the laparoscope can be used and passed directly into the cystotomy to visualize the calculi. If a cystoscope is not used, it is helpful to place a urinary catheter through the prepuce/vulva to provide retrograde flushing.

Calculi can be retrieved in a variety of ways. A basket retrieval catheter can be placed down the working channel of a cystoscope to capture individual stones. Other instruments can be placed alongside the cystoscope such as grasping forceps, or laparoscopic graspers. Large-volume, high-pressure retrograde flushing can be a very time-efficient way of expelling a large number of stones through the cystotomy incision. It is also helpful in those cases with large numbers of very small stones or sandy debris.

Upon removal of all the calculi, the bladder should again be thoroughly inspected. In females, a rigid laparoscope can usually be passed down the majority of the length of the urethra to look for any remaining urethal calculi. In male dogs, a small flexible bronchoscope/urethroscope, if available, can be passed down the entire length of the urethra to check that no remaining calculi are present. In all cases with radiodense calculi, the author recommends that postoperative radiographs be taken to rule out the presence of residual calculi within the bladder. After completion of the procedure the cystotomy incision is released from the skin and closed routinely (usually with a single layer of simple interrupted appositional sutures of 1.5–3 metric (4/0–2/0 USP) polydioxanone, depending on patient size).

Gastropexy

Case selection

This is a prophylactic procedure for the prevention of gastric dilatation and volvulus and is appropriate for use in any dog considered at high risk for the condition.

Laparoscopic instrumentation

Two trocar–cannula assemblies or a single-port device, 5 or 10 mm Babcock or Duval forceps and a blunt probe.

Patient positioning

Dogs are positioned in dorsal recumbency.

Surgical technique

A subumbilical camera portal is established and a laparoscope is used to examine the cranial abdominal structures. Under direct visualization, an instrument port is established at the intended location of the gastropexy, just lateral to the margin of the rectus abdominus muscle and 2–4 cm caudal to the last rib on the right-hand side. Consideration should be given to the size of this cannula because, especially in larger breeds, it can be helpful to use 10 mm Babcock or Duval forceps to grasp the gastric antrum. If 10 mm forceps are to be used, a cannula large enough to accommodate the instrument needs to be inserted.

Upon examination of the cranial abdomen, in some cases an unobstructed view of the gastric antrum will already be available, whereas in others organs may lie over the stomach. Using either a blunt probe or the grasping forceps the overlying tissues are retracted out of the way until the antrum is clearly in view and can be grasped. The antrum is usually held midway between the greater and lesser curvatures, approximately 5–7 cm oral to the pylorus (Figure 3.28). Once a firm hold on the antrum is achieved, the pneumoperitoneum is evacuated by opening the side-valves on one of the cannulae.

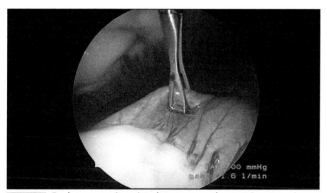

3.28 For laparoscopic-assisted gastropexy the gastric antrum is grasped midway between the greater and lesser curvatures of the stomach.

The Babcock forceps and antrum are exteriorized by removing the right-sided cannula and extending the port incision to 4–5 cm in an orientation parallel to the last rib. During this dissection a muscle-splitting approach to the external and internal abdominal oblique muscles may result in less pain postoperatively. During exteriorization of the stomach, care should be taken to avoid gastric rotation. After exteriorization, two stay sutures are placed in the stomach wall at opposing ends of the proposed gastropexy site and the grasping forceps are released (Figure 3.29). An incision at least 4 cm long is made through the seromuscular layer of the antrum along the long axis of the stomach, avoiding the larger blood vessels emerging from the greater and lesser curvatures. The seromuscular and mucosal layers of the stomach wall are gently separated and care should be taken not to penetrate full-thickness into the stomach lumen. Two simple continuous lines of 2–3 metric (3/0–2/0 USP) monofilament absorbable sutures are placed to appose both margins of the seromuscular layer of the stomach to the transversus abdominis muscle.

Prior to closure it is important to remove the full-thickness stay sutures that were placed initially. The oblique abdominal muscles are closed with interrupted or continuous sutures of a synthetic absorbable material, and the remainder of the incision is closed in routine fashion. After

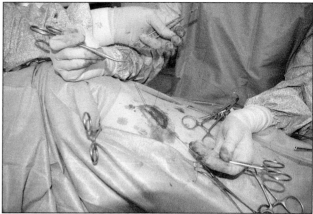

3.29 After exteriorization, stay sutures are used to elevate the gastric wall prior to creation of the gastric seromuscular incision.

completion, the pneumoperitoneum should be re-established briefly and the gastropexy viewed laparoscopically to ensure that optimal positioning and orientation have been achieved and that excessive haemorrhage or body wall defects are not present (Figure 3.30). After once more evacuating the pneumoperitoneum, the midline cannula can be removed and the incision closed.

A single-incision approach to laparoscopic-assisted gastropexy can be used if either an operating laparoscope or a single-port device is available. In either case the single port site is established at the location of the gastropexy. In the case of the operating laparoscope, 5 mm grasping forceps can be placed through the working channel of the laparoscope. In the case of the single-port device, the laparoscope and the grasping forceps are placed through two of the available port sites within the device. The procedure continues as described for the two-port approach once the antrum has been grasped and exteriorized through the incision. In both single-port approaches, the only disadvantage lies in the inability to inspect the gastropexy from within the abdominal cavity at the termination of the procedure.

Laparoscopic assisted gastropexy can easily be combined with ovariectomy or ovariohysterectomy. In this case, the most cranial instrument port is made at the site of the gastropexy and used to aid in completion of the ovariectomy, prior to its enlargement for completion of the gastropexy.

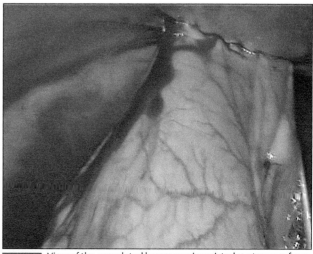

3.30 View of the completed laparoscopic-assisted gastropexy from the peritoneal cavity.

Gastrointestinal surgery

Laparoscopic instrumentation

Two trocar–cannula assemblies or a single-port device, Babcock forceps, blunt probe and a wound retraction device (optional).

Patient positioning

Patients are positioned in dorsal recumbency.

Surgical technique

A camera port can be established at a subumbilical location and used to perform a cursory examination of the abdominal cavity. The need to obtain biopsy samples from other organs, in many of these cases, may influence subsequent instrument port location. If gastrointestinal tract access alone is required, a small 3–4 cm 'assist' incision can be created at the umbilicus, incorporating the incision that was created for the camera portal. This incision can be carefully retracted using small Gelpi retractors or a disposable minimally invasive surgical wound retractor (e.g. Alexis®, Applied Medical Inc.). Grasping forceps or a gloved finger can then be used to grasp a section of duodenum, jejunum or ileum and exteriorize it through the 'assist' incision.

Once a small area has been exteriorized, the bowel can be examined by running it in both oral and aboral directions. Biopsies can be performed in standard fashion (Figure 3.31). Depending on the species and animal size, access to various abdominal organs will be possible. In the author's experience, excellent access to the ascending duodenum, jejunum, ileum and ileocaecocolic junction can be achieved. The base of the mesentery, mesenteric lymph nodes and the right limb of the pancreas are usually also readily accessible. If access to the stomach for biopsy is necessary, the 'assist' incision may be positioned slightly more cranially (midway between the umbilicus and xiphoid cartilage). Areas that are usually not readily accessible include the descending colon, pylorus and cardia of the stomach.

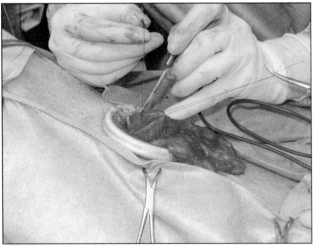

3.31 Harvesting of a small intestinal biopsy sample through a small 'assist' incision that has been created using a wound retraction device.

After closure of the biopsy sites is complete, local lavage can be performed away from the abdominal incision site, thus preventing any contamination of the peritoneal cavity with lavage solution. After completion of all procedures, all abdominal wall incision sites can be closed routinely.

Enterotomy and intestinal resection and anastomosis have also been described using a laparoscopic-assisted approach (Figure 3.32). Case selection needs to be carefully considered to make sure that pathology is not missed and to ensure that any intestinal lesions can be resected in a way that preserves oncological principles. A small case series of laparoscopic-assisted intestinal resection has been described in which successful resection of modestly sized intestinal masses was performed in dogs and cats (Gower and Mayhew, 2011).

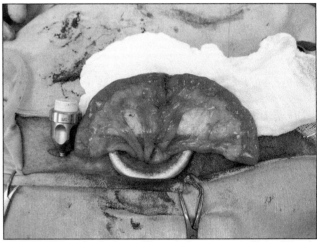

3.32 This cat has had a small intestinal mass resected in traditional fashion extraperitoneally through a small 'assist' incision.

References and further reading

Barnes RF, Greenfield CL, Schaeffer DJ *et al.* (2006) Comparison of biopsy samples obtained using standard endoscopic instruments and the Harmonic scalpel during laparoscopic and laparoscopic-assisted surgery in normal dogs. *Veterinary Surgery* **35**, 243–251

Culp WTN, Mayhew PD and Brown DC (2009) The effect of laparoscopic *versus* open ovariectomy on postsurgical activity in small dogs. *Veterinary Surgery* **38**, 811–817

Devitt CM, Cox RE and Hailey JJ (2005) Duration, complications, stress, and pain of open ovariohysterectomy *versus* a simple method of laparoscopic-assisted ovariohysterectomy in dogs. *Journal of the American Veterinary Medical Association* **227**, 921–927

Gower SB and Mayhew PD (2011) A wound retraction device for laparoscopic-assisted intestinal surgery in dogs and cats. *Veterinary Surgery* **40**, 485–488

Mayhew PD, Freeman L, Kwan T *et al.* (2012) Comparison of surgical site infection rates in clean and clean-contaminated wounds in dogs and cats after minimally invasive *versus* open surgery: 179 cases (2007–2008). *Journal of the American Veterinary Medical Association* **240**, 193–198

O'Donnell E, Mayhew PD, Culp WTN *et al.* (2013) Laparoscopic splenectomy: operative technique and outcome in three cats. *Journal of Feline Medicine and Surgery* **15**, 48–52

Rawlings CA, Mahaffey MB, Barsanti JA *et al.* (2003) Use of laparoscopic-assisted cystoscopy for removal of urinary calculi in dogs. *Journal of the American Veterinary Medical Association* **222**, 759–762

Runge JJ (2012) The cutting edge: introducing reduced port laparoscopic surgery. *Today's Veterinary Practice* **2**, 14–21

Vasanjee SC, Bubenik LJ, Hosgood G *et al.* (2006) Evaluation of hemorrhage, sample size, and collateral damage for five hepatic biopsy methods in dogs. *Veterinary Surgery* **35**, 86–91

Chapter 4

The body wall

Davina Anderson

The body wall consists of sheets of muscle that maintain abdominal integrity, provide support and strength for movements such as jumping and twisting and, when tense, are rigid enough to protect the abdominal contents (Figure 4.1). Open surgery on intra-abdominal structures involves breaching this well designed system, and it is important to ensure a robust and long-lasting repair of any approach to the abdominal cavity.

Name	Abbreviation	Description
External abdominal oblique	EAO	Caudoventral fibres
Internal abdominal oblique	IAO	Cranioventral fibres
Transversus abdominis	TA	Dorsoventral fibres
Rectus abdominis	RA	Craniocaudal fibres

4.1 Muscle layers of the abdominal wall.

Muscle	Origin	Insertion
External abdominal oblique	Lateral surface of ribs 4 or 5 to 12; thoracolumbar fascia	Aponeurosis is always lateral to RA
Internal abdominal oblique	Caudal thoracolumbar fascia and tuber coxae	Aponeurosis is lateral to RA except in the cranial third where the fibres pass on both sides
Transversus abdominis	Thoracolumbar fascia and transverse processes of the lumbar vertebrae, also the medial surface of the last 4–5 ribs and costal cartilages	Aponeurosis is medial to RA in the cranial two-thirds and then passes lateral to the RA
Rectus abdominis	First costal cartilage	Pubis

4.2 Origins and insertions of the abdominal wall musculature.

Anatomy

The ventral abdominal wall of most dogs and cats has sparse hair and thinner skin than the rest of the trunk. The midline is identified by the linea alba, which is a tough fibrous band joining the two halves of the abdominal muscle wall together. It is usually in a slight trough between the rectus abdominis (RA) muscles, and it is thinner and wider in the cat than in the dog. The fibres of the aponeuroses of the abdominal wall muscles all converge on the linea alba. The internal surface of the transversus abdominis (TA) muscle is lined by fascia and peritoneum.

The origins and insertions of these muscles indicate that each muscle runs in a different direction (Figure 4.2). This arrangement contributes to the overall strength of the abdominal wall. It is important to understand the relative contribution of each of these muscles and their aponeuroses in maintaining the integrity of the body wall when considering surgical approaches to the abdomen, and for its subsequent repair (Figure 4.3).

Prepubic tendon

The prepubic tendon is made up mostly of the tendons of the RA and pectineus muscles, with some contribution from the external abdominal oblique (EAO) muscle. The

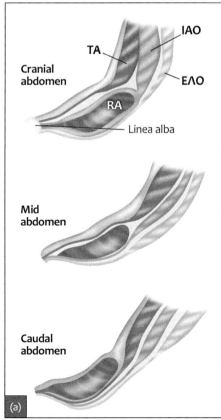

4.3 (a) Cross-section of the abdominal wall muscles, showing aponeuroses inserting on the linea alba. EAO = external abdominal oblique; IAO = internal abdominal oblique; RA = rectus abdominis; TA = transversus abdominis. (continues) ▶

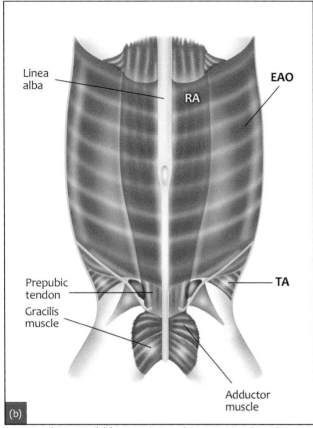

eminence. In both sexes, the external pudendal artery and vein pass through the canal to give rise to the caudal superficial epigastric vessels and the labial/scrotal vessels. The genital branch of the genitofemoral nerve also passes through the canal. A blind pouch of peritoneum passes through the inguinal canal into a subcutaneous position and is called the vaginal tunic in the male and the vaginal process in the female. In the male dog, the vaginal tunic encloses the route of testicular descent and in the adult contains the spermatic cord. In the female, the vaginal process contains the round ligament and a variable amount of fat. The cranial part of the external opening of the inguinal canal is the weakest point.

4.3 (continued) (b) External view of the ventral surface of the abdomen and abdominal wall openings. EAO = external abdominal oblique; RA = rectus abdominis; TA = transversus abdominis.

tendon is palpable as a firm structure extending from the iliopubic eminence to the pubic tubercle, and attaches the caudal end of the linea alba to the pelvis (see Figure 4.3b). The iliopubic cartilages incorporated in the tendon may or may not ossify.

Natural openings

Femoral canals

These are bilaterally symmetrical vascular lacunae caudolateral to the superficial inguinal ring, bounded cranially by the internal abdominal oblique (IAO) muscle and the inguinal ligament and medially by the RA muscle, and thus separated from the internal ring of the inguinal canal by only the inguinal ligament. The femoral artery and vein, lymphatics and saphenous nerve pass through the canal.

Inguinal canals

These bilaterally symmetrical openings in the caudoventral abdominal wall form a natural slit, lateral to the RA muscle in the aponeuroses of the IAO and EAO muscles. Technically there are internal and external openings (Figure 4.4) with a short oblique canal between them, but this is not obvious on superficial dissection (Figure 4.5). The lateral wall is formed by the EAO muscle alone, while the medial wall is formed by the aponeuroses and borders of the other abdominal muscles. The caudal boundary is formed by the inguinal ligament at the internal end and the EAO ligaments at the external end. The inguinal ligament is the caudal border of the EAO muscle and consists of fibres running from the tuber coxae to the iliopubic

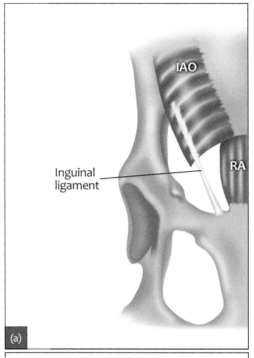

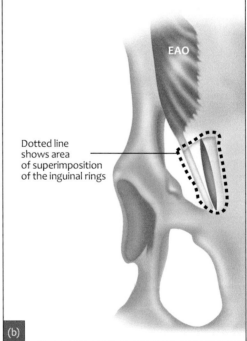

4.4 Anatomy of the inguinal ring in the dog. (a) Internal inguinal ring. (b) External inguinal ring. EAO = external abdominal oblique; IAO = internal abdominal oblique; RA = rectus abdominis.

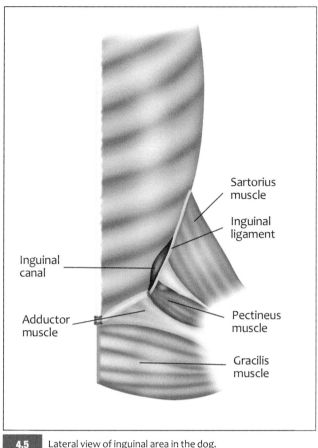

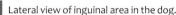
4.5 Lateral view of inguinal area in the dog.

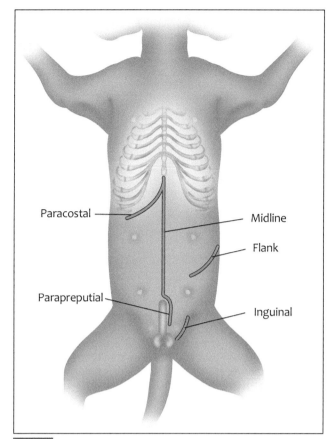
4.6 Surgical approaches to the abdomen.

Umbilicus

This is a scar in the middle of the linea alba where the umbilical vessels, vitelline duct and allantoic stalk pass in the fetus. The falciform fat is found immediately inside the abdomen at the level of the umbilicus.

Surgical approaches

Coeliotomy *versus* laparotomy

Technically, a *laparotomy* refers to a flank approach to the abdomen and a *coeliotomy* refers to the common ventral midline approach in dogs and cats. However, it is accepted practice to refer to the ventral approach as a laparotomy.

Individual approaches

The different approaches to the abdomen are illustrated in Figure 4.6.

- The *midline approach* is the commonest technique used for abdominal surgery in dogs and cats (see Operative Technique 4.1). It allows a bilaterally symmetrical view of the abdomen and can be extended cranially into the sternebrae, or caudally into the pelvic symphysis if necessary. It is also the easiest approach to repair.
- The *paramedian approach* uses a craniocaudal incision lateral to the lateral border of the RA muscle. It is occasionally used for a limited caudal approach in the male dog to dispense with

dissection underneath the prepuce. However, it is difficult to explore the opposite side of the abdomen and the repair is more painful postoperatively than a midline incision. Bleeding and bruising are common complications.

- The *flank laparotomy* is commonly used in the UK for ovariohysterectomy in the cat (see Operative Technique 4.2 and Chapter 17).
- The *paracostal approach* is an incision through the body wall parallel and caudal to the last rib. It is sometimes described for a minimal approach to gastropexy or decompressive gastrotomy (see Chapter 6), or access to the kidney and adrenal gland.

A *gridiron dissection* is usually recommended for both the flank and paracostal approaches in order to minimize muscle trauma, but in dogs and cats this significantly limits the size of the opening that is possible. It is not possible to examine the contralateral organs, and exposure of the rest of the abdomen is limited. These approaches may be quite painful, owing to constant postoperative movement of the incision site with respiration.

Combined approaches

Combined midline and paracostal incisions, or combined paralumbar and paracostal incisions, have been described for greater access to the costal recess or retroperitoneal space for hepatic or vascular surgery. This is a complex approach and should be reserved for major surgeries; it is probably best suited to referral centres and tends to be very painful postoperatively.

Closure

Closure of surgical incisions has become much safer with the development of reliable synthetic absorbable suture materials. Clinical research on closure of the midline in dogs and cats has also shown that incorporation of the peritoneum may increase the risk of postoperative adhesions, and that the only tissue layer with suture-holding strength is the external fascial sheath of the RA muscle and the combined aponeuroses of the other abdominal muscles. This has simplified the repair techniques used for midline approaches and greatly improved healing and postoperative morbidity (see Operative Technique 4.1 and Figure 4.7). Cranial to the umbilicus, it may be necessary in dogs to incorporate the internal rectus sheath in the repair, as there is less contribution to the external sheath (see Figure 4.3). In the cat, the linea alba is wider than in the dog and this is less likely to be an issue. Repair of non-midline approaches aims to reconstruct the muscle layers individually with short continuous patterns, followed by routine skin repair.

Generally, a repair causing minimal trauma and inflammatory responses will promote more rapid healing and resolution of the damage caused by the incision. To this end, monofilament absorbable or non-absorbable materials are recommended for the linea alba. Long-lasting absorbable materials, such as polydioxanone, are ideal and more cosmetic, particularly in thin-skinned animals where the permanent materials may be palpable or visible through the skin even after the wound is fully healed. Suture materials that cause irritation may increase the risk of patient interference with the wound, and therefore infection, followed by a delayed period of healing.

- Historically it was thought important to include the external fascial sheath, a portion of the RA muscle, the internal fascial sheath, and the peritoneum for a secure abdominal closure. It is now well established that the strongest layer is the external fascial sheath and inclusion of the peritoneum may increase the risk of adhesions
- There is no indication to include a portion of the RA muscle as this has no suture-holding strength, ultimately loosening the suture repair as the suture tears through or tissue regresses within the suture bites. In the cranial part of the abdomen, the external fascial sheath is thinner and inclusion of the internal fascial sheath is advisable here, particularly in obese or very large dogs
- Continuous sutures of synthetic absorbable material are strong enough to repair the abdomen in all dogs and cats where healing is expected to proceed normally
- All owners should be given written instructions to limit the activity of the animal until healing and collagen remodelling are established

4.7 Closure of the abdominal midline incision.

Complications

Wound dehiscence or herniation

Incisional hernia should be extremely rare if the guidelines for good surgical technique and adequate closure are followed. Failure of the midline laparotomy is more common than that of flank laparotomy, but herniation of flank laparotomy sites can occur, particularly if repair of long muscle incisions is incomplete at the ventral aspect. Incisional hernias can result in self-trauma, as a consequence of the discomfort, and ultimately evisceration.

Acute incisional hernias are usually identified within a few days of surgery or at the time of suture removal. There may be evidence of wound swelling, skin discoloration or a serosanguineous discharge. Often they are not painful, though the animal may lick at any discharge. Skin healing is delayed by the presence of herniated abdominal contents (Figure 4.8) and there is a high risk of sudden skin rupture and evisceration if the skin sutures are removed.

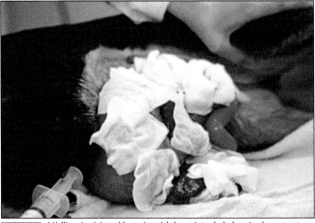

4.8 Midline incisional hernia with herniated abdominal contents (evisceration).

Chronic incisional hernias usually present weeks to months after the original surgery and rarely cause evisceration as the skin edges have fully healed. The hernia may be due to a failure of collagen remodelling of the scar if the animal develops other systemic diseases, such as hyperadrenocorticism, where the scar widens and thins as the abdomen sags. Clinical findings are typically a variably sized doughy swelling over the site of the original surgery, which may or may not be reducible. Deep palpation may reveal the defect in the abdominal wall or it may be possible to palpate subcutaneous abdominal contents.

Cause of failure	Examples
Technical error	Suture pull-out due to incorrect placement Poor knot tying Incomplete closure (especially flank laparotomy) Fat trapped between sutured edges Inappropriate suture material Introduction of infection
Concurrent therapy	Corticosteroids
Concurrent disease	Hyperadrenocorticism Cachexia/hypoalbuminaemia Obesity
Postoperative management	Failure to restrict activity Failure to prevent interference with sutures Postoperative pain resulting in abdominal tensing

4.9 Causes of postoperative incisional hernia.

In some circumstances, poor holding strength of the wound is an important contributory factor. Where fascial tissues are damaged or thin, a simple interrupted repair or mattress or cruciate pattern sutures may be considered. Excessive force on the incision will also cause suture pull-out or breakage; causes include violent coughing, straining or struggling in the postoperative period, as well as excessive activity and obesity.

Any wound showing signs of delayed healing should be carefully examined for evidence of incisional dehiscence. Sometimes deep palpation is sufficient to identify a midline defect or demonstrate reduction of the hernia. In obese animals, or where there is postoperative inflammation or infection, radiography or ultrasound examination may be necessary. Chronic hernias can be managed as an elective procedure as long as abdominal contents are not incarcerated or obstructed. Acute incisional hernias should be explored and repaired immediately, because of the risk of evisceration.

Treatment of incisional hernia

A careful clinical examination should confirm whether the hernia can be treated by an elective procedure. A light abdominal bandage may help to support the hernia in the interim, and the animal's activity should be restricted.

- Animals that are unstable with incarcerated or obstructed hernias should be stabilized and treated for shock.
- Acute hernias where the skin appears unhealed should have a protective bandage placed immediately and the animal should be hospitalized with constant supervision until surgery is performed.
- The veterinary surgeon (veterinarian) should try to determine the causal factors for the dehiscence and herniation (see Figure 4.9).
- The hernia should be approached through the original wound and all suture material removed. Organs should be examined closely for evidence of strangulation or vascular compromise prior to reducing the hernia. The condition of the fascial edges should be carefully noted. A photographic record may be helpful in case of dispute later.
- Minimal debridement should be used to trim torn edges or inflamed fat. If infection is suspected, the debrided tissue should be submitted for culture prior to administering any antibiotics. Primary musculofascial repair is carried out using a standard technique unless

the reason for failure is suspected to be other than technical error. Horizontal mattress or cruciate suture patterns may be used to supplement the repair if poor tissue quality is suspected. Suture bites of fascial layers should be a *minimum* of 5 mm from the edges.
- Subcutaneous and skin closures are routine. Postoperative instructions (verbal and written) are reiterated to the owner and the importance of vigilance and strict activity restriction in the healing period should be emphasized.

Management of evisceration

Evisceration is a true emergency. Animals may just lick at the abdominal contents, but often may be found having chewed parts of the intestine or spleen.

- The viscera should be covered immediately with sterile materials (e.g. saline-soaked swabs (sponges)). Restrain the animal and provide constant supervision.
- Blood and fluid loss results in severe shock. Rapid fluid resuscitation, intravenous antibiotics and immediate surgical intervention are required.
- The animal is prepared for surgery with skin antiseptic solutions that do not contain detergent or alcohol. Body temperature should be carefully monitored. Waterproof drapes are essential.
- Abdominal contents are carefully examined and washed thoroughly with warm sterile saline. Where possible, all contaminated or non-viable organs are removed prior to returning the tissues into the abdomen.
- The abdomen should be thoroughly lavaged prior to closure and the need for a closed suction drain or management as an open abdomen should be considered (see Chapter 18).
- The condition of the sutures and state of the linea alba edges should be carefully noted at surgery (it may even be advisable to save the suture material for the purposes of the record). The linea alba should be debrided, decontaminated and carefully repaired. Some surgeons recommend interrupted cruciate sutures for the second repair, as the tissues are inflamed and possibly infected. The owners should be warned of a guarded prognosis, particularly if large segments of bowel have been removed.

> **PRACTICAL TIP**
>
> If there has been contamination of the abdominal cavity a sample should be taken and submitted for bacterial culture and sensitivity testing

Haemorrhage

Rarely, excessive haemorrhage or bruising may be noted in the few hours postoperatively when little haemorrhage had been noted during surgery. Screening for coagulopathies may be indicated, particularly for certain breeds (e.g. Dobermann, German Shepherd Dog). Poor technique may also be the cause if the major vessels encountered in specific approaches have not been adequately ligated.

Suture abscess and reactions

Sutures rarely cause abscesses unless there has been contamination or poor sterile technique during surgery or the wound is infected. With appropriate use of good technique and modern sterile suture materials, these reactions should not be common. However, some animals seem more prone to tissue reaction around the knots than others, and this is another advantage of the continuous suture patterns where there is less suture material left in the repair.

Suture reactions can be palpated as small nodules over the knot long after tissue healing is complete. They can be removed for cosmetic reasons, though they will generally resolve. If infection is found to be present, it should be managed with antibiotics, based on the results of *in vitro* sensitivity testing, and the knot may have to be removed. It must be remembered that the presence of purulent material need not necessarily indicate infection.

Postoperative care

Abdominal surgery causes postoperative stress and pain to the animal regardless of the complexity of the surgery performed. Postoperative ileus is seen in cats and dogs as a consequence of both abdominal surgery and operative stress. Perioperative analgesia for any abdominal procedure should be routine. Pre-emptive analgesic techniques should be used, incorporating opiates and non-steroidal anti-inflammatory drugs in the premedication protocol. Postoperative assessment should include the animal's mobility and response to gentle palpation of the sides of the wound. *Any* pain response should be treated with appropriate parenteral or oral drugs.

Postoperative appetite, mobility and healing will progress more quickly if adequate analgesic support is provided.

At the time of patient discharge, the owner should be given written instructions (Figure 4.10) advising them on management of their pet with regard to protecting the coeliotomy repair: prevention of excessive activity or jumping up; prevention of trauma to sutures; and daily monitoring.

Abdominal wall hernias

A hernia is the protrusion of an internal organ through a defect in the wall of the anatomical cavity in which it normally lies. The hernia is lined by peritoneum, which forms the hernial sac.

* A *true hernia* is the protrusion of abdominal contents through an existing or potential opening in the body wall that has become pathologically enlarged or disrupted.
* A *false hernia* is the protrusion of abdominal contents through a rupture in the body wall. True hernias will therefore have a peritoneal lining, whereas false hernias will not.
* Most *acquired* hernias are false hernias resulting from trauma.
* Many true hernias are *congenital* defects of embryogenesis. These animals may have other congenital defects, such as cryptorchidism.

DISCHARGE INSTRUCTIONS SPAY/CASTRATION

PRACTICE ADDRESS AND PHONE NUMBER

Name of Veterinary Surgeon/Veterinary Nurse

Client: _____
Animal's Name:_____
Breed: _____
Age: _____ Sex: _____

Discharge date:_____

1. <u>Please check the incision daily for the next 10 days.</u> The incision should look better each day and any bruising should gradually subside. If you notice increasing redness, swelling or any discharge, please contact us.

2. <u>Please restrict activity for the next 10 days.</u> Cats should remain indoors and be confined to a small room or cage. Dogs should go outside on a lead when passing motions or urine but should not be allowed to run off the lead until the stitches have been removed.

3. Your pet should not lick at its incision. If it is licking excessively a plastic Elizabethan collar should be placed around the animal's neck to prevent trauma to the wound.

4. If the animal seems depressed or is not eating, please telephone the practice.

5. ☐ Sutures need to be removed in 10 days.
   ☐ Suture removal is not required. The stitches will dissolve over time and re-evaluation is not needed unless problems arise.

6. Additional instructions:
   _____
   _____
   _____
   _____

Please do not hesitate to call if you have any problems or concerns

4.10 An example of postoperative discharge instructions.

Incidence and heredity

There is probably a polygenic determined threshold character involved in the heredity of some hernias, because there are breed predispositions for certain types of congenital hernia. General recommendations are that animals with congenital hernias may not be suitable for breeding. However, exposure to some toxins during pregnancy can also induce hernias in animals. The likelihood of inheritance must be considered in conjunction with breed evidence, clinical history and evidence of other abnormalities in the litter.

Clinical presentation

Hernias present as subcutaneous swellings on the abdominal wall (Figure 4.11). They may be non-painful or very painful, swollen, bruised or ulcerated. The hernia may or may not be reducible. There are a number of differential diagnoses for an abdominal wall swelling (Figure 4.12). Hernias seen in dogs and cats include: umbilical, inguinal (Figure 4.13), scrotal, femoral, paracostal, prepubic (false), sciatic and perineal (see Chapter 8), pericardioperitoneal, pleuroperitoneal, diaphragmatic and hiatal (see Chapter 5).

Pathophysiology

Herniation occurs when the body wall is breached and fat, omentum or abdominal organs protrude through the hole. In the case of true hernias, herniation occurs when the natural opening fails to close adequately during embryogenesis or enlarges during adulthood.

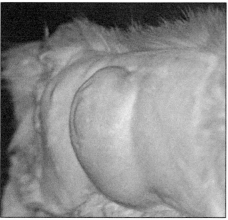

4.11 Abdominal wall (paracostal) hernia in a cat.

Possible diagnosis
• Hernia
• Abscess
• Cyst
• Haematoma
• Neoplasia
• Granuloma
• Seroma

Clinical information for differentiation
• Clinical history and signalment
• Site of swelling
• Palpate swelling
• Number of swellings
• Other clinical signs
• Aspirate swelling
• Ultrasound examination of swelling

4.12 Differential diagnoses for body wall masses.

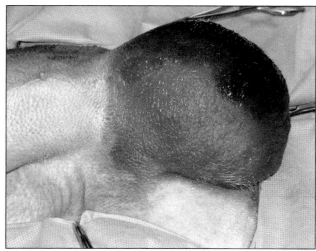

4.13 Inguinal hernia in a 5-year-old male hound. Note the dramatic scrotal swelling.
(Courtesy of J Niles)

Small hernias may have only a small amount of omentum or fat protrusion and in these cases clinical findings are unremarkable, other than a small swelling. Larger hernias allow abdominal contents to migrate into the hernial sac; if the neck of the hernia is narrow, the blood supply to these organs may become restricted or twisted. In certain circumstances, the organ itself may become obstructed and dilated, with specific clinical consequences. Which organs enter the hernia depends on the site of the hernia and the condition of the animal; for example, a gravid uterus might migrate into a large inguinal hernia.

Strangulation or vascular torsion of hernia contents results in tissue necrosis and organ rupture. These hernias are often painful and very swollen and rapidly result in shock, septicaemia and collapse. The animal may present with vomiting, abdominal pain or depression.

Diagnosis

Clinical examination is an important part of the diagnostic procedure for hernias, particularly hernias that reduce. Gentle palpation finds that the herniated contents 'pop' back into the abdomen, leaving a flat surface with a palpable hole in the body wall. More complex cases may require identification of hernia contents, and diagnostic imaging can be very useful. Ultrasonographic investigation of the mass is usually diagnostic, allowing identification of abdominal wall defects, intestines and/or specific organs. Plain radiographs may show loss of abdominal wall continuity, the presence of gas-filled loops of small intestine on the outside of the abdominal wall or loss of definition of the caudal abdominal strip. A gravid uterus may be obvious after 43 days of gestation, owing to the presence of fetal skeletons. Contrast studies of the gastrointestinal or urinary tract may confirm the presence of intestine or bladder in the hernia.

Umbilical hernias

An umbilical hernia is usually a congenital defect of embryogenesis and is occasionally associated with other defects such as peritoneopericardial hernias, sternal defects or cryptorchidism. Most umbilical hernias are thought to be inherited and they are the most common abdominal hernia in small animals. The overall incidence has been reported as 0.6%, and breed predispositions have been reported in the Cornish Rex (10.7%), Abyssinian (10.7%), Airedale, Basenji, Pekingese, Pointer and Weimeraner. It is thought to be more common in bitches. Small umbilical hernias in puppies may resolve spontaneously during the first 6 months, but can recur at a later age if they suffer increased abdominal pressure (e.g. with an enlarging abdominal mass or acute organ distension).

Inguinal hernias

An inguinal hernia is the result of a defect in the inguinal canal, allowing herniation of abdominal contents, and is usually non-traumatic in origin. The reported incidence of *congenital* inguinal hernia is 1.6%, with females and males equally affected, and the defect is probably heritable (particularly in Golden Retrievers, Cocker Spaniels and Dachshunds). There is often a concurrent umbilical hernia. Predisposed breeds include Basenji, Pekingese, Cairn Terrier, Basset Hound and West Highland White Terrier. Congenital inguinal hernias in males may be associated with delayed testicular descent, and sometimes the hernia resolves spontaneously as the inguinal rings decrease in size over the first few months of life.

Acquired inguinal hernias occur most often in middle-aged intact bitches but have been seen occasionally in male dogs and there are a few reports of inguinal hernias in cats. The exact aetiology of acquired hernias is unclear, but sex hormones play an important role and one study indicated a link to perineal hernia in the male dog. Oestrogen production may be a key element because most inguinal hernias present during oestrus or pregnancy. An intrinsic weakness of the inguinal canal, particularly in the female, may play a contributory role in those dogs that present with obesity or poor metabolic (e.g. hyperadrenocorticism) or nutritional status.

Herniation may occur within the vaginal process (termed *indirect*) or alongside the vaginal process (termed *direct*) (Figure 4.14). Direct hernias are more common in both sexes. They can occur unilaterally or bilaterally; unilateral hernias may be more common on the left. The swelling can be extremely large and may extend into the scrotum in males (see Figure 4.13) and all the way along the round ligament to the vulva in females. As the hernias are often large, strangulation is less common but they may contain urinary, reproductive or gastrointestinal structures (Figure 4.15). Careful investigation of these hernias is important, as they may be confused with mammary gland masses, lipomas, enlarged lymph nodes or abscesses. Both inguinal canals should be investigated in order to determine the surgical requirements. Inguinal hernias are best repaired at the time of diagnosis (see Operative Technique 4.3).

Indirect hernias allow herniation of organs within the vaginal process and are seen as *scrotal hernias* in the male. These hernias are rare, usually unilateral and seen in young large-breed dogs. There is an increased risk of strangulation of the hernia contents and they may be associated with testicular neoplasia. Some hernias only protrude a small way down the vaginal process; they are not always associated with gross scrotal enlargement, but a widened spermatic cord can be palpated just distal to the inguinal canal. Scrotal inflammation, orchitis, testicular neoplasia or torsion should be ruled out prior to surgery. Surgical repair should be carried out as soon as possible, because of the high risk of strangulation. Where the sac contains strangulated viscera, a midline approach may be preferable to allow decontamination and removal of tissue prior to replacement in the abdomen.

The hernia may be repaired with or without castration, but castration is strongly recommended to prevent recurrence and the development of neoplasia. When castration is

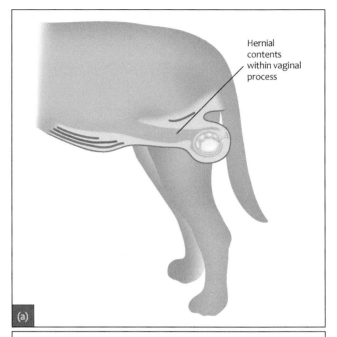

Hernial contents within vaginal process

(a)

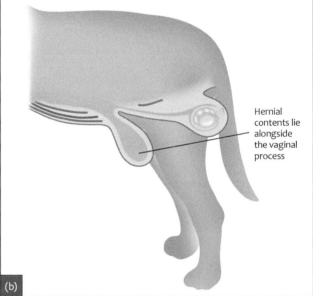

Hernial contents lie alongside the vaginal process

(b)

4.14 Inguinal hernia. (a) Indirect herniation and (b) direct herniation in the male dog.

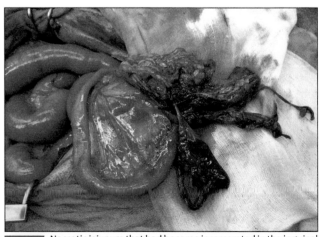

4.15 Necrotic jejunum that had become incarcerated in the inguinal canal of the dog in Figure 4.13. Note: a scrotal ablation and abdominal exploratory were performed in this dog.
(Courtesy of J Niles)

not carried out, the hernia is reduced and the vaginal tunic (hernial sac) is reduced as much as possible, using mattress sutures. The inguinal ring is then closed, leaving room for the genital and pudendal vessels on the caudal edge. When castration is planned, the hernial sac is opened, castration is carried out and the external inguinal ring is closed.

Femoral hernias

Femoral hernias are rare in cats and dogs. Abdominal fat is seen protruding caudomedial to the femoral artery and vein, next to the pectineus muscle. Herniation may be a consequence of trauma, prepubic ligament rupture or a complication of pectineal myectomy. It is important to distinguish this from herniation through the adjacent inguinal canal, which is cranial to the inguinal ligament. Careful placement of sutures between the inguinal ligament and the pectineal fascia may be used to close the femoral canal, but it is important to avoid the neurovascular structures in this area. The animal should be monitored postoperatively for progressive oedema, excessive pain or femoral nerve deficits.

Principles of surgical repair

The main aims of hernia repair are:

- Reduction of hernia contents
- Anatomical reconstruction of the defect without tension
- Closure of the dead space resulting from reduction of the hernia, and high amputation of the hernial sac.

Most hernias are approached by a direct incision over the sac of the hernia. This enables assessment of the hernia contents and excision of necrotic or ischaemic tissue in strangulated hernias prior to reduction. However, sometimes it is useful to have simultaneous access to the abdominal cavity. The hernial ring may need to be enlarged to allow reduction of organs, though aspiration may assist in stabilization of obstructed organs such as the stomach or bladder. Devitalized loops of bowel may be resected and re-anastomosed prior to return to the abdomen. In these cases, a concurrent midline approach may assist in assessing bowel viability after enterectomy; it is important that the abdominal cavity is not contaminated by necrotic hernia contents during the procedure. Once the hernia is reduced, the hernial sac may be ligated and/or transected and sutured closed.

> **PRACTICAL TIP**
>
> It is essential that organs are thoroughly evaluated prior to return into the abdomen, because they may not be visible from a direct approach after hernia reduction

The hernial ring is usually closed by direct appositional suture repair. The specific recommendations depend on the anatomy and the presence of suture-holding tissue adjacent to the ring. Knowledge of local anatomy is essential to avoid strangulation of vital structures that pass through the normal opening. Very large or chronic hernias may be difficult to repair with primary sutures, and muscle flaps or tissue mobilization techniques may be used to augment repair of the hernial ring. Where this is not possible, polypropylene meshes or porcine small intestine submucosa (SIS) can be used to strengthen the repair and close the defect (Figure 4.16). Although there

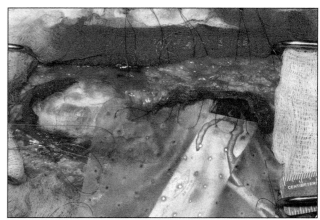

4.16 A sheet of porcine SIS being used to repair a chronic abdominal wall hernia. Note how the polypropylene mattress sutures have been pre-placed.
(Courtesy of J Niles)

are successful reports of the use of meshes or SIS in hernia repair, there is an increased risk of postoperative pain, infection and seroma formation, and considerable experience is needed to use these techniques successfully.

Animals with traumatic hernias or strangulated contents may need stabilization and assessment of other injuries prior to anaesthesia for the surgical repair. Assessment should be made of the hernia contents in order to determine the urgency of repair (e.g. stomach, bladder or uterus herniation may result in progressive clinical deterioration if not resolved rapidly). If the hernia is painful or cannot be easily reduced, then it is not suitable for elective surgery.

Complications of hernia repair

Seroma

The commonest complications of hernia repair are seroma and haematoma due to excessive tissue dissection or inadequate haemostasis. Diagnosis is best made by ultrasound-guided aspiration of the postoperative swelling. Aspiration of fluid is rarely helpful in terms of resolving the fluid accumulation, and there is an increased risk of infection and ultimately repair breakdown. Most seromas will resolve without the need for drainage, though some cases may require further exploratory surgery and the placement of drains.

Infection

Infection of the repair causes delayed healing, or chronic fistulation if implants have been used, and is most common where there has been poor technique or where severely devitalized tissue has been inadequately excised. Ruptured intestine or other organs will also increase the risk of postoperative infection. Early recognition of infection is extremely important in ensuring rapid resolution and preventing hernia dehiscence. The surgical site must be reopened for debridement and lavage. A swab for bacteriology taken at this point will assist in the rational choice of antibiotic therapy.

Recurrence

Contralateral herniation may occur when early hernias are missed at the time of surgery. Hernia dehiscence occurs when there is excessive straining, poor technique, or poor postoperative management (Figure 4.17). Second and subsequent repairs carry a worse prognosis and may be best carried out by experienced surgeons.

Cause	Comments
Poor technique	Inappropriate suture material Inappropriate use of tissue layers Poor tissue handling on reduction of hernia Tension on the repair Poor suture placement Poor anchoring of implants
Infection	Increased risk with use of implants Increased risk with necrotic hernia
Postoperative strain on repair	Poor postoperative restraint Tenesmus or vomiting Barking, coughing Abdominal enlargement (pregnancy)

4.17 Causes of failure of hernia repair.

Abdominal trauma

The most common sites for traumatic abdominal hernia are the paracostal (especially in cats) and the ventrocaudal or prepubic regions (Figure 4.18). If there is evidence of abdominal trauma, other organs are often involved. It is helpful to determine the aetiology, as this helps with planning and determining likely associated injuries (e.g. gunshot wounds *versus* dog bites *versus* road accidents). Most traumatic hernias are due to blunt trauma such as road accidents, falls or kicks.

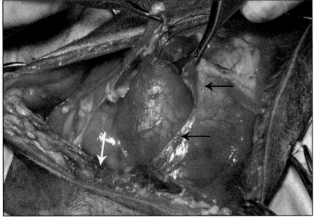

4.18 Prepubic tendon rupture in a Domestic Shorthaired cat following a road traffic accident. The cat's head is to the right of the photograph. The abdominal wall (black arrows) has been avulsed from the pubis (white arrow). The bladder can be seen in the centre of the picture.
(Courtesy of J Niles)

Stabilization and assessment

- The patient is triaged, stabilized and given analgesia as necessary and then steps are taken towards a diagnosis.
- The patient should be assessed for orthopaedic, spinal, thoracic or diaphragmatic injury, as up to 75% of patients will have concurrent injuries.
- The abdominal cavity should be assessed for visceral and parenchymatous organ damage (e.g. spleen, liver), crush injury or avulsion injury (e.g. vascular avulsion, urinary tract) (see Figures 4.18 and 4.19).
- Evidence of the function of each abdominal organ system should be systematically obtained: urinalysis, packed cell volume, total protein, albumin, electrolytes (especially sodium and potassium), ultrasonography and radiography for evidence of fluid or gas in the peritoneal cavity.

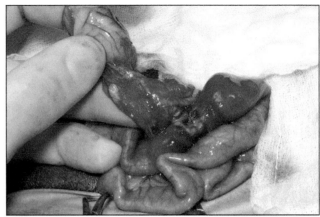

4.19 Devitalized area of jejunum found on abdominal exploration prior to repair of the prepubic tendon in the cat in Figure 4.18. An intestinal resection and anastomosis were performed.
(Courtesy of J Niles)

- Paracentesis or diagnostic peritoneal lavage may also be necessary for diagnosis (see Chapter 18).
- The hernia should be assessed using clinical examination and ultrasonography to determine optimal management. It is important to assess:
  - The degree of disruption to the body wall
  - Incarceration or obstruction/strangulation of organs
  - Which organs are involved
  - Penetrating wounds or tears in open hernias.

Clinical examination and diagnosis

Clinical examination may allow immediate diagnosis of body wall rupture. Severe bruising, haematoma formation, loss of abdominal contour or obvious herniation of abdominal contents through a non-anatomical opening may be detectable with simple palpation and examination. Clipping the hair of the ventral abdomen may reveal bruising (Figure 4.20) and small skin injuries. Ultrasonographic or radiographic examination may confirm loss of the body wall continuity, and plain radiographs may also demonstrate loops of gas-filled intestine in the subcutaneous space. Where penetrating injuries, such as ballistic injuries or dog bites, are suspected, exploratory surgery will be required to rule out injury to internal organs.

Management and repair

Management of a hernia depends on the immediate presentation and injury. Hernias with incarcerated obstructed organs or strangulated organs require immediate surgical repair. If the patient is stable and there is no risk of organ obstruction, it may be sufficient to provide analgesia and

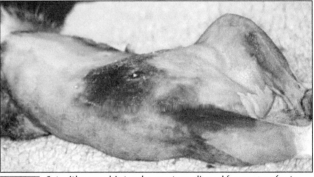

4.20 Cat with prepubic tendon rupture clipped for surgery (note extensive bruising).

support the body wall using a broad, well padded bandage. Caudal abdominal hernias require use of an indwelling urinary catheter and collection bag in order to prevent soiling of the bandage. This is particularly important in animals where there are open wounds associated with the hernia or injury.

> **WARNING**
>
> Approximately 50% of body wall ruptures that are contaminated at the time of injury (e.g. dog bite injuries) become infected

Repair of the hernia is often best left as an elective procedure to allow adequate stabilization and resolution of haemorrhage and bruising prior to attempting repair. Many surgeons recommend hernia repair 3–5 days after injury. Longer delays are sometimes necessary in the interest of patient stabilization, but abdominal wall contracture will make the repair more difficult. Chronic hernias may develop if the animal has severe injuries and the acute hernia is missed. With time, the muscle edges retract and the muscle contracts to become shorter and less compliant. Loss of abdominal domain (space) occurs as the abdomen adapts to permanently herniated abdominal contents. Ultimately, the hernia becomes difficult to repair with primary closure, and complex techniques, such as the use of mesh, SIS or vascular pedicle muscle grafts, may be necessary. Muscle flaps using EAO, cranial sartorius and pectineus muscles have been described (see *BSAVA Manual of Canine and Feline Wound Management and Reconstruction*). These procedures can be difficult to perform after trauma and are usually only performed at referral institutions. Multilayered SIS material may be more physiological than mesh, because it is biologically incorporated with the development of skeletal muscle in the defect over time, whereas the mesh only fills in with scar tissue.

Paracostal hernias

Paracostal hernias (see Figure 4.11) involve the origin of the EAO and TA muscles, and the insertion of the IAO muscle. The defect is probably always traumatic, and rib fractures, intercostal muscle tears or concurrent diaphragmatic rupture may be found. Cats may present with chronic paracostal hernias and these appear to be more common than in dogs. Abdominal contents can migrate under the skin or through into the thorax. Defects that only involve one or two muscle layers (TA and/or IAO) may be difficult to palpate as the EAO muscle flattens the hernia, and diagnostic imaging techniques may be necessary to identify the abdominal wall defect.

The defect is repaired using the ribs to anchor the muscle layers, ensuring that each layer is identified and repaired specifically (Figure 4.21). Recurrence may be common, owing to the constant movement of the site with breathing.

Prepubic tendon rupture

Prepubic tendon rupture (see Operative Technique 4.4) is usually an avulsion injury following a road traffic accident. The animal should be carefully assessed for other avulsion injuries such as inguinal or dorsolateral avulsion. Given that many of these animals will also have concurrent orthopaedic injuries, the insertion of the RA muscle may be completely separated from the pelvis and may be associated with fractures of the pelvic floor. In such cases it is

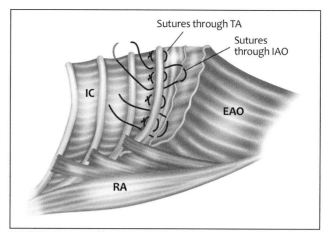

4.21 Paracostal hernia repair. Muscle layers are attached to the costal arch sequentially, using mattress sutures anchored to the ribs. EAO = external abdominal oblique muscle; IAO = internal abdominal oblique muscle; IC = intercostalis muscles; RA = rectus abdominis; TA = transversus abdominis.

essential that the animal is carefully assessed for urethral damage and managed accordingly (see Chapter 16).

Chronic prepubic tendon ruptures often require the use of mesh, SIS graft or a vascular myofascial flap (e.g. EAO muscle). Early diagnosis is important, as these ruptures can be very difficult to repair once they become chronic.

Lateral wall ruptures

Lateral abdominal wall ruptures are occasionally seen with or without prepubic disruption. The tear may extend from the lateral prepubic area through the inguinal canal and caudal aponeuroses up to the origin of the abdominal muscles on the transverse processes of the lumbar vertebrae. In this situation repair of the prepubic tendon will be insufficient and herniation occurs dorsally and lateral to the RA muscle. A sound understanding of the abdominal wall anatomy is required in order to appose the body wall to the correct structures. The same materials and techniques are used as for prepubic repair.

Inguinal seromas

Inguinal seromas are occasionally seen in cats that have suffered a traumatic event and, much like prepubic tendon rupture, they present with inguinal bruising and swelling. Trauma to the inguinal fat pad causes fat necrosis and an inflammatory exudate, together with disruption of the regional vascular and lymphatic vessels. Ultrasonography can be used to confirm the integrity of the abdominal wall; it shows an area of diffuse hypoechoic subcutaneous fluid accumulation and areas of fat necrosis. Most cases will resolve over 5–7 days with strict rest and judicious use of non-steroidal anti-inflammatory medication.

Persistent cases may require surgical exploration to place a drain or omentalization of the inguinal area, and this is usually successful (Figure 4.22) (Charlesworth and Moores, 2012).

> **Editors' note:**
>
> The Editors would like to emphasize that the choice of non-steroidal anti-inflammatory drug rests with the veterinary surgeon; use of these agents should be governed by clinical judgement and national licensing laws

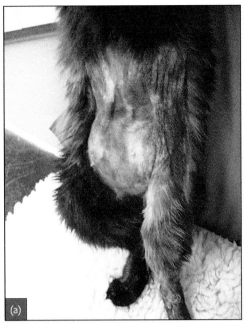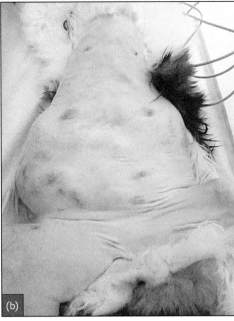

4.22 (a) Inguinal seromas usually present with a non-painful soft fluctuant swelling in the inguinal area. This cat has a bilateral swelling that is predominantly situated in the inguinal area, even when the forelimbs are elevated. (b) In dorsal recumbency, during preparation for surgery, palpation of the caudal abdominal wall is unremarkable and the seroma spreads bilaterally over the inguinal area.
(a, Reproduced from Charlesworth and Moores (2012) with permission from the *Journal of Small Animal Practice*; b, © Tim Charlesworth)

References and further reading

Alexander LG, Pavletic MM and Engler SJ (1991) Abdominal wall reconstruction with a vascular external abdominal oblique myofascial flap. *Veterinary Surgery* **20**, 379–384

Alimoglu O, Akcakaya A, Sahin M *et al.* (2003) Prevention of adhesion formations following repair of abdominal wall defects with prosthetic materials (an experimental study). *Hepatogastroenterology* **50**, 725–728

Bellenger CR (2003) Abdominal wall. In: *Textbook of Small Animal Surgery*, ed. D Slatter, pp.405–424. WB Saunders, Philadelphia

Charlesworth TM and Moores AL (2012) Post trauma inguinal seroma formation in the cat. *Journal of Small Animal Practice* **53**, 301–303

Hayes HM (1973) Congenital umbilical and inguinal hernias in cattle, horses, swine, dogs and cats: risk by breed and sex among hospitalised patients. *American Journal of Veterinary Research* **35**, 839–842

Hoer J, Junge K, Schachtrupp A, Klinge U and Schumpelick V (2002) Influence of laparotomy closure technique on collagen synthesis in the incisional region. *Hernia* **6**, 93–98

Robinson R (1977) Genetic aspects of umbilical hernia incidence in cats and dogs. *Veterinary Record* **100**, 9–10

Ruble RP and Hird DW (1993) Congenital abnormalities in immature dogs from a pet store: 253 cases (1987–1988). *Journal of the American Veterinary Medical Association* **202**, 633–636

Schachtrupp A, Hoer J, Tons C *et al.* (2002) Intra-abdominal pressure: a reliable criterion for laparostomy closure? *Hernia* **6**, 102–107

Smeak DD (2012) Abdominal wall reconstruction and hernias. In: *Veterinary Surgery: Small Animal*, ed. KM Tobias and SA Johnston, pp.1353–1379. Elsevier Saunders, Philadelphia

Waldron DR, Hedlund CS and Pechman R (1986) Abdominal hernias in dogs and cats: a review of 24 cases. *Journal of the American Animal Hospital Association* **22**, 817–823

Waters DJ, Roy RG and Stone EA (1993) A retrospective study of inguinal hernia in 35 dogs. *Veterinary Surgery* **22**, 44–49

Williams J and Moores A (2009) *BSAVA Manual of Canine and Feline Wound Management and Reconstruction, 2nd edn.* BSAVA Publications, Gloucester

Ziv Y, Brosh T, Lushkov G and Halevy A (2001) Effect of electrocautery vs. scalpel on fascial mechanical properties after midline laparotomy incision in rats. *Israeli Medical Association* **3**, 566–568

OPERATIVE TECHNIQUE 4.1

Midline laparotomy (coeliotomy)

PREPARATION AND POSITIONING

Hair on the ventral surface is clipped from the mid sternum to the ventral perineum. The clip should be wide, up to one-third of the way up the costal arch. The skin should be prepared for surgery and draped (see Chapter 1). In male dogs, the urethra may be catheterized prior to preparation and the end stopped to prevent urine leakage during surgery. The prepuce may be moved to one side and secured to the ventral abdominal skin with a towel clamp to ensure that the preputial opening is out of the surgical site. The patient is secured in dorsal recumbency using troughs, sandbags or leg ties. It is usual for a right-handed surgeon to stand on the patient's right side and for a left-handed surgeon to stand on the patient's left side.

EQUIPMENT EXTRAS

Self-retaining retractors (Gelpi or Gosset if an assistant is available, otherwise Balfour, or baby Balfour for cats and small dogs); hand-held retractors (Army–Navy, malleable, Langenbeck).

ASSISTANT

Routine elective procedures are usually performed without assistance, but inexperienced surgeons may need a surgical assistant until they have developed strategies for retraction and ligation of structures without help. Obese or deep-chested dogs can be extremely difficult to operate on without assistance.

SURGICAL TECHNIQUE

Surgical manipulations

1   Use a No. 10 or 15 scalpel blade to make a smooth long incision centred on the part of the abdomen that is most important to the approach (for exploratory surgery, the whole abdomen should be opened from the sternum to the pubis).

2   Gently dissect the underlying fat using scissors or the scalpel to minimize trauma. Avoid creating excessive dead space and do not disrupt the fascial blood vessels.

3   In the male dog, deviate the incision laterally to avoid the prepuce. Sever the preputial muscle; caudally a medial branch of the caudal superficial epigastric artery and vein may be encountered. Ligate these vessels (or use diathermy) and transect. Continue the dissection on to the midline underneath the prepuce for abdominal access via the linea alba.

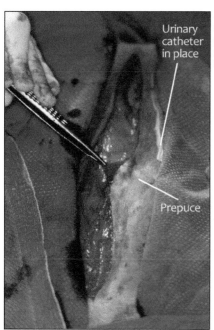

Urinary catheter in place

Prepuce

Midline laparotomy with incision deviating laterally around the prepuce (the forceps are grasping the severed preputial muscle).

→ **OPERATIVE TECHNIQUE 4.1 CONTINUED**

4 Make a small nick in the linea alba using a scalpel blade in the region of the umbilicus. Alternatively, use forceps to elevate the linea alba to allow a small incision to be made. Before enlarging the wound, slide a finger cranially and caudally along the inside of the abdominal surface to ensure that there are no adhesions of organs to the midline. Once the tissues are clear, the linea alba incision is usually enlarged using a 'slide-cut' with straight Mayo scissors to the required length. Alternatively, a scalpel can be used as long as the underlying organs are protected by forceps.

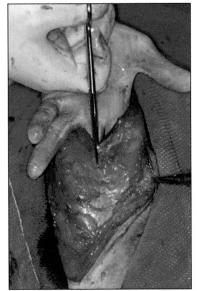

Mayo scissors being used to enlarge incision in linea alba.

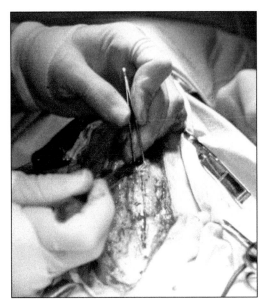

Scalpel being used to extend linea alba incision. Underlying organs are protected by elevating the linea alba prior to incision.

5 In some dogs and cats the falciform fat may be large and difficult to retract during examination of the cranial abdomen. Complete transection and removal of the falciform fat will facilitate exposure of the abdominal contents.

6 Protect the wound edges from desiccation, contamination or bruising with moistened surgical swabs during the surgery. Stretching or tearing of the cranial or caudal ends of the incision will contribute to bruising and postoperative pain, as well as increase the risk of delayed healing.

PRACTICAL TIP
Self-retaining retractors are essential when a surgical assistant is not available

PRACTICAL TIP
Tilting the table can sometimes help to move abdominal contents out of the way when trying to access the cranial compartment

PRACTICAL TIP
It is essential to establish a routine for counting surgical swabs before and after abdominal surgery

Wound closure

WARNING
If a contaminated viscus has been entered during surgery (e.g. enterotomy) the surgeon should change their contaminated gloves, remove all contaminated materials from the surgical site and use fresh sterile instruments for closure. It is essential that suture material used for intestinal closure is discarded and not used for repair of the external tissues

→ **OPERATIVE TECHNIQUE 4.1 CONTINUED**

1   Repair the midline with a single continuous suture of moderate to long-lasting synthetic absorbable material (e.g. polydioxanone). Start the suture at the caudal end, taking care to take wide (0.5–1 cm) bites of the external fascial sheath. With large and giant-breed dogs it may be useful to use a looped suture; this reduces the diameter of suture required and only requires a secure knot at the cranial end of the incision. It is not necessary to incorporate the RA muscle, the internal fascial sheath or the peritoneum. Pull up the suture at each bite to ensure that the suture bites are snug but not over-tightened. As the suture approaches the cranial end of the wound, the external fascial sheath is less obvious and the linea alba is wider. It is acceptable at this point to use the thick fibrous edges of the abdominal wall aponeuroses where they join the linea alba.

2   Subcutaneous fat is closed carefully to ensure closure of dead space, using absorbable suture materials in a simple continuous pattern. In the male dog, the preputial muscle should be repaired to stabilize the prepuce back into the midline, and the fat should be closed underneath the prepuce to prevent fluid accumulation in the dead space. Take care not to penetrate the caudal superficial epigastric vessels accidentally during this repair, particularly in the male dog.

3   Skin closure is routine. A subcuticular continuous suture with a fine absorbable material may be used. There is no specific indication to place skin sutures on top of this suture as well, unless there are anticipated complications with wound healing. Skin sutures can also be placed in a continuous fashion using an appositional pattern, such as Ford interlocking. It is important to place skin sutures loosely to ensure that they do not become tight and begin to irritate the patient as postoperative swelling occurs. Alternatively, skin staples may be used.

POSTOPERATIVE MANAGEMENT AND COMPLICATIONS

Postoperative management and complications vary according to the intra-abdominal procedure performed and are discussed in the relevant chapters.

OPERATIVE TECHNIQUE 4.2

Flank laparotomy

This technique is usually used in the UK for feline ovariohysterectomy (see also Operative Technique 17.3). *It cannot be recommended for canine ovariohysterectomy.*

POSITIONING

If the surgeon is right-handed, a left flank approach is performed with the cat in right lateral recumbency and the hindlimbs drawn caudally and stabilized. Left-handed surgeons usually prefer to approach the right flank with the cat in left lateral recumbency.

EQUIPMENT EXTRAS

None. Synthetic absorbable suture material is recommended. The author and editors *do not* recommend the use of spay hooks.

ASSISTANT

Not necessary.

SURGICAL TECHNIQUE

Surgical manipulations

1   Palpate the anatomical landmarks; identify the transverse processes of the lumbar vertebrae, the iliac crest, the coxofemoral joint and the cranial aspect of the quadriceps muscle group.

→

→ **OPERATIVE TECHNIQUE 4.2 CONTINUED**

2   The site of the incision may be identified by various techniques. One text describes a 2.5 cm incision ventral to the transverse processes and cranial to the iliac crest. Another method is to visualize an ipsilateral triangle using the coxofemoral joint, iliac crest and the dorsal point of the incision, when the hindlegs are drawn well caudally (see Operative Technique 17.3).

> **PRACTICAL TIP**
>
> The most common mistake is to make the incision too far dorsally or too far caudally. The incision must start ventral to the fixed fat of the retroperitoneal space under the transverse processes. It must be well cranial to the front of the hindleg, and in the soft part of the flank

3   Make a vertical incision in the flank skin and extend into the subcutaneous fat and on to the abdominal wall muscle. In fat animals, a small lump of fat may be removed to ease visualization.

4   Ideally, the abdominal wall muscles are separated as a gridiron along the lines of origin/insertion of each layer. Less experienced surgeons may cut the EAO muscle with scissors, and sometimes all the layers may be cut vertically in line with the skin incision. This technique is more traumatic and may result in more bleeding as the branches of the circumflex iliac artery are encountered. As the fibres of the TA muscle are separated, the peritoneum may be visualized as a very fine membrane. This is punctured with atraumatic forceps or Metzenbaum scissor tips and the abdomen is entered; the pale loose 'yellowish' lobular fat of the omentum should be seen.

> **PRACTICAL TIP**
>
> If the incision is made too far dorsally, the retroperitoneal fat is seen under the muscle layers. This fat is whiter than omental fat and less mobile. The peritoneum should be identified intact ventral to this fat, and then the omental fat is found, confirming entry to the abdomen

Wound closure

Where the gridiron approach has been used, the muscles may completely overlap and a single suture should be placed across the centre of the gridiron to prevent the risk of herniation. Where the muscles have been cut it is important to suture the defect closed with a simple continuous suture, taking care to identify and include all muscle layers, which will have retracted in opposite directions during the procedure. This can be difficult for inexperienced surgeons, particularly if the muscle incisions are longer than the skin incision. The subcutaneous fat should be closed to reduce dead space with a single interrupted suture, and the skin is closed with simple interrupted sutures.

> **PRACTICAL TIP**
>
> Where the muscle layers have retracted it may be helpful to pull the suture material through each layer one at a time

OPERATIVE TECHNIQUE 4.3

Inguinal hernia repair

> **POSITIONING**
>
> Dorsal recumbency with the hindlimbs drawn gently caudally.

> **EQUIPMENT EXTRAS**
>
> Mesh implants or porcine SIS may be useful.

> **ASSISTANT**
>
> Extremely helpful.

→ **OPERATIVE TECHNIQUE 4.3 CONTINUED**

Approach

The inguinal canal is carefully palpated under general anaesthesia to determine whether a bilateral approach is necessary. Bilateral hernias are routinely approached with a midline incision, but it is possible to approach a unilateral hernia with an incision over the lateral aspect of the swelling. A midline approach enables exploration of the contralateral inguinal canal (and closure if necessary) and allows intra-abdominal visualization of the reduced hernia contents, and ovariohysterectomy if required. The midline is a more versatile and reliable approach and is described here.

Surgical manipulations

1 Make a midline skin incision from the umbilicus to midway along the pelvic symphysis or to the end of the hernia.

2 Gently dissect the subcutaneous tissues (mammary glands in the female) from the fascial surface of the RA muscle and reflect laterally until the inguinal canal and external inguinal ring are exposed.

3 For an uncomplicated hernia, gently reduce the hernia by palpation and twisting of the hernial sac to push the contents through the inguinal canal. If the hernia cannot be reduced, enlarge the inguinal canal by incising through the inguinal ring on the craniomedial aspect (taking care to avoid the genital and pudendal vessels).

4 Amputate the neck of the hernial sac and ligate once all structures are reduced. Close the inguinal ring using synthetic monofilament absorbable or non-absorbable suture material from the cranial aspect. Leave space for the passage of the genital and pudendal structures. Where the fascial tissue is weakened or very thin, placement of sutures between the inguinal ligament and the external rectus fascia may help security of closure.

- Ovariohysterectomy may be performed simultaneously through the midline approach, using a midline coeliotomy.
- In a breeding bitch, successful replacement of the gravid uterus and repair of the hernia to allow delivery of the litter have been accomplished at up to 7 weeks' gestation. After this time, ovariohysterectomy is recommended.
- Where the hernia contents are incarcerated or strangulated, exploratory surgery may be carried out first and then the hernia repaired extra-abdominally after the devitalized tissue has been removed.

WARNING

Never reduce hernias with devitalized or necrotic tissue prior to resection

5 Carefully assess the opposite side. Inguinal ring closure may be augmented with one or two sutures even if there is no evidence of current herniation.

6 Very large hernias may benefit from placement of a subcutaneous drain to prevent seroma formation. Closed suction drains are preferred, to prevent urinary or faecal soiling and contamination of the surgical site.

Wound closure

Closure of the dead space is achieved with simple interrupted sutures, and skin closure is routine.

The prognosis associated with uncomplicated inguinal hernia repair is excellent. However, this depends on the initial presentation and the presence of strangulated or necrotic hernia contents. Analgesia is extremely important and postoperative hospitalization may be necessary in order to administer effective analgesic agents. Gentle on-lead exercise is started as soon as possible postoperatively to encourage resolution of oedema. The incision must be closely monitored for signs of infection or hernia recurrence. Bandaging is unnecessary. Exercise is restricted to lead walks only for at least 3–4 weeks postoperatively, until scar remodelling is complete.

OPERATIVE TECHNIQUE 4.4

Prepubic tendon rupture repair

POSITIONING

Dorsal recumbency with the hindlimbs relaxed and able to be manipulated through the drapes by the surgeon.

EQUIPMENT EXTRAS

Drill and K-wire; surgical wire or 3.5 metric (0 USP) polypropylene; mesh or porcine SIS; polytetrafluroethylene (PTFE) pledgets.

ASSISTANT

Often beneficial, especially in chronic cases.

SURGICAL TECHNIQUE

Approach

A large area of the ventral abdomen is prepared for surgery (see Figure 4.20). A midline approach is used, and the ventral abdominal wall musculature is examined. The surgeon should be prepared for the possibility that there is more than one abdominal wall defect or indeed that the defect is not prepubic.

Surgical manipulations

1 Remove fibrinous adhesions and haematoma from the site of the rupture. Sterile saline lavage of the tissues may help in identification of muscle layers and structures. Reduce herniated tissues into the abdomen.

2 Repair prepubic ligament avulsion with sutures placed through the ligament and into small holes drilled in the pubis. This may not be possible if there are pelvic floor fractures. If this is not possible, use PTFE pledgets in the muscles to reduce the risk of suture pull-out.

3 Pre-place synthetic monofilament non-absorbable (preferably) or absorbable material (polydioxanone) sutures along the caudal edge of the torn RA muscle and into the holes in the pubis or the prepubic ligament if it is still attached to the pelvis. Strict attention to detail is necessary for correct anatomical reconstruction of the deficit.

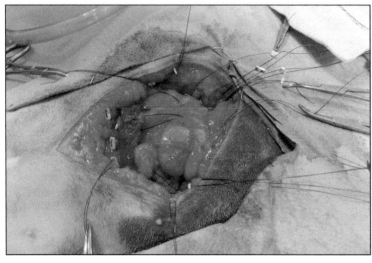

Sutures are pre-placed using PTFE pledgets to reduce the risk of them tearing through when tightened.
(© J Williams)

4 Place simple interrupted sutures if the external fascial sheath of the RA muscle is intact. Where the muscle and fascial sheath are torn, use interrupted vertical mattress sutures to augment the repair and decrease the risk of suture pull-out on tightening.

→ **OPERATIVE TECHNIQUE 4.4 CONTINUED**

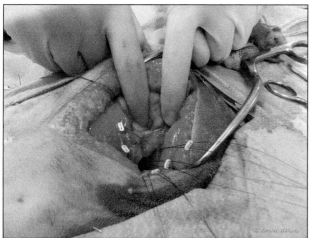

(© J Williams)

PRACTICAL TIP

Pre-placing all the sutures before tying them may facilitate the repair, particularly when a mesh is being sutured in to fill the defect

---

5 At this stage, mesh may be used in a 'sandwich' on each side of the muscle to help to anchor the sutures or to augment repair where the tension is too great.

6 Tie the sutures, ensuring snug apposition of tissues but not crushing of muscle edges. It is essential that the repair is not under tension.

Wound closure

- Before closure, the femoral and inguinal canals should be examined for concurrent avulsion injury.
- Dead space is closed meticulously, using simple interrupted sutures. In contaminated wounds, it may be necessary to use a postoperative drain.
- Skin closure is routine.

POSTOPERATIVE MANAGEMENT AND COMPLICATIONS

Many animals have multiple injuries and require intensive care, continuous nursing and monitoring postoperatively. Animals with pelvic fractures may be recumbent and require frequent turning, physiotherapy and cleaning. As with repair of other hernias, restriction of exercise is important, particularly with regard to healing of ligamentous tissue on the pelvis in the presence of avulsion fractures.

PRACTICAL TIP

Complex contaminated abdominal wall injuries can be extremely difficult to repair and the patient difficult to stabilize and nurse postoperatively. These cases benefit from specialist intensive care and surgical techniques

---

Hernia dehiscence

As described in the text, this is usually due to poor surgical technique, poor nursing or patient overactivity.

Infection

This is extremely common in cases of dog bites, ballistic injuries or overlying skin wounds. Infections should be managed with bacteriological testing, aggressive lavage, debridement of the wounds and appropriate antibiotic therapy. Skin sloughs are common following dog bite wounds, but do not appear to increase the likelihood of hernia dehiscence.

Abdominal compartment syndrome

This is a rare but life-threatening complication. It is possible that those animals with poor recovery from abdominal hernia have undiagnosed increased intra-abdominal pressure, increased central venous pressure and decreased urine output; such conditions may be more common than is thought after repair of chronic hernias or body wall defects. Abdominal pressure can be measured from intra-abdominal sites, or intravesical or intragastric catheters. Postoperative vomiting with decreased urination may be a warning sign.

Chapter 5

The stomach

Gary W. Ellison

The stomach serves as a reservoir for food and initiates digestion. Grinding or trituration of large food particles into small ones (i.e. <2 mm) occurs, and the latter flow through the pylorus passively. The large oropharynx and indiscriminate eating habits of small animal patients allow for the swallowing of sizeable foreign bodies, which are often not retrievable endoscopically and require gastrotomy. Gastric outflow obstruction is another common reason for gastric surgery. The large lumen size and rich vascular supply of the stomach promote successful healing without much danger of stenosis or leakage. The antimicrobial population of the gastric lumen is often insignificant, owing to the acidic pH of 2–3, making the risk of septic peritonitis lower than with intestinal or colonic surgery and often obviating the need for perioperative antibiosis.

Anatomy

The empty stomach often cannot be palpated because it is bordered cranioventrally by the liver and laterally by the costal arches. It is fixed proximally at the oesophageal–diaphragmatic hiatus, and distally at the pylorus by the hepatogastric ligament and common bile duct. Additional mesenteric attachments include the greater and lesser omentum. The greater omentum contains the gastrosplenic ligament, which attaches the spleen to the greater curvature of the stomach.

The stomach is divided into five regions (Figure 5.1a). The cardia marks the entrance of the intra-abdominal oesophagus into the stomach and contains primarily mucous cells to provide lubrication for ingesta. The fundus lies to the left and dorsal to the cardia. Food fills the fundus first and then passes into the body, which is the largest region of the stomach and most capable of dilatation. The fundus and body contain primarily chief cells for the production of pepsinogen and parietal cells that produce hydrochloric acid (HCl). The antrum is the distal portion of the stomach and is directed cranially. The antrum serves in mechanical digestion and contains many mucous cells as well as gastrin-secreting cells (G-cells), which stimulate HCl secretion from the parietal cells. The pylorus serves as the anatomical sphincter between the stomach and duodenum. It controls gastric outflow as well as prevents duodenal reflux. The stomach wall is composed of four distinct layers; from internal to external they are the mucosa, submucosa, muscularis and serosa. The mucosa is composed of columnar surface epithelium, a glandular lamina propria and a lamina muscularis mucosa, and is thrown up into large folds known as rugae. The submucosa is composed of a thin elastic layer of connective tissue and is the critical holding layer during surgical closure of incisions through the stomach wall. The muscularis consists of outer longitudinal and inner circular smooth muscle fibres which are thicker in the region of the

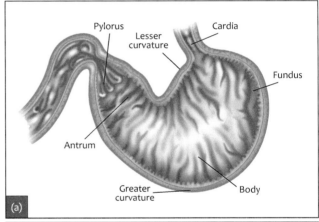

(a)

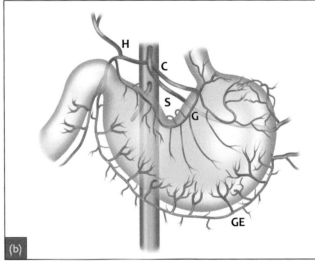

(b)

5.1 (a) Anatomical regions of the stomach. The stomach is divided into a greater and a lesser curvature with five distinct regions: the cardia, the fundus, the body (or corpus), the antrum and the pylorus. The pyloric 'sphincter' has a thicker inner circular muscle. (b) Blood supply to the stomach. Major arterial blood vessels to the stomach arise from the coeliac (C) artery, which gives rise to the hepatic (H), splenic (S), gastric (G) and gastroepiploic (GE) vessels.

pylorus. The outer serosa is a smooth membrane consisting of a thin layer of epithelial cells which offer a layer of minimal holding power for sutures.

The blood supply to the stomach is primarily via the coeliac artery, which branches into the hepatic, left gastric and splenic arteries. The right gastric artery branches off the hepatic artery and anastomoses with the left gastric artery to supply the lesser curvature of the stomach. The hepatic artery then continues as the gastroduodenal artery and gives rise to the right gastroepiploic artery. The left gastroepiploic artery arises from the splenic artery and arborizes with the right gastroepiploic artery to supply the greater curvature of the stomach (Figure 5.1b). Venous drainage of the stomach is via the gastrosplenic vein on the left and the gastroduodenal vein on the right, which then empty into the portal vein. Innervation is via parasympathetic fibres from the vagus nerves and sympathetic fibres from the coeliac plexus. Lymphatic drainage of the stomach is through the gastric and splenic lymph nodes to the hepatic lymph nodes.

The stomach is capable of rapid healing, due its rich blood supply and paucity of intraluminal bacteria. During the first 3–4 days after gastric surgery, inflammation predominates with infiltration of neutrophils and macrophage clean-up of cellular debris. A fibrin seal along the serosa typically prevents leakage but surgical sutures are responsible for maintaining wound approximation during this period. Migration of mucosal epithelium across the open wound bed also occurs during the first few days. Rapid acceleration of wound strength occurs during the following week, with the collagen-rich submucosa being the main source of fibroblasts for this proliferative phase. Maturation of the gastrotomy scar occurs in the weeks thereafter. Long-term complications after gastrotomy are uncommon.

Presurgical considerations

Preoperative fasting for 8 12 hours has been traditionally recommended for dogs and cats. However, for dogs, withholding food does not reliably empty the stomach, lowers the pH and actually increases the risk of oesophagitis and postoperative stricture from gastro-oesophageal reflux. Small amounts of canned food fed at least 3 hours before the procedure have been shown to reduce gastric acidity and even the incidence of reflux. Since oesophageal reflux is common during gastric surgery, a properly sized endotracheal tube with a functional inflatable cuff must be established at the time of induction to minimize the possibility of postoperative aspiration pneumonia. Antibiotics are not typically given perioperatively with gastric surgery unless gastric perforation is present or spillage occurs during the procedure.

Clinical signs and fluid therapy

Gastric disease is usually accompanied by vomiting, which may be either acute or chronic, and intermittent or continuous in nature. Vomiting of gastric fluid may precipitate dehydration, electrolyte, acid–base and cardiovascular abnormalities. Since gastric contents are high in sodium chloride and potassium, hypochloraemia and occasionally metabolic acidosis may exist prior to surgery. Adequate correction of dehydration with isotonic lactated Ringer's (Hartmann's) solution will often correct these sodium and bicarbonate deficiencies. Occasionally

a foreign body lodges in the pylorus, causing acute profuse projectile vomiting and rapid dehydration. In these cases loss of fluids rich in K^+, Na^+, H^+ and Cl^- sometimes results in a hypokalaemic hypochloraemic metabolic alkalosis. Once dehydration is corrected and effective circulation is restored, the kidneys generally re-establish homeostasis. However, electrolyte values should be monitored carefully during the perioperative and immediate postoperative period.

Technical considerations

* The stomach cannot usually be exteriorized from the abdomen and there is a risk of contamination of the abdominal cavity with spilled ingesta.
* Visualization of the stomach requires an abdominal incision of adequate length that should extend from the xiphoid process of the sternum to a point caudal to the umbilicus. This may require a parapreputial skin incision in the male dog.
* Excision of the falciform ligament facilitates visualization of the stomach, especially in overweight and deep-chested dogs.
* Use of Balfour retractors maximizes exposure of the stomach (see Chapter 2). In smaller dogs and cats large Gelpi retractors can be used as a substitute.

PRACTICAL TIP

Stay sutures should be placed in the stomach wall to elevate it out of the laparotomy incision before a gastrotomy incision is made. Gastrointestinal forceps, such as Babcock forceps, can also be used for this purpose

Laparotomy swabs (sponges) are essential absorbent barriers to contamination. The swabs should be moistened with saline prior to application to reduce the degree of gastric serosal abrasion. Even with a clean procedure, intra-abdominal contamination should be assumed. Therefore, liberal lavage of the abdominal cavity with sterile 0.9% saline or Hartmann's solution, at 37–39°C, should be performed prior to closure. As a rule of thumb, a minimum of 1 litre should be used in a medium-sized dog and 500 ml in a cat. Several litres should be used in large and giant-breed dogs. The fluid should be suctioned from the abdominal cavity, because residual blood, exudates or irrigation fluid may interfere with clearance of microorganisms and debris.

PRACTICAL TIP

Most gastric surgical procedures are clean–contaminated or contaminated. Gloves should be changed prior to closure and uncontaminated instruments should be used for abdominal closure to avoid the inadvertent introduction of gastric contents into the abdomen

Unless gastric spillage has occurred during the procedure, perioperative antibiotics are not usually necessary with gastric procedures because the bacterial flora population in the stomach is inherently quite low.

Closure

The large luminal diameter, abundant blood supply and rapid healing of the stomach provide many different options for gastric closure.

- The *lag* or *reparative* phase lasts from day 1 to day 3. During this time, the wound is held together by sutures.
- The *proliferative* phase of rapid fibroplasia occurs from day 3 to day 14 and wound strength accelerates greatly, reaching about 80% of normal.
- Lastly, the *maturation* phase takes place from day 14, during which time the stomach increases in wound strength to 90% of normal bursting strength.

Therefore the risk of leakage is usually greatest in the first 72–96 hours postoperatively.

> **PRACTICAL TIP**
>
> The submucosa is the layer of greatest vascularity, collagen content and tensile strength. It must be included in at least one of the two layers of closure

Engaging the submucosa and mucosa with a Cushing or Connell continuous inverting pattern in the first layer will generally ensure adequate healing of the stomach. It is permissible for the suture material to enter the lumen of the stomach. The second layer should engage the serosa, muscularis and submucosa. Most textbooks recommend a continuous Cushing or Lembert pattern for the second layer but this author prefers a simple continuous approximating pattern, since less tissue is inverted.

> **Editors' note:**
>
> An alternative method of gastric closure consists of a simple continuous approximating pattern for the first layer, followed by a continuous Cushing or Lembert or approximating pattern for the second layer

Suture materials and needles

Many suture materials have been used successfully to close the stomach. The synthetic monofilament absorbable suture materials are preferable. They have little tissue drag and reasonably good knot security, and do not collect particulate food matter. Monofilament absorbable suture materials, such as poliglecaprone 25, polydioxanone, polyglyconate and glycomer 631, all have the advantage of a tensile strength half-life that lasts into the proliferative phase of healing. They are also resistant to dissolution by gastric juices. Braided suture materials, such as polyglactin 910, lactomer 9–1 and polyglycolic acid, have the disadvantage of tissue drag and also allow particulate matter to lodge within the interstices of the suture material.

In terms of needle selection, a tapered needle or taper-point needle is more suitable for closure than a cutting needle, which might lacerate the muscularis or submucosa during passage through those tissues.

> **WARNING**
>
> Chromic catgut must be avoided for gastric closure because it loses tensile strength rapidly when exposed to gastric acid

Staples

Thoracoabdominal (TA) and *gastrointestinal anastomosis (GIA) auto staplers* apply two rows of overlapping titanium or stainless steel staples that safeguard against leakage and allow for rapid resection of gastric tissue. Although these auto staplers cause eversion of the wound edge, they provide good protection against leakage. Stapler cartridges come in various lengths and staple sizes to accommodate varying tissue thickness (see Chapter 2). Auto staplers also offer the advantage of being able to overlap two staple lines if one cartridge is too short. The end-to-end anastomosis (EEA) stapling system can be used to perform a gastroduodenostomy (Billroth I procedure).

Gastrotomy

Gastric foreign bodies

The most common reason for performing gastrotomy is to remove gastric foreign bodies. Common gastric foreign bodies seen in dogs include bones, chew toys, corn cobs, fabric clothing, sticks and cellophane wrappers. Linear foreign bodies, such as fishing line, yarn, tinsel or string meat-wrappings, are more common in cats, but hairballs (trichobezoars) may also be seen (Figure 5.2). Linear foreign bodies pass down into the small intestine, resulting in 'plication' of the small bowel (see Chapter 7), although the proximal anchor point is often located in the stomach.

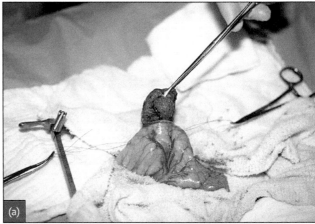
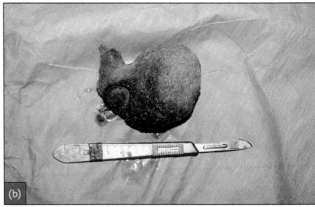

5.2 Gastrotomy for removal of a hairball in a cat. (a) Stay sutures are used to elevate the stomach out of the abdomen, and the stomach is packed off using laparotomy swabs. Allis tissue forceps are used to retrieve the foreign body. (b) The hairball assumes the shape of the gastric lining.

Sharp foreign bodies such as nails, straight pins and bones will often pass spontaneously through the entire intestinal tract without causing perforation. In such cases the animal should be fed a high-fibre diet and carefully monitored for the onset of vomiting, abdominal tenderness or fever. Radiographs should be repeated daily to ensure that aboral passage has occurred. Complete passage usually takes 3–4 days. Radiolucent objects, such as cellophane wrappers, often require administration of iodinated contrast medium to be visualized adequately. In cases that are difficult to diagnose, injecting air into the stomach lumen after contrast administration may help to delineate the object.

Flexible endoscopes have become invaluable in diagnosing gastric foreign bodies, ulceration and neoplasms that are not apparent radiographically. Endoscopes are often useful for removing smaller foreign bodies, such as coins, which may be retrieved with basket forceps. Rubber balls, bones or abrasive foreign bodies such as corn cobs cannot usually be removed in this manner. With linear foreign bodies such as string, exploratory surgery and gastrotomy should be performed quickly because the proximal anchor point must be released or plication and perforation of the intestine may occur. Tights or stockings also tend to lodge distally in the duodenum, making gastrotomy necessary.

Surgical technique

1. A cranial abdominal incision is made from the xiphoid to the umbilicus.
2. The stomach is mobilized with either stay sutures or Babcock intestinal forceps.
3. Moistened laparotomy swabs are placed around the stomach to prevent spillage.
4. The gastrotomy is made with a No. 10, 15 or 11 blade and extended with Metzenbaum scissors.
5. Retrieval of foreign bodies is done with swab-holding forceps (e.g. Rampley's) or Allis tissue forceps.
6. Gastric closure is performed in two layers (see Operative Technique 5.1).

Gastric biopsy

The differential diagnoses for any vomiting dog or cat include gastritis, foreign bodies, ulcers and inflammatory processes such as lymphocytic–plasmacytic or eosinophilic gastritis, chronic hypertrophic gastropathy, fungal granulomas and neoplasia. Most of these gastric conditions can be diagnosed via endoscopic biopsy. However, many lesions, such as leiomyoma, leiomyosarcoma and gastric carcinoma, do not fully extend into the lumen of the stomach and therefore require full-thickness biopsy (see Operative Technique 5.2).

Partial gastrectomy

Indications

Partial gastrectomy of the gastric fundus is indicated to resect areas of gastric necrosis secondary to gastric dilatation and volvulus (GDV) (Figure 5.3; see also Chapter 6), or to remove neoplasms involving the body or fundus. Determination of devitalized areas in cases of GDV is done

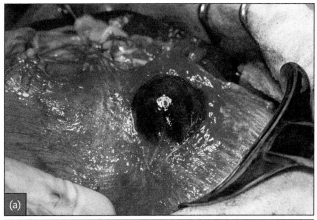
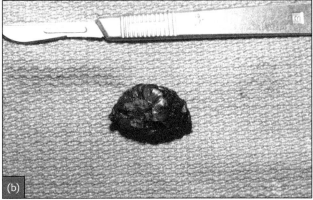

5.3 (a) Intraoperative view of a 4-year-old Chinese Shar Pei who underwent gastric decompression for gastric dilatation and volvulus 12 hours earlier. Note the circular area of gastric necrosis protruding from the gastric fundus. (b) A partial gastrectomy was performed and the excised tissue is shown.

visually and via palpation of the tissue. Black, grey or green tissue is usually non-viable and feels thin on palpation, whereas viable tissue may be discoloured but still has good thickness upon palpation.

Surgical considerations

Partial gastrectomy involves ligation of branches of the left gastroepiploic arteries and veins, allowing areas along the greater curvature of the stomach to be resected. The stomach is resected back to areas of healthy tissue with good bleeding. Spillage is prevented through the use of Doyen intestinal forceps and packing with laparotomy swabs. After resection is complete, the stomach is closed in two layers (see Operative Technique 5.3).

Alternatively, surgical stapling allows for rapid gastrectomy with minimum risk of spillage. The TA55 or TA90 auto stapler (see Chapter 2) is used with the green (4.8 mm) or blue (3.5 mm) staple cartridge. Often several end-to-end staple lines have to be placed, because each staple line is at most 9 cm in length (for the TA90; the TA55 has a staple line of 5.5 cm). The staple lines need to be overlapped by a few millimetres to prevent leakage between the staples. The 60 mm GIA instrument can also be used for the same purpose. This instrument fires four rows of staples and then transects between the middle two rows. The stomach and the resected tissue are then both sealed, thus preventing spillage of gastric ingesta.

Following gastric resection the abdomen is thoroughly lavaged with saline. An omental patch can be sutured on to the suture line in order to assist in wound healing.

Pyloroplasty

Indications, diagnosis and techniques

Pyloric stenosis due to mucosal hypertrophy is usually seen in toy breeds of dog and results in chronic hypertrophic gastropathy. Pyloric stenosis may also result from mast cell tumours, which secrete histamine, and from pancreatic gastrinomas causing excessive secretion of gastrin (Zollinger–Ellison syndrome). This hormone not only causes thickening of the gastric muscularis but also lowers intragastric pH, causing mucosal hyperplasia.

Other causes of pyloric stenosis include neoplasia, hepatic or pancreatic abscesses, inflammatory lesions (histoplasmosis and phycomycosis, both seen in the USA) and gastroduodenal ulcers. These latter conditions must be dealt with by gastrotomy, gastrectomy or abscess drainage.

Diagnosis of pyloric stenosis is often made with contrast radiography. Liquid contrast medium is a poor indicator of gastric emptying time, but filling defects can sometimes be seen. Fluoroscopy is often useful for assessing gastric motility and demonstrating a filling defect at the pylorus. Endoscopy is often the easiest way to diagnose pyloric stenosis due to gastric mucosal hypertrophy (Figure 5.4) or a polyp.

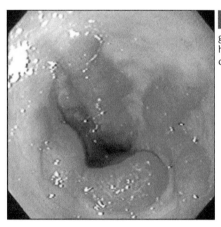

5.4 Endoscopic view of gastric mucosal hyperplasia in the area of a dog's pylorus.

> **PRACTICAL TIP**
>
> The intraluminal presence of gastric contrast medium for more than 12–24 hours is usually considered a sign of gastric retention

Surgical considerations

For all pyloric procedures a cranial midline laparotomy is made, a Balfour abdominal retractor is placed and the hepatogastric ligament is incised (Figure 5.5) to allow better mobility of the pylorus. Stay sutures or Babcock forceps are used to provide traction and elevate the pylorus into the surgical field. Moistened laparotomy swabs are placed around the pylorus to guard against spillage.

The *Heineke–Mikulicz transverse pyloroplasty* and *Y–U antral advancement flap* techniques allow access to the lumen, which is needed to resect mucosal lesions. They are slightly more time-consuming to perform than the *Fredet–Ramstedt pyloromyotomy* and carry the risk of postoperative leakage. Occasionally, pyloric mucosal hypertrophy goes 360 degrees around the perimeter of the pylorus and a full-thickness pyloric resection is indicated (see Billroth I procedure). The relative efficacy of one technique over the other in increasing gastric outflow has not been determined.

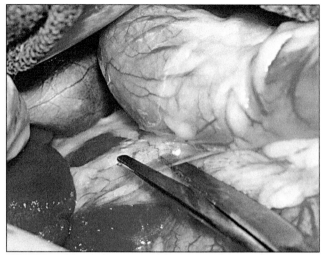

5.5 Incising the hepatogastric ligament with Metzenbaum scissors increases mobility of the pylorus prior to performing any of the pyloric procedures. Care should be taken to avoid the common bile duct when incising the ligament.

Heineke–Mikulicz transverse pyloroplasty with submucosal resection

If the lesion is intraluminal an open pyloroplasty procedure is indicated. With a transverse pyloroplasty, the incision is made in a location similar to that for a pyloromyotomy and for a length of 3–4 cm, depending on the size of the animal. It is usually easiest to make a stab incision into the duodenal lumen and to extend the incision with Metzenbaum scissors by cutting through the pyloric sphincter into the antrum (Figure 5.6a). Closure is somewhat difficult, because the gastric and duodenal mucosae tend to evert. When this occurs it is often best to use an interrupted Gambee-type suture pattern. The needle is passed full thickness into the lumen and then reversed to pick up the submucosa on the way out. The suture is tied down with gentle tissue apposition without crushing the tissue. The first suture is placed at the proximal and distal margins of the longitudinal incision and then sutures are placed every 3–4 mm on either side until closure is complete (Figure 5.6b). The main disadvantage of the transverse pyloroplasty is that 'dog ears' tend to occur at the cranial and caudal wound edges (see Operative Technique 5.4).

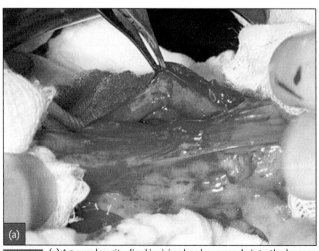

(a)

5.6 (a) A 3 mm longitudinal incision has been made into the lumen of the pylorus. (continues) ▶

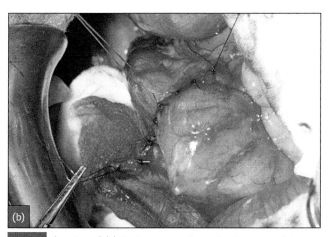

5.6 (continued) (b) The transverse closure has been completed.

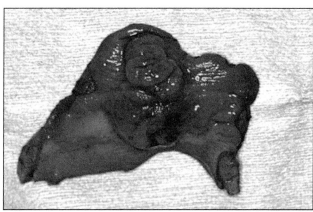

5.8 Intraoperative photograph of a resected hypertrophic mucosal lesion removed during pyloroplasty.

Pyloric submucosal resection

It is often necessary to remove hyperplastic mucosal lesions from the pylorus during either the Heineke–Mikulicz pyloroplasty or the Y–U procedure. With either technique, the hyperplastic mucosa can be undermined and excised using Metzenbaum scissors (Figure 5.7a). The resultant wound bed can then be closed with a simple continuous or Cushing pattern of 2 metric (3/0 USP) poliglecaprone, polydioxanone or glycomer 631, which is used to approximate the edges of the mucosal and submucosal layers (Figure 5.7b). The pyloroplasty incision is then closed as previously described. The excised mucosa should be submitted for histopathology (Figure 5.8).

Y–U antral advancement flap

The Y–U antral advancement flap, also known as the Y–U pyloroplasty or the U–U pyloroplasty, is a useful technique for the excision of large pyloric mucosal lesions as well as for relief of severe pyloric stenosis. A Y-shaped incision is created at the pylorus (Figure 5.9a). The gastric antrum is advanced to fill the defect and sutured in a U-shaped configuration (Figure 5.9b; see Operative Technique 5.5). The technique also allows for the resection of hyperplastic mucosa. The end result is to increase the diameter of the pyloric lumen by transposing the larger diameter antrum over the smaller diameter duodenum.

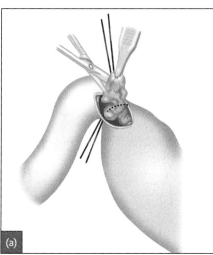

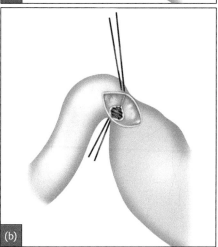

5.7 (a) The hyperplastic mucosa is incised, undermined and resected using Metzenbaum scissors. (b) The open bed is closed by re-opposing mucosa and submucosa with a simple continuous or Cushing pattern.

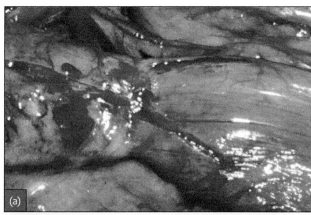

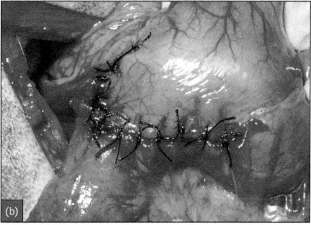

5.9 (a) The pylorus has been scored with a surgical blade, showing the tail of the Y towards the duodenum and the arms towards the stomach. (b) Finished U-shaped configuration, which widens the pyloric outflow tract.
(Courtesy of R M Bright)

Pyloromyotomy (Fredet–Ramstedt procedure)

Congenital pyloric stenosis secondary to muscular hypertrophy is a rarely reported condition in brachycephalic breeds of dog, especially the Boxer, and also in the Siamese cat. The muscular coat of the stomach comprises two muscle layers: an outer longitudinal and an inner circular layer. At the pylorus the circular muscle layer is several times thicker than the outer longitudinal layer. This circular muscle 'sphincter' is continuous with that of the antrum but is completely separated from that of the duodenum by a thin fibrous septum. The pylorus functions both as a sphincter and as an anti-reflux organ. In all cases of pyloric muscle hypertrophy, it is the circular muscle layer that becomes affected. With the pyloromyotomy procedure this muscle is transected, leading to relaxation of the stenosis. When all the muscle bands have been severed, the submucosa and mucosa will bulge out between the seromuscular layers (Figure 5.10; see Operative Technique 5.6).

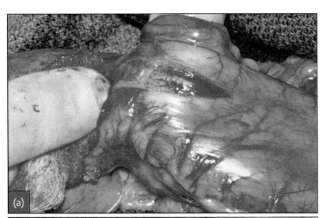

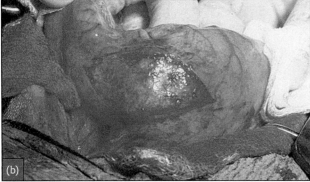

5.10 (a) The pylorus is incised through the outer longitudinal and (b) inner circular musculature to allow protrusion of the submucosa.

The advantage of the pyloromyotomy technique is that it is safe, easy and rapid to perform. The gastroduodenal lumen is not entered and so there is no risk of gastric leakage and peritonitis. The disadvantage is that the mucosa is not examined. There are also reports that the pyloric myotomy incision may heal after a few weeks, resulting in recurrent stenosis.

> **WARNING**
>
> Pyloric stenosis due to hypertrophy of the circular muscle sphincter is much less common than stenosis caused by mucosal hypertrophy

Gastric neoplasia and ulceration of the outflow tract

Severe outflow obstruction requiring gastropyloric resection may be caused by neoplasia, infiltrative lesions or fungal granulomas (USA), or may result from gastroduodenal ulcers. Although rare, fungal granulomas due to histoplasmosis, cryptococcosis or phycomycosis may require a combination of surgery and antifungal therapy.

Gastric neoplasia

The most common benign neoplasms of the canine stomach are adenomatous polyps and leiomyomas. Benign adenomatous polyps are also common in cats.

- *Polyps* occur as pedunculated or polypoid nodules of mucosal origin that protrude from the gastric surface. They range from a few millimetres to a few centimetres in size and usually occur as single masses or as several solitary nodules. *Benign adenomatous polyps* often occur at the gastroduodenal junction in older cats. These lesions can be removed in most cases via submucosal resection, with good results.
- *Leiomyomas* are the second most common canine gastric tumour after gastric adenocarcinoma and are usually seen in aged dogs. They arise from the smooth muscle wall and vary in size and shape but are often polypoid in appearance.

Most benign adenomatous polyps and gastric leiomyomas (Figure 5.11) do not cause overt clinical signs and are found incidentally at necropsy. Occasionally, they will be located adjacent to the pylorus and result in signs consistent with pyloric obstruction. In these cases surgical excision may be required.

- *Gastric adenocarcinoma* is the most common canine gastric malignancy. The mean age at presentation is 8 years, and males are afflicted more often than females. These tumours are most commonly located in the pyloric antrum and appear grossly as raised plaques

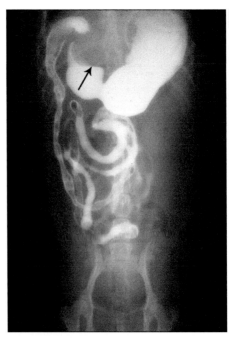

5.11 Contrast study of a 13-year-old Beagle with a golf ball-sized filling defect located at the pylorus (arrowed). This was caused by a leiomyoma, which was successfully removed surgically.

with central ulcers or as diffuse infiltrating masses, which impair distension of the stomach. They are seen less frequently in cats.

* *Lymphosarcoma* (LSA) is the most common feline gastric tumour. These tumours can occur either as raised nodular masses or as diffuse infiltrations of the gastric wall. Gastric ulceration is sometimes present. The majority of cats with gastric LSA are feline leukaemia virus (FeLV) negative.
* *Leiomyosarcomas* and *fibrosarcomas* are two less frequently seen tumours of the stomach in the dog and cat. The *c-kit* gene was first identified as the cellular homologue of the feline sarcoma oncogene *v-kit*. Mutations of this gene are thought to be associated with gastrointestinal stromal tumours and mast cell tumours.

Given that the majority of gastric malignancies have metastasized at the time of surgery, the role of surgery in cases of gastric neoplasia is often to perform a biopsy of the lesion and regional lymph node in order to confirm the diagnosis. The treatment of choice for gastric neoplasia without evidence of metastatic disease is partial gastrectomy or segmental resection of the stomach. Since most malignant neoplasms involve the pylorus and antral area, resection of both areas is often required.

Dogs with adenocarcinoma, leiomyosarcoma or LSA treated with antrectomy, pylorectomy and Billroth I or Billroth II procedures often have a poor prognosis, with short survival times ranging from only 17 days for LSA to 9 weeks for gastric carcinoma. Cats with gastric lymphoma have a variable prognosis, with intermediate- and high-grade types having short survival times but those with low-grade small cell types having median survival times of up to 100 weeks.

Gastric ulceration and perforation

Gastroduodenal ulceration in dogs often occurs secondary to diseases such as chronic renal failure, liver disease, mast cell tumours and gastrin-secreting tumours. More commonly, ulcers may be drug induced with combination non-steroidal anti-Inflammatory drug (NSAID) and glucocorticoid therapy. NSAIDs inhibit cyclooxygenase (COX) activity and subsequent prostaglandin E production, which leads to reduced mucosal blood flow, mucus production, bicarbonate production and epithelial turnover rate. Glucocorticoids are also thought to reduce mucus production and cell turnover rate and thus increase the risk of gastric haemorrhage. COX-2 inhibiting agents do not spare dogs from either ulceration or perforation. Treatment of dogs with meloxicam and dexamethasone in combination results in a much higher rate of pyloric ulceration than with either drug alone. The spiral bacterium *Helicobacter* may also play a role. Although a normal inhabitant of the stomach, it has been implicated as possibly leading to lymphocytic–plasmacytic infiltration and ulceration, and as a cause of spontaneous gastric perforation.

Clinical signs of ulceration *versus* perforation

Anorexia and vomiting are commonly reported in animals with gastric ulceration. There is often digested blood with a 'coffee ground appearance' present in the vomitus. While signs of gastric ulceration in dogs and cats may be periodic and vague, once perforation occurs they become severe, with 90–100% of cases showing signs of progressive lethargy, anorexia, vomiting and weight loss. Acute abdominal discomfort consistent with peritonitis eventually ensues.

Diagnosis of ulceration *versus* perforation

Animals with gastric ulceration may merely have evidence of anaemia and elevated blood urea nitrogen due to the digestion of blood. Dogs and cats with perforation also typically have an elevated white blood cell count, hypoproteinaemia and hypocalcaemia. Definitive diagnosis of gastric ulceration usually requires gastric endoscopy; however, this method has low sensitivity for distinguishing between ulceration alone and ulceration with perforation. Pyloric thickening may be detectable on abdominal ultrasonography but this also may not distinguish between the two conditions. Abdominal radiographs are often unremarkable with ulceration alone but the presence of pneumoperitoneum is highly suggestive of gastric perforation.

Medical management of ulceration

Gastric ulcers are initially managed medically unless perforation has occurred. Histamine (H2) receptor antagonists such as ranitidine and famotidine, proton pump antagonists such as omeprazole and pantoprazole, and oral binding agents such sulphated disaccharide–aluminium hydroxide complex (sucralfate) have all been successfully used for the medical treatment of ulcers in small animals (see the *BSAVA Manual of Canine and Feline Gastroenterology*).

Surgical management of ulceration and perforation

Surgical management of gastric ulceration is indicated when medical therapy is ineffective or in certain cases of intractable bleeding with or without gastric perforation. With small peripherally located ulcers, elliptical incisions around the ulcer can be made and primary closure performed. Frequently ulcers are more extensive, requiring pylorectomy with gastroduodenostomy. Duodenal ulcers commonly interfere with the openings of the common bile duct, requiring cholecystoduodenostomy in combination with partial gastric resection.

> **WARNING**
>
> Gastropyloric gastrectomy techniques are technically difficult to perform and have numerous complications associated with them, such as gastric dumping syndrome, marginal ulceration developing at the anastomosis site, and ascending cholecystitis. Once gastric resection has been performed, the surgeon may consider placement of a jejunostomy tube in order to bypass the surgical site and provide enteral alimentation

Pylorectomy and gastroduodenostomy

Pylorectomy and gastroduodenostomy (Billroth I procedure; see Operative Technique 5.7) is indicated for management of gastric neoplasms, granulomas, 360-degree mucosal hyperplasia and severe gastroduodenal ulceration. A complete pylorectomy is performed and the duodenum is anastomosed to the remaining gastric stump. In cases of neoplasia, 1–2 cm of normal tissue should be removed with the tumour and the margins should be evaluated on histopathology. If the common bile duct is involved, a chole-cystoduodenostomy may be necessary (see Chapter 9). After ligation of the appropriate vessels, Doyen intestinal forceps are placed and the diseased tissues are resected. The gastric stump is oversewn until the opening of the stomach is equal in diameter to the duodenal lumen. The duodenum is then anastomosed to the stomach with 2 metric (3/0 USP) monofilament suture material using an interrupted suture pattern.

Gastrojejunostomy

Wide resection of the gastric outflow tract for neoplasia often precludes closure via gastroduodenostomy. Gastrojejunostomy (Billroth II procedure) may be performed, with or without the creation of a blind duodenal loop (Roux-en-Y procedure). The Billroth II technique is usually performed for resection of gastric adenocarcinoma. This disease carries a grave prognosis and surgery should be considered palliative and never curative. Additionally, owners should be warned of the very high incidence of postoperative complications (see later). Chemotherapy has not been very effective with respect to increasing longevity. Conversely, chemotherapy (vincristine, cyclophosphamide and prednisolone in combination) has been effective in treating LSA in cats after surgical removal of the mass(es). The Billroth II procedure is associated with significantly more complications than the Billroth I procedure.

> **WARNING**
>
> The Billroth II technique is a very technically demanding procedure with many postoperative complications. It requires a surgical assistant and is best performed with some specialized equipment available. The surgical approach, instruments and postoperative care are similar to those discussed for the Billroth I technique (Operative Technique 5.7)

Postoperative considerations after gastric and pyloric surgery

Selection of analgesia

Most of the opioids reduce gastric emptying, and drugs such as morphine or hydromorphone have a tendency to induce postoperative vomiting. Drugs less likely to induce emesis, such as methadone, oxymorphone, butorphanol, buprenorphine or fentanyl, are good alternatives for postoperative analgesia.

NSAIDs must be used with care after gastric surgery, because their antiprostaglandin effects adversely affect gastromucosal circulation and may predispose to ulceration. Other alternatives for postoperative analgesia include epidural morphine or an intravenous continuous rate infusion (CRI) of lidocaine (30–50 µg/kg/min). Both of these regimens have little negative effect on gastrointestinal motility, though CRI lidocaine can reduce appetite.

Restoration of motility

Restoration of normal gastrointestinal motility often enhances postoperative patient outcome and shortens hospitalization. General anaesthesia, incision through the peritoneum and handling of the gastrointestinal tract reduce the normal peristaltic activity of the stomach and intestine, thereby resulting in postoperative ileus. Early postoperative feeding is recommended because it has a positive role in restoring gastrointestinal motility and early return to function. Drugs that increase gastric motility include metoclopramide, erythromycin and cisapride. Of these, cisapride and erythromycin are more effective. Although cisapride was withdrawn from the human market because of the induction of fatal cardiac arrhythmias, these effects have not been reported in dog or cats, and cisapride is now readily available from compounding pharmacies. Metoclopramide has a powerful antiemetic property and works well clinically. The H2 blocker ranitidine also increases motility. It is prudent to assess potassium levels and to supplement intravenous fluids if hypokalaemia is present. In cases of refractory gastric atony, a nasogastric tube is an effective method of providing either intermittent or continuous decompression of the stomach.

Treatment of emesis

Emesis is a common postoperative occurrence with all types of gastropyloric surgery, especially with procedures involving the gastric outflow tract. Postoperative gastritis and/or oesophagitis secondary to reflux are common, and medical treatment with H2 blockers is often warranted. Of the commonly used H2 blockers, famotidine is available as an injectable preparation or, alternatively, can be used once daily as an oral preparation. Ranitidine, on the other hand, possesses more promotility activity but must be given orally twice daily. The centrally acting antiemetic maropitant citrate is also a very useful drug. Maropitant is a neurokinin (NK1) receptor antagonist that blocks the pharmacological action of substance P in the central nervous system (CNS). This drug can be given at a dose of 1 mg/kg s.c. q24h for up to 5 days. An oral formulation is also available, dosed at 2 mg/kg q24h.

Feeding

Sporadic vomiting is often seen during the first 24–72 hours following pyloric surgery, usually due to gastric atony or reflux of bile into the stomach. The vomit is often tinged with bile or blood. The patient is usually allowed to lick ice chips and eat small amounts of low-fat gruel from 12 hours after surgery. Small amounts of food (e.g. meatballs or gruel) are offered thereafter. The volume of food is gradually increased and feeding intervals are lengthened over a period of 7–10 days. Most animals can be safely released from the hospital within 48–72 hours after surgery.

> **PRACTICAL TIP**
>
> Consideration should be given to placement of a feeding tube in animals that were anorexic before surgery or are anticipated to have prolonged anorexia postoperatively

A serious potential complication with all types of pyloric surgery is the development of pancreatitis, and this should be suspected in animals with persistent postoperative vomiting and abdominal pain (see Chapter 11 and the *BSAVA Manual of Canine and Feline Gastroenterology*).

Clinical syndromes following antrectomy

Almost all patients vomit periodically following antrectomy. Postoperatively this may be due to something as simple as gastritis caused by bile reflux, or from the development of pancreatitis, or it might originate from suture-line dehiscence and leakage with associated peritonitis. There are also several long-term pathophysiological complications that occur after antrectomy in dogs and cats.

- *Chronic vomiting* is reportedly more common in animals undergoing a Billroth II procedure, especially if the stoma length exceeds 3 cm, and may be due to reflux gastritis, marginal (anastomotic) ulcers or gastric dumping syndrome.
- *Alkaline reflux gastritis* results from reflux of bile into the gastric remnant. In small animals this can often be managed with prokinetic agents and H2 blockers. (In humans, unrelenting alkaline reflux gastritis is usually managed surgically with a Roux-en-Y procedure, creating a blind duodenal loop which diverts bile away from the stomach.)
- *Marginal (anastomotic) ulcer* development is more common after gastrojejunostomy (Billroth II procedure) and may lead to melaena and chronic vomiting. Ulcers may develop either because the protective mucus-secreting cells in the antrum have been removed or because the remaining antral gastrin-secreting cells are bathed in alkaline media, increasing the secretion of gastrin, which lowers the pH at the anastomotic site.
- *Gastric dumping syndrome* results from the sudden emptying of the hyperosmolar gastric contents into the duodenum and jejunum. Clinical signs including postprandial vomiting, diarrhoea, syncope and pallor may be seen. Weight loss, anaemia and malnutrition may ultimately result.
- *Afferent loop syndrome*, either acute or chronic, may result after Billroth II techniques when accumulation of bile and pancreatic juice in the blind loop causes abdominal discomfort, nausea and bilious vomiting. The affected limb can also rupture, causing peritonitis. Creation of an afferent limb that is as short as possible may prevent this problem from occurring.

Oesophageal hiatal hernia

Hiatal hernias (HHs) are occasionally reported in the dog and cat. The hernias are thought to be congenital in most cases but they also can be acquired. Occasionally, a paraoesophageal HH (rolling or fixed HH) is seen, but the sliding variety (axial HH) is more common (Figure 5.12). The Chinese Shar Pei and English Bulldog are predisposed to sliding hernias. The cardio-oesophageal junction and part of the stomach may slide up into the thoracic cavity. Reflux oesophagitis is usually associated with HH. Regurgitation of mucus (sometimes blood-tinged), hypersalivation, dysphagia and weight loss are prominent clinical signs.

Diagnosis of HH is usually made on survey or contrast radiography (Figure 5.13) and endoscopy. The presence of the gastric shadow cranial to the diaphragm suggests HH. With contrast radiography, gastric rugae may be identified. A dilated caudal mediastinal oesophagus with mucosal erosions indicates reflux oesophagitis. Oesophagitis can

be verified with oesophagoscopy. The endoscope can also be reversed to look at the gastro-oesophageal junction and a large diaphragmatic hiatus may be noted. Fluoroscopy may be necessary to diagnose hernias that undergo spontaneous reduction.

Medical management for HH includes mucosal protectants, such as sucralfate, as well as H2 blocking agents. Since medical therapy is usually only palliative, surgical correction is often necessary. Surgical management of HH

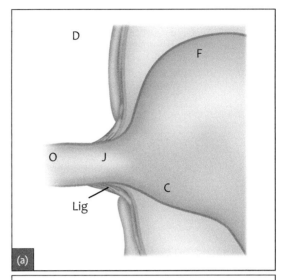

(a)

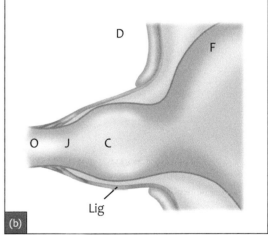

(b)

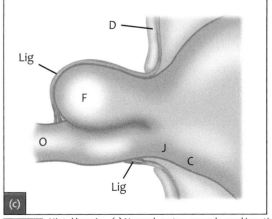

(c)

5.12 Hiatal hernias. (a) Normal gastro-oesophageal junction. (b) Axial or sliding hiatal hernia; the junction slides into the thorax. (c) Paraoesophageal or rolling hiatal hernia; the junction remains fixed at the diaphragm but the cardia rolls into the thorax. C = cardia; D = diaphragm; F = fundus; J = gastro-oesophageal junction; Lig = phrenico-oesophageal ligament; O = oesophagus.

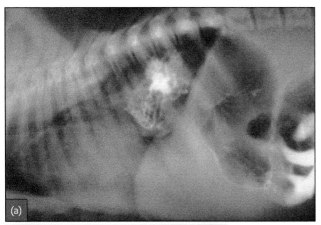

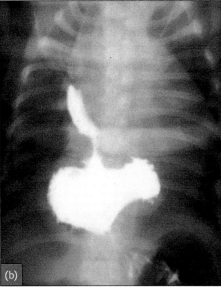

5.13 (a) Lateral and (b) ventrodorsal radiographs of a 9-month-old Shar Pei with a paraoesophageal hiatal hernia. Note the large soft tissue opacity cranial to the diaphragm and dorsal to the vena cava.

entails surgical reduction of the oesophageal hiatus, pexy of the cardia of the stomach to the diaphragm and a left-sided tube or incisional gastropexy to place caudal traction on the stomach and reduce the chances of re-herniation (see Operative Technique 5.8). However, even with correction of HH up to 50% of patients may experience continued regurgitation.

References and further reading

Bellenger CR, Maddison JE, MacPherson GC and Ilkiw JE (1990) Chronic hypertrophic pyloric gastropathy in 14 dogs. *Australian Veterinary Journal* **67**, 317–320

Bright RM, Richardson DC and Stanton ME (1988) Y-U antral advancement flap pyloroplasty in dogs. *Compendium on Continuing Education for the Practicing Veterinarian* **10**, 139–145

Brockman D and Holt D (2005) *BSAVA Manual of Canine and Feline Head, Neck and Thoracic Surgery*. BSAVA Publications, Gloucester

Clark GN (1994) Gastric surgery with surgical stapling instruments. *Veterinary Clinics of North America: Small Animal Practice* **24**, 279–303

Cornell K (2012) The stomach. In: *Veterinary Surgery Small Animal, 1st edn*, ed. KB Tobias, pp.1496–1498. Elsevier Saunders, St Louis

Dulisch ML (1998) Pyloromyotomy, pyloroplasty and pyloric resection. In: *Current Techniques in Small Animal Surgery, 4th edn*, ed. MJ Bojrab, pp.207–212. Williams and Wilkins, Baltimore

Ellison GW (2000) Gastric dilatation volvulus. *Compendium: Standards of Care: Emergency and Critical Care Medicine* **2**, 6–12

Hall E, Simpson J and Williams DA (2005) *BSAVA Manual of Canine and Feline Gastroenterology, 2nd edn*. BSAVA Publications, Gloucester

MacDonald JM, Mullen HS and Moroff SD (1993) Adenomatous polyps of the duodenum in cats: 18 cases (1985–1990). *Journal of the American Veterinary Medical Association* **202**, 647–651

Matthiesen DT (1987) Indications and techniques of partial gastrectomy in the dog. *Seminars in Veterinary Medicine and Surgery* **2**, 248–256

Matthiesen DT and Walter MC (1986) Surgical treatment of chronic hypertrophic pyloric gastropathy in 45 dogs. *Journal of the American Animal Hospital Association* **22**, 241–246

Papageorges M, Bonneau NH and Breton L (1987) Gastric drainage procedures: effects in normal dogs. Clinical observations and gastric emptying. *Veterinary Surgery* **16**, 332–340

Rasmussan L (2003) Stomach. In: *Textbook of Small Animal Surgery, 3rd edn*, ed. D Slatter, pp.592–635. WB Saunders, Philadelphia

Rimback G (1990) Treatment of postoperative paralytic ileus by intravenous lidocaine infusion. *Anesthesia and Analgesia* **70**, 414–419

Savvas I, Rallis D and Raptopoulis D (2009) The effect of pre-anaesthetic fasting time and type of food on gastric content volume and acidity in dogs. *Veterinary Anaesthesia and Analgesia* **36**, 539–546

Smith KR (1996) *Helicobacter* sp. infection in a dog in association with gastric perforation. *Australian Veterinary Practice* **26**, 140–143

Stanton ME and Bright RM (1989) Gastroduodenal ulceration in dogs. Retrospective study of 43 cases and literature review. *Journal of Veterinary Internal Medicine* **3**, 238–244

Stanton ME, Bright RM, Toal R et al. (1987) Effects of the Y-U pyloroplasty on gastric emptying and duodenogastric reflux in the dog. *Veterinary Surgery* **16**, 392–397

Sullivan M, Lee R, Fisher EW, Nash AS and McCandlish IA (1987) A study of 31 cases of gastric carcinoma in dogs. *The Veterinary Record* **120**, 79–83

Walter MC, Matthiesen DT and Stone EA (1985) Pylorectomy and gastroduodenostomy in the dog: technique and clinical results in 28 cases. *Journal of the American Veterinary Medical Association* **187**, 909–914

Welsh JA and Henderson RA (1998) Surgery for gastric neoplasia. In: *Current Techniques in Small Animal Surgery, 4th edn*, ed. MJ Bojrab, pp.214–222. Williams and Wilkins, Baltimore

Wilson DV, Evan AT and Mauer WA (2006) Influence of metoclopramide on gastroesophageal reflux in anesthetized dogs. *American Journal of Veterinary Research* **67**, 26–31

OPERATIVE TECHNIQUE 5.1

Gastrotomy

POSITIONING

Dorsal recumbency with all four limbs secured.

ASSISTANT

Recommended to prevent spillage.

EQUIPMENT EXTRAS

Self-retaining abdominal retractors; swab-holding forceps or Allis tissue forceps for foreign body retrieval; suction; Babcock forceps (optional).

SURGICAL TECHNIQUE

Approach

A routine ventral midline incision is performed from the xiphoid process to caudal to the umbilicus. Moistened laparotomy swabs are placed over the incision and Balfour abdominal retractors are applied.

Surgical manipulations

1   Inspect and palpate the stomach and place either sutures or Babcock forceps 10 cm apart on the ventral surface. Pack off the area with laparotomy swabs.

2   Locate the gastrotomy incision in the ventral aspect of the stomach between the greater and lesser curvatures at its most avascular point. Make a stab incision with either a No. 10 or 11 scalpel blade into the lumen of the stomach and extend it 5–7 cm with Metzenbaum scissors.

3   Use stay sutures to open the gastric lumen for foreign body removal.

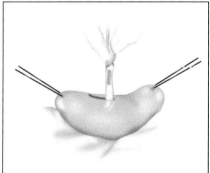 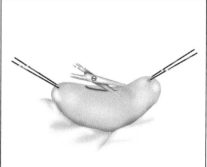 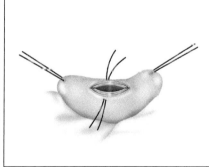

Stab incision.　　　　Extending the incision.　　　　Stay sutures to open the lumen.

PRACTICAL TIP

Once a gastric foreign body has been removed, the stomach should be suctioned and gently palpated to ensure that no additional foreign material remains

PRACTICAL TIP

Stay sutures or Babcock forceps can be used to retract the wound edge for better visualization of the lumen. The fingers are kept out of the gastric lumen if possible. Foreign bodies can be removed using swab-holding forceps or Allis tissue forceps

→ **OPERATIVE TECHNIQUE 5.1 CONTINUED**

Wound closure

Any instruments that were used inside the gastric lumen should be discarded. If any contamination with gastric contents has occurred, gloves should be changed.

* Monofilament absorbable materials such as poliglecaprone 25, polydioxanone, polyglyconate or glycomer 631 (3 metric (2/0 USP) for larger dogs; 2 metric (3/0 USP) for small dogs or cats) are used. Chromic catgut should not be used because it loses its tensile strength rapidly when exposed to gastric juices.
* Gastrotomy closure is performed in two layers, with the submucosa engaged in both layers:
  * The first layer consists of a continuous Cushing pattern, which primarily engages the submucosa and mucosa
  * The second layer is closed with either a continuous Cushing or continuous approximating pattern that engages the serosa muscularis and submucosa but does not enter the lumen.
* The body wall is closed routinely (see Chapter 4).

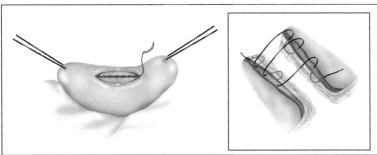

Closure of the first layer with a continuous Cushing pattern (inset).

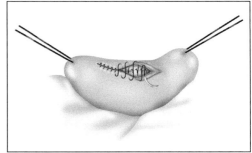

Closure of the second layer with a continuous Cushing or continuous approximating pattern.

POSTOPERATIVE MANAGEMENT

Dogs are usually fed small amounts of a low-fat gruel three to four times a day beginning 12 hours after gastrotomy and, if vomiting does not occur, are released from the hospital within 24 hours. Antibiotic therapy is not necessary unless spillage has occurred, but H2 blockers, such as ranitidine (2 mg/kg orally q12h) or famotidine (0.5 mg/kg orally q24h), can be prescribed.

OPERATIVE TECHNIQUE 5.2

Gastric biopsy

POSITIONING

Dorsal recumbency with all four limbs secured.

ASSISTANT

Often unnecessary.

EQUIPMENT EXTRAS

Self-retaining abdominal retractors; Babcock forceps (optional).

SURGICAL TECHNIQUE

Approach

A routine ventral midline incision is performed from the xiphoid process to cranial to the umbilicus. Moistened laparotomy swabs are placed over the incision and Balfour abdominal retractors are applied.

→ **OPERATIVE TECHNIQUE 5.2 CONTINUED**

Surgical manipulations

1 Inspect and palpate the stomach for the area to be biopsied.

2 Pack off the area with laparotomy swabs.

3 A 10 mm × 5 mm full-thickness biopsy can be performed with a No. 10 or 11 scalpel blade, or with Metzenbaum scissors.

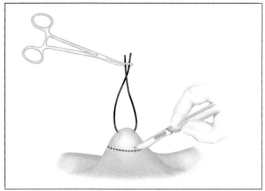

A gastric biopsy is performed by tenting the stomach wall with a stay suture. An elliptical sample 10 mm long by 5 mm wide is taken.

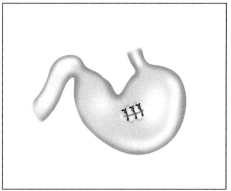

The gastric wall is closed with three simple interrupted sutures that engage the submucosa, the muscularis and the serosa.

PRACTICAL TIP
Alternatively a circular biopsy can be performed using a 6 mm skin biopsy punch

Wound closure

- Closure is made with two or three simple interrupted or Gambee sutures that engage the serosa, muscularis and submucosa. The mucosa should be pushed inwards during tying of the sutures and should not be allowed to evert between sutures.
- Monofilament absorbable materials such as poliglecaprone 25, polydioxanone, polyglyconate or glycomer 631 (3 metric (2/0 USP) for larger dogs; 2 metric (3/0 USP) for small dogs or cats) are used. Chromic catgut should not be used because it loses its tensile strength rapidly when exposed to gastric juices.
- Any instruments that were used inside the gastric lumen should be discarded. If any contamination with gastric contents has occurred, gloves should be changed.
- The body wall is closed routinely (see Chapter 4).

OPERATIVE TECHNIQUE 5.3

Partial gastrectomy of the gastric fundus

POSITIONING

Dorsal recumbency with all four limbs secured.

ASSISTANT

Required for retraction and to prevent spillage.

EQUIPMENT EXTRAS

Self-retaining abdominal retractors; Babcock forceps; Doyen bowel forceps; suction; TA or GIA auto stapling equipment, if available.

→ **OPERATIVE TECHNIQUE 5.3 CONTINUED**

Approach

A routine ventral midline incision is performed from the xiphoid process to just cranial to the pubis. Moistened laparotomy swabs are placed over the incision and Balfour abdominal retractors are applied. The approach for gastric resection is similar to that described for gastrotomy (see Operative Technique 5.1).

Surgical manipulations

1   Identify the area of gastric tumour, ischaemia or necrosis.

2   Ligate and divide corresponding vessels along the greater curvature. These include the left gastroepiploic vessels and sometimes some of the short gastric vessels. Apply Doyen bowel forceps to the stomach and excise the necrotic tissue.

3   Alternatively, resect the necrotic area using a TA55 or TA90 auto stapler. Apply Doyen bowel forceps to the devitalized tissue to prevent spillage during transection and removal.

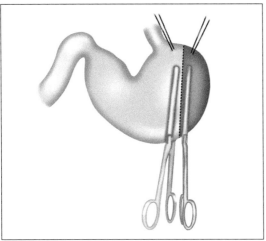

Identification of necrotic area.

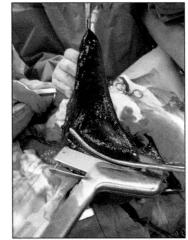

A TA90 stapling device is used to resect the necrotic portion of the stomach.

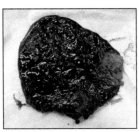

Resected portion of the stomach.

PRACTICAL TIP

If the area of necrosis is longer than a single staple line, a second line of staples can be added to overlap the first line

Wound closure

* The stomach is closed in two layers: the mucosa and submucosa are closed with an inverting continuous or interrupted suture pattern, and the seromuscular layer is closed with a simple interrupted pattern.
* Suture materials are similar to those described for gastrotomy (see Operative Technique 5.1).

PRACTICAL TIP

Placement of a gastrostomy tube (see Chapter 6) allows postoperative gastric decompression and is recommended following major gastric resection

→ **OPERATIVE TECHNIQUE 5.3 CONTINUED**

• The body wall is closed routinely (see Chapter 4).

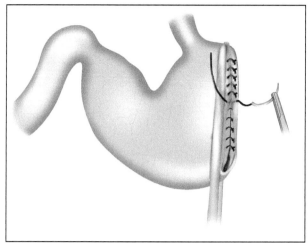

Closure.

POSTOPERATIVE MANAGEMENT

The animal is kept *nil per os* (NPO) for a period of 24 hours. Maintenance fluids should be given at a rate of 40–60 ml/kg per day. With GDV patients, a total body potassium deficit may exist because of the NPO status, vomiting, oral gastric intubation and removal of gastric secretions. Therefore, 20 mmol/l (20 mEq/l) of potassium chloride is usually added to each litre of fluids to help maintain total body potassium. Ideally, potassium levels should be monitored and the dose and rate of potassium tailored to the patient's needs. Hypokalaemia can also contribute to the development of cardiac arrhythmias and gastrointestinal ileus.

Antibiotic therapy is not necessary unless spillage has occurred but H2 blockers, such as ranitidine (2 mg/kg orally q12h) or famotidine (0.5 mg/kg orally q24h), are often prescribed to counteract gastritis. Promotility agents may also be considered.

OPERATIVE TECHNIQUE 5.4

Transverse pyloroplasty (Heineke–Mikulicz procedure)

POSITIONING

Dorsal recumbency with all four limbs secured.

ASSISTANT

Recommended to prevent spillage.

EQUIPMENT EXTRAS

Self-retaining abdominal retractors; Babcock forceps; suction.

SURGICAL TECHNIQUE

Approach

A routine ventral midline incision is performed from the xiphoid process to the umbilicus. Moistened laparotomy swabs are placed over the incision and Balfour abdominal retractors are applied.

→ **OPERATIVE TECHNIQUE 5.4 CONTINUED**

Surgical manipulations

1 Incise the hepatogastric ligament to mobilize the pylorus (see Figure 5.5).

2 Inspect and palpate the pylorus and place two stay sutures 10 cm apart, the first anchored in the duodenum and the second in the ventral surface of the stomach. Alternatively, use Babcock forceps instead of stay sutures.

3 Make a stab incision into the duodenal lumen and extend the incision with Metzenbaum scissors by cutting through the pyloric sphincter into the antrum. The incision is made in a location similar to that for a pyloromyotomy and for a length of 3–4 cm.

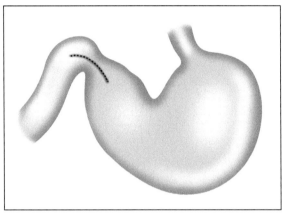

A 3–4 cm incision is centered over the pylorus and made into the lumen.

4 Evaluate the pyloric mucosa. The hyperplastic mucosa should be undermined and resected using Metzenbaum scissors. Any excised mucosa should be sent for histopathological evaluation (see Figure 5.7a).

5 The open bed is closed by re-opposing the mucosa with a simple continuous pattern (see Figure 5.7b).

Wound closure

1 Use a simple interrupted or Gambee suture pattern for the closure. Use synthetic monofilament absorbable suture materials, such as poliglecaprone 25, polydioxanone, polyglyconate or glycomer 631, in 3 metric (2/0 USP) for larger dogs and 2 metric (3/0 USP) for cats or small dogs. The first suture is placed in the centre of the wound.

2 Place the sutures every 3–4 mm on either side of the centre.

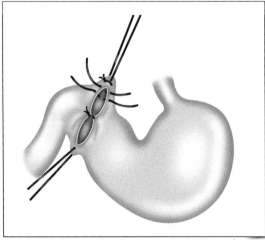

The wound edges are closed transversely using a simple interrupted pattern.

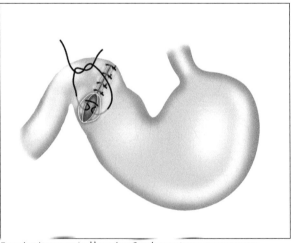

Eversion is prevented by using Gambee sutures as necessary.

→ **OPERATIVE TECHNIQUE 5.4 CONTINUED**

3   The completed closure significantly widens the pyloric outflow tract.

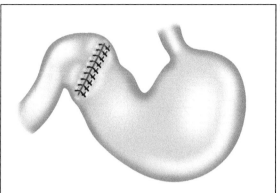
Final closure.

> **PRACTICAL TIP**
>
> After completion of the transverse pyloroplasty procedure, an omental wrap should be sutured over the surgical site to guard against leakage

OPERATIVE TECHNIQUE 5.5

Y–U antral advancement flap

POSITIONING

Dorsal recumbency with all four limbs secured.

ASSISTANT

Recommended to prevent spillage.

EQUIPMENT EXTRAS

Self-retaining abdominal retractors; Babcock forceps; suction.

SURGICAL TECHNIQUE

Approach

A routine ventral midline incision is performed from the xiphoid process to the umbilicus. Moistened laparotomy swabs are placed over the incision and Balfour abdominal retractors are applied.

Surgical manipulations

1   Incise the hepatogastric ligament to mobilize the pylorus (see Figure 5.5).

2   Inspect and palpate the pylorus and place two stay sutures 10 cm apart, the first anchored in the duodenum and the second in the ventral surface of the stomach. Alternatively, use Babcock forceps instead of stay sutures.

→ **OPERATIVE TECHNIQUE 5.5 CONTINUED**

3   The incisions are usually etched in the seromuscular layer with a No. 15 blade; make a stab incision into the lumen and extend the incision with Metzenbaum scissors. Direct the tail of the Y towards the duodenum and extend the two arms of the Y at an angle of about 45 degrees into the pyloric antrum. Both the arms and the tail of the Y should be approximately 2 cm in length with the pylorus serving as the midpoint.

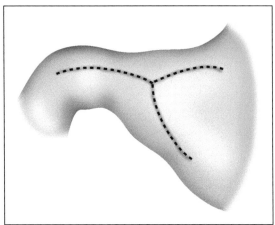

A Y-shaped full-thickness incision is centred over the pylorus with the tail of the Y towards the duodenum and the arms towards the antrum.

4   Once the incision is complete, trim off the point of the antral flap to prevent necrosis.

5   Evaluate the pyloric mucosa and undermine and excise the hyperplastic tissue using Metzenbaum scissors (see Figure 5.7). Any excised mucosa should be sent for histopathological evaluation.

Wound closure

1   Advance the flap aborally and suture transversely to the distal part of the duodenal incision.

2   Suture the sides of the flap to the sides of the duodenal incision, thereby creating a U-shaped closure, which greatly widens the gastric outlet.

3   Use a simple interrupted or Gambee suture pattern for the closure. Use synthetic monofilament absorbable materials, such as poliglecaprone 25, polydioxanone, polyglyconate or glycomer 631, in 3 metric (2/0 USP) for larger dogs and 2 metric (3/0 USP) for cats or small dogs.

4   Perform a routine abdominal closure.

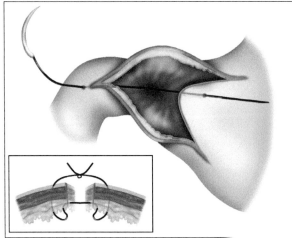

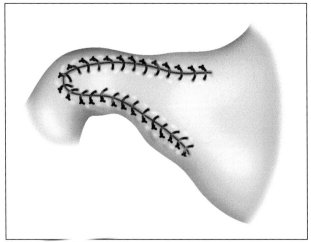

The point of the Y is trimmed to round it and the resultant flap is advanced distally and sutured to the end of the Y with a simple interrupted or modified Gambee suture pattern.

The two sides of the antral flap are sutured to the sides of the duodenum, resulting in a U-shaped closure.

→ **OPERATIVE TECHNIQUE 5.5 CONTINUED**

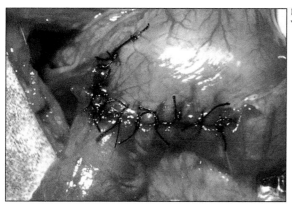

Intraoperative photograph of a completed Y–U antral advancement flap.

> **WARNING**
>
> Chromic catgut is not recommended because it loses its tensile strength rapidly when exposed to gastric juices

> **PRACTICAL TIP**
>
> After completion of the Y–U procedure, an omental wrap should be sutured over the surgical site

POSTOPERATIVE MANAGEMENT

Vomiting is common following this procedure, owing to duodenal gastric reflux of bile. Antibiotic therapy is not necessary unless spillage has occurred but prokinetic agents, such as metoclopramide (0.2–0.4 mg/kg orally or intravenously q6–8h, or preferably as a CRI at 1–2 mg/kg/24 h), sometimes reduce reflux and help to minimize vomiting. H2 blockers, such as ranitidine (2 mg/kg orally q12h) or famotidine (0.5 mg/kg orally q24h), are often prescribed to offset the gastritis. Dogs are usually fed small amounts of a low-fat gruel 3–4 times a day beginning 12 hours after surgery. Feeding is increased in amount if vomiting does not occur. Unrelenting vomiting may indicate either leakage with peritonitis or the development of pancreatitis.

OPERATIVE TECHNIQUE 5.6

Pyloromyotomy (Fredet–Ramstedt procedure)

POSITIONING

Dorsal recumbency with all four limbs secured.

ASSISTANT

Often unnecessary.

EQUIPMENT EXTRAS

Self-retaining abdominal retractors.

SURGICAL TECHNIQUE

Approach

A routine ventral midline incision is performed from the xiphoid process to cranial to the umbilicus. Moistened laparotomy swabs are placed over the incision and Balfour abdominal retractors are applied.

➜ **OPERATIVE TECHNIQUE 5.6 CONTINUED**

Surgical manipulations

1   Incise the hepatogastric ligament to mobilize the pylorus (see Figure 5.5).

2   For pyloromyotomy, a 3–4 cm longitudinal incision is extended from the ventral hypovascular area of the antrum to the antimesenteric border of the duodenum, with the pylorus serving as the midpoint of the incision.

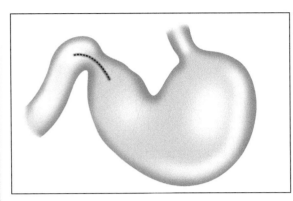

The pyloromyotomy procedure involves a 3–4 cm incision through the serosa and pyloric muscle.

3   The incision extends through the serosa and superficial longitudinal muscle layer. The deeper circular muscle bands are gently transected with a scalpel or Metzenbaum scissors, taking care not to penetrate the tough submucosa.

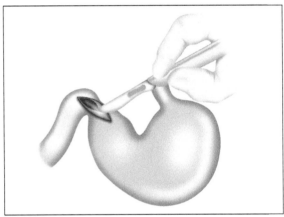

Care is taken not to enter the lumen of the stomach.

4   When all the muscle bands have been severed, the submucosa and mucosa will bulge out between the seromuscular layers.

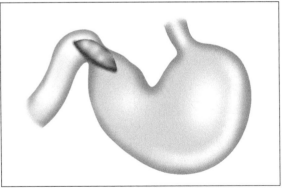

Note how the submucosa bulges out through the muscularis.

Wound closure

- If the technique is performed properly no contamination should occur and routine abdominal closure is performed.

PRACTICAL TIP

If the submucosa is inadvertently incised, it can be closed with simple interrupted sutures of 2 or 3 metric (3/0 or 2/0 USP) monofilament absorbable suture material

---

Pylorectomy and gastroduodenostomy (Billroth I procedure)

> **WARNING**
>
> This technically demanding procedure requires proper instrumentation, an assistant and a good understanding of the regional anatomy. In some of these cases the disease process will extend into the common bile duct and a biliary diversion procedure may be required (see Chapter 9). If the surgeon does not feel comfortable performing the resection and anastomosis, it is prudent to obtain a full-thickness biopsy sample from the lesion for histopathological diagnosis and to close the abdomen

POSITIONING

Dorsal recumbency with all four limbs secured.

ASSISTANT

Essential.

EQUIPMENT EXTRAS

Balfour abdominal retractors; Doyen intestinal forceps; haemostatic clips; Babcock forceps; suction (recommended); TA instrumentation (if available).

SURGICAL PROCEDURE

Approach

A routine ventral midline incision is performed from the xiphoid process to the pubis. Moistened laparotomy swabs are placed over the incision and Balfour abdominal retractors are applied.

Surgical manipulations

1. Mobilize the pylorus by transecting the hepatogastric ligament (see Figure 5.5).

2. Fix areas to either side of the lesion with stay sutures of 3 metric (2/0 USP) monofilament suture material or with Babcock forceps.

3. Inspect and palpate the pyloric lesion for depth and extent. Sometimes the lumen needs to be examined through a pyloric incision. Spillage is controlled by cross-clamping with Doyen forceps. Patency of the common bile duct can be established by gentle compression of the gallbladder.

4. Ligate and divide the branches of the right gastric and gastroepiploic artery and vein, using 2 metric (3/0 USP) suture material or small haemostatic clips.

5. Clamp the area to be resected with Doyen forceps and divide.

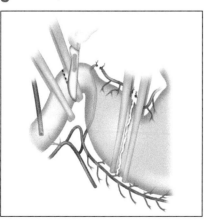

Branches of the right gastric and gastroepiploic arteries are ligated around the pylorus. Forceps are placed and the pylorus and antrum are resected between Doyen forceps to prevent spillage.

→ **OPERATIVE TECHNIQUE 5.7 CONTINUED**

Wound closure

After resection, the gastric stump is reduced in size with a two-layer closure.

1. Use a simple interrupted or Cushing pattern to invert the submucosa, followed by a simple interrupted approximating pattern which apposes the seromuscular layer.

2. The stomas of the stomach and duodenum are now similar in diameter. Anastomose using a simple interrupted or a modified Gambee suture pattern. Use synthetic monofilament absorbable materials such as poliglecaprone 25, polydioxanone, polyglyconate or glycomer 631, in 3 metric (2/0 USP) for larger dogs and 2 metric (3/0 USP) for cats or small dogs.

3. Cover the anastomosis with an omental wrap after completion.

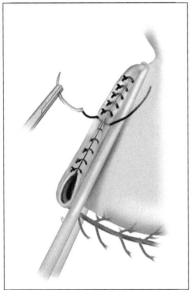

The submucosa and mucosa are inverted with an interrupted pattern and the seromuscular layer is approximated with a simple interrupted Lembert pattern.

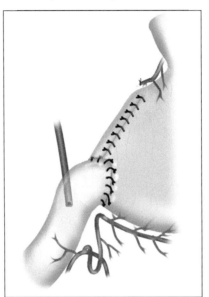

Two similar lumens are established and the anastomosis is completed with simple interrupted or Gambee sutures.

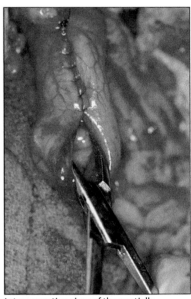

Intraoperative view of the partially oversewn gastric stump with haemostats placed in the gastric stoma.

PRACTICAL TIP

It is *strongly* recommended that an enterostomy (jejunostomy) tube (see Chapter 7) be placed after completion of the Billroth I procedure. This provides for enteral feeding of the patient while bypassing the surgical site. In addition to resting the surgical site, jejunostomy tubes are very useful for treating patients who have developed postoperative pancreatitis

---

4. Perform a routine abdominal closure.

POSTOPERATIVE MANAGEMENT

Vomiting is common following this procedure due to chronic gastric atony or duodenal gastric reflux of bile.

- Intravenous prophylactic antibiotics, such as cefazolin (20 mg/kg i.v. q2h during surgery and q6–8h thereafter; not authorized in the UK), amoxicillin/clavulanate (co-amoxiclav; 20–22 mg/kg i.v. q2h during surgery and q6–8h thereafter) or cefuroxime (15 mg/kg i.v. q3h during surgery) are warranted if spillage has occurred.
- Prokinetic agents are often helpful to reduce gastric atony and postoperative vomiting.
- Metoclopramide (0.2–0.4 mg/kg orally, i.v. q6–8h or 1–2 mg/kg/24 h as a CRI) has weak prokinetic properties but strong antiemetic properties and often works well.
- For dogs only, cisapride (0.1 0.5 mg/kg orally q12h) is a powerful prokinetic agent.
- H2 blockers, such as ranitidine (2 mg/kg orally q12h), famotidine (0.5 mg/kg orally q24h) or nizatidine (5 mg/kg orally q24h), are often prescribed to offset the gastritis. Ranitidine and nizatidine have an added advantage, because they increase gastric motility.
- The antiemetic maropitant may be used at a dose of 1 mg/kg s.c. q24h for up to 5 days. An oral formulation is also available and dosed at 2 mg/kg q24h.

OPERATIVE TECHNIQUE 5.8

Oesophageal hiatal hernia repair

POSITIONING

Dorsal recumbency with all four limbs secured.

ASSISTANT

Required for retraction. Second assistant for anaesthesia ventilation.

EQUIPMENT EXTRAS

Balfour self-retaining abdominal retractors; malleable abdominal (ribbon) retractors; Babcock forceps; thoracostomy tube; three-way stopcock and 50 or 60 ml syringe.

SURGICAL TECHNIQUE

Approach

A routine ventral midline incision is performed from the xiphoid process to the pubis. Moistened laparotomy swabs are placed over the incision and Balfour abdominal retractors are applied.

Surgical manipulations

1 Extend the ventral midline incision from the xiphoid to 10 cm caudal to the umbilicus.

2 Retract the liver caudally with malleable retractors.

3 Place a Penrose drain around the oesophagus to facilitate caudal oesophageal retraction.

4 Incise the phrenico-oesophageal ligament to freshen the edges of the diaphragm.

WARNING

Pneumothorax occurs after incision of the phrenico-oesophageal ligament. When this occurs the patient must be assisted with ventilation and a thoracostomy tube must be placed

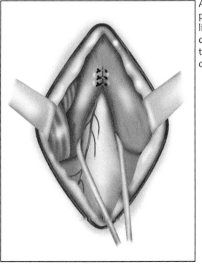

After incising the phrenico-oesophageal ligament, the diaphragm is apposed to reduce the oesophageal hiatus.

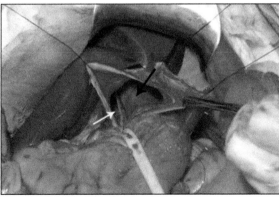

The phrenico-oesophageal ligament has been cut and is retracted with stay sutures, freeing the oesophagus (black arrow) from the diaphragm. A Penrose drain had been placed caudally around the distal oesophagus to retract it caudally into the abdomen. The dorsal branch of the vagus nerve can be seen (white arrow).
(Courtesy of J. Niles)

➜ **OPERATIVE TECHNIQUE 5.8 CONTINUED**

5 Reduce the diameter of the hiatus with simple interrupted sutures of 0 polypropylene or nylon suture material, taking care to spare the ventral branch of the vagus nerve.

> **PRACTICAL TIP**
>
> A large diameter orogastric tube is placed into the stomach during reconstruction of the oesophageal hiatus. This ensures that the hiatus is not closed too much, resulting in postoperative gas-bloat syndrome

6 Perform a cardio-oesophagopexy to the diaphragm, and perform a left-sided tube gastropexy to further prevent herniation of the stomach into the thorax. Alternatively, use a left-sided incisional gastropexy (see Chapter 6).

7 Place a thoracostomy tube (see the *BSAVA Manual of Canine and Feline Head, Neck and Thoracic Surgery*).

> **PRACTICAL TIP**
>
> Pre-place all the sutures for the cardio-oesophagopexy before tying them. The sutures should penetrate the muscular layers but not the mucosa

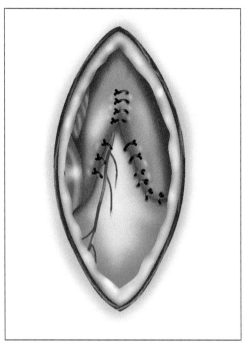

The oesophagus and cardia can also be sutured to the diaphragm.

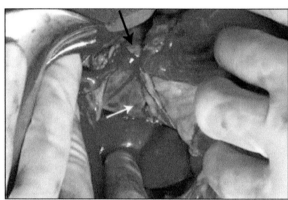

The diaphragm has been closed around a large orogastric tube to reduce the diameter of the hiatus (black arrow), and simple interrupted sutures have been placed to pexy the distal oesophagus and cardia to the margin of the diaphragmatic hiatus (white arrow).
(Courtesy of J. Niles)

Wound closure

Routine abdominal closure is performed.

POSTOPERATIVE MANAGEMENT

Sucralfate, ranitidine, famotidine or nizatidine can be used to reduce the clinical signs secondary to continued reflux. Follow-up studies indicate that only about 50% of dogs treated surgically become clinically normal.

Chapter 6

Gastric dilatation and volvulus

John M. Williams

Gastric dilatation and volvulus (GDV) is an acute life-threatening abnormal accumulation of gastric gas (dilatation), which may be complicated by rotation of the stomach (volvulus) about its mesenteric axis (Figure 6.1). A series of peracute pathophysiological changes occur that are responsible for the high reported mortality rate associated with this condition. Though GDV has been recognized as a condition affecting dogs for many decades, the course of events and aetiopathogenesis are still not fully understood, as many risk factors may predispose an individual to this potentially fatal condition. Although historically GDV has been associated with a high mortality rate, a recent study reported an overall mortality rate of 10% (Mackenzie *et al.*, 2010).

Risk factors

A number of risk factors, both environmental and 'host'-related, have been implicated in GDV. These include breed, age, sex, chest conformation, diet, stress/anxiety and exercise patterns (Glickman *et al.*, 1994; Elwood, 1998; Pipan *et al.*, 2012). Determining the relative importance of the various risk factors is an ongoing process, and the results of various studies in the UK and USA are shown in Figure 6.2. Large-breed dogs are reported to have a 24% lifetime risk of developing GDV, compared with 21.6% for giant-breed dogs (Glickman *et al.*, 2000). A recent internet-based study involving over 2500 dogs suggested that dogs fed solely on a commercial dry diet were at higher risk of developing GDV and, interestingly, showed that moderate immediate postprandial exercise lowered the risk (Pipan *et al.*, 2012).

Higher risk
• Large and giant breeds
• Dogs with a close relative (parent or sibling) who has had GDV
• Large thoracic depth to width ratio (deep narrow chest)
• Underweight for breed
• Increasing age
• Previous splenomegaly or splenectomy
• Aerophagia or 'gulping' food
• Eating from a raised bowl
• Stress (e.g. being kennelled, car journey or dog show)
• Feeding once a day, particularly dry food
• Small food particle size (<30 mm in diameter)

Lower risk
• 'Happy' dogs
• Dogs fed 'table scraps'
• Supplementing diet with egg or fish
• Feeding more than once a day
• Large food particle size (>30 mm in diameter)
• Moderate daily and postprandial exercise

6.2 Risk factors associated with GDV.

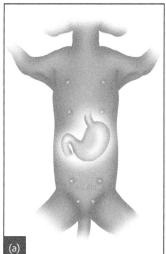 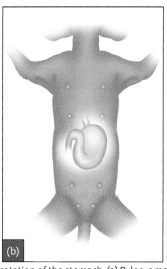 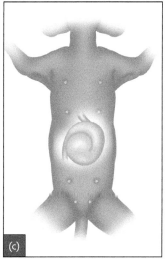 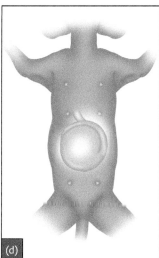

(a) (b) (c) (d)

6.1 Ventral view of 180-degree rotation of the stomach. (a) Pylorus moves ventrally from right to left. (b) Pylorus and body of stomach move clockwise. (c) Pylorus lies to left of stomach. (d) Pylorus moves more dorsally.

Pathophysiology

GDV may be acute or chronic; the latter is discussed later in the chapter.

The initial presenting signs are identical for both acute gastric dilatation (GD) and acute GDV. Both cause cardiorespiratory dysfunction due to the distended gas-filled stomach. There is still much debate as to which occurs first, the dilatation or the volvulus; the consensus is that it is likely that volvulus is secondary. This theory is backed by the evidence that gastropexy reportedly prevents recurrence (Glickman *et al.*, 1998; Dujowich *et al.*, 2010).

The reason for failure of the stomach to release air (mostly swallowed) is still unclear. The mechanism for eructation fails, and air, gas and fluids all combine to exacerbate distension. There is no experimental or clinical evidence that associates delayed gastric emptying with GDV. As the stomach becomes more distended, the pylorus is displaced from right to left across the floor of the abdomen and comes to lie dorsally on the left (see Figure 6.1). This distension and movement of the stomach causes a number of deleterious effects on the body systems, which lead to the life-threatening nature of this condition.

Respiratory system

The primary effect of the distended stomach on the respiratory system results from the fact that it puts pressure on the diaphragm, resulting in reduced excursion of the diaphragm and thereby reducing the functional reserve capacity of the lungs. This will lead to alveolar hypoventilation, which will in turn cause a ventilation/perfusion mismatch and arterial hypoxaemia as the degree of respiratory dysfunction worsens. The subsequent rise in partial pressure of carbon dioxide (pCO_2) will result in a respiratory acidosis (which further compromises the patient's acid–base status; see below).

Cardiovascular system

The low pressure venous structures (caudal vena cava, hepatic portal vein and splanchnic vessels) of the cranial abdomen are readily compressed by the rapidly distending stomach. This compression has a twofold effect, greatly reducing venous return (compounded by splanchnic pooling) and causing portal hypertension.

- *Reducing venous return* leads to a reduced cardiac output, with a resultant fall in systemic blood pressure.
- *Portal hypertension* leads to interstitial oedema (which may in severe cases lead to tissue ischaemia) and fluid leaking from the vascular spaces. This will further compromise circulating volume, with a consequence of reduced tissue perfusion and hypovolaemic shock.
- *Reduced tissue perfusion* during acute GD/GDV may lead to myocardial injury, and there is the risk of reperfusion injury occurring when circulation is re-established during treatment. Detectable concentrations of cardiac troponin I and cardiac troponin T have been found in the serum of dogs with GDV, suggesting cardiomyocyte degeneration and necrosis (Schober *et al.*, 2002)

Cardiac arrhythmias, particularly premature ventricular contractions and ventricular tachycardia, are a probable consequence of reduced tissue perfusion, though their precise aetiology is uncertain. They may occur as a consequence of subendocardial ischaemia and necrosis

together with reduced coronary flow, as a result of both reduced venous return and tachycardia. The situation may also be compounded by *metabolic acidosis*, which can further decrease cardiac muscle contractility and hence cardiac output.

A further factor in reducing cardiac contractility is *myocardial depressant factor* (MDF). This factor is thought to be secreted as a result of reduced tissue perfusion in other organ systems, particularly the pancreas and intestines. The true nature of MDF has not been fully identified, but nitrous oxide is thought to play a leading role in causing the cellular damage associated with the arrhythmias. MDF may also be released as a consequence of endotoxaemia and the systemic inflammatory response syndrome (SIRS).

Cardiovascular effects are further compromised by the release of *catecholamines*, which increase peripheral resistance in order to compensate for the reduced systemic blood pressure. Though effective in the short term, they cause a further reduction in tissue perfusion, which can ultimately lead to a severe reduction in renal perfusion together with loss of the intestinal mucosal barrier. If not checked, this process will lead to irreversible shock and death.

Gastric and splenic ischaemia and necrosis

Gastric necrosis develops as a result of the torsion, occlusion and avulsion of the short gastric arteries supplying the greater curvature and fundus of the stomach. This will often result in ischaemia, which frequently leads to necrosis of large areas of the stomach that subsequently leak gastric contents.

During volvulus of the stomach, the spleen will also move with the greater curvature of the stomach. This can lead to splenic infarcts and necrosis, due to compromise of the splenic vasculature during volvulus.

Metabolic effects
Acid–base and potassium abnormalities

Acid–base and electrolyte problems in GDV are multifactorial, arising as a combination of ischaemic events (Figure 6.3) and ventilation/perfusion mismatching (see above). Though a large base excess may be present at presentation, it cannot be used as a predictor for either gastric necrosis or outcome (Beer *et al.*, 2013). The complex nature of these events in GDV indicates that it is particularly important to monitor potassium levels as well as acid–base status during treatment, because they can change rapidly. If monitoring is not feasible, it is probably best to use large volumes of intravenous fluids that are low in potassium. If renal perfusion is re-established, it will not only help in potassium homeostasis but also greatly aid in establishing a normal acid–base balance by maintaining a normal circulating bicarbonate concentration.

Glucose abnormalities

Glucose production is increased early on in GDV by the release of catecholamines but, as poor tissue perfusion occurs, glucose metabolism changes from aerobic to anaerobic. The anaerobic pathway is far less efficient and leads to high consumption of glucose, just as glucose availability becomes reduced as a result of hepatic congestion and underperfusion. The finding of hypoglycaemia in GDV indicates a poor prognosis.

Event	Cause	Effect
Cell hypoxia	Increased lactic acid	Metabolic acidosis
Endotoxin	Increased lactic acid	Metabolic acidosis
Poor liver/kidney perfusion	Reduced lactate recycling	Exacerbated metabolic acidosis
Ventilation/perfusion mismatch	Increased pCO_2 Large hydrogen ion (H^+) loss into the lumen	Respiratory acidosis Metabolic acidosis
Compensatory intracellular shift of H^+	Potassium ion (K^+) loss into extracellular fluid	Hyperkalaemia (this may be a minor event, as intracellular lactate shift may minimize movement of K^+ from cells)
GD with fluid pooling	Potassium ion (K^+) loss into lumen	Hypokalaemia
Reduced renal perfusion	Activation of renin–angiotensin system	Sodium ion resorption with loss of K^+ in urine (this helps to compensate for any hyperkalaemia)

6.3 Summary of acid–base and electrolyte abnormalities in GDV.

Reperfusion injury

Reperfusion injury occurs when tissue that has been deprived of blood is exposed to blood flow as the circulation returns to a more normal state upon treatment of a condition.

Cellular hypoxia, in addition to causing acidosis, disturbs the ion gradient, leading particularly to an increase in intracellular calcium ions. This leads to cell membrane breakdown and acceleration of the conversion of xanthine dehydrogenase to xanthine oxidase. This pathway is a precursor to oxygen free-radical formation once tissue reperfusion occurs. Free-radical scavengers, such as deferoxamine, have been shown to be effective in lowering morbidity in experimental cases. It has been suggested that lidocaine may have a positive effect in preventing reperfusion injury, in addition to its anti-arrhythmic properties. The reported lidocaine dose used was 2 mg/kg intravenously, followed by a continuous rate infusion (CRI) of 0.05 mg/kg/min for at least 3 hours (8 out of 51 dogs), or just a CRI of lidocaine (0.05 mg/kg/min) for at least 3 hours (Buber *et al.*, 2007).

Disseminated intravascular coagulopathy

Disseminated intravascular coagulopathy (DIC) is a secondary phenomenon with a multifactorial aetiology. Poor tissue perfusion causes microthrombus formation, which leads to further vascular occlusion, thus promoting further tissue hypoxia and becoming part of a vicious cycle. Both tissue ischaemia and sepsis (particularly associated with bacterial endotoxin) cause the release of tissue thromboplastin (factor III), which has the potential to activate both the intrinsic and extrinsic pathways of coagulation. In acute cases, spontaneous bleeding may be seen from mucosal surfaces and into body cavities, and may cause organ ischaemia due to vascular occlusion by thrombi.

Diagnosis of suspected DIC is based on prolonged prothrombin time (PT) and activated partial thromboplastin time (aPTT) together with the presence of fibrin degradation products (FDP). Plasma fibrinogen concentration, serum concentrations of fibrin and fibrinogen-related antigens (FRAs), and particularly plasma antithrombin III, can also be used to confirm a diagnosis.

Endotoxaemia and bacteraemia

In GDV there is thought to be a physical breakdown of the mucosal barrier that normally prevents bacterial translocation; this is exacerbated by the local acidosis. The development of portal hypertension greatly reduces the effectiveness of the hepatic reticuloendothelial system in removing bacteria from the portal system. However, Winkler *et al.* (2003) cast doubt on this widely held hypothesis. In their study, only 43% of clinical GDV cases had a detectable bacteraemia, as did 40% of their controls, although all but one case had been given intravenous perioperative antibiotics. In this particular study the presence of bacteraemia did not have a negative effect on case outcome.

Despite these findings, endotoxaemia remains a real concern, particularly as endotoxin may be released when the intestines, pancreas and spleen are reperfused. Endotoxin exerts its effects in many ways, but particularly by:

- Damaging endothelial cells
- Inducing release of histamine, bradykinin and tumour necrosis factor
- Activating the complement system
- Activating platelets and the clotting cascade
- Stimulating neutrophils.

These mechanisms in turn have widespread systemic effects, including reduced vascular resistance, increased cardiac output, renal tubular damage, microvascular occlusion, and initiation of DIC and pyrexia, all of which contribute to and accelerate the systemic inflammatory response.

Renal effects

The kidneys have an inbuilt mechanism, via local production of prostaglandins E2 and I2, to limit the effects of reduced perfusion. The effect of these prostaglandins is to produce severe vasoconstriction of afferent vessels. If perfusion is not improved, this mechanism can be overwhelmed if circulation pressures are not normalized. Initially the glomerular filtration rate will be reduced, with a resultant oliguria, but if the reduced perfusion persists, acute renal failure will ensue. Nephrons may also be damaged by the effects of the factors involved in reperfusion injury.

Clinical signs

Typical clinical signs of GDV are summarized as follows:

- Retching
- Unproductive vomiting
- Cranial abdominal distension
- Circulatory collapse (weak peripheral pulse and tachycardia)
- Hypersalivation
- Dyspnoea.

The most common clinical sign is non-productive vomiting, associated with rapid abdominal distension. There is no 'typical' history for this condition, although the episode of dilatation may be associated with an episode of stress, as noted above. GDV is seen more commonly in large and giant breeds of dog and tends to be commoner in older dogs (see Figure 6.2). There is no sex predilection but a recent internet survey of over 2500 patients suggested that intact females may be at higher risk (Pipan *et al.*, 2012).

Findings on physical examination will vary depending on the extent and severity of the condition at presentation.

- Most commonly, patients will have a distended painful abdomen which is hyper-resonant on percussion.
- Patients tend to be tachycardic and tachypnoeic, with slightly pale mucous membranes and a slow capillary refill time (CRT).
- As shock progresses from the compensatory phase, patients may also exhibit evidence of hypotension, muddy mucous membranes and pyrexia.
- In non-compensatory shock, patients may become bradycardic and have weak pulses, a poor CRT, white mucous membranes and hypothermia.

Diagnosis

A presumptive diagnosis is made on the basis of the clinical findings. As adjuncts to the physical examination, blood samples may be taken and radiography carried out. Emergency management of a suspected GDV case should not be delayed by carrying out tests and waiting for the results. They are useful in the ongoing management but do not alter the need to stabilize the patient.

Blood sampling

The results of blood tests will not provide a definitive diagnosis of GDV but will give an indication of the status of the patient at the time of presentation (Figure 6.4). Repeated samples will allow monitoring of the progression of the condition.

Plasma lactate concentrations

Preoperative plasma lactate concentrations have been shown to be a good predictor of gastric necrosis and the outcome for dogs with GDV. In a study by De Papp *et al.* (1999), 99% of dogs with a plasma lactate concentration <6.0 mmol/l survived, compared with only 58% of dogs with a plasma lactate concentration of >6.0 mmol/l. In addition, the median plasma lactate concentration in dogs with gastric necrosis (6.6 mmol/l) was significantly higher than the concentration in dogs without gastric necrosis (3.3 mmol/l). There has been some debate in recent work as to the absolute value for prediction of necrosis, with values ranging from 6 to 9 mmol/l (Zacher *et al.*, 2010; Green *et al.*, 2011; Beer *et al.*, 2013). Two recent studies have suggested that assessing the reduction in lactate levels during acute treatment, particularly the first 12 hours, may give a better indication of the outcome. When the percentage change in lactate concentration was ≤42.5%, survival was 15%, compared with 100% when the percentage change was >42.5% (Zacher *et al.*, 2010; Green *et al.*, 2011).

Urinalysis

Measuring urinary thromboxane metabolites following surgery may be useful in predicting postoperative complications. One of the consequences of intestinal reperfusion is production of thromboxane A2; this is metabolized via thromboxane B2 to the stable metabolite 11-dehydro-thromboxane B2, which can be measured in the urine (Baltzer *et al.*, 2006). An increase in the ratio of urinary 11-dehydro-thromboxane B2 to creatinine following surgery for GDV was shown to correlate with an increased incidence of postoperative complications.

Radiography

> **WARNING**
>
> Radiography is a useful diagnostic tool but no patient with suspected GDV should have radiographs taken until they have been clinically stabilized

Test	Finding	Interpretation
Haematology	Increased packed cell volume (and total protein)	Haemoconcentration
	Increased neutrophils, increased monocytes and decreased lymphocytes	Stress or inflammatory response
	Decreased neutrophils	Exhausted inflammatory response or endotoxic shock
	Decreased platelet count	Hypercoagulation (possible DIC)
Biochemistry	Increased alanine aminotransferase	Hepatocellular hypoxia
	Increased blood urea nitrogen and creatinine	Renal dysfunction (prerenal, renal, post-renal)
	Low total protein/albumin	Transudation or blood loss
	Normal to low potassium	Potassium loss (see text)
	Increased lactate	Anaerobic cellular metabolism or endotoxic effects
	Prolonged PT and aPTT	DIC
	Prolonged aPTT, high FDP (antithrombin III) and increased lactate	Suggests gastric necrosis
	Hypoglycaemia	End-stage shock
Blood gases	Variable pH, variable total carbon dioxide or bicarbonate	Acid–base abnormality
	Increased arterial pCO_2	Impaired ventilation

6.4 Laboratory findings and interpretation in GDV.

Radiography can help to differentiate between 'simple' dilatation and GDV, but it must be used with care. Many patients will become stressed by radiographic procedures. If it is to be used, the patient must be stabilized medically and the benefits must outweigh the risks involved.

PRACTICAL TIP

If radiography is used, a right lateral view should be taken. If there is a volvulus, the gas-filled pylorus is seen dorsal to the gas-filled gastric shadow (compartmentalization) (Figure 6.5)

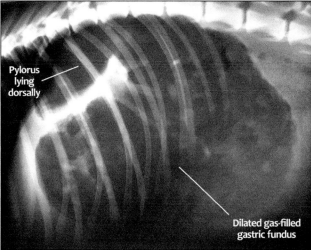

Pylorus lying dorsally

Dilated gas-filled gastric fundus

6.5 Right lateral radiograph showing gastric volvulus. (© John Williams)

Radiographs should be carefully scrutinized for the presence of free abdominal air. Unless air has leaked during gastrocentesis, this indicates gastric rupture and is associated with a much higher mortality rate.

Thoracic radiography

Preoperative thoracic radiographs have been shown to be of benefit, despite the critical nature of these cases. The presence of cardiomegaly on preoperative radiographs carries a poor prognosis for dogs with GDV (Green et al., 2012).

Initial management (stabilization)

The initial aim of management is to stabilize the patient, primarily by restoring the cardiovascular system. This in turn will aid renal function and the respiratory system. In order to achieve this, it is necessary to reduce the restricting effects of the dilated stomach on the cranial abdominal veins and on the respiratory system. In addition, it is essential to provide supportive fluid therapy. Gastric decompression should not be carried out without providing fluid support for the patient.

There is some debate as to whether gastric decompression should be carried out before initiating intravenous fluid support, or *vice versa*. It has been shown that continued dilatation of the stomach (with or without volvulus) is the major cause of gastric necrosis and therefore decompression should not be delayed. The author prefers to start fluid therapy and then decompress the stomach, though decompression should not be delayed by more than 10–15 minutes if vascular access is difficult.

Fluid therapy

The aim of fluid therapy (Figure 6.6) is to aid in restoring the circulation and thus to improve tissue and organ perfusion. Fluid can be administered rapidly if two large-bore intravenous catheters are placed in the cephalic or jugular veins. It is most effective to combine a crystalloid with a colloid, because colloids have the advantages of a prolonged effect and of raising oncotic pressure, thereby enhancing the effect of the crystalloids. Hypertonic saline solution has been used successfully in the treatment of GDV-induced shock. Following the administration of hypertonic saline, crystalloids should be given at 20 ml/kg/h (Schertel et al., 1997).

Fluid type	Rate
Crystalloids	
Lactated Ringer's solution (Hartmann's)	Initially: 90 ml/kg/h Monitor response and reduce as needed
Colloids	
Succinated gelatine (4%) (Gelofusine®, Braun)	20 ml/kg/24 h
Hetastarch (6% solution)	10–20 ml/kg
Combinations	
Hypertonic (7%) saline solution combined with a colloid	5 ml/kg over 15 minutes
Hypertonic (7%) saline solution given simultaneously with a crystalloid	10–40 ml/kg

6.6 Fluid administration in GDV.

WARNING

Fluid administered via the saphenous veins will be ineffective for restoring circulating volume, owing to the reduced venous return caused by gastric compression of the vena cava

---

Response to therapy is assessed on the basis of changes in heart rate, pulse rate and quality, and respiratory rate. With large-volume infusions it is essential to ensure that urine is being produced; this should be at a rate of at least 0.5–1 ml/kg/h.

Antibiotics

It is generally accepted that antibiotics given intravenously are beneficial in reducing the incidence of bacteraemia and consequently endotoxaemia. The paper by Winkler et al. (2003) would support this hypothesis; although 43% of their clinical cases developed bacteraemia, the bacteria isolated did not adversely affect the outcome of the cases, and all but one of their cases had been given antibiotics at presentation. When choosing an antibiotic it is best to use an agent that can be given intravenously, is bactericidal and has a broad spectrum of activity.

Suitable antibiotics are amoxicillin/clavulanate (co-amoxiclav; 15–25 mg/kg), cefuroxime (10–15 mg/kg) or cefazolin (20 mg/kg, USA only) given intravenously every 8 hours. If surgery is prolonged (over 90 minutes) then a repeat dose of intravenous antibiotic should be administered. There is no positive benefit in continuing antibiotic cover beyond 24 hours.

Anti-arrhythmia therapy

The common arrhythmias, as noted above, are premature ventricular contractions and ventricular tachycardia (Figure 6.7). They may be detected shortly after presentation, but commonly begin intra- or postoperatively.

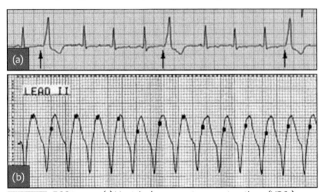

6.7 ECG traces. (a) Ventricular premature contractions (VPCs). Note that every fourth beat is a VPC (arrowed). (b) Ventricular tachycardia. Note wide 'bizarre' QRS complexes.

Anti-arrhythmic drugs are indicated if ventricular premature contractions (VPCs) interfere with cardiac output. If VPCs occur in runs of >20, if ventricular tachycardia (heart rate >160 beats per minute) is evident or peripheral pulse quality is poor, or if the echocardiogram (ECG) shows multiform VPCs or R-on-T phenomenon, treatment should be instituted:

* Slow intravenous bolus of lidocaine (initial bolus is usually 2 mg/kg i.v.), repeated if sinus rhythm does not develop (up to a total dose of 8 mg/kg)
* Continuous lidocaine drip (25–75 µg/kg/min) to maintain a normal rhythm
* Monitoring for signs of lidocaine toxicity (including muscle tremors, vomiting and seizures).

> **PRACTICAL TIP**
>
> Ideally the potassium level should be checked prior to lidocaine administration. This drug is ineffective if the animal is hypokalaemic

> **WARNING**
>
> Care should be taken to ensure that only lidocaine *without* adrenaline (epinephrine) is used

Corticosteroids

There is no published evidence that gives a definitive view on the use of corticosteroids in patients with shock or GDV. The perceived benefits include an antioxidant effect, increased vascular tone and a positive inotropic effect. On the negative side, they may impair the immune system and may predispose to gastrointestinal ulceration.

If a glucocorticoid is to be administered, methylprednisolone succinate should be given intravenously at 30 mg/kg over 5–10 minutes.

> **Editors' note:**
>
> Neither of the editors routinely uses corticosteroids in patients with GDV

Free-radical scavengers

Although drugs such as deferoxamine and allopurinol have been shown to be useful experimentally in GDV, there is as yet no evidence that they are beneficial in clinical cases.

Non-steroidal anti-inflammatory drugs

> **WARNING**
>
> Non-steroidal anti-inflammatory drugs (NSAIDs) should not be used in animals in shock owing to their deleterious effect on renal perfusion and their potential for causing gastrointestinal ulceration

Sedation and analgesia

Care must be taken with sedation in these patients and in most cases sedation is not required in order to pass an orogastric tube. Phenothiazine derivatives (e.g. acepromazine maleate) and alpha agonists (e.g. medetomidine) should be avoided, owing to their effect of further lowering blood pressure in a compromised patient. Opioid analgesics should be used in these patients; the author uses methadone (0.25–0.5 mg/kg; see *BSAVA Manual of Canine and Feline Anaesthesia and Analgesia*).

Gastric decompression

Stomach tubing (orogastric intubation)

A wide-bore stomach tube is measured from the dog's rhinarium to its 11th rib and marked. It must not be passed beyond this length, in order to minimize the risk of rupturing a potentially compromised gastric wall.

1. Attempts should be made to pass the tube with the patient in the 'sitting' position.
2. An adhesive bandage roll 7.5 cm wide with a hollow plastic core (Figure 6.8a) is inserted end-on between the teeth, and the mouth is taped closed over this improvised gag (Figure 6.8b).
3. The stomach tube is then passed down the core of the roll.

Sedation should be avoided, so as not to exacerbate hypotensive changes. If it is impossible to intubate the stomach with the dog in the 'sitting' position, right lateral recumbency may prove more useful. Rotating the stomach tube gently about its long axis may aid entry into the stomach if there is a partial volvulus.

Care must be taken not to be over-vigorous in passing the tube, because this may lead to rupture. If the tube cannot be passed, percutaneous needle decompression can be carried out (see Figure 6.10 and below) followed by a further attempt to pass a stomach tube. This latter technique is particularly useful in that it helps to lower pressure at the gastro-oesophageal junction, making passing of a stomach tube easier.

Once the tube has been passed into the stomach, gastric lavage (Figure 6.9) is carried out with copious volumes of warm normal (0.9%) saline or lactated Ringer's (Hartmann's) solution.

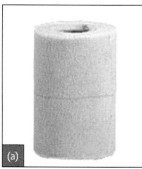

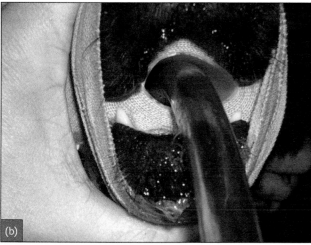

6.8 (a) A 7.5 cm adhesive bandage roll with plastic core. (b) The roll placed 'end-on' orally with similar tape wrapped around the dog's muzzle to facilitate passage of a stomach tube.
(© John Williams)

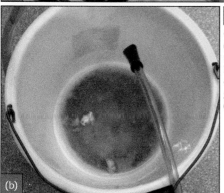

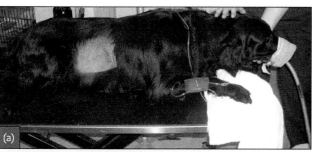

6.9 Gastric lavage. (a) Recumbent dog undergoing gastric lavage. (b) 'Typical' contents from gastric lavage.
(© John Williams)

Percutaneous needle decompression

A 14, 16 or 18 G over-the-needle catheter is introduced through a clipped sterilized area over the tympanitic right flank (Figure 6.10). The author routinely carries out this procedure prior to or instead of orogastric intubation. The rationale for this is that it allows for rapid decompression which quickly relieves pressure on the caudal vena cava.

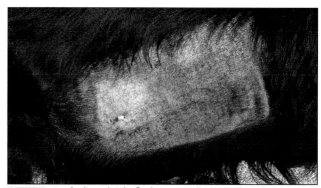

6.10 Dog's clipped right flank, prepared aseptically and with a 16 G intravenous needle inserted.
(© John Williams)

Temporary paracostal (flank) gastrostomy

Though this can be a useful technique, its use is no longer widespread with the advent of aggressive fluid therapy and safer anaesthetic techniques. Most surgeons prefer to stabilize the patient and to carry out derotational surgery sooner rather than later. The major disadvantage of this procedure is that it does not allow assessment of gastric wall viability.

Surgery

Surgical exploration is indicated in *all* cases of GD and GDV. The controversial aspect is the timing of the laparotomy to ensure that the chance of patient survival is optimal. In cases of simple dilatation, surgery can be delayed so as to minimize the risk to the patient; nevertheless, a gastropexy procedure should be performed in all cases of GD and GDV.

Dogs that have had one episode of gastric dilatation are at an increased risk of repeated episodes and a gastropexy aids in prevention of future volvulus. If volvulus has occurred, surgery can be delayed once decompression has been achieved to allow further stabilization of the patient. Laparoscopic management of GDV has been described; such cases would need careful evaluation to rule out the benefits of a full surgical procedure.

If gastric decompression cannot be achieved, or if gastric necrosis is suspected (any blood that appears in the stomach tube at the time of decompression is suggestive of gastric necrosis), surgery should be performed without delay. In general, laparotomy should be carried out once the signs of shock have been adequately treated; usually this will be between 2 and 4 hours after treatment starts.

Circulatory and respiratory compromise should not be further aggravated by general anaesthesia. Sedatives and barbiturate drugs should be used with great care, and avoided if possible, because of their respiratory depressive and arrhythmogenic side effects. Intravenous induction with a short-acting agent, such as propofol or alfaxalone (UK and AUS only), is viewed as appropriate in these high-risk cases (Psatha *et al.*, 2011).

> **WARNING**
>
> Nitrous oxide must be avoided because of the risk of creating additional gastric distension

The goals of surgery are threefold and are summarized in Figure 6.11.

Goal	Surgical procedure(s)
Restore the anatomy	Gastric derotation
Assess gastric and splenic viability	If non-viable, carry out gastric invagination; partial gastrectomy or splenectomy as required
Prevent/minimize risk of recurrence	Permanent right-sided gastropexy

6.11 Goals of surgery in GDV.

Approach and derotation

A midline laparotomy is performed and the direction of gastric rotation must be established. Greater omentum covering the stomach (Figure 6.12) suggests a clockwise rotation, but this must be confirmed by palpation of the gastro-oesophageal junction. The stomach must be repositioned with great care, and in the correct direction, to avoid perforation of any devitalized areas. The pylorus is gently lifted across to the right whilst the fundus is pushed down and to the left (Figure 6.13). Further decompression by stomach tube may be necessary to allow the stomach to be manipulated successfully; further lavage can also be carried out at this stage if required.

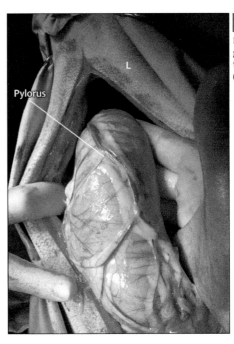

6.13 Pylorus being lifted gently from left (L) to right.
(© John Williams)

Gastrotomy for the removal of the gastric contents is contraindicated, owing to the risk of abdominal contamination and the added surgical time. Current evidence suggests that there is no indication to perform pyloric surgery to improve gastric outflow.

Assessing gastric and splenic viability

The greater curvature and fundus are most likely to be ischaemic; any area that is erythematous (Figure 6.14) or discoloured (purple, blue or black) should be regarded as suspect. It is better to assume the worst and deal with it rather than leave a suspect area unmanaged. However, gastric resection (see Chapter 5) is time-consuming, can add to hypovolaemia and should preferably not be undertaken unless a linear thoracoabdominal (TA) stapling instrument is available. It has been shown that, if gastrectomy is performed, mortality is only 10% with a stapling device compared with 60% if manual suturing is carried out.

Gastric invagination is an effective, safe and quick alternative to resection (Figure 6.15). Devitalized areas of the fundus and body are inverted into the gastric lumen

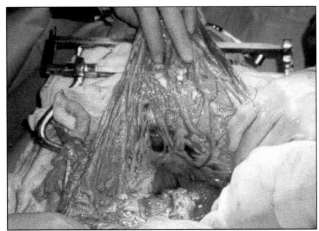

6.12 Omentum 'covering' a clockwise-rotated stomach. The stomach serosa is inflamed and potentially ischaemic.
(© John Williams)

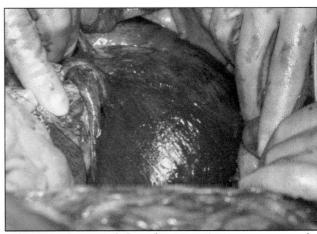

6.14 Erythematous (inflamed) serosa on the greater curvature of stomach following GDV.
(© John Williams)

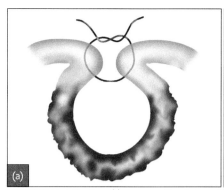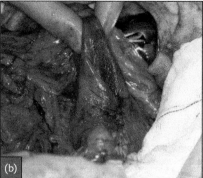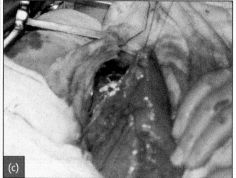

6.15 Invagination. (a) Cross-sectional view of the greater curvature to show invagination (the stippled area is the non-viable area). (b) Invagination in process, using a continuous suture pattern. (c) Invagination completed.
(Photographs © John Williams)

and serosa, and sutured in position with absorbable interrupted Lembert sutures. The non-viable tissue will slough into the lumen, whilst any viable tissue will survive without major complication once inverted. Patients who do slough necrotic tissue will show melaena postoperatively.

Splenectomy (see Chapter 12) should only be performed where extensive infarction and necrosis of the spleen is seen. Splenectomy is associated with high mortality because it adds considerably to the surgical time (Mackenzie *et al.*, 2010).

Gastropexy

Gastropexy to anchor the stomach in a normal anatomical position is an integral and essential part of the surgery for both GD and GDV. Recurrence rates can be as high as 80% if gastropexy is not carried out, whilst gastropexy reduces the risk of recurrence to less than 10% (Glickman *et al.*, 1998). There is a dramatic increase in median survival time for gastropexy patients (547 days) compared with non-gastropexy patients (188 days). A number of gastropexy techniques have been described and are summarized in Figure 6.16.

Tube gastropexy/gastrostomy

Tube gastropexy (see Operative Technique 6.1) has the advantage of being quick to perform and allowing gastric

decompression postoperatively. Though the tube is easy to place, increased morbidity and longer hospitalization periods are associated with this technique. Tube gastropexy is recommended after major gastric resection.

Belt loop gastropexy

Belt loop gastropexy provides excellent adhesions and is the author's technique of choice both for acute cases and for elective gastropexy (see Operative Technique 6.2). It is also technically feasible for the unassisted surgeon.

Incisional gastropexy

Incisional gastropexy is a straightforward technique that relies on healing between the edges of a peritoneum–transversus abdominis muscle incision and a seromuscular incision in the pyloric antrum (see Operative Technique 6.3).

Circumcostal gastropexy

Circumcostal gastropexy is a technically difficult procedure, for which an assistant is required. Although it produces strong adhesions, there is the potential to fracture the rib or induce a pneumothorax if it is carried out incorrectly. Its use is more appropriate for a prophylactic gastropexy, rather than on an emergency basis.

Technique	Adhesions	Probability of recurrence	Other advantages	Other disadvantages
Simple suturing	Poor	High	Relatively quick	
Tube gastropexy	Adequate	Low	Relatively quick	Patient interference Increased morbidity Increased hospitalization
Incisional gastropexy	Strong	Low		
Belt loop gastropexy	Strong	Low		
Circumcostal gastropexy	Strong (probably the most secure)	Low		Technically demanding Risk of rib fracture Risk of pneumothorax
Incorporating (linea alba) gastropexy	Strong	Low		Not generally suitable as gastric fundus is sutured into midline laparotomy closure Risk of gastric perforation if any further laparotomies carried out
Gastrocolopexy		Low		Possibly higher potential for recurrence
Laparoscopic gastropexy	Strong	Low	Minimally invasive	Generally not suitable for acute cases Specialist equipment required

6.16 Gastropexy techniques.

Postoperative considerations

Analgesia and fluid therapy should be continued for 24–48 hours after surgery, until the patient is comfortable and is eating and drinking adequately. Water can be offered by mouth after 12 hours and if there is no evidence of vomiting a small amount of food should be offered. Patients should have their electrolyte status checked and be assessed for cardiac arrhythmias for up to 72 hours after surgery. Any abnormality in electrolytes should be corrected as necessary. If arrhythmias are still significant in the postoperative period, oral procainamide (10–15 mg/kg q8h) or sotalol (0.5–2 mg/kg q12h) can be used.

If there is vomiting or evidence of ileus after surgery, potassium levels should be carefully checked and corrected. In addition, a suitable intravenous prokinetic agent can be used (e.g. metoclopramide 0.25–0.5 mg/kg). If gastric mucosal damage is suspected, sucralfate and an H2 receptor antagonist, such as ranitidine or famotidine, can be given.

It is generally recommended that post-GDV patients should be fed three to four times a day. It is preferable to feed rapidly digested food. Longer term precautions must also be taken, with advice to reduce stress and to reduce the speed at which some dogs will eat. This will help to minimize aerophagia.

Consideration should also be given to using long-term prokinetic agents to aid gastric motility in these patients, such as metoclopramide (0.25–0.5 mg/kg orally, s.c. q8h), ranitidine (2 mg/kg orally, s.c. q12h), cisapride (0.1–0.5 mg/kg orally q8–12h) or low-dose erythromycin (0.5–1.0 mg/kg orally q8h with food).

The key to successful management of acute GDV is prompt stabilization followed by surgery to create a gastropexy. Failure to create a gastropexy will almost inevitably lead to recurrence.

Prophylactic gastropexy

As a consequence of the success of gastropexy in preventing recurrence of GD and GDV, it would appear logical to offer prophylactic gastropexy in those breeds or lines that are most at risk from GD/GDV. In bitches, such a procedure could be readily carried out at the same time as a routine ovariectomy or ovariohysterectomy.

However, the risks of occurrence of GDV need to be weighed against the risks of anaesthesia and elective surgery in an otherwise healthy animal. From a surgeon's and an anaesthetist's point of view, there is less risk in carrying out an elective procedure than emergency surgery on a GDV patient. Some concerns have been expressed that gastropexy may significantly alter gastric motility, owing to the repositioning of the stomach. The work by Mathon *et al.* (2009) showed that there was minimal disruption to gastric motility and emptying 10 weeks post surgery.

Ward *et al.* (2003) sought to quantify the risks *versus* benefits of prophylactic gastropexy. The data presented only pertained to the USA and considered the lifetime probability or risk of a dog dying from GDV, against the expected cost-effectiveness of prophylactic gastropexy. The conclusion was that, although prophylactic gastropexy reduced mortality from GDV, it was a cost-effective procedure only in very high-risk patients. There are also ethical issues when considering carrying out such a prophylactic procedure but these are beyond the scope of this chapter.

Laparoscopic and laparoscopic-assisted gastropexy have gained popularity (Hardie *et al.*, 1996; Rawlings *et al.*, 2002; Runge *et al.*, 2009). These minimally invasive techniques offer an alternative to open abdominal surgery, with a lower postoperative morbidity (Runge *et al.*, 2009).

Chronic gastric dilatation

Chronic GD is an increasingly recognized condition in the GDV 'at risk' breeds. The clinical signs are often vague and varied. The problems arise as a result of chronic dilatation, with or without partial volvulus. The degree of dilatation and volvulus does not cause the acute crisis discussed above, but some cases will proceed to develop acute GDV.

This condition is often seen in underweight dogs suffering from excessive borborygmi and flatulence; they may also have intermittent bouts of vomiting and diarrhoea. Clinical examination is often unrewarding but patients may have borborygmi, and gastric tympany may be noted on percussion of the cranial abdomen. Diagnosis is usually made using radiography: these patients have large gastric shadows filled with gas and fluid; occasionally the pylorus is noted to be displaced dorsally. Barium studies show delayed gastric outflow in some cases (Paris *et al.*, 2011).

Treatment

Management of chronic GD requires derotation (there is often a 90-degree rotation of the stomach) and a right-sided gastropexy. If the patient's stomach is grossly distended and flaccid, the author carries out partial gastric resection (with some success). Recurrence following these procedures is rare (Paris *et al.*, 2011). Postoperatively these patients should be fed three to four times a day and placed on a prokinetic agent.

References and further reading

Baltzer WI, McMichael MA, Ruaux CG *et al.* (2006) Measurement of urinary 11-dehydro-thromboxane B2 excretion in dogs with gastric dilatation-volvulus. *American Journal of Veterinary Research* **67(1)**, 78–83

Beer KAS, Syring RS and Drobatz KJ (2013) Evaluation of plasma lactate concentration and base excess at the time of hospital admission as predictors of gastric necrosis, and outcome and correlation between those variables in dogs with gastric dilatation–volvulus: 78 cases (2004–2009). *Journal of the American Veterinary Medical Association* **242(1)**, 54–58

Buber T, Saragusty J, Ranen E *et al.* (2007) Evaluation of lidocaine treatment and risk factors for death associated with gastric dilatation and volvulus in dogs: 112 cases (1997–2005). *Journal of the American Veterinary Medical Association* **230(9)**, 1334–1339

De Papp E, Drobatz KJ and Hughes D (1999) Plasma lactate concentrations as a predictor of gastric necrosis and survival among dogs with gastric dilatation-volvulus: 102 cases (1995–1998). *Journal of the American Veterinary Medical Association* **215**, 49–52

Dujowich M, Keller ME and Reimer SB (2010) Evaluation of short- and long-term complications after endoscopically assisted gastropexy in dogs. *Journal of the American Veterinary Medical Association* **236(2)**, 177–182

Elwood CM (1998) Risk factors for gastric dilatation in Irish Setter dogs. *Journal of Small Animal Practice* **39**, 185–190

Glickman LT, Glickman LW, Perez CM, Schellenberg DB and Lantz GC (1994) Analysis of risk factors for gastric dilatation and dilatation-volvulus in dogs. *Journal of the American Veterinary Medical Association* **204**, 465–471

Glickman LT, Glickman NW, Schellenberg DB *et al.* (2000) Incidence of and breed-related risk factors for gastric dilatation-volvulus in dogs. *Journal of the American Veterinary Medical Association* **216(1)**, 40–45

Glickman LT, Lantz GC, Schellenberg DB and Glickman NW (1998) A prospective study of survival and recurrence following the acute gastric dilatation-volvulus syndrome in 136 dogs. *Journal of the American Animal Hospital Association* **34**, 253–259

Green JL, Cimino Brown D and Agnello KA (2012) Preoperative thoracic radiographic findings in dogs presenting for gastric dilatation-volvulus (2000–2010): 101 cases. *Journal of Veterinary Emergency and Critical Care* **22(5)**, 595–600

Green TI, Tonozzi CC, Kirby R and Rudloff E (2011) Evaluation of initial plasma lactate values as a predictor of gastric necrosis and initial and subsequent plasma lactate values as a predictor of survival in dogs with gastric dilatation–volvulus: 84 dogs (2003–2007). *Journal of Veterinary Emergency and Critical Care* **21(1)**, 36–44

Hardie RJ, Flanders JA, Schmidt P *et al.* (1996) Biomechanical and histological evaluation of a laparoscopic stapled gastropexy technique in dogs. *Veterinary Surgery* **25**, 127–133

Mackenzie G, Barnhart M, Kennedy S, DeHoff W and Schertel E (2010) A retrospective study of factors influencing survival following surgery for gastric dilatation-volvulus syndrome in 306 dogs. *Journal of the American Animal Hospital Association* **46(2)**, 97–102

Mathon DH, Dossin O, Palierne S *et al.* (2009) A laparoscopic-sutured gastropexy technique in dogs: mechanical and functional evaluation. *Veterinary Surgery* **38(8)**, 967–974

Paris JK, Yool DA, Reed N *et al.* (2011) Chronic gastric instability and presumed incomplete volvulus in dogs. *Journal of Small Animal Practice* **52(12)**, 651–655

Pipan M, Brown DC, Battaglia CL and Otto CM (2012) An Internet-based survey of risk factors for surgical gastric dilatation-volvulus in dogs. *Journal of the American Veterinary Medical Association* **240(12)**, 1456–1462

Psatha E, Alibhai HIK, Jimenez-Lozano A, Armitage-Chan E and Brodbelt DC (2011) Clinical efficacy and cardiorespiratory effects of alfaxalone, or diazepam/fentanyl for induction of anaesthesia in dogs that are a poor anaesthetic risk. *Veterinary Anaesthesia and Analgesia* **38(1)**, 24–36

Rawlings CA, Mahaffey MB, Bement S and Canalis C (2002) Prospective evaluation of laparoscopic-assisted gastropexy in dogs susceptible to gastric dilatation. *Journal of the American Veterinary Medical Association* **221**, 1576–1581

Runge J, Mayhew P and Rawlings C (2009) Surgical views – laparoscopic-assisted and laparoscopic prophylactic gastropexy: indications and techniques. *Compendium on Continuing Education for the Practicing Veterinarian* **31(2)**, 58–65

Schertel ER, Allen DA, Muir WW, Brourman JD and DeHoff WD (1997) Evaluation of a hypertonic saline-dextran solution for treatment of dogs with shock induced by gastric dilatation-volvulus. *Journal of the American Veterinary Medical Association* **210**, 226–230

Schober KE, Cornand C, Kirback B, Apperle H and Oechtering G (2002) Serum cardiac troponin I and cardiac troponin T concentrations in dog with gastric dilatation–volvulus. *Journal of the American Veterinary Medical Association* **221**, 381–388

Seymour C and Duke-Novakovski T (2007) *BSAVA Manual of Canine and Feline Anaesthesia and Analgesia, 2nd edn.* BSAVA Publications, Gloucester

Ward MP, Patronek GJ and Glickman LT (2003) Benefits of prophylactic gastropexy for dogs at risk of gastric dilatation-volvulus. *Preventive Veterinary Medicine* **60**, 319–329

Winkler KP, Greenfield CL and Schaeffer DJ (2003) Bacteremia and bacterial translocation in the naturally occurring canine gastric dilatation–volvulus patient. *Journal of the American Animal Hospital Association* **39**, 361–368

Zacher LA, Berg J, Shaw SP and Kudej RK (2010) Association between outcome and changes in plasma lactate concentration during presurgical treatment in dogs with gastric dilatation–volvulus: 64 cases (2002–2008). *Journal of the American Veterinary Medical Association* **236(8)**, 892–897

OPERATIVE TECHNIQUE 6.1

Tube gastropexy

POSITIONING

Dorsal recumbency.

ASSISTANT

Not required but useful.

EQUIPMENT EXTRAS

Balfour abdominal retractor; large abdominal swabs; Crile forceps.

SURGICAL TECHNIQUE

Approach

Routine midline abdominal incision.

Surgical manipulations

1 Make a subcutaneous tunnel by means of blunt dissection with long artery forceps, from a stab incision in the skin lateral to the laparotomy wound and caudal to the last rib on the right.

2 Draw a Foley catheter through the tunnel into the abdominal cavity.

3 Pre-place a purse-string suture (2 metric (3/0 USP) polydioxanone or glycomer 610) in the wall of the pyloric antrum and make a stab incision within the suture into the gastric lumen.

4 Place the Foley catheter into the stomach, inflate the balloon and tighten the purse-string suture.

5 Wrap the omentum around the Foley catheter.

6 Apply traction to the Foley catheter to draw the pyloric antrum into firm contact with the abdominal wall and use an absorbable synthetic suture material to suture the gastric serosa to the abdominal wall.

7 Fix the Foley catheter in place with a Roman Sandal suture pattern or zinc oxide butterfly tapes.

→ **OPERATIVE TECHNIQUE 6.1 CONTINUED**

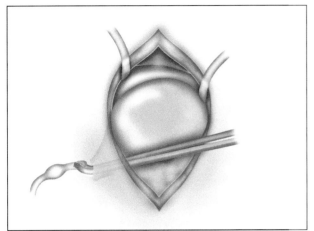

Foley catheter being drawn into the abdominal cavity.

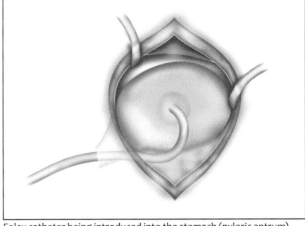

Foley catheter being introduced into the stomach (pyloric antrum) after pre-placing a purse-string suture.

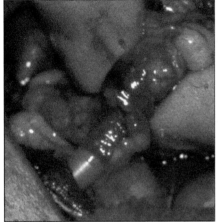

Omentum wrapped around the catheter.
(© John Williams)

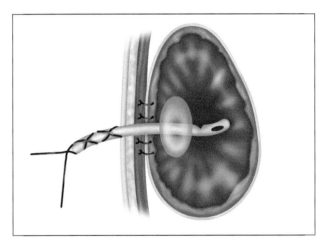

Relative positions of the catheter, stomach and body wall.

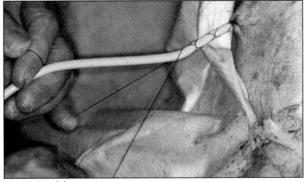

Roman Sandal suture.
(© John Williams)

Wound closure

Routine abdominal closure is performed.

POSTOPERATIVE MANAGEMENT

The tube can be removed 5–7 days after placement. The bulb of the Foley catheter is deflated and the tube is pulled out. The small hole in the body wall will granulate closed in 24 hours.

• Complications include premature dislodgement and inflammation around the stoma.

OPERATIVE TECHNIQUE 6.2

Belt loop gastropexy

POSITIONING

Dorsal recumbency.

ASSISTANT

Not essential, but useful until the surgeon becomes experienced with the technique.

EQUIPMENT EXTRAS

Balfour abdominal retractor; large abdominal swabs.

SURGICAL TECHNIQUE

Approach

Routine midline abdominal incision.

Surgical manipulations

1 Create a tongue of seromuscular tissue from the stomach wall over the pyloric antrum (the author tries to incorporate at least two short gastric arteries).

2 Make two parallel incisions in the transversus muscle of the abdominal wall, caudal to the costal arch.

3 Create a tunnel, wider than the flap, by blunt dissection with long artery forceps.

4 Gently draw the seromuscular pedicle through the tunnel by means of stay sutures or Babcock forceps, and suture it into its original bed in the gastric wall. Anchor the pedicle in place with simple interrupted 2 or 3 metric (3/0 or 2/0 USP) sutures using a monofilament synthetic suture material. Absorbable suture materials such as polydioxanone, glycomer 631 or polyglyconate, or non-absorbable polypropylene are suitable choices.

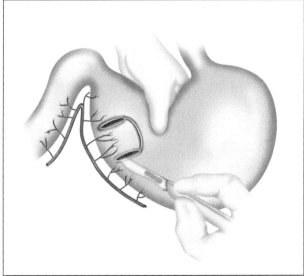

A tongue of seromuscular tissue is created from the stomach wall over the pyloric antrum, incorporating two short gastric arteries.

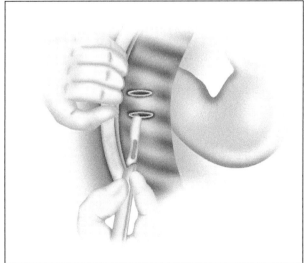

Two parallel incisions are made in the transversus muscle of the abdominal wall, caudal to the costal arch; a tunnel, wider than the flap, is created by blunt dissection with artery forceps.

→ **OPERATIVE TECHNIQUE 6.2 CONTINUED**

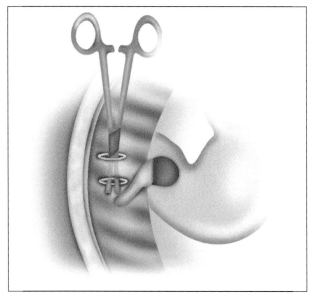

The seromuscular pedicle is drawn gently through the tunnel with Babcock forceps.

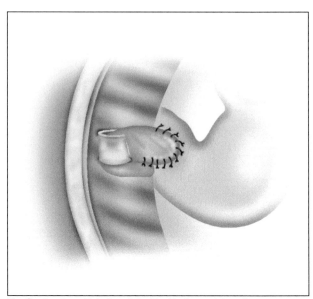

The flap is sutured into its original bed in the gastric wall.

Wound closure

Routine abdominal closure is performed.

OPERATIVE TECHNIQUE 6.3

Incisional gastropexy

POSITIONING

Dorsal recumbency.

ASSISTANT

Not essential but useful until the surgeon becomes experienced with the technique.

EQUIPMENT EXTRAS

Balfour abdominal retractor; large abdominal swabs.

SURGICAL TECHNIQUE

Approach

Routine midline abdominal incision.

Surgical manipulations

1   An incision 4–5 cm long is made through the seromuscular layer of the pyloric antrum (taking care not to penetrate through the submucosa) and a similar incision is made through the peritoneum into the transversus abdominis muscle 6–8 cm from the laparotomy wound edge on the right.

→

➜ **OPERATIVE TECHNIQUE 6.3 CONTINUED**

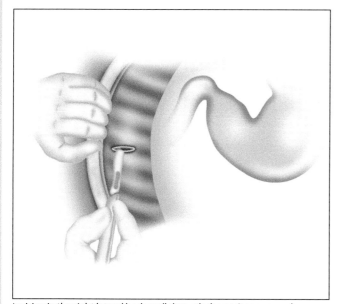

Incision in the right lateral body wall through the peritoneum and transversus abdominis muscle.

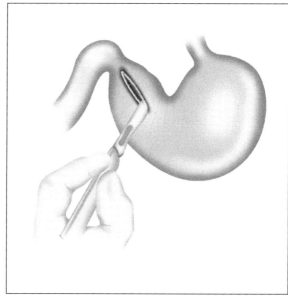

Partial thickness incision in the pyloric antrum.

2   The wound edges are sutured together using 2 or 3 metric (3/0 or 2/0 USP) monofilament absorbable suture material. The two cranial incisions are sutured together first and then the two caudal incisions.

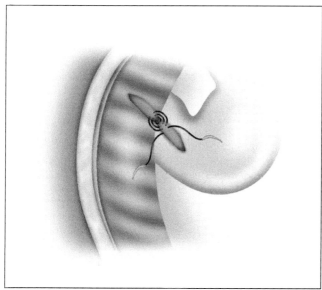

Suturing the gastric incision edges to the edges of the body wall incision with a simple continuous suture pattern (the caudal edges are sutured in the same manner).

Wound closure

Routine abdominal closure is performed.

Chapter 7

The small intestine

Alison Moores

Surgery of the small intestine is commonly performed in small animals. Both the oesophagus and stomach are larger and more distensible than the small intestine, so foreign bodies are more likely to become lodged in the small intestine, particularly the duodenum and jejunum. The greater size of the large intestine means that a foreign body that can pass through the small intestine is likely to be excreted. Enterotomy is more commonly performed that enterectomy. Whilst tumours are less common than foreign bodies, they are almost exclusively treated by enterectomy. Intestinal surgery is also performed for diagnostic purposes (full-thickness biopsy) in animals with intestinal disease, for the placement of feeding tubes and for treating other intestinal diseases (e.g. intussusception and torsion).

Anatomy

A thorough knowledge of all the anatomy within the abdominal cavity is essential as exposure is usually limited. A systematic exploration of the entire abdominal cavity should be carried out whenever intestinal surgery is performed. The small intestine, the longest part of the digestive tract, measures approximately three and a half times the body length, in both dogs and cats. The small intestine is tethered by mesentery arising from the mesenteric root, from which the cranial mesenteric artery and vein, intestinal lymphatics and a large mesenteric nerve plexus arborise. The small intestine grossly comprises the relatively immobile duodenum, the long and mobile jejunum and the short ileum.

Duodenum

The duodenum is approximately 25 cm long. It is a continuation of the pylorus of the stomach, the first portion being the cranial duodenal flexure in the right cranial quadrant of the abdomen at the ninth intercostal space. The duodenum courses caudally before turning in a cranial direction at the caudal duodenal flexure, at the level of the fifth or sixth lumbar vertebra, although its position changes depending upon colonic and bladder filling. Cranially the duodenum lies adjacent to the liver and pancreas, with the right limb of the pancreas lying within the short mesoduodenum adjacent to the duodenum. The duodenocolic ligament attaches the duodenum at the caudal duodenal flexure to the colon, and it must be transected for the caudal duodenum to be mobilized. Pancreatic ducts and the common bile duct enter the duodenum. Two pancreatic ducts are present in 75% of dogs. The larger accessory duct opens into the

duodenum, 8 cm caudal to the pylorus, at the minor duodenal papilla. The smaller pancreatic duct may be absent, but where present, opens with the common bile duct on the major duodenal papilla, 3 cm cranial to the minor duodenal papilla. In cats, the pancreatic duct and common bile duct open on the major duodenal papilla; only about 20% of cats have an accessory pancreatic duct, which opens at a minor duodenal papilla 2 cm caudal to the major papilla. The duodenal blood supply is from the cranial and caudal pancreaticoduodenal arteries, arising from the coeliac and cranial mesenteric arteries, respectively.

Jejunum

The duodenum continues as the jejunum to the left of the root of the mesentery in the cranial abdomen. The jejuno-ileum is the longest part of the small intestine (250 cm in an average sized dog) and forms a series of loops around the root of the mesentery. The mesentery is long, allowing relative jejunal and ileal mobility. It contains the cranial mesenteric vessels, lymphatics and the mesenteric nerve plexus. The jejunum is in contact with the majority of abdominal organs, but rarely extends to the pelvic cavity. It is covered ventrally and laterally by the omentum. The cranial mesenteric artery gives off the ileocolic and caudal pancreaticoduodenal arteries before branching into 12–15 jejunal arcadial arteries, which in turn branch into terminal arcadial arteries (Figure 7.1). The latter supply the jejunum via multiple vasa recti that penetrate and supply all layers of the intestinal wall.

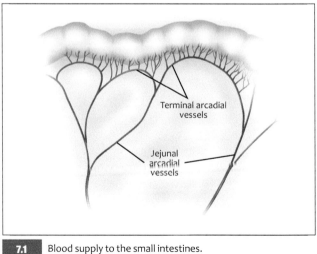

Terminal arcadial vessels

Jejunal arcadial vessels

7.1 Blood supply to the small intestines.

Ileum

The ileum is the terminal 15 cm of the small intestine. Its only gross characteristic is an antimesenteric ileal vessel within the ileocolic fold, the artery arising from the ileocaecal artery and anastomosing with the last jejunal artery. The mesenteric ileal artery is a branch of the ileocolic and last jejunal arteries. The ileum is otherwise grossly the same as the jejunum. It joins the large intestine at the ileocolic valve.

Blood supply, lymphatic drainage and innervation

The blood supply is from the pancreaticoduodenal arteries (the cranial pancreaticoduodenal artery is a branch of the hepatic artery from the coeliac artery; the caudal pancreaticoduodenal artery is from the cranial mesenteric artery) and the jejunal and ileal arteries (both from the cranial mesenteric artery), which branch to form a network of interconnecting blood vessels, and the corresponding veins.

Lymphatic drainage from the duodenum is to the hepatic and duodenal lymph nodes. Drainage from the jejunum and ileum is into the right and left mesenteric lymph nodes, with additional drainage from the ileum to the colic lymph nodes. Innervation of the duodenum is via the thoracolumbar ganglia and distal ganglia. Nerve supply to the jejunoileum is via the vagus nerve (from the coeliac plexus) and splanchnic nerve (from the cranial mesenteric plexus).

Layers of the intestinal wall

The wall of the intestine comprises the mucosa, submucosa, muscularis and serosa. The mucosa consists of columnar and goblet cells that form a protective barrier, glands and lymphoid tissue, including lymphoid follicles (Peyer's patches), which appear as circumscribed elevations visible at the serosal surface. They can be quite prominent and are more numerous in the duodenum and proximal jejunum. The mucosa has tight enterocyte junctions and a layer of mucus along the brush border. Enterocyte health is critical to the maintenance of this mucosal barrier, as well as for secretion and absorption. The presence of the villi mean there is an 8.5 times greater area of mucosa than serosa, which contributes to mucosal eversion during enteric surgery. The submucosa consists of loose but strong connective tissue, which binds the mucosa and muscularis together and contains blood vessels and nerves.

> **PRACTICAL TIP**
>
> The submucosa is the strongest layer of the intestinal wall and it is essential that it is incorporated in sutures for maximal wound strength

The muscularis consists of longitudinal and circular muscle layers that contract sequentially to give peristaltic waves for the propulsion of intestinal chyme. The serosa consists of peritoneum but is not present at the mesenteric attachments, on the antimesenteric side of the terminal ileum, the duodenocolic ligament or the reflection to the pancreas.

Intestinal healing

Intestinal wounds rapidly gain strength, though healing can be delayed by a number of factors in compromised animals (Figure 7.2). The surgeon must recognize and address these factors or risk high morbidity and mortality due to wound dehiscence and subsequent peritonitis.

Factor	Examples
Hypovolaemia/shock	Major trauma
Hypoproteinaemia/hypoalbuminaemia	Peritonitis, protein-losing enteropathy
Severe anaemia	Haemoabdomen
Massive blood transfusion (reported)	
Concurrent infection	Peritonitis
Immunosuppression	Exogenous corticosteroids, hyperadrenocorticism
Metabolic/endocrine disorders	Diabetes mellitus, hepatic disease, renal disease
Malnutrition	

7.2 Host factors affecting wound healing in the intestine.

Healing in the gastrointestinal tract is relatively fast and is arbitrarily divided into three phases, but as with all physiological events there is overlap between these, and the divisions are there for ease of understanding:

- **Lag phase:** Begins on the first day and continues for 3 to 4 days. During this phase, macrophages invade the wound. These are essential for wound debridement and for delivering and stimulating the cytokines that facilitate fibroplasia and angiogenesis. The resulting fibrin clot has minimal strength in holding wound edges together, but does help to minimize leakage. By day 3, epithelial migration will have occurred, sealing the wound. This is the most critical phase of healing and dehiscence/breakdown are most likely to occur during the first 72–96 hours, as the fibrin seal is weakened by fibrinolysis. All support and strength of the wound at this stage comes from the sutures
- **Proliferative phase:** Occurs from day 3 or 4 through to day 14. During this phase there is a proliferation of fibroblasts and a marked increase in the production of immature collagen, resulting in a rapid gain in wound-bursting strength. By day 14 post-suturing, wound strength will have reached normal levels
- **Maturation phase:** This phase is of little clinical importance and continues from day 14 to about day 180, during which time there is reorganization and remodelling as the collagen fibres are selectively resorbed or form important crosslinks; this process is dependent on intramural tension.

Omentum

Omental pedicle wraps (omentoplasty) have long been used to reinforce gastrointestinal wounds and their use in veterinary surgery has been well described. The primary benefit of omentum is to stimulate and augment angiogenesis. It also helps to reduce wound 'leak rates' and increase wound-bursting strength. However, recent human studies have cast some doubts on the value of omentum in augmenting wound healing (Williams, 2012). Despite doubts, the potential benefits of omentoplasty outweigh the potential risks, and it remains prudent to reinforce any intestinal wound with omentum.

Pathophysiology of obstruction

Obstruction may be partial or complete and involve the proximal or distal small intestine. It may be intraluminal (e.g. foreign body or intramural neoplasia) or extramural (e.g. extraluminal neoplasia or strangulation). Most clinical cases are due to intraluminal obstruction. Distensibility of the intestinal wall may be reduced in the presence of intramural tumours, contributing to obstruction. Clinical signs are more acute and severe for proximal and/or complete obstructions than distal or partial obstructions.

Complete obstruction leads to the accumulation of fluid and gas within the intestinal lumen, due to the retention of ingested fluid and gas, production of upper gastrointestinal tract secretions and failure of fluid absorption in the distal small intestine (Figure 7.3). Increased intestinal intraluminal pressure from fluid and gas interferes with blood flow within the intestinal wall and mucosal ischaemia occurs, although full-thickness necrosis does not typically occur in dilated small intestine proximal to an obstruction. Blood flow to the intestine at the site of the obstruction may be sufficiently compromised by marked distension and direct pressure to cause full-thickness necrosis. Bacterial overgrowth occurs due to stasis of the small intestine. In the presence of mucosal injury, there may be migration of bacteria and bacterial toxins into the blood and peritoneum, leading to septicaemia or septic peritonitis.

> **WARNING**
>
> Just 6 hours of stasis leads to a dramatic increase in the bacterial population of the small intestine

In addition, strangulated small intestine is associated with obstruction or thrombosis of one or both of the venous and arterial blood supply (Figure 7.4). It may occur due to intussusception, mesenteric avulsion, entrapment within a diaphragmatic or body wall hernia, mesenteric tear or between intestinal adhesions. Large areas of intestine will be involved if the cranial mesenteric or multiple jejunal vessels are affected. Venous obstruction initially results in intestinal wall oedema, haemorrhage and mucosal epithelial sloughing, before progressing to full-thickness wall necrosis. Necrosis occurs rapidly with arterial occlusion. Bacterial overgrowth and toxin production is rapid and loss of the mucosal barrier is more complete and rapid than with simple obstruction, leading to earlier toxaemia, septicaemia and septic peritonitis. Following the correction of strangulation, the release of oxygen-derived free radicals leads to reperfusion injury, with the majority of tissue damage occurring within 5 minutes.

Vomiting is the most common clinical sign of obstruction and intestinal hyperactivity may lead to abdominal pain. Animals with complete or proximal obstruction are more likely to be dehydrated or hypovolaemic. Untreated obstructions will lead to hypovolaemia and/or septic shock with death occurring after 3–4 days. For partial or distal obstructions, clinical signs are milder and may comprise intermittent vomiting, inappetence, weight loss and diarrhoea.

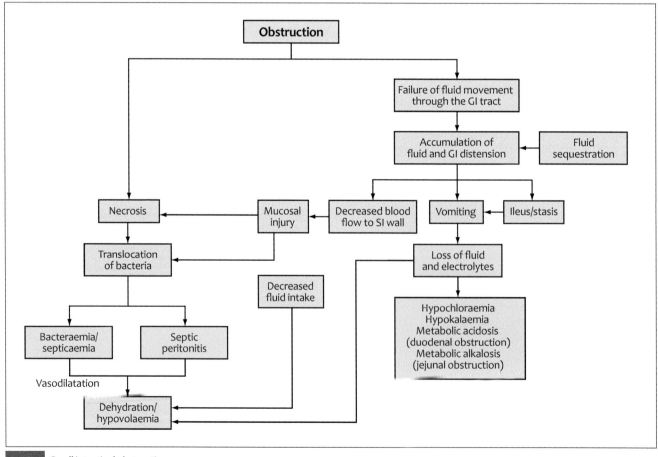

7.3 Small intestinal obstruction.

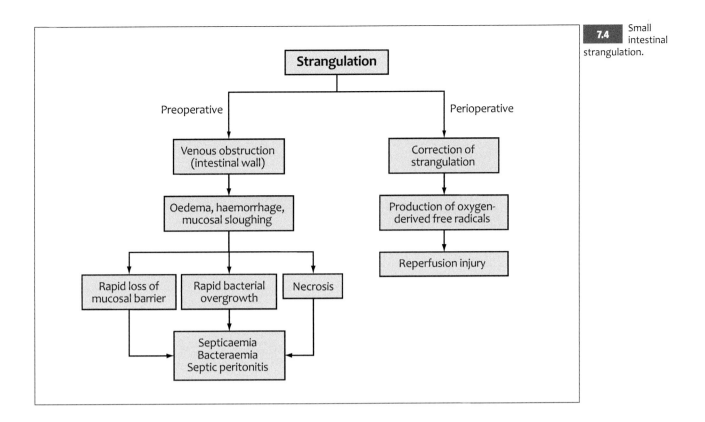

7.4 Small intestinal strangulation.

Diagnostic techniques

Obtaining a good history is an essential diagnostic tool for small intestinal disease. The veterinary surgeon (veterinarian) should ask specific questions relating to recent dietary changes, character of the stool or vomitus, any current medications, access to toys, rubbish or laundry, and the character of the dog (e.g. tendency to chew), which may help indicate a cause for the current problem. The severity and timescale of the clinical signs should be noted; this may distinguish between a partial obstruction or a complete proximal or distal obstruction.

Clinical signs of small intestinal disease include vomiting, anorexia, dehydration, abdominal pain or discomfort, weight loss, depression/lethargy and shock (Figure 7.5). These signs are variable, non-specific and similar in presentation to many other diseases (Figure 7.6).

Abdominal auscultation and palpation are useful diagnostic tools. Decreased borborygmi and abdominal pain may be noted or a palpable lesion located. However, many animals with small intestinal obstruction will not have any detectable abnormality on abdominal palpation and auscultation.

> **WARNING**
>
> A patient presenting with clinical signs of an acute abdomen (including intractable, persistent vomiting or retching, abdominal pain, abdominal distension, weakness, recumbency or signs of circulatory shock) is suggestive of a crisis that requires simultaneous diagnostic testing and aggressive stabilizing management, followed by surgery

Signs	Complete proximal obstruction	Complete distal obstruction	Partial obstruction
Onset of signs	Within 24 hours	Several days	Several days
Vomiting	Frequent, severe	Less frequent	Occasional
Anorexia	Yes	Variable initially	Variable
Dehydration	Yes; severe	Yes; variable	Variable
Weight loss	No (unless due to dehydration)	Often	Often
Diarrhoea	No	No	Often; may be mucoid; melaena
Depression/lethargy	Yes	Yes	Usually; mild
Shock	Yes	Variable	Not usually
Abdominal discomfort	Often	Variable	Not usually; may be mild
Electrolytes; acid–base	Hypokalaemia, hypochloraemia, acidosis (very proximal obstructions may have alkalosis initially)	Variable; usually acidosis	Variable; may be normal

7.5 Clinical signs of small intestinal obstruction. Note: Intestinal volvulus, strangulation and ischaemia of the small intestine present with acute signs and impending cardiovascular collapse due to shock. Early perforation may not manifest acutely for several hours but will then deteriorate rapidly.

Disease	Examples
Partial obstruction	Neoplasia; foreign body; intussusception
Malabsorption/maldigestion	Lymphoma; irritable bowel disease; lymphangiectasia
Hepatic disease	Neoplasia; portosystemic shunts
Renal disease	Pyelonephritis; renal failure
Pancreatic disease	Insufficiency; inflammation
Hyperadrenocorticism	Adrenal cortical carcinoma or pituitary adenoma
Hypoadrenocorticism	Atrophy or immune-mediated destruction
Intoxication	Lead

7.6 Differential diagnoses for cats and dogs presenting with vomiting, diarrhoea and weight loss.

Minimum database

Routine haematology, serum biochemistry, blood gas analysis (if available) and urinalysis should be performed. These tests will help rule out other conditions that present with gastrointestinal signs such as vomiting, diarrhoea and weight loss (see Figure 7.6). Initial laboratory data also establish baselines and provide guidance for therapy to correct fluid, electrolyte and acid–base abnormalities.

Classically described changes on biochemistry include hypokalaemia, hypochloraemia and metabolic alkalosis for proximal complete obstruction (e.g. in the proximal duodenum) and mild metabolic acidosis for mid and distal small intestinal obstruction. However, hypokalaemia, hypochloraemia and metabolic alkalosis are common findings regardless of the site of obstruction. Dehydration is typical but will be more rapid and severe with proximal and complete obstruction.

Imaging
Radiography

Abdominal radiography is a useful and commonly used technique in general practice for the diagnosis of small intestinal disease. Survey radiographs (lateral and ventrodorsal (VD) views) must be taken before using any contrast medium. Plain radiographs may demonstrate distended gas-filled loops of intestine, a mass effect (displacement of viscera by a space-occupying lesion), herniation through the body wall, presence of peritoneal fluid (ground glass effect), the presence of free gas in the abdomen or a radiopaque foreign body. Small intestinal obstruction is confirmed radiographically by comparing the luminal diameter to the height of the body of the fifth lumbar vertebra at its narrowest point (Graham *et al.*, 1998) (Figure 7.7). A ratio of 1.6 is considered the upper limit for normal small intestinal diameter, and a ratio of ≥1.95 gives a >80% chance of an obstruction being present.

When plain radiographs are inconclusive, contrast radiography can be considered. Barium sulphate suspension (10 ml/kg of a 1:3 barium:water dilution) is routinely used as a contrast agent, unless intestinal perforation is suspected. A barium study can reveal information with respect to transit time and changes to the intestine wall (e.g. mucosal integrity, thickening of the wall, luminal occlusion), although ultrasonography is now regarded as more sensitive for assessing mural anatomy. Radiographs should be obtained immediately after administration of the contrast

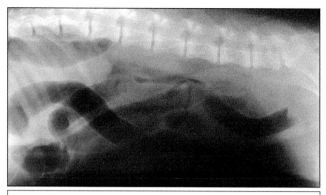
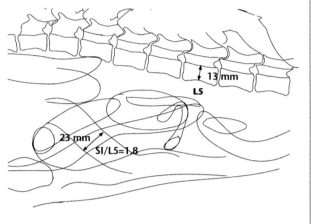

7.7 Radiographic diagnosis of small intestinal obstruction. (Reproduced from Graham *et al.* (1998) with permission from the *Journal of Small Animal Practice*)

medium and then every 15 minutes for the first hour, then every 45–60 minutes until the contrast medium reaches the colon. The frequency of radiography can be changed according to the rate of passage of contrast medium in each case.

Gastric emptying should begin within 30 minutes and the stomach should be fairly empty within 1–2 hours. The contrast medium should have reached the colon within 4–6 hours following oral administration. It is often useful to take a 24-hour post-administration radiograph to confirm that all the contrast medium has reached the colon. A water-soluble positive contrast agent, such as iohexol, can be used if the integrity of the bowel is debatable, although its efficacy is questionable. However, it is better practice to use ultrasonography and peritoneal fluid analysis in cases of suspected perforation (see Chapter 18).

Ultrasonography

Abdominal ultrasonography is extremely useful in diagnosing conditions of the small intestines. It allows assessment of intestinal wall thickness and is now recognized as a more precise modality for identifying obstructive lesions in the hands of an experienced diagnostic imager, than radiography. It is particularly sensitive in identifying linear foreign bodies. Intestinal masses can be isolated and aspirated under ultrasound guidance. Intussusceptions demonstrate characteristic repeated concentric rings, giving a 'target' or 'bull's eye' effect on ultrasonography.

Advanced imaging

Computed tomography (CT) and magnetic resonance imaging (MRI) can also be used to investigate small intestinal disease.

Endoscopy

Endoscopy can be used to assess duodenal lesions and, very occasionally, proximal jejunal conditions; biopsy samples are limited to the mucosa. The ileum can be examined via colonoscopy, by an experienced endoscopist. The reader is referred to the *BSAVA Manual of Canine and Feline Endoscopy and Endosurgery* for more information.

Abdominocentesis

Abdominocentesis may be useful for diagnosing conditions of the small intestine (see Chapter 18 for further details).

Preoperative considerations

Small intestinal surgery may be contaminated or clean-contaminated, depending upon whether there is leakage of gastrointestinal contents into the peritoneal cavity. Intestinal surgery is dirty if there is intestinal perforation, in the presence of abscesses or if there is septic peritonitis.

Antibiotic therapy

Antibiotic prophylaxis is not necessary for clean-contaminated surgery (i.e. incision of the small intestinal wall without spillage) of <90 minutes. Examples include small intestinal biopsy and simple solid foreign body removal, where the intestinal wall is not compromised. Spillage of intestinal contents is more likely to occur during removal of larger solid foreign bodies, linear foreign bodies, tumours, intussusceptions, where there is dilated intestine or when enterectomy is anticipated for another reason, so prophylactic antibiotics are indicated. Antibiotic use is therapeutic in the face of infection, such as septic peritonitis after intestinal rupture, and is indicated in cases of mesenteric volvulus or intestinal strangulation. The small intestine contains both Gram-negative and Gram-positive bacteria, so antibiotics must be broad-spectrum and appropriate for the bacteria of the small intestine. More information on antibiotic use is given in Chapter 1.

Anaesthesia and analgesia

The use of non-steroidal anti-inflammatory drugs (NSAIDs) is controversial in gastrointestinal surgery. Their use is typically avoided where mucosal vascularity is abnormal (e.g. after intestinal dilation or in the presence of gastrointestinal ulceration) or in hypovolaemic animals. However, NSAIDs may be initiated several days after surgery when the intestinal mucosal viability has improved. Alternative analgesia options include the use of opioids, lidocaine and ketamine (see the *BSAVA Manual of Canine and Feline Anaesthesia and Analgesia*).

Fluid therapy

Prior to surgery, fluids are used to replace fluid loss to the gastrointestinal tract and losses from vomiting. The goal of fluid therapy is to correct the fluid imbalance, which depends upon the severity of dehydration and hypovolaemia. Further information on the correction of fluid, electrolyte and acid–base abnormalities is given in Chapter 1.

Surgical techniques

Enterotomy and enterectomy

Enterotomy may be performed for the removal of solid or linear foreign bodies, or for intestinal biopsy. Indications for enterectomy and anastomosis include intestinal perforation, neoplasia, non-reducible intussusception and poor intestinal viability and/or necrosis. Surgical biopsy specimens may be preferred to endoscopic biopsy samples to differentiate neoplasia from inflammatory bowel disease, but are typically only obtained if the endoscopic samples are non-diagnostic. Biopsy incisions should be longitudinal or circular, and full-thickness, ensuring that an adequate amount of each intestinal wall layer is obtained. Enterotomy incisions for foreign body removal are longitudinal and on the antimesenteric border. Handling of the small intestine should be performed with care as inflamed or dilated intestinal wall may be more easily damaged than normal intestine.

Suturing techniques

The submucosa is the strongest layer of the intestinal wall and must therefore be incorporated by sutures to maximize wound healing. Simple appositional suture patterns (Figure 7.8) should be used as they lead to good submucosal apposition and primary healing, and whilst there is a degree of eversion and inversion seen histologically following appositional suturing, clinical results are good. Crushing or double-layer closures narrow the intestinal lumen and have poor submucosal apposition, so they heal by second intention, which is slower. Everting patterns

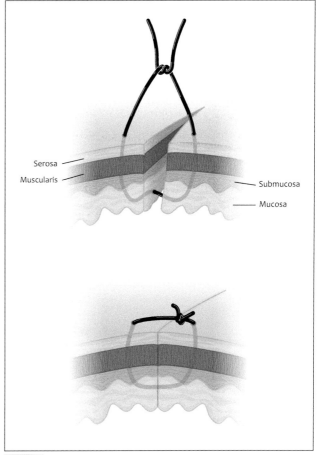

Serosa
Muscularis
Submucosa
Mucosa

7.8 Simple appositional suture pattern.

should be avoided as they may cause adhesions. A modified Gambee pattern (Figure 7.9) can help to evert the mucosa and avoid mucosal penetration by suture material. A continuous appositional suture pattern for closure of enterotomy or enterectomy incisions is a recognized alternative to simple interrupted sutures.

Sutures must be placed in viable intestine. There are no well described objective measurements of viability (Figure 7.10). The appearance of the intestine can improve following relief from an obstruction, so a period of 10–15 minutes should be allowed before making a definitive decision about resection. Obviously necrotic tissue is dark purple (Figure 7.11), brown, black or white, may be very thin, tears easily and does not bleed from cut surfaces. It is more difficult to assess intestine that has suffered minor vascular injury. Intestine that is haemorrhagic, deep red and has serosal tearing will actually be viable in most cases, and viable intestine will usually bleed from cut surfaces. Surgeons should be aware that seemingly viable tissue (Figure 7.12) may suffer ongoing vascular injury following surgery and may become non-viable, leading to

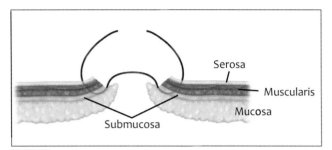

7.9 Modified Gambee suture.

Type of assessment	Parameters
Bowel wall colour	Pink, with refill = normal Deep red, purple = vascular compromise: reassess in 10 minutes and look at other parameters White, black or greenish = necrotic
Arterial pulsations	Prominent; pulsing of jejunal arcade should be easily detected Veins should fill immediately upon release of compression
Peristalsis	Sections of tightened white bowel, slowly transitioning back to normal Not a reliable parameter as ileus may be present
Bleeding from cut edge	Bright red brisk bleeding = normal Dark and sluggish oozing = vascular compromise: reassess in 10 minutes and look at other parameters
Intravenous fluorescein (10% solution): give 20 mg/kg i.v. and wait 2–3 minutes; view intestines with Wood's lamp in darkened room	Smooth green–yellow or fine granular pattern = adequate perfusion Patchy, blotchy, with areas >3 mm of non-fluorescence = inadequate perfusion Very accurate for detecting non-viable bowel; less accurate for detecting viable bowel (err on the side of caution, resect viable bowel rather than leave non-viable bowel behind) This test should be used only once in 24 hours
Doppler ultrasonic flow probe	Detects pulsatile blood flow within the intestinal wall Very accurate
Pulse oximetry	Measure oxygen saturation reliably and reproducibly

7.10 Assessment of intestinal viability.

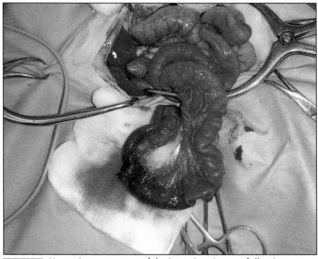

7.11 Necrotic appearance of the intestines in a cat following an intussusception and strangulation.

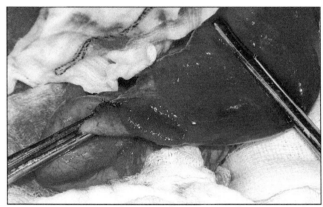

7.12 Enterotomy with suspected necrotic areas later converted to enterectomy.

intestinal wound dehiscence (see below). Given that failure to resect non-viable intestine will lead to wound dehiscence and septic peritonitis, it may be prudent to overestimate the length of intestine to be resected, unless there are concerns about short bowel syndrome (see below).

PRACTICAL TIP

Serosal tearing may occur when tying sutures in inflamed small intestine. It is not likely to lead to dehiscence as long as the submucosa is engaged, so can be left if the intestine is so inflamed that serosal tearing occurs in all portions of the small intestine. However, if submucosal tearing occurs, further resection of the affected intestine may be necessary to locate healthier tissues

Healing and gain in tensile strength is reduced in the presence of inflammation, which also degrades collagen, leading to weakening of sutured tissues.

Enteric closure is traditionally performed using small gauge (1.5–2 metric; 4/0–3/0 USP) simple interrupted appositional sutures on a swaged-on taper or taper-cut needle. Sutures are placed 3–5 mm from the wound edge to ensure that they engage the submucosa and to minimize the risk of tearing through the tissue, which would lead to dehiscence. Sutures are placed 3–5 mm apart. They are pulled tightly enough to appose the wound edges without crushing (Figure 7.13). Additional sutures are

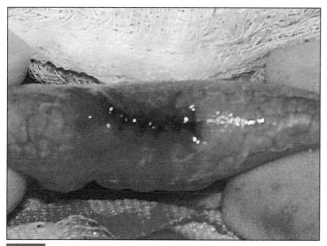

7.13 Sutured enterotomy.

placed as necessary. There is no difference in the gross or histological appearance of the jejunum sutured with monofilament or multifilament suture material, except that monofilament suture material tends to cause a more fibrous tissue reaction in the muscularis layer.

Typically, monofilament absorbable suture materials with prolonged tensile strength (i.e. the tensile strength of the suture material is maintained for longer than the time taken for the healing intestinal tissues to gain adequate tensile strength), such as polydioxanone, polyglyconate and poliglecaprone 25, are used. Multifilament suture materials may increase tissue drag, potentiate infection and increase inflammation. Permanent sutures can lead to foreign body attachment. Closure of enterotomy incisions using skin staples has been described experimentally, but is not routinely used and has not replaced suturing techniques. (For further information on suture materials, the reader is referred to Chapter 2.)

Stapling techniques

Surgical stapling techniques have been described for the resection and anastomosis of the small intestine, as well as for anastomosis of the small to the large intestine. The most common clinically used technique is the modified functional end-to-end anastomosis using either a gastrointestinal anastomosis (GIA) stapler or a thoracoabdominal (TA) stapler (see Operative Technique 7.6).

The main advantages of using a stapling technique are the ease with which intestine of different diameters can be anastomosed (e.g. when the oral portion is dilated

after intestinal obstruction or when anastomosing the small intestine to the colon), less manipulation, high reproducibility, high bursting strength and better strength during healing compared with suture material. The disadvantages of using a stapling technique are similar to those described for sutured anastomosis, with leakage, abscess formation and late foreign body obstruction at the stapled site having all been reported. Use of the GIA stapler is restricted to larger dogs in which the forks can enter the intestinal lumen; an endoscopic linear cutting stapler can be used in smaller dogs and cats. Cost may also limit the use of staplers, although this may be offset by reduced surgical times, especially where there is luminal disparity.

Jejunostomy tube placement

Jejunostomy tube placement (Figure 7.14) has been suggested for patients with pancreatic disease or where feeding into or oral to the stomach, duodenum or pancreas is contraindicated. Feeding directly into the jejunum may also allow earlier absorption of fluid than gastric feeding. Tubes can be used in the presence of septic peritonitis. Red rubber jejunostomy tubes are more secure than silicone tubes in cadaver models, but silicone is preferable in clinical cases as it is associated with less inflammation (Song *et al.*, 2008). Laparoscopic-assisted jejunostomy tube placement or a limited right flank approach for duodenotomy can be performed in dogs not requiring a coeliotomy.

The liquid diet can be fed intermittently or continuously through the tube. Liquid medication can also be administered via the tube. Tubes should be flushed regularly with water to prevent blockage, including before and after bolus feeds and the administration of liquid medication. Dressings should be changed daily and antibiotic ointment used if inflammation is noted. Animals should be prevented from interfering with the tube with the use of dressings and Elizabethan collars. Tubes should be removed when they are no longer needed, but ideally are left in place for at least 10 days to minimize the risk of peritonitis on tube removal. Tubes can be removed by traction following removal of the skin suture, and the tube site left to heal by second intention.

PRACTICAL TIP

Carbonated drinks can help to unblock tubes that cannot be cleared using water

---

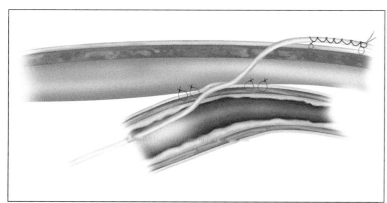

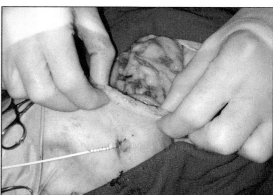

7.14 Final positioning for a jejunostomy tube.

Complications

Complication rates of 15–40% are reported in animals. Minor tube complications include patient interference with the tube, tube obstruction and difficulty in administering liquid food through the tube. Localized inflammation and/or cellulitus can be managed with local wound care, or tubes can be removed if they are no longer needed. Major complications include separation of the jejunum from the body wall, due to failure of the jejunopexy, leading to leakage of intestinal contents into the body wall (causing inflammation) or peritoneal cavity (leading to septic peritonitis), but rates of occurrence are low. Major complications may be related to inexperience with the technique.

Surgical conditions

Foreign bodies

Small intestinal foreign bodies account for 37–63% of all gastrointestinal obstructions in dogs and cats. Complete obstruction occurs in 70% of dogs and 42% of cats.

Solid foreign bodies

Solid foreign bodies, found in 63–84% of dogs and 67% of cats, are more common than linear foreign bodies. Over-represented breeds of dogs include English and Staffordshire Bull Terriers, Springer Spaniels, Border Collies and Jack Russell Terriers; affected dogs and cats are typically young. Most animals present with gastrointestinal signs, although some patients are presented after being seen to ingest foreign objects. Gastrointestinal foreign bodies or gastrointestinal abnormalities are reportedly palpable in 76% of dogs and 58% of cats (Hayes, 2009).

Ultrasonography is an appropriate diagnostic tool in the hands of an experienced ultrasonographer, as foreign bodies are visible within the small intestine and can be differentiated from intestinal masses. However, for most veterinary surgeons, radiography remains the main diagnostic tool. Enterectomy is required in 1–28% of cases, with fewer enterectomies being performed in a study from first-opinion practice than referral practice (Hayes, 2009). Mortality rates are higher with a longer duration of clinical signs, linear foreign bodies and the need for multiple intestinal incisions. Survival is not affected by the location of the obstruction or whether it is complete or partial. Survival rates for dogs and cats with solid foreign bodies was 94% and 100%, respectively, compared with 80% of dogs and 63% of cats surviving surgery for linear foreign bodies (Hayes, 2009). Another study reported a 99% survival rate for dogs and cats (Boag et al., 2005). The dehiscence rate is low (<5%) in animals treated in first-opinion practice and complications are rare and often minor.

> **PRACTICAL TIP**
>
> Some animals may have multiple sites of foreign body obstruction; the entire gastrointestinal tract must be examined at surgery

Linear foreign bodies

Linear foreign bodies may occur due to the ingestion of any long foreign material, ranging from thin pieces of cotton to thick material. Cats are more likely to ingest cotton and string, and the foreign body is more likely to anchor under the tongue (63% of cases). Dogs often ingest wide foreign bodies, such as fabric and plastic, and 67–78% of cases anchor at the pyloric antrum (Hayes, 2009). Normal peristaltic movements occur in an attempt to move what is perceived as intestinal contents in an aboral direction. Due to the anchored site, the intestine becomes bunched up around the foreign material (Figure 7.15). The length of intestine involved reflects the length of the foreign body and the time since ingestion.

> **PRACTICAL TIP**
>
> It is possible for linear foreign bodies to anchor in the small intestine

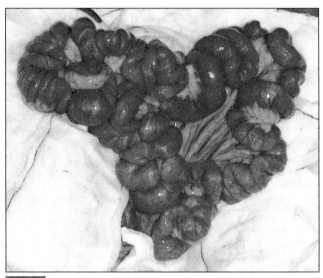

7.15 Plication of small intestines containing a linear foreign body.

Radiographic and ultrasonographic findings include intestinal plication and tapered gas bubbles. Pathophysiological consequences include partial or complete intestinal obstruction, perforation (often multiple) along the mesenteric border of the small intestine and adhesions. Repair of small defects can be performed. Enterectomy is required for large areas of perforation or adhesions that leave the small intestines plicated even after foreign body removal. A single enterotomy technique, using a catheter to 'feed' the foreign body along the intestine has been described (Anderson et al., 1992). This technique does not appear to be used commonly in practice, and is not suitable for wide linear bodies or those embedded in the mesenteric mucosa.

Intussusception

Intussusception is the invagination of a portion of the intestine (the intussusceptum) into the lumen of another (the intussuscipiens) (Figure 7.16). Small intestinal intussusception has been described in a retrograde direction (duodenogastric intussusception) or, more commonly, a normograde direction either into another portion of the small intestine or the large intestine. Gastroduodenal intussusception has been reported. The majority of intussusceptions involve the enterocolic junction in dogs and the small intestine in cats (Figure 7.17). A double intussusception may occur.

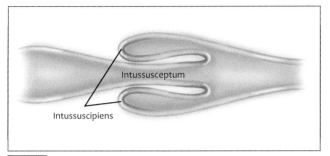

7.16 Intussusception.

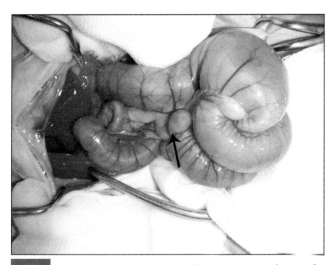

7.17 Intussusception at the enterocolic junction in a cat (arrowed).

Predisposing causes cannot always be established and most cases are idiopathic, although intussusceptions may be seen with intestinal masses or gastroenteritis. Cats have a bimodal age distribution, with underlying neoplasia (especially lymphoma) a common finding in older cats, whereas dogs are generally young and more likely to have inflammatory disease. Animals typically present with vomiting, haemorrhagic diarrhoea and abdominal pain. Diagnosis is based on clinical examination findings of a palpable abdominal mass and imaging findings (signs of an intestinal mass and/or obstruction on radiography, a 'target-like' mass on transverse ultrasonography and multiple hyperechoic or hypoechoic parallel lines on longitudinal ultrasonography). Spontaneous resolution of intussusceptions may occur, therefore repeat ultrasound examination is recommended after anaesthesia but before surgery. Colour Doppler ultrasonography in experienced hands is a useful measure for predicting reducibility, as blood flow is more likely with reducible intussusceptions.

At surgery, reduction should be attempted by pushing the intussusceptum from the intussuscipiens. However, it should be noted that pulling in reverse can lead to tearing. Recent intussusceptions can be manually reduced, but the affected intestine must be examined for viability of the intestinal wall and blood supply. More chronic intussusceptions have adhesions between the serosal surfaces, along part or all of their length, and cannot be reduced. Adhesions are more common in cats. Resection and anastomosis is therefore necessary in the majority of cases. Underlying causes, such as a mass, must be ruled out. Recognition of underlying intestinal disease can be improved by obtaining intestinal biopsy samples at the time of surgery.

Some surgeons perform enteroplication (see Figure 7.18 and Operative Technique 7.7) in an attempt to reduce recurrence, although this has not been conclusively proven to be preventative and complications can be life-threatening (Applewhite et al., 2001). Recurrence rates are reported as 10–30%, regardless of location of the intussusception and whether it was reduced or resected. Prognosis for survival is good.

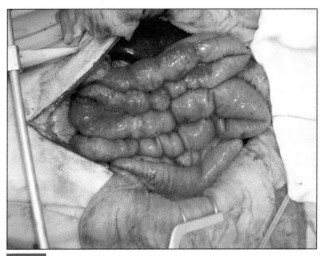

7.18 Enteroplication.

Mesenteric volvulus and intestinal strangulation

Volvulus is a rare condition that may occur spontaneously in dogs and cats, but has also been reported following jejunal entrapment, after treating intussusception with enteroplication (Figure 7.19), and following treatment for worm infestation. It may also be associated with activity, trauma or dietary indiscretion. German Shepherd Dogs and large-breed dogs are over-represented. Rotation around the root of the mesentery occludes the cranial mesenteric artery, leading to ischaemia and necrosis of part or all of the intestine from the distal duodenum to the proximal descending colon (Figure 7.20). The volvulus may be complete or segmental, and chronic torsion has been reported. Gastric dilatation and volvulus may also be present. Clinical signs include acute abdominal distension, abdominal pain and hypovolaemic shock.

Diagnosis is based on radiographic findings of markedly distended intestinal loops lying parallel to each other. Diagnosis may be more difficult in cats. Following medical stabilization, an immediate laparotomy should be performed to untwist the volvulus, as strangulation can lead to full-thickness intestinal wall necrosis within 8–12 hours. Intestinal viability should be assessed. In some cases intestinal viability is not compromised and normal circulation and motility resume. Resection and anastomosis should be performed if there is necrosis of part of the intestine; however, short bowel syndrome can occur if too much small

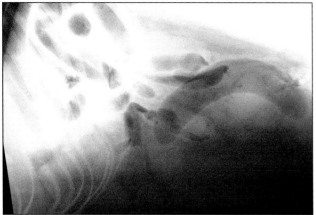

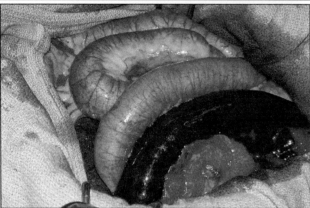

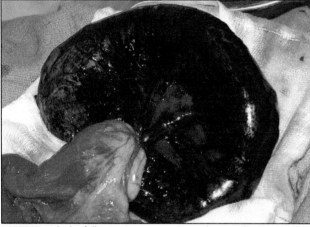

7.19 Volvulus following intussusception and enteroplication in a dog. (Reproduced from Jasani *et al.* (2005) with permission from the *Journal of Small Animal Practice*)

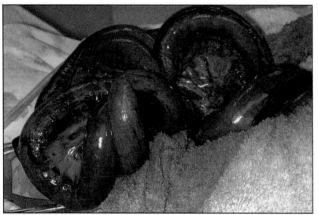

7.20 Severe mesenteric volvulus. The bowel is strangulated and necrotic.
(Courtesy of B. Stanley)

intestine is resected (see below). Euthanasia is necessary if the majority of the intestine is necrotic. Approximately 40% of dogs survive with death rates attributable to hypovolaemia, sepsis, exotoxaemia and endotoxaemia.

Rarely, incarceration of small intestine can occur into hernias or ruptures. Entrapment occurs if the defect is small and constricts the intestine. Strangulated portions of intestine should be released where possible. Contracted hernias may need to be incised and adhesions may need to be broken down. Intussusceptions should be gently pushed apart. Depending upon viability, the affected portion of small intestine may require resection.

Neoplasia

Gastrointestinal tumours are rare and generally affect older animals. Tumours are less common in the small intestine than the large intestine in dogs, with the exception of lymphoma which occurs more commonly in the stomach and small intestine. In cats, small intestinal tumours are more common than tumours at other intestinal sites. Small intestinal tumours are more likely to be malignant than benign. Tumours can arise in any layer of the intestinal wall and may therefore be:

- Epithelial – e.g. adenocarcinoma
- Neuroendocrine
- Haemopoietic – e.g. lymphoma, mast cell tumour
- Mesenchymal – e.g. leiomyoma, leiomyosarcoma.

The most common small intestinal tumours in dogs are adenocarcinomas, leiomyosarcomas/gastrointestinal stromal tumours (GISTs) and lymphomas, which occur with similar frequency. Canine leiomyomas and leiomyosarcomas have been reclassified as smooth muscle tumours and GISTs using immunohistochemistry (the latter expresses c-kit). Male dogs are over-represented for smooth muscle tumours and lymphoma. Typically, adenocarcinomas occur in the duodenum and leiomyosarcomas in the jejunum of dogs. Other reported malignant tumours include fibrosarcomas, mast cell tumours, haemangiosarcomas, carcinomatosis and carcinoid tumours. Benign tumours include polyps and leiomyomas.

Lymphoma is the most common tumour in cats (75% of cases), followed by adenocarcinoma; Siamese cats are over-represented for both tumour types. Feline leukaemia virus (FeLV) and feline immunodeficiency virus (FIV) may have a role in lymphoma development, with 80% of cats being FeLV positive. It can be difficult to differentiate lymphoma from inflammation in biopsy samples, particularly those obtained via endoscopy (Evans *et al.*, 2006).

Clinical signs are more common with small intestinal tumours compared with large intestinal tumours, as they are more likely to interfere with normal gastrointestinal function. Clinical signs include lethargy, vomiting, inappetence and weight loss. Bleeding from an adenocarcinoma may cause haematemesis, melaena and anaemia. Tumours are easier to palpate in cats (50–86% of cases) than dogs (20–50% of cases).

Masses may be difficult to see with radiography, although there may be evidence of obstruction or peritonitis in some cases. Obstruction may be more common with adenocarcinomas, which tend to form annular lesions, than with mesenchymal tumours. Tumours tend to be readily visible on ultrasonography, averaging 4 cm in length and with loss of wall layering, which differentiates them from non-neoplastic lesions, which tend to have normal layering. However, some tumours may be diffuse and infiltrative (e.g. mast cell tumours and some lymphomas) and appear normal on ultrasonography. Animals may present with septic peritonitis if the mass has perforated. Diagnosis can be made preoperatively by ultrasound-guided fine-needle aspiration, although it can be difficult to perform in large or obese animals. Ultrasound-guided biopsy is rarely performed due to the risk of intestinal wall perforation.

> **PRACTICAL TIP**
>
> Endoscopy is a useful tool in the diagnosis of some mucosal tumours. However, it may not add much additional information to that provided by ultrasonography, except the ability to obtain biopsy samples from mucosal lesions. Mural lesions are not typically seen on endoscopy

Disease is usually advanced at the time of diagnosis, with metastatic rates varying from 16–50%. Metastasis is more common with small intestinal rather than large intestinal adenocarcinomas. Metastasis is most likely to occur to the mesentery and omentum via local extension, local lymph nodes (especially adenocarcinoma) and liver (particularly leiomyosarcoma). Other sites of metastasis may be seen, but thoracic metastasis is less common than abdominal metastasis. Small intestinal tumours are treated by resection and anastomosis. Resection of 4-8 cm of normal intestine oral and aboral to the mass should be performed (Figure 7.21), as tumour cells will be present in grossly normal tissue some distance from the mass. Any omentum adhered to the mass should also be resected as it may contain tumour cells. The presence of residual tumour cells may affect healing or lead to recurrence. Aspirates and biopsy samples should be obtained from regional lymph nodes and the liver for staging.

Varying survival times after surgical resection of small intestinal tumours have been reported, but information regarding survival times can be difficult to interpret as case series may include both small and large intestinal tumours. The overall median survival time in dogs with small intestinal tumours is 10 months, with a 1-year and 2-year survival rate of 40% and 33%, respectively. In the presence of metastasis, the median survival time is 3 months and the 1-year survival rate is 20%. Reported survival rates for adenocarcinoma are between 5 and 10 months. For GISTs and leiomyosarcomas, the 1-year and 2-year recurrence free periods are reported as 80% and 67%, respectively, with a median survival time of 10 months to 2 years. There is no statistically significant difference in survival times between dogs with adenocarcinomas and leiomyosarcomas, or dogs with GISTs and leiomyosarcomas. Large tumour size and not being neutered were poor prognostic factors in dogs with mesenchymal tumours. Adjunctive chemotherapy is reported for adenocarcinomas and sarcomas, but its benefit has not been proved. Recurrence after resection of benign tumours is rare.

Surgical resection of small intestinal adenocarcinomas significantly improves the median survival time in cats, and survival can be prolonged even in the face of advanced disease. In one report (Green *et al.*, 2011) the median survival time was 27 months for those patients without metastatic disease and 13 months for those patients with metastatic disease (although shorter survival times are also reported). There is a high metastatic rate (at least 70%) for cats with mast cell tumours and survival time is poor (<4 months). These cats may also have concurrent lymphoma.

Surgery may be performed as an adjunct to chemotherapy for nodular lymphoma (e.g. where there is obstructive disease, where the tumour has perforated, where clinical signs are marked, or where there are concerns of intestinal rupture during treatment). Median survival times for cats with intestinal lymphoma are between 6 and 9 months. Canine small intestinal lymphoma has a poor prognosis and is worse for diffuse compared with nodular lymphoma.

Small intestinal and mesenteric trauma

Trauma can occur secondary to penetrating trauma (e.g. ballistics, bite wounds), blunt force trauma (e.g. road traffic accidents) or incarceration in hernias and ruptures. There may be direct penetration of the small intestine, leading to leakage of intestinal contents and rapid onset of septic peritonitis. Damage to individual mesenteric vessels (e.g. by mesenteric avulsion) will not have a clinical effect, but intestinal necrosis will occur if a larger number of vessels are damaged. Loss of integrity of the intestinal barrier will lead to bacterial translocation and septic peritonitis. Peritonitis will be more rapid if the intestinal wall perforates. Small penetrating injuries can be surgically repaired if the intestinal wall is not compromised. Large penetrating wounds and necrosis secondary to mesenteric avulsion must be treated by enterectomy.

Congenital malformations

Failure of embryonic development can lead to intestinal diverticula (herniation of the intestinal wall with luminal communication) and duplication (additional segments of intestine next to or within the intestinal wall but without luminal communication). The presence and degree of clinical signs is related to the size and location of the malformation and whether it causes intestinal obstruction. Intestinal bleeding has been described secondary to mucosal ulceration. Surgical resection should be performed if the malformation causes clinical signs and usually requires enterectomy.

Intestinal infarction

Acute mesenteric thromboembolism and intestinal ischaemia is a rare complication of feline hypertrophic cardiomyopathy. Affected segments of intestine have reduced motility, leading to vomiting and abdominal pain. Full-thickness wall necrosis can occur, leading to septic peritonitis. Abnormal areas of intestine require resection.

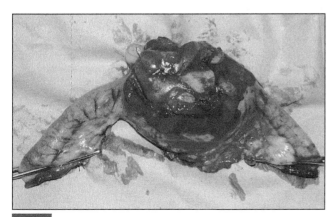

7.21 Mass resected with 4–8 cm margins.

Postoperative care

Analgesia

Postoperative analgesia should be tailored to the individual patient and should routinely include the use of an opioid. For further discussion on analgesia please see the *BSAVA Manual of Anaesthesia and Analgesia.*

Fluid therapy

Fluid therapy should be continued postoperatively to correct losses from vomiting and diarrhoea. Blood gas and electrolyte abnormalities may also need to be corrected. Blood gas and electrolyte analysis should be performed to assess the need for electrolyte supplementation. Information on the use of fluids during routine small intestinal surgery and in animals with small intestinal obstruction is given in Chapter 1.

Enteral nutrition

Animals should be fed as soon as is feasible following recovery from small intestinal surgery. Enteral feeding promotes mucosal cell proliferation, gastrointestinal barrier integrity, improved healing and decreased septic complications. In addition, glutamate absorbed from the intestinal lumen is used directly by the enterocytes.

Imaging

Ultrasonography can be used to assess enterotomy or enterectomy healing. Approximately 50% of enterotomy sites and all enterectomy sites can be visualized in the immediate postoperative period. On day 1 following surgery, there is loss of intestinal wall layering and this remains absent or altered on day 10. Twenty percent of dogs have normal wall thickness by day 10. Peritoneal effusion, pneumoperitoneum and hyperechoic omental and mesenteric fat do not hamper visualization and resolve in 80–90% of dogs by 3–10 days following surgery (Matthews *et al.*, 2008). In the long term, 78% of enterectomy sites are visible (Mareschal *et al.*, 2010).

Complications

Dehiscence and septic peritonitis

Dehiscence rates following small intestinal surgery are 2–16%. Dehiscence is most commonly seen following enterotomy or enterectomy for foreign body removal, although this is not shown in all studies. Dehiscence is three times more likely to occur if there is pre-existing septic peritonitis, as healing is impaired (Allen *et al.*, 1992). Other risk factors include low serum albumin or plasma protein concentration and intraoperative hypotension. It occurs most commonly 3–5 days after surgery, but may occur within the first 24 hours or after more than a week following the procedure. Dehiscence may occur as a result of poor surgical technique (e.g. placing sutures too close to the wound edge, too far apart, or failing to engage the submucosa). However, dehiscence can occur even with good surgical technique, as there is often a delay between removal of the fibrin seal by fibrinolysis and the deposition of collagen across the wound. A small area of dehiscence (several millimetres) can become plugged by omentum, leading to local peritonitis or abscess formation. More typically, there is a larger gap

between the wound edges with leakage of large volumes of intestinal contents and generalized septic peritonitis (see Chapter 18). Risk factors for dehiscence after enterectomy and anastomosis include preoperative peritonitis, low serum albumin or plasma protein concentration, and intraoperative hypotension. Intestinal foreign body was a risk factor in some studies (Ralphs *et al.*, 2003), but another study failed to demonstrate this association and showed that dogs with foreign bodies were conversely less likely to die than dogs having small intestinal surgery for other reasons (Grimes *et al.*, 2011). Dogs may be at greater risk of dehiscence than cats. Septic peritonitis may occur despite enteric surgery sites being intact. This may occur due to contamination or insufficient lavage at the time of the original surgery, translocation of bacteria across the intestine or haematogenous spread.

> **PRACTICAL TIP**
>
> The major clinical sign of septic peritonitis is vomiting. Further information on peritonitis is provided in Chapter 18

Short bowel syndrome

Short bowel syndrome may occur if there is extensive small intestinal resection, leading to nutritional and metabolic disturbances, including weight loss and diarrhoea. Resection of 50–90% of small intestine in a group of dogs and cats resulted in most animals (85%) surviving to discharge, of which there was a good eventual outcome in 80% of animals (Gorman *et al.*, 2006). Diarrhoea tends to resolve following intestinal adaptation after weeks or a few months, and can be controlled using dietary modification and medication whilst this occurs. No risk factors, including percentage of intestine removed, are associated with outcome.

Adhesions

Adhesions are uncommon in dogs and cats due to an active fibrinolytic system, but may occur in response to ischaemia, inflammation or foreign material. Abdominal lavage at the end of surgery does not offer any protection against adhesion formation. Adhesions can lead to en-trapment of other abdominal organs, including the small intestine.

Ileus

Ileus may occur within the first 24 hours of surgery. It may be induced by laparotomy, manipulation of the gastrointestinal tract, gastrointestinal dilation, sepsis or electrolyte disorders. Clinical signs may be confused with those of septic peritonitis (abdominal pain and distension, vomiting) but can be differentiated with ultrasonography. Treatment includes correction of electrolyte abnormalities, treatment of sepsis and administration of a prokinetic agent (e.g. metoclopramide or ranitidine).

References and further reading

Allen DA, Smeak DD and Schertel ER (1992) Prevalence of small intestinal dehiscence and associated clinical factors: a retrospective study in 121 dogs. *Journal of the American Animal Hospital Association* **28**, 70–76

Anderson S, Lippincott CL and Gill PJ (1992) Single enterotomy removal of gastrointestinal linear foreign bodies. *Journal of the American Animal Hospital Association* **28**, 487–490

Applewhite AA, Hawthorne JC and Cornell KK (2001) Complications of enteroplication for the prevention of intussusception recurrence in dogs: 35 cases (1989–1999). *Journal of the American Veterinary Medical Association* **219(10)**, 1415–1418

Basher AW and Fowler JD (1987) Conservative *versus* surgical management of gastrointestinal linear foreign bodies in the cat. *Veterinary Surgery* **16(2)**, 135–138

Boag AK, Coe RJ, Martinez TA and Hughes D (2005) Acid-base and electrolyte abnormalities in dogs with gastrointestinal foreign bodies. *Journal of Veterinary Internal Medicine* **19**, 816–821

Bone DL, Duckett KE, Patton CS and Krahwinkel DJ Jr (1983) Evaluation of anastomoses of small intestine in dogs: crushing versus noncrushing suturing techniques. *American Journal of Veterinary Research* **44**, 2043–2048

Brockman DJ, Pardo AD, Conzemius MG, Cabell LM and Trout NJ (1996) Omentum-enhanced reconstruction of chronic nonhealing wounds in cats: techniques and clinical use. *Veterinary Surgery* **25(2)**, 99–104

Burkitt JM, Drobatz KJ, Saunders HM and Washabau RJ (2009) Signalment, history and outcome of cats with gastrointestinal tract intussusception: 20 cases (1986–2000). *Journal of the American Veterinary Medical Association* **234(6)**, 771–776

Carobbie B, Foale RD and White RA (2009) Trichobezoar obstruction after stapled jejunal anastomosis in a dog. *Veterinary Surgery* **38(3)**, 417–420

Cohen M, Post GS and Wright JC (2003) Gastrointestinal leiomyosarcoma in 14 dogs. *Journal of Veterinary Internal Medicine* **17**, 107

Church EM, Mehlhaff CJ and Patnaik AK (1987) Colorectal adenocarcinoma in dogs: 78 dogs (1973–1984). *Journal of the Veterinary Medical Association* **191**, 727–730

Coolman BR, Ehrhart N and Maretta SM (2000) Healing of intestinal anastomoses. *Compendium on Continuing Education for the Practising Veterinarian* **22**, 363–372

Crawshaw J, Berg J, Sardinas JC *et al.* (1998) Prognosis for dogs with nonlymphomatous, small intestinal tumors treated by surgical excision. *Journal of the American Animal Hospital Association* **34(6)**, 451–456

Crowe DT and Devey JJ (1997) Clinical experience with jejunostomy feeding tubes in 47 small animal patients. *Journal of Veterinary Emergency and Critical Care* **7**, 7–19

Ellison GW (2011) Complications of gastrointestinal surgery in companion animals. *Veterinary Clinics of North America: Small Animal Practice* **41(5)**, 915–934

Ellison GW, Jokinen MP and Park RD (1982) End-to-end approximating intestinal anastomosis in the dog: a comparative fluorescein dye, angiographic and histopathologic evaluation. *Journal of the American Animal Hospital Association* **18**, 729–736

Ellison GW (2011) Complications of gastrointestinal surgery in companion animals. *Veterinary Clinics of North America: Small Animal Practice* **41(5)**, 915–934

Evans SE, Bonczynski JJ, Broussard JD, Han E and Baer KE (2006) Comparison of endoscopic and full-thickness biopsy specimens for diagnosis of inflammatory bowel disease and alimentary tract lymphoma in cats. *Journal of the American Veterinary Medical Association* **229(9)**, 1447–1450

Frank JD, Reimer SB, Kass PH and Kiupel M (2007) Clinical outcomes of 30 cases (1997–2004) of gastrointestinal lymphoma. *Journal of the American Animal Hospital Association* **43(6)**, 313–321

Graham JP, Lord PF and Harrison JM (1998) Quantitative estimation of intestinal dilation as a predictor of obstruction in the dog. *Journal of Small Animal Practice* **39(11)**, 521–524

Green ML, Smith JD and Kass PH (2011) Surgical *versus* non-surgical treatment of feline small intestinal adenocarcinoma and the influence of metastasis on long-term survival in 18 cats (2000–2007). *The Canadian Veterinary Journal* **52(10)**, 1101–1105

Grimes JA, Schmiedt CW, Cornell KK and Radlinsky MA (2011) Identification of risk factors for septic peritonitis and failure to survive following gastrointestinal surgery in dogs. *Journal of the American Veterinary Association* **238(4)**, 486–494

Gorman SC, Freeman LM, Mitchell SL and Chan DL (2006) Extensive small bowel resection in dogs and cats: 20 cases (1998–2004). *Journal of the American Veterinary Medical Association* **228(3)**, 403–407

Harvey HJ (1990) Complications of small intestinal biopsy in hypoalbuminemic dogs. *Veterinary Surgery* **19(4)**, 289–292

Hayes G (2009) Gastrointestinal foreign bodies in dogs and cats: a retrospective study of 208 cases. *Journal of Small Animal Practice* **50(11)**, 576–583

Jardel N, Hidalgo A, Leperlier D *et al.* (2011) One stage functional end-to-end stapled intestinal anastomosis and resection performed by nonexpert surgeons for the treatment of small intestinal obstruction in 30 dogs. *Veterinary Surgery* **40(2)**, 216–222

Jasani S, House AK and Brockman DJ (2005) Localised mid-jejunal volvulus following intussusception and enteroplication in a dog. *Journal of Small Animal Practice* **46(8)**, 398–401

Junius G, Appeldoorn AM and Schrauwen E (2004) Mesenteric volvulus in the dog: a retrospective study of 12 cases. *Journal of Small Animal Practice* **45(2)**, 104–107

Kapatkin AS, Mullen HS, Matthiesen DT and Patnaik AK (1992) Leiomyosarcoma in dogs: 44 cases (1983–1988). *Journal of the American Veterinary Medical Association* **201(7)**, 1077–1079

Kirpensteijn J, Maarschalkerweerd RJ, van der Gaag I, Kooistra HA and van Sluijs FJ (2001) Comparison of three closure methods and two absorbable suture materials for closure of jejunal enterotomy incisions in healthy dogs. *Veterinary Quarterly* **23(2)**, 67–70

Knell SC, Andreoni AA, Dennler M and Venzin CM (2010) Successful treatment of small intestinal volvulus in two cats. *Journal of Feline Medicine and Surgery* **12(11)**, 874–877

Kosovsky JE, Matthiesen DT and Patniak AK (1988) Small intestinal adenocarcinoma in cats: 32 cases (1978–1985). *Journal of the American Veterinary Medical Association* **192(2)**, 233–235

Laurenson MP, Skorupski KA, Moore PF and Zwingenberger AL (2011) Ultrasonography of intestinal mast cell tumors in the cat. *Veterinary Radiology and Ultrasound* **52(3)**, 330–334

Levien AS and Baines SJ (2011) Histological examination of the intestine from dogs and cats with intussusception. *Journal of Small Animal Practice* **52(11)**, 599–606

Lhermette P and Sobel D (2008) *BSAVA Manual of Canine and Feline Endoscopy and Endosurgery.* BSAVA Publications, Gloucester

Maas CP, ter Haar G, van der Gaag I and Kirpensteijn J (2007) Reclassification of small intestinal and cecal smooth muscle tumors in 72 dogs: clinical, histologic and immunohistochemical evaluation. *Veterinary Surgery* **36(4)**, 302–313

Mareschal A, Penninck D and Webster CR (2010) Ultrasonographic assessment of long-term enterectomy sites in dogs. *Veterinary Radiology and Ultrasound* **51(6)**, 652–655

Matthews AR, Penninck DG and Webster CR (2008) Postoperative ultrasonographic appearance of uncomplicated enterotomy or enterectomy sites in dogs. *Veterinary Radiology and Ultrasound* **49(5)**, 477–483

Oakes MG, Lewis DD, Hosgood G and Beale BS (1994) Enteroplication for the prevention of intussusception recurrence in dogs: 31 cases. *Journal of the American Veterinary Medical Association* **205(1)**, 72–75

Paoloni MC, Penninck DG and Moore AS (2002) Ultrasonographic and clinicopathologic findings in 21 dogs with intestinal adenocarcinoma. *Veterinary Radiology and Ultrasound* **43(6)**, 562–567

Papazoglou LG, Tontis D, Loukopoulos P *et al.* (2010) Foreign body-associated intestinal pyogranuloma resulting in intestinal obstruction in four dogs. *Veterinary Record* **166(16)**, 494–497

Patsikas MN, Papazoglou LG and Adamama-Moraitou KK (2008) Spontaneous reduction of intestinal intussusception in five young dogs. *Journal of the American Animal Hospital Association* **44(1)**, 41–47

Patsikas MN, Papazoglou LG, Jakovljevic S and Dessiris AK (2005) Color Doppler ultrasonography in prediction of the reducibility of intussuscepted bowel in 15 young dogs. *Veterinary Radiology and Ultrasound* **46(4)**, 313–316

Patsikas MN, Jakovljevic S, Moustardas N *et al.* (2003) Ultrasonographic signs of intestinal intussusception associated with acute enteritis or gastroenteritis in 19 young dogs. *Journal of the American Animal Hospital Association* **39(1)**, 57–66

Ralph SC, Jessen CR and Lipowitz AJ (2003) Risk factors for leakage following intestinal anastomosis in dogs and cats: 115 cases (1991–2000). *Journal of the American Veterinary Medical Association* **223(1)**, 73–77

Russell KN, Mehler SJ, Skorupski KA *et al.* (2007) Clinical and immunohistochemical differentiation of gastrointestinal stromal tumors from leiomyosarcomas in dogs: 42 cases (1990–2003). *Journal of the American Veterinary Medical Association* **230(9)**, 1329–1333

Saile K, Boothe HW and Boothe DM (2010) Saline volume necessary to achieve predetermined intraluminal pressures during leak testing of small intestinal biopsy sites in the dog. *Veterinary Surgery* **39(7)**, 900–903

Seymour C and Duke-Novakovski (2007) *BSAVA Manual of Canine and Feline Anaesthesia and Analgesia, 2nd edn.* BSAVA Publications, Gloucester

Shealy PM and Henderson RA (1992) Canine intestinal volvulus. A report of nine new cases. *Veterinary Surgery* **21(1)**, 15–9

Smith AL, Wilson AP, Hardie RJ, Krick EL and Schmiedt CW (2011) Perioperative complications after full-thickness gastrointestinal surgery in cats with alimentary lymphoma. *Veterinary Surgery* **40(7)**, 849–852

Song EK, Mann FA and Wagner-Mann CC (2008) Comparison of different tube materials and use of Chinese finger trap or four friction suture technique for securing gastrostomy, jejunostomy and thoracostomy tubes in dogs. *Veterinary Surgery* **37(3)**, 212–221

Swann HM, Sweet DC and Michel K (1997) Complications associated with use of jejunostomy tubes in dogs and cats: 40 cases (1989–1994). *Journal of the American Veterinary Medical Association* **210(12)**, 1764–1767

Tyrell D and Beck C (2006) Survey of the use of radiography vs. ultrasonography in the investigation of gastrointestinal foreign bodies in small animals. *Veterinary Radiology and Ultrasound* **47(4)**, 404–408

Ullman SL, Pavletic MM and Clark GN (1991) Open intestinal anastomosis with surgical stapling equipment in 24 dogs and cats. *Veterinary Surgery* **20**, 385–391

Weisman DL, Smeak DD, Birchard SJ *et al.* (1999) Comparison of a continuous suture pattern with a simple interrupted pattern for enteric closure in dogs and cats: 83 cases (1991–1997). *Journal of the American Veterinary Medical Association* **214**, 1507–1510

White RN (2008) Modified functional end-to-end stapled intestinal anastomosis: technique and clinical results in 15 dogs. *Journal of Small Animal Practice* **49(6)**, 274–281

Williams JM (2012) Colon In: *Veterinary Surgery: Small Animal*, ed. KM Tobias and SA Johnson, pp. 1542–1563. Elsevier, St. Louis

Wylie KB and Hosgood G (1994) Mortality and morbidity of small and large intestinal surgery in dogs and cats: 74 cases (1980–1992). *Journal of the American Animal Hospital Association* **30**, 469–474

OPERATIVE TECHNIQUE 7.1

Approach to small intestinal surgery

POSITIONING

Dorsal recumbency.

ASSISTANT

Optional – most useful when performing enterectomy and anastomosis.

EQUIPMENT EXTRAS

Abdominal retractors (e.g. Balfour, Gosset); non-crushing intestinal forceps (e.g. two pairs of Doyen clamps (optional if an assistant is available to digitally occlude the intestine)); suction unit with suction tubing and Poole suction tip; moistened laparotomy swabs with radiographic marker; water-impermeable drape; diathermy (optional).

SURGICAL TECHNIQUE

Approach

1   Sufficient aseptic preparation should be performed to allow incision from the xiphoid to the pubis if necessary. Perform a midline coeliotomy.

2   Removal of the falciform fat by sharp dissection is useful to improve exposure. Use of diathermy or placement of ligatures is necessary for haemostasis, especially cranially.

3   Moistened laparotomy swabs (or small swabs in small dogs and cats) are placed over the edges of the incision to protect the tissues from trauma and desiccation.

> **PRACTICAL TIP**
>
> Use swabs with radiographic markers. If there is doubt as to whether a swab has been retained in the abdomen during or after surgery, it can be verified with radiography or fluoroscopy

4   Self-retaining retractors are placed over the abdominal wall edges and swabs and opened, taking care not to trap the abdominal contents between the retractor and the abdominal wall.

5   Additional moistened laparotomy swabs can be placed cranial and caudal to the incision if exteriorization of the small intestine is planned.

Surgical manipulations

1   Note the presence of peritoneal fluid (e.g. blood, pus). Collect samples for cytology, fungal and bacteriological culture and sensitivity testing, packed cell volume and biochemistry. See Chapter 18 for more information on the management of septic peritonitis.

2   Identify the area of intestine requiring enterotomy or enterectomy (e.g. site of foreign body obstruction).

3   Perform a complete exploratory laparotomy, preferably before small intestinal surgery, to recognize concurrent pathology. In particular, note other areas of intestinal pathology, such as additional foreign bodies, perforation etc.

4   Exteriorize the small intestine by gentle retraction. Handling with moistened swabs can limit tissue damage, especially for inflamed intestine. Exteriorized small intestine can be placed on additional moistened swabs.

5   Recognize areas where exteriorization is limited, including the oral portion of the duodenum.

> **PRACTICAL TIP**
>
> Transect the duodenocolic ligament to improve exposure of the caudal flexure of the duodenum if necessary. Transection close to the duodenum limits the size of the defect in the mesocolon. Repair of the defect in the mesocolon will be necessary

→ **OPERATIVE TECHNIQUE 7.1 CONTINUED**

6 Place moistened laparotomy swabs around and deep to the affected intestine to protect the rest of the abdomen in case of spillage of intestinal contents.

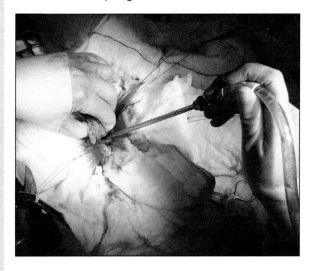

PRACTICAL TIP

Place multiple layers of swabs so that the superficial swabs can be removed if they become contaminated by spillage of intestinal contents and replaced without contaminating the peritoneal cavity

7 See the relevant Operative Technique for the small intestinal procedure required.

8 At the end of the surgery, discard all contaminated swabs. Perform a swab count.

9 Perform abdominal lavage and remove residual fluid using suction. The volume of lavage fluid needed depends upon the degree of contamination.

Wound closure

1 Perform omentalization or serosal patching as needed (see Operative Technique 7.8).

2 Change contaminated surgical gloves ± gowns. Place an additional surgical drape over the operative field to minimize contamination of the peritoneum during abdominal closure.

3 Perform abdominal closure using new instruments that have not been used for intestinal surgery to minimize contamination.

POSTOPERATIVE MANAGEMENT AND COMPLICATIONS

See main text.

OPERATIVE TECHNIQUE 7.2

Enterotomy for removal of a solid foreign body

POSITIONING

Dorsal recumbency.

ASSISTANT

Optional.

EQUIPMENT EXTRAS

Abdominal retractors (e.g. Balfour, Gosset); non-crushing intestinal forceps (e.g. two pairs of Doyen clamps (optional if an assistant is available to digitally occlude the intestine)); suction unit with suction tubing and Poole suction tip; moistened laparotomy swabs with radiographic marker; water-impermeable drape; diathermy (optional).

SURGICAL TECHNIQUE

Approach

See Operative Technique 7.1.

Surgical manipulations

1 Identify the part of the small intestine for enterotomy. Look for evidence of intestinal damage (oedema, change of colour (red, purple, black) or serosal petechiation upon handling) that in combination may suggest enterectomy may be more appropriate. See the main text for further information on intestinal viability. Note the presence of dilatation proximal to obstructive lesions.

2 In the presence of a solid foreign body, aim to make the incision in normal, non-dilated intestine, just aboral to the foreign body. This will allow sutures to be placed in healthier intestine and decrease the risk of dehiscence.

3 Manually express intestinal contents away from the proposed incision site.

4 Place atraumatic clamps (e.g. Doyen) oral and aboral to the proposed incision site, leaving sufficient room for sutures to be placed in the enterotomy (e.g. 2–5 cm). In the absence of intestinal forceps an assistant's fingers can be used to manipulate and occlude the small intestine at a similar position.

PRACTICAL TIP

Ensure that there are sufficient laparotomy swabs beneath the small intestine in case of spillage of intestinal contents. If mesenteric length allows, perform the enterotomy with the intestine exteriorized to one side of the abdominal incision over drapes and swabs

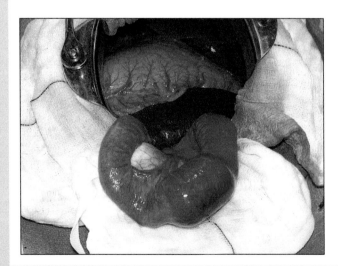

→ **OPERATIVE TECHNIQUE 7.2 CONTINUED**

5   Make a longitudinal incision in the antimesenteric border of the small intestine using a scalpel blade.

PRACTICAL TIP

Ensure the incision is long enough to allow the solid foreign body to be removed without tearing the intestine. Torn intestine is harder to suture accurately than planned incisions

6   Milk out the foreign body on to a swab and place to one side of the instrument trolley or hand to a non-scrubbed assistant. Wipe away any small intestinal contents with a swab and discard.

PRACTICAL TIP

Keep count of all swabs that are discarded from the operative field

7   Replace moistened laparotomy swabs underneath the small intestine if there has been spillage of intestinal contents on to the swabs, to prevent peritoneal contamination.

8   If there was questionable viability of small intestine prior to foreign body removal, allow the intestine 10 minutes to recover from distension and reassess. If there is doubt about viability, perform enterectomy instead (see Operative Technique 7.5).

9   Small intestinal mucosa is not routinely resected, but this can be performed if there is eversion that will make suture placement difficult.

PRACTICAL TIP

Excess mucosa is trimmed using Metzenbaum scissors. Take care not to resect submucosa as it makes accurate placement of sutures more difficult

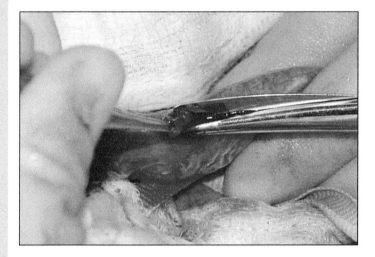

10   Most longitudinal incisions are closed in the same orientation, although very small incisions can be closed transversely.

11   Sutures are placed using an absorbable monofilament synthetic suture material with a prolonged absorption time (e.g. polydioxanone or glycomer 631).

PRACTICAL TIP

Avoid using sutures of an excessively large size as they are hard to place accurately and lead to larger knots. Suture material of 1 metric (5/0 USP) and 1.5 metric (4/0 USP) is suitable for small and large breeds, respectively

12   Sutures should incorporate the submucosa, which is the strongest layer of the intestinal wall. It is visible as a white line between the mucosa and serosa, although it can sometimes be hard to see.

→ **OPERATIVE TECHNIQUE 7.2 CONTINUED**

> **PRACTICAL TIP**
>
> Should it prove impossible to see the submucosa, ensure that the sutures are placed symmetrically through both the serosa and mucosa in order to incorporate it

13 Sutures are placed 3–5 mm from the edge of the incision and 3–5 mm apart (see Figure 7.13). Sutures are usually full-thickness and appositional, although a Gambee pattern can be used to avoid incorporating the mucosa. Inverting and everting patterns should be avoided (particularly inverting patterns), as they can lead to intestinal narrowing and stricture formation. The suture pattern can be interrupted or continuous; care should be taken with the latter to place the suture tight enough to appose the wound edges, but not so tight to cause puckering.

14 The suture line should be examined for large gaps and additional sutures placed as necessary. Saline can be injected into the lumen using a 23 G needle and syringe to help look for leaks.

> **PRACTICAL TIP**
>
> If injecting saline to look for leaks, avoid applying too much pressure to the suture line as all sutures will leak at high pressure. This technique is used to look for obvious leakage between sutures during moderate distension. For the canine jejunum, saline volumes of 16.3–19 ml (where digital occlusion is carried out) or 12.1–14.8 ml (where Doyen clamps are employed for occlusion) can be used to achieve an intraluminal pressure of around 34 cm of water for leak testing of a 10 cm segment of intestine containing a closed incision site

15 Perform abdominal lavage and suction away residual fluid.

16 Complete examination of the remainder of the abdominal contents if not already performed.

Wound closure

1 Wrap the small intestine in omentum (see Operative Technique 7.8). Consider serosal patching in patients with a high risk of dehiscence or in the absence of omentum.

2 Perform routine abdominal closure.

> **POSTOPERATIVE MANAGEMENT AND COMPLICATIONS**
>
> See main text.

OPERATIVE TECHNIQUE 7.3

Small intestinal biopsy

> **POSITIONING**
>
> Dorsal recumbency.

> **ASSISTANT**
>
> Optional.

> **EQUIPMENT EXTRAS**
>
> Abdominal retractors (e.g. Balfour, Gosset); non-crushing intestinal forceps (e.g. two pairs of Doyen clamps (optional if an assistant is available to digitally occlude the intestine)); suction unit with suction tubing and Poole suction tip; moistened laparotomy swabs with radiographic marker; water-impermeable drape; diathermy (optional).

→ **OPERATIVE TECHNIQUE 7.3 CONTINUED**

Approach

See Operative Technique 7.1.

Surgical manipulations

1 Identify the part of the small intestine for biopsy. Look for grossly abnormal lesions. Otherwise, select one to three biopsy sites in the duodenum, jejunum and/or ileum, as determined by the clinical signs of gastrointestinal disease. Commonly a biopsy sample is obtained from the duodenum, jejunum and ileum. It is rare to obtain a biopsy sample from the colon, unless there is a specific indication, due to the potential complication of dehiscence and the high morbidity associated with faecal peritonitis.

2 Using a new scalpel blade, make a 5–10 mm full-thickness longitudinal (but slightly curved) incision along the antimesenteric border of the small intestine. Make a second incision 3–4 mm adjacent to it to complete an elliptical biopsy.

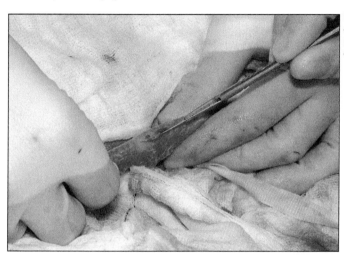

Use of a scalpel blade to take a full-thickness elliptical biopsy sample: 3–4 mm wide and 5–10 mm long. An assistant's fingers are occluding the intestine orally and aborally.

3 Alternatively, use a new skin biopsy punch to take a full-thickness sample of small intestine from the antimesenteric border. Avoid penetrating the opposite intestinal wall.

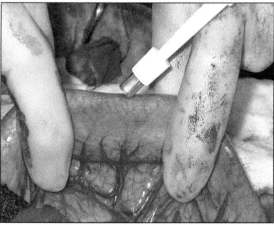
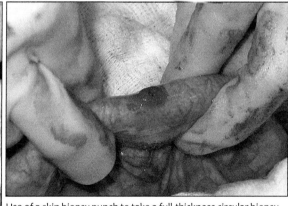

Use of a skin biopsy punch to take a full-thickness circular biopsy sample.

Handle the biopsy sample with care and avoid the use of crushing thumb forceps, in order to prevent crushing artefacts that can interfere with histological interpretation. It can be more difficult to close the circular wound created by the biopsy punch, but this technique makes it easier to obtain a specimen without crushing artefacts

➔ **OPERATIVE TECHNIQUE 7.3 CONTINUED**

4 Suture closed the biopsy site as for enterotomy (see Operative Technique 7.2).

5 Take further biopsy samples as appropriate.

6 Perform abdominal lavage and suction away residual fluid.

7 Complete examination of the remainder of the abdominal contents if not already performed.

Wound closure

1 Wrap the small intestine in omentum (see Operative Technique 7.8). Consider serosal patching in patients with a high risk of dehiscence or in the absence of omentum.

2 Perform routine abdominal closure.

POSTOPERATIVE MANAGEMENT AND COMPLICATIONS

See main text.

OPERATIVE TECHNIQUE 7.4

Combined gastrotomy and enterotomy for removal of a linear foreign body

POSITIONING

Dorsal recumbency.

ASSISTANT

Optional.

EQUIPMENT EXTRAS

Abdominal retractors (e.g. Balfour, Gosset); non-crushing intestinal forceps (e.g. two pairs of Doyen clamps (optional if an assistant is available to digitally occlude the intestine)); suction unit with suction tubing and Poole suction tip; moistened laparotomy swabs with radiographic marker; water-impermeable drape; diathermy (optional).

SURGICAL TECHNIQUE

Approach

See Operative Technique 7.1.

Surgical manipulations

1 A wide surgical field is required and the laparotomy incision should extend from the xiphoid as far caudally as needed, typically between the umbilicus and the pubis.

2 Careful examination will reveal the extent of gastrointestinal involvement. In dogs, there is often foreign material in the stomach, typically blocking the pylorus; whereas cats are more likely to have the linear foreign body anchored at the tongue with no large gastric component. The extent of small intestinal plication should be noted and whether the foreign body is thick (e.g. clothing or material) or thin (e.g. sewing cotton).

3 With thick foreign bodies, surgery can begin at any location, but it is easiest to start with gastrotomy in order to remove the anchored portion (see Chapter 5). The gastrotomy incision should be close enough to the pylorus to

➜ **OPERATIVE TECHNIQUE 7.4 CONTINUED**

reach the foreign body, typically located within the pyloric antrum, but not compromise the function of the pylorus. The gastric portion of the foreign body is cut from the portion entering the pylorus and is removed on to a swab and discarded. The gastrotomy incision is closed routinely. Typically, the small intestinal plication will reduce or disappear as tension is taken off the linear foreign body.

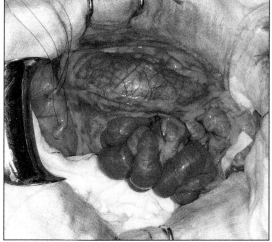

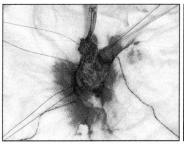 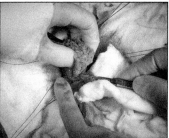

The stomach has been isolated with laparotomy swabs and stay sutures. A gastrotomy has been performed and the gastric portion of the foreign body is being removed.

Linear foreign body in the stomach (left) and pylorus of a dog. The intestines are plicated.

4 Perform an enterotomy halfway between the pylorus and the most aboral extent of the foreign body (see Operative Technique 7.2).

5 Pull gently on the foreign body in both directions and remove it if possible to do so without exerting excess tension.

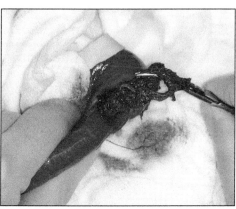

Enterotomy of the small intestine to remove the residual linear foreign body. Note the intestine has been isolated from the abdomen and swabs have been placed in a layered fashion to contain the spillage of intestinal contents.

> **WARNING**
>
> Do not pull hard on linear foreign bodies, especially thin ones, as this may cause full thickness laceration of the mesenteric border of the intestine

6 If the foreign body cannot be removed from either or both directions through the enterotomy, further incisions will be needed. Cut the foreign body at the first enterotomy incision and close the incision (see Operative Technique 7.2). Attempt to remove the foreign body through subsequent enterotomy incisions, made halfway between the pylorus and first enterotomy and/or halfway between the first enterotomy and the caudal extent of the foreign body. Repeat as necessary.

> **WARNING**
>
> There is an increased risk of contamination when performing multiple incisions. Care is needed to avoid spillage and initial incisions should be closed before subsequent incisions are made

→ **OPERATIVE TECHNIQUE 7.4 CONTINUED**

Most linear foreign bodies can be removed via a gastrotomy incision and one to three enterotomy incisions

7 Very thin foreign bodies can become embedded in the small intestinal mucosa along the mesenteric border and can be hard to locate after the anchored portion has been cut. It is preferable to make the first enterotomy incision and clamp the foreign body whilst it is under tension, before cutting the anchored part, either from under the tongue or in the stomach. In this situation, a gastrotomy and enterotomy will be open simultaneously and great care is needed to avoid contamination.

8 Examine the mesenteric border of the affected intestine. Bruising is common. Small lacerations can be repaired as for enterotomy. Large or multiple defects necessitate enterectomy and anastomosis (see Operative Techniques 7.5 and 7.6).

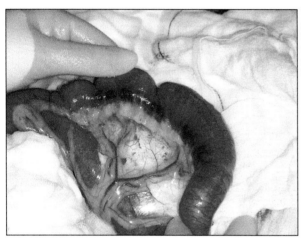

The intestine is being examined following removal of a linear foreign body. Note the bruising and change in intestinal colour along the mesenteric border. The presence of necrosis or any large perforations would necessitate enterectomy.

PRACTICAL TIP

After performing enterectomy, carefully examine the mesenteric portion of the small intestine that is to be anastomosed. Laceration of the mesenteric mucosa and submucosa by the foreign body may have occurred and will make it difficult to achieve anastomosis. Either resect a longer length of intestine or place additional sutures longitudinally on the mesenteric border. Be extra vigilant in ensuring that the suture line is complete and consider leak testing

9 Perform abdominal lavage and suction away residual fluid.

10 Complete examination of the remainder of the abdominal contents if not already performed.

Wound closure

1 Wrap the small intestine in omentum (see Operative Technique 7.8). Consider serosal patching in patients with a high risk of dehiscence or in the absence of omentum.

2 Perform routine abdominal closure.

POSTOPERATIVE MANAGEMENT AND COMPLICATIONS

See main text.

OPERATIVE TECHNIQUE 7.5

Enterectomy and anastomosis (sutured anastomosis)

POSITIONING

Dorsal recumbency.

ASSISTANT

Optional.

EQUIPMENT EXTRAS

Abdominal retractors (e.g. Balfour, Gosset); non-crushing intestinal forceps (e.g. two pairs of Doyen clamps (optional if an assistant is available to digitally occlude the intestine)); suction unit with suction tubing and Poole suction tip; moistened laparotomy swabs with radiographic marker; water-impermeable drape; diathermy (optional).

SURGICAL TECHNIQUE

Approach

See Operative Technique 7.1.

Surgical manipulations

1   Identify the part of the small intestine for enterectomy. Look for evidence of intestinal damage (e.g. necrosis, perforation). Ensure that there is a good blood supply to the residual small intestine.

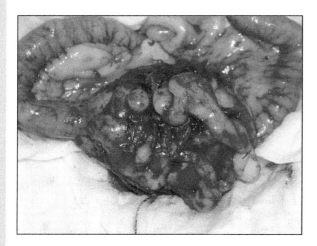

PRACTICAL TIP

Plan the enterectomy incision between vessels supplying the small intestine. Avoid making the incision a long distance from a vessel, as the anastomotic site may have a poor blood supply

---

2   Identify the proposed incision site.

   a. For necrotic intestine, the necrotic area and a margin of grossly normal tissue are removed to avoid placing sutures in abnormal tissue. Where small intestine is dilated, for example following torsion or an obstructive lesion, it may be inflamed (red in colour) and it can be difficult to assess what is viable.
   b. For neoplastic tumours, a 4–8 cm margin of normal tissue oral and aboral to the mass is removed.

→ **OPERATIVE TECHNIQUE 7.5 CONTINUED**

3　Manually express intestinal contents away from the proposed enterectomy site.

4　Place atraumatic clamps (e.g. Doyen intestinal clamps) oral and aboral to the proposed enterectomy site, leaving sufficient room so that when the intestinal ends retract they do not slip out of the forceps (e.g. 5–10 cm). In the absence of intestinal clamps, an assistant's fingers can be used to manipulate and occlude the small intestine, although this is more difficult to perform than with enterotomy.

5　Place additional Doyen intestinal clamps or crushing forceps adjacent to the proposed enterectomy sites on the portion of intestine that is to be resected.

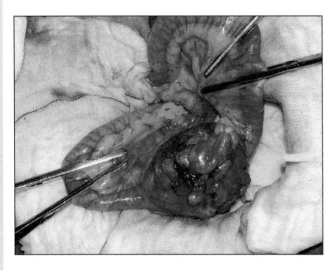

6　Place two ligatures on each vessel that supplies the length of small intestine to be resected (e.g. the jejunal arcadial vessels) and transect between them. Incise the mesentery between the vessels and continue the mesenteric incision towards the proposed enterectomy incisions orally and aborally.

7　Ligate the terminal arcadial vessel at each enterectomy site.

8　Ensuring that laparotomy swabs are positioned deep to the small intestine, incise the small intestine along each of the Doyen clamps/crushing forceps at the proposed enterectomy sites, leaving the forceps on the intestine to be resected. The other Doyen clamps, placed a small distance away on the retained intestine, will minimize spillage. The incision is transverse if each portion of the small intestine is the same size.

→ **OPERATIVE TECHNIQUE 7.5 CONTINUED**

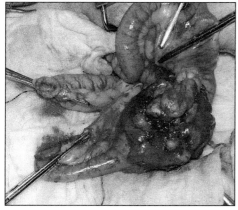
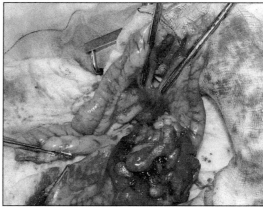

For minor size disparity, the smaller side can be transected at an angle to create a larger diameter. Alternatively, sutures can be placed closer together on the smaller portion of the intestine and further apart on the large portion, as long as the sutures can be placed 3–5 mm apart. This technique may be preferred in cases where the large diameter is due to dilatation of a normal portion of intestine, as inherent elasticity means that the intestinal ends will return to the same diameter in a short period of time. Finally, an incision can be made along the antimesenteric border of the smaller diameter intestine to create a greater cut edge to suture to the larger diameter portion of intestine.

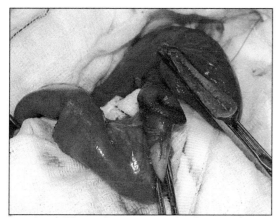
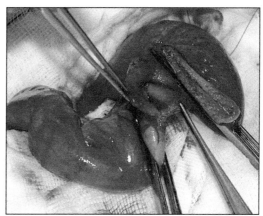

Intestine of different diameters. Note that the Doyen forceps on the larger diameter intestine could be moved further from the cut edge to aid suturing.

The mesenteric border of the smaller diameter intestine has been incised to increase the circumference and aid in suturing to the larger diameter intestine.

9 Sutures are placed using an absorbable monofilament synthetic suture material with a prolonged absorption time (e.g. polydioxanone or glycomer 631).

PRACTICAL TIP

Avoid using sutures of an excessively large size as they are hard to place accurately and lead to larger knots. Suture material of 1 metric (5/0 USP) and 1.5 metric (4/0 USP) is suitable for small and large breeds, respectively

10 Sutures should incorporate the submucosa, which is the strongest layer of the intestinal wall. It is visible as white line between the mucosa and serosa, although it can sometimes be hard to see.

PRACTICAL TIP

The mucosa can be trimmed if it is excessively everted and preventing visualization of the submucosa and placement of sutures

PRACTICAL TIP

Should it prove impossible to see the submucosa, ensure that the sutures are placed symmetrically through both the serosa and mucosa in order to incorporate the submucosa

→ **OPERATIVE TECHNIQUE 7.5 CONTINUED**

11 Initial sutures are placed at the mesenteric border, as the presence of mesenteric fat makes the sutures difficult to place, making it the most common site of suture failure. One to three sutures are placed (as stay sutures if multiple sutures are to be used) before tying. Knots are placed on the external surface rather than in the lumen.

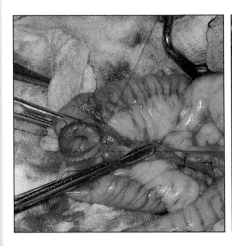 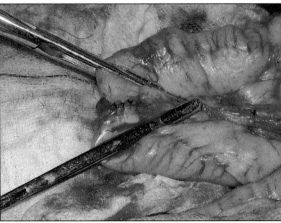

12 Subsequent sutures are placed 3–5 mm from the edge of the incision and 3–5 mm apart. After placement of the antimesenteric suture(s), it may be helpful to place a suture at the antimesenteric border to help plan accurate suture placement. Sutures are usually appositional, although a Gambee pattern is described to avoid incorporating the mucosa. Inverting and everting patterns should be avoided (particularly inverting patterns), as these can lead to stricture formation.

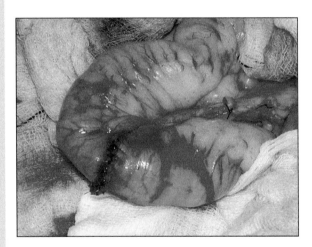

13 For continuous sutures, an initial suture line is placed around half of the intestinal circumference, from the mesenteric border to the antimesenteric border, and a second suture line is placed along the opposite circumference. Care should be taken to place the sutures tight enough to appose the wound edges, but not so tight as to cause puckering or narrowing of the lumen.

PRACTICAL TIP

Placement of two continuous suture lines minimizes the risk of pulling the suture too tight, which can lead to stricture formation

---

14 The suture line is examined for large gaps and additional sutures are placed as necessary. Saline can be injected into the lumen using a 23 G needle and syringe to gently distend the intestine between the atraumatic clamps to help look for leaks (see Operative Technique 7.2).

15 Suture the defect in the mesentery with an absorbable suture material, using a simple continuous or interrupted pattern. Avoid damaging or ligating adjacent blood vessels.

→ **OPERATIVE TECHNIQUE 7.5 CONTINUED**

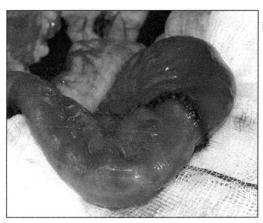

Enterectomy completed with simple interrupted sutures.

16 Perform abdominal lavage and suction away the residual fluid.

17 Complete examination of the remainder of the abdominal contents if not already performed.

For anastomosis using surgical staples, see Operative Technique 7.6.

PRACTICAL TIP

Resection of small intestine, caecum and colon necessitates anastomosis of small intestine to colon. A small size disparity can occasionally be overcome by incising the small intestine at an angle and placing sutures at different distances, as long as they are 3–5 mm apart. Alternatively, the antimesenteric border of the colon can be sutured transversely, until the residual diameter matches that of the small intestine. Care should be taken in placing the sutures at the antimesenteric edge to avoid leaving gaps between the anastomotic site and the sutured end of the colon. Never transversely close part of the small intestine to overcome size disparity. Most large diameter small intestine is due to dilatation and it will return to its normal diameter. Transversely closing part of the antimesenteric border will narrow the intestinal diameter and may lead to obstruction.

WARNING

Enterectomy of the proximal duodenum is difficult due to the entry of the pancreatic and common bile ducts and the shared vasculature of the pancreas and duodenum. If it is required, it must be accompanied by cholecystoenterostomy to allow flow of bile into the small intestine. Exocrine and endocrine pancreatic functions must be controlled medically. Surgery is technically challenging, postoperative recovery is difficult and complication rates are high

---

Wound closure

1 Wrap the small intestine in omentum (see Operative Technique 7.8). Consider serosal patching in patients with a high risk of dehiscence or in the absence of omentum.

2 Perform routine abdominal closure.

POSTOPERATIVE MANAGEMENT AND COMPLICATIONS

See main text.

OPERATIVE TECHNIQUE 7.6

Functional end-to-end anastomosis using surgical staples

POSITIONING

Dorsal recumbency.

ASSISTANT

Optional.

EQUIPMENT EXTRAS

Abdominal retractors (e.g. Balfour, Gosset); non-crushing intestinal forceps (e.g. two pairs of Doyen clamps (optional if an assistant is available to digitally occlude the intestine)); suction unit with suction tubing and Poole suction tip; moistened laparotomy swabs with radiographic marker; water-impermeable drape; diathermy (optional).

Linear cutting staplers	
DST Series™ GIA™ stapler (Covidien Inc.) Linear cutter® stapler (Ethicon Inc.)	• Used for transecting, resecting and creating anastomosis in gastrointestinal tissue • Stapler length and height combinations vary between manufacturers • Available stapler lengths: 55 mm, 75 mm and 100 mm (Ethicon Inc.); 60 mm, 80 mm and 100 mm (Covidien Inc.) • Available staple heights (closed): 1.0 mm, 1.5 mm, 1.8 mm and 2.0 mm (Ethicon Inc.); 1.0 mm, 1.5 mm and 2.0 mm (Covidien Inc.) • Delivers two double staggered rows of titanium staples and cuts the tissue between the two double rows • The stapler comes loaded and can be reloaded seven times for a total of eight firings • Endoscopic versions of the stapler are available for endoscopic procedures or for open surgery in smaller animals
Linear staplers	
DST Series™ TA™ stapler (Covidien Inc.) PROXIMATE® reloadable linear stapler (Ethicon Inc.)	• Used for approximating tissues and haemostasis during thoracic and alimentary tract procedures • There is no cutting blade • Stapler length and height combinations vary between manufacturers • Available stapler lengths: 30 mm, 60 mm and 90 mm (Ethicon Inc.); 30 mm, 45 mm, 60 mm and 90 mm (Covidien Inc.) • Available staple heights (closed): 1.0 mm, 1.5 mm and 2.0 mm • Delivers two staggered rows of titanium staples (vascular cartridges deliver three staggered rows) • The stapler comes loaded and can be reloaded three or seven times for a total of four or eight firings (depending upon the type) • Endoscopic versions of the stapler are available for endoscopic procedures or for open surgery in smaller animals

SURGICAL TECHNIQUE

Approach

See Operative Technique 7.1.

Surgical manipulations

This procedure can be used to anastomose small intestine to either small or large intestine and can be used for intestine of similar or different diameters.

1   Identify the proposed incision site.

→ **OPERATIVE TECHNIQUE 7.6 CONTINUED**

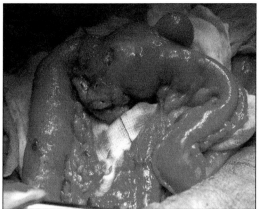

Perforation of the caecum due to sharp foreign bodies in the small and large intestine. Vessels to the distal small intestine, caecum and proximal large intestine have been ligated and transected.

2 Manually express intestinal contents away from the proposed enterectomy site.

3 Place Doyen intestinal clamps oral and aboral to the proposed enterectomy site, leaving sufficient room to allow placement of the stapling equipment (e.g. 10–15 cm). In the absence of intestinal forceps, an assistant's fingers can be used to manipulate and occlude the small intestine, although this is more difficult to perform than with enterotomy.

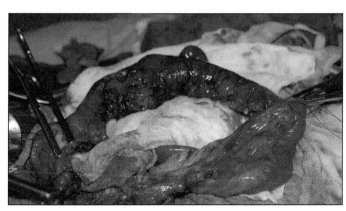

Two pairs of Doyen (bowel) clamps have been placed at the planned sites of transection. Note that the current position of the clamps will need to be adjusted to allow placement of the arms of the stapler. Stay sutures have been placed for manipulation of the intestine into the stapler.

4 Place two ligatures on each vessel that supplies the length of intestine to be resected (e.g. the jejunal arcadial vessels) and transect between them. Incise the mesentery between the vessels and continue the mesenteric incision towards the proposed enterectomy incisions orally and aborally.

PRACTICAL TIP

When incising the mesentery from the ligated blood vessels towards the intestine, leave a portion of mesentery intact adjacent to the residual blood vessels, so that the sutures can be placed easily without damaging the blood vessels

5 Ligate the terminal arcadial vessel at each incision site.

PRACTICAL TIP

The terminal arcadial vessel is not usually visible within the mesenteric fat. Sutures can be placed without direct visualization by placing a suture around the mesenteric fat to the edge of the mesenteric border of the small intestine. Ensure that the suture is placed in the portion of small intestine to be retained

6 Ensuring that laparotomy swabs are positioned deep to the small intestine, incise the small intestine along each of the Doyen clamps/crushing forceps at the proposed enterectomy sites, leaving the forceps on the intestine to be resected. The other Doyen clamps placed a small distance away on the retained intestine will minimize spillage. Place a stay suture on the antimesenteric border of each, close to the transected end, for manipulation.

→ **OPERATIVE TECHNIQUE 7.6 CONTINUED**

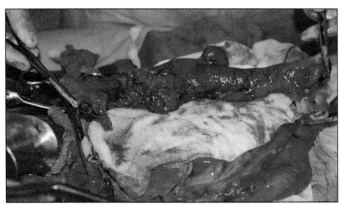

The small and large intestine have been transected between the bowel clamps. Note the swab under the intestine to prevent abdominal contamination.

7 Alternatively, make a transverse incision in each portion of the intestine to be anastomosed prior to resecting any intestine, wide enough to allow placement of the blade of the stapler.

8 Ensuring that the small intestine is not twisted, place the oral and aboral portions of intestine to be anastomosed adjacent to each other along the antimesenteric borders.

9 Place one limb of the GIA stapler in each lumen of intestine, ensuring that the limbs are inserted to their full length or at least 6–7 cm of their length, to avoid creating a narrow anastomosis.

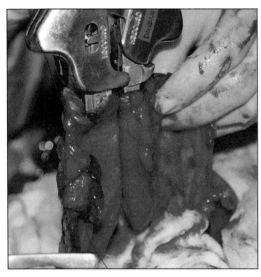

The two cut ends of intestine have been placed with the anti-mesenteric borders adjacent to each other. Each fork of a linear cutting stapler has been placed into each lumen of intestine.

PRACTICAL TIP

Use the stay sutures to ensure that the loops of intestine remain adjacent to each other along the antimesenteric borders

---

10 Engage and lock the stapler, checking that the limbs remain correctly inserted. Fire the stapler. The GIA stapler places two double staggered rows of staples through the adjacent portions of intestine. Each double row of staples lies either side of a blade, which simultaneously cuts the intestine longitudinally. The incision creates a stoma between the oral and aboral portions of intestine, which have been anastomosed on either side of the incision.

11 Remove the stapler and examine the intestine to ensure creation of the stoma and to check that the anastomosis has been performed correctly and the staples have been deployed. Haemorrhage is negligible.

→ **OPERATIVE TECHNIQUE 7.6 CONTINUED**

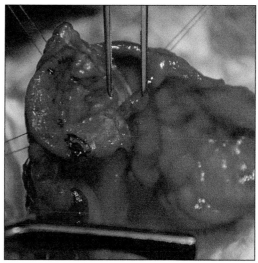

After firing the stapler, an anastomosis has been formed between the two segments of intestine. The staple lines will be offset from each other when the next stapler is placed to avoid them healing together and closing or narrowing the anastomosis.

12 A second GIA or a TA stapler is placed transversely across the open ends of the intestine, typically 5–10 mm from the cut edges. If the anastomosis was created through enterotomy incisions, the second stapler is placed across the first staple line adjacent to the enterotomy incisions.

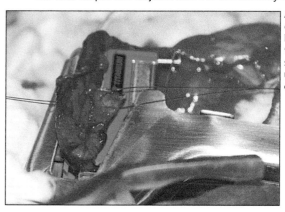

A linear stapler has been placed across the open ends of the intestine. The stay sutures have been used for manipulation to ensure the intestinal wall is fully incorporated in the stapler. A linear cutting stapler could be used, but the first line of staples may impede cutting by the blade.

PRACTICAL TIP

The stay sutures and forceps are used to manipulate the open ends of intestine to ensure that the stapler incorporates the full circumference of the cut ends of intestine

13 The cut ends of intestine are placed into the second stapler such that the first staple lines are slightly offset (by approximately 1 cm) to avoid them forming an adhesion that could close the anastomosis site. Fire the stapler. Use of a GIA stapler will result in the intestine being incised. Incision along the edge of the stapler is required when using a TA stapler to remove the end of the intestine not included in the anastomosis. Examine the staple line to ensure that the staples have deployed correctly.

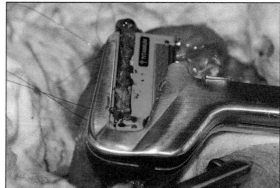

After firing the stapler, residual tissue has been resected by cutting along the stapler.

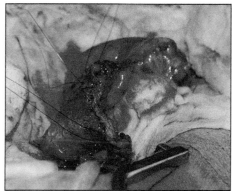

Complete staple line closing the intestinal lumen.

→ **OPERATIVE TECHNIQUE 7.6 CONTINUED**

PRACTICAL TIP

In the absence of a second stapler, the open ends of the intestine can be closed with sutures, although this is more difficult to perform

14 Place a simple interrupted suture (e.g. 2 metric (3/0 USP) absorbable suture material) at the junction of the first staple line, at the opposite end of the anastomosis from the second staple line and on the antimesenteric edges, to reduce tension on the staple line. Incorporate the submucosa.

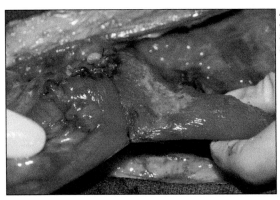

A stay suture has been placed at the opposite end of the completed anastomosis for additional security, although this is not necessary.

15 Suture the defect in the mesentery with an absorbable suture material, using a simple continuous or interrupted pattern. Avoid damaging or ligating adjacent blood vessels.

16 Perform abdominal lavage and suction away residual fluid.

17 Complete examination of the remainder of the abdominal contents if not already performed.

Wound closure

1 Wrap the small intestine in omentum (see Operative Technique 7.8). Consider serosal patching in patients with a high risk of dehiscence or in the absence of omentum.

2 Perform routine abdominal closure.

POSTOPERATIVE MANAGEMENT AND COMPLICATIONS

See main text.

OPERATIVE TECHNIQUE 7.7

Reduction of intussusception and enteroplication

POSITIONING

Dorsal recumbency.

ASSISTANT

Optional.

EQUIPMENT EXTRAS

Abdominal retractors (e.g. Balfour, Gosset); non-crushing intestinal forceps (e.g. two pairs of Doyen clamps (optional if an assistant is available to digitally occlude the intestine)); suction unit with suction tubing and Poole suction tip; moistened laparotomy swabs with radiographic marker; water-impermeable drape; diathermy (optional).

→ **OPERATIVE TECHNIQUE 7.7 CONTINUED**

Approach

See Operative Technique 7.1.

Surgical manipulations

1 Perform a complete abdominal and intestinal examination to locate the intussusception. Note which part and the length of small intestine is involved, and whether the intussusceptum passes into the colon.

> **PRACTICAL TIP**
>
> Multiple sites of intussusception may be noted

2 If omental adhesions are present, remove them by blunt dissection if the adhesions are immature or by ligating the omentum if the adhesions are mature.

3 Place moistened laparotomy swabs around and deep to the affected intestine to protect the rest of the abdomen in case of perforation or spillage of intestinal contents (see Figure 7.17).

4 Gently squeeze the contents of the intussuscipiens in an oral direction to reduce the intussusception. Avoid pulling on the intussusceptum from an oral direction, as this is more likely to lead to tearing.

5 Complete reduction of the intussusception may be achievable in early cases where there are no serosal adhesions present. Assuming there are no areas of decreased viability, enterectomy is not required. Enteroplication can be subsequently performed.

6 With increasing chronicity, serosal adhesions will form, and complete reduction of the intussusception will not be achievable. Attempting forcible reduction will lead to serosal tearing and possibly intestinal perforation. Identify non-viable intestine and perform resection and anastomosis (see Operative Techniques 7.5 and 7.6).

7 Examine the affected intestine carefully for predisposing causes such as neoplasia, especially in older animals.

8 Enteroplication is performed for cases that are considered high risk for recurrence. Enteroplication is performed between loops of jejunum. The part of the small intestine with short mesenteric attachments (proximal duodenum up to the caudal flexure) does not require enteroplication as it does not typically undergo intussusception. The small intestine is placed into approximately 15–20 cm lengths, allowing gentle loops to form at each turn to avoid luminal obstructive episodes. Intermittent sutures are placed between adjacent lengths using non-penetrating submucosal sutures (see Figure 7.18). Some surgeons place serosal sutures in the knowledge that they may only last a short time before they pull through, thus minimizing the risk of obstructive episodes.

9 Perform abdominal lavage and suction away residual fluid.

10 Complete examination of the remainder of the abdominal contents if not already performed.

Wound closure

1 Wrap the small intestine in omentum (see Operative Technique 7.8). Consider serosal patching in patients with a high risk of dehiscence or in the absence of omentum.

2 Perform routine abdominal closure.

See main text.

OPERATIVE TECHNIQUE 7.8

Omentalization of the small intestine

POSITIONING

Dorsal recumbency.

ASSISTANT

Optional.

EQUIPMENT EXTRAS

Abdominal retractors (e.g. Balfour, Gosset); moistened laparotomy swabs with radiographic marker; water-impermeable drape; diathermy (optional).

SURGICAL TECHNIQUE

Approach

See Operative Technique 7.1.

Surgical manipulations

Omentalization can be performed to augment small intestinal suture lines following biopsy, enterotomy or enterectomy (Brockman et al., 1996).

1   Following surgery and abdominal lavage, return the small intestine to its normal anatomical position.

2   Replace the free distal end of the omentum in its normal position in the abdomen, ventral to the small intestine.

3   Identify a portion of omentum and carefully and completely wrap it around the small intestinal suture line, taking care to avoid omental tearing.

4   Sutures can be placed between the omentum and small intestine, taking care not to ligate the omental vasculature, if the omentum does not remain in place after it has been wrapped around the small intestine, or if multiple suture lines need to be omentalized.

For multiple gastrointestinal incisions, or for omentalization of other organs at a more distant site (such as the prostate gland or subcutaneous sites), an omental pedicle can be created to increase its length.

1   Divide the dorsal leaf of the omentum from the pancreas, dorsal gastric and splenic attachments, using diathermy or ligating blood vessels.

2   Gently open the dorsal and ventral leaves of the omentum.

3   The omentum can be further lengthened by creating an L-shaped incision; however, this is rarely necessary in practice.

WARNING

Omentum is very fragile and will easily tear. Handle it gently and avoid pulling on it. Omentum can be wrapped in a moistened swab if it needs to be handled a lot

PRACTICAL TIP

Note in all abdominal surgery reports whether the omentum was ligated, resected or used to augment any suture lines. This information will be important should be patient need to be considered for omentalization procedures in the future

Wound closure

Perform routine abdominal closure.

POSTOPERATIVE MANAGEMENT AND COMPLICATIONS

See main text.

Chapter 8

The large intestine and perineum

Jacqui D. Niles and John M. Williams

Differentiation of large bowel disease from small intestinal disorders is based on history and clinical examination. The clinical signs are a result of disruption of the functions of the large bowel – namely, absorption of water and electrolytes from luminal contents, and storage and periodic expulsion of faecal material.

- Clinical features of large intestinal disease include diarrhoea, constipation, tenesmus, haematochezia and dyschezia.
- Other clinical signs may include depression, vomiting, anorexia, abdominal pain, abdominal enlargement, abnormal faecal shape and rectal prolapse.

During the physical examination, particular attention should be given to caudal abdominal palpation and examination of the anus and perineum; the investigation should always include digital rectal examination.

- Shape and symmetry of the pelvic canal should be noted on rectal examination. Strictures as well as intra- and extraluminal masses may be detected.
- The anus and anal sacs should be evaluated and in a male dog the prostate gland should be assessed.
- Enlargement of the sublumbar lymph nodes can sometimes be detected by rectal examination or caudal abdominal palpation and may be suggestive of metastatic neoplasia.

Plain abdominal radiographs rarely contribute significantly to diagnosis, but are useful in animals with megacolon. Radiographs may also provide information on extraluminal masses, and may show enlarged sublumbar lymph nodes or malaligned pelvic fractures causing compression of the colon or rectum. Luminal masses may be identified if the colon contains gas. Additional information may be obtained by the use of contrast radiography, ultrasonography, proctoscopy, colonoscopy and endoscopy.

Barium enemas can reveal dilatations, constrictions, filling defects, infiltrative disease, intraluminal masses, extraluminal compression, intussusceptions and caecal inversion. To perform a barium enema:

1. Insert a Foley catheter into the rectum and inflate the balloon to create a tight seal.
2. Administer 10 ml barium/kg bodyweight per rectum, following colonic preparation (see *BSAVA Manual of Canine and Feline Gastroenterology*).

Ultrasonography is most helpful for evaluation of masses and intussusceptions in the large intestine, but gas in the intestine can limit the usefulness of this technique. When a mass lesion is detected, the mesenteric and sublumbar lymph nodes should be evaluated and ultrasound-guided aspirates or biopsy samples should be obtained prior to definitive surgery.

Colonoscopy is more sensitive than radiography, allowing for direct visualization of the lumen, and enables samples to be obtained for culture and histopathology, although significant preparation is required prior to scoping to ensure that the colon is sufficiently clean to allow thorough visualization of the mucosa.

The large intestine

Anatomy

The large intestine is divided into the caecum, colon (ascending, transverse and descending), rectum and anus. Most surgeons consider the colorectal junction to be at the pelvic inlet. Histologically the colon and rectum are composed of four distinct layers: mucosa, submucosa, muscularis and serosa.

- The mucosa of the colon consists of columnar and cuboidal epithelial cells as well as numerous mucus-secreting goblet cells.
- The submucosa has a rich neurovascular and lymphatic supply and a high collagen and elastin content, making it the important suture-holding layer.
- The muscularis is composed of an inner circular smooth muscle layer and an outer longitudinal layer.
- The serosa consists of loose connective tissue covered with a layer of squamous mesothelial cells.

The proximal portion of the colon receives its blood supply from branches (colic, right colic and middle colic arteries) of the ileocolic artery, a branch of the cranial mesenteric artery (Figure 8.1). The descending colon is supplied by the left colic artery, which is the cranial branch of the caudal mesenteric artery (Figure 8.2). The cranial rectal artery is the caudal branch of the caudal mesenteric artery and primarily supplies the cranial rectum.

In addition to the blood vessels supplying it, the large intestine is anchored in the sublumbar region by the mesocolon. As a consequence of the short length of the mesocolon, the large intestine is less mobile than the small intestine and its position in the abdomen is less variable.

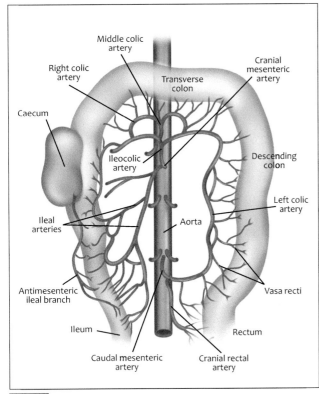

8.1 Anatomy and vascular supply of the large intestine.

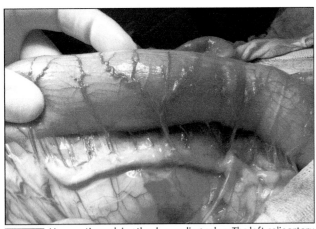

8.2 Vasa recti supplying the descending colon. The left colic artery anastomoses with the middle colic artery and supplies the descending colon by numerous vasa recti, and not the anastomosing arcades seen in the small intestines.

Healing of the large intestine

The large intestine heals similarly to the small intestine but return of tensile strength is slower than for the small intestine, reaching 75% of normal strength at 4 months post surgery (Williams, 2012). As with any surgical wound, optimal healing depends on gentle tissue handling, accurate mucosal apposition, a tension-free closure and preservation of blood supply. In particular, the blood supply should be maintained at the colorectal junction, where it is important to preserve the cranial rectal artery to avoid ischaemic necrosis. Local and systemic factors that delay gastrointestinal healing are summarized in Figure 8.3.

Surgical closure of the colon requires a thorough understanding of the healing process so that the most

Local factors
• Poor tissue perfusion
• Wound tension
• Poor wound apposition
• Infection
• Distal intestinal obstruction

Systemic factors
• Hypovolaemia
• Blood transfusion
• Chemotherapeutic agents (e.g. cisplatin)
• Immunodeficiency
• Poorly controlled diabetes mellitus
• Icterus
• Zinc deficiency
• Iron deficiency

8.3 Local and systemic factors that delay gastrointestinal healing.

appropriate technique is used. Failure to maximize healing potential may lead to catastrophic life-threatening complications. The colonic lumen contains high numbers of aerobic and anaerobic bacteria (10^{10} to 10^{11} bacteria per gram of faeces) and leakage from a colonic incision can result in severe and rapidly fatal peritonitis. The large bacterial population and high intraluminal pressures generated during passage of faecal material mean that the risk of dehiscence is high for the first 4 days after surgery. In humans, colonic anastomoses are more likely to leak than those of the small intestine, with a complication rate of 7–40% reported; such a high complication rate has not been reported in dogs and cats (Williams, 2012).

Preoperative considerations

- Correct electrolyte and acid–base imbalances before surgery.
- Ensure adequate hydration.
- Perioperative antibiotics effective against Gram-negative aerobes and anaerobes should be given at the time of anaesthetic induction (e.g. second-generation cephalosporins, such as cefoxitin (20–30 mg/kg), which is particularly effective against Gram-negative organisms) and then every 90 minutes throughout surgery to reduce the risk of postoperative sepsis.

WARNING

The routine use of enemas prior to colotomy or colectomy cannot be recommended. Owing to the liquid slurry created, enemas are associated with a greatly increased risk of leakage and gross abdominal contamination

---

General surgical considerations

- Perform a complete abdominal exploration.
- Evaluate and perform biopsy on the liver, spleen and lymph nodes in cases of suspected neoplasia.
- Isolate the colon from the rest of the abdominal cavity by packing off with laparotomy swabs.
- Use a slowly absorbed or permanent suture material for colonic surgery (i.e. polydioxanone, glycomer 631 or polypropylene).
- Change gloves and instruments after closure of the colon.
- Omentalize the incision site.

Colotomy

Colotomy (see Operative Technique 8.1) is performed most commonly to obtain a full-thickness biopsy sample when other diagnostic procedures (e.g. colonoscopic biopsy) have failed. Rarely, colotomy is performed to remove a foreign body, but foreign bodies that have reached the large intestine are usually expelled with the faeces unless the object has sharp points or the distal colon or rectum is obstructed.

Large intestinal intussusception

Intussusception of the large intestine usually occurs at the ileocolic junction and can progress to a point where small intestine protrudes from the anus. This can be differentiated from a rectal prolapse by passing a blunt probe between the prolapsed segment and the rectum. These animals often have a history of tenesmus and haematochezia. Treatment involves a complete abdominal exploration, manual reduction if possible, or resection, anastomosis and enteroplication (see Chapter 7).

Caecal inversion

Caecal inversion is an uncommon condition that tends to affect dogs younger than 4 years of age, though it has been reported in older dogs. Clinical signs include diarrhoea, haematochezia, tenesmus, weight loss and vomiting. Occasionally animals present with acute signs of intestinal obstruction (see Chapter 7). Plain radiographs may reveal a small fluid-dense intraluminal mass in the proximal colon, but contrast radiography or colonoscopy is often required to confirm the diagnosis. Treatment involves typhlectomy (caecal resection).

Typhlectomy (caecal resection)

Indications for resecting the caecum include impaction, perforation, inversion, severe inflammation and neoplasia (Figure 8.4). Depending on the type and extent of the disease process, the caecum can either be removed from the colon or be removed in conjunction with the distal ileum and proximal colon (see Operative Technique 8.3). It is preferable to preserve ileocolic anatomy and function if possible.

Caecal impaction

Rarely, the caecum becomes impacted with faeces or foreign material (Wells *et al.*, 1995; White, 1997). Non-specific clinical signs include vomiting, diarrhoea, anorexia, haematochezia and tenesmus. A firm mass may be detected on abdominal palpation. Abdominal radiographs may show loss of the gas-filled caecal silhouette or foreign material in the caecum (Figure 8.5). Treatment is via typhlectomy (see Operative Technique 8.3).

Caecal–colic volvulus

Small intestinal volvulus is the pathological twisting of the small bowel around its mesenteric axis (see Chapter 7). Volvulus of the small intestine is uncommon and most frequently reported in German Shepherd Dogs, often in association with exocrine pancreatic insufficiency (Westermarch and Rimaila-Parnanen, 1989). Volvulus of the large intestine is reported even less frequently, with one report describing the condition in two middle-aged

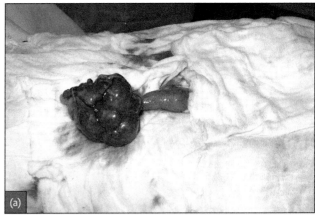
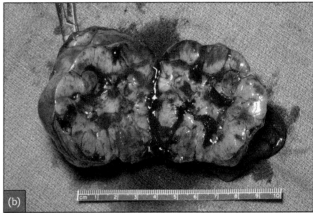

8.4 (a) Caecal leiomyosarcoma in a cat. (b) Cross-section of removed tumour.

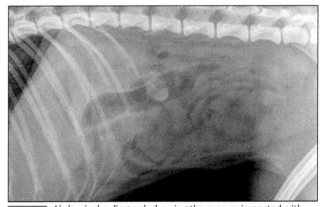

8.5 Abdominal radiograph showing the caecum impacted with mineralized material, immediately caudal to rib 13.

male Great Danes (Carberry and Flanders, 1993) and one reported case in a cat (Drobatz, 1996). In addition, one of the authors [JN] has seen one case in a Rottweiler bitch. Caecal–colic and colonic volvulus have been reported in dogs that have had gastric dilatation and volvulus (GDV) episodes managed by gastropexy, or intussusception and exocrine pancreatic insufficiency (Carberry and Flanders, 1993; Halfacree *et al.*, 2006).

The cause of this condition is unknown. Clinical signs include depression, anorexia, diarrhoea, vomiting, mild abdominal distension, tenesmus and lack of faeces. Abdominal radiographs may reveal a severe gas- and fluid-distended large bowel with an abrupt constriction just proximal to the pelvic inlet (Figure 8.6). The diagnosis is confirmed by abdominal exploratory surgery. The distal ileum, caecum and ascending, transverse and proximal

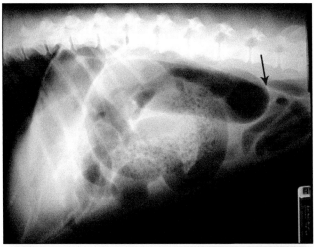

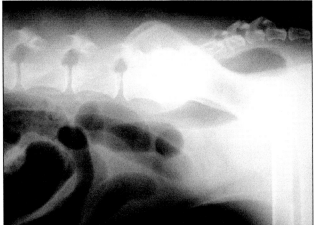

8.6 Abdominal radiographs of a 4-year-old Rottweiler bitch with caecal–colic volvulus. Note the dilated colon, ending abruptly cranial to the pelvic inlet (arrowed).

descending colon are found to be rotated around the root of their mesenteric arterial supply. Before and after derotation, intestinal viability should be assessed. If the intestine is viable, a colopexy to the left body wall should be performed. Non-viable bowel should be resected.

Incisional colopexy

Colopexy (see Operative Technique 8.4), or fixation of the colon to the adjacent abdominal wall, is performed for the treatment of severe or recurrent rectal prolapse (where rectal tissue is viable) or as an adjunctive procedure for correcting rectal sacculation prior to perineal herniorrhaphy. Rarely, colopexy may also be performed following successful identification and reduction of colonic volvulus or torsion. Gastrocolopexy has been reported as a technique to prevent recurrence of GDV (Eggertsdottir *et al.*, 2001).

> **WARNING**
>
> Every effort should be made to identify and treat underlying causes of tenesmus predisposing to recurrent rectal prolapse

> **PRACTICAL TIP**
>
> An epidural anaesthetic can help to minimize postoperative pain and straining but is not essential

Megacolon

Megacolon is characterized by severe and irreversible dilatation of the colon, colonic hypomotility and chronic constipation. In humans, the syndrome of megacolon encompasses a variety of diseases that result in colonic dilatation. The syndrome is usually classified into two categories: congenital megacolon (Hirschsprung's disease) and acquired megacolon. In most affected humans with congenital megacolon, the pathological lesion that causes faecal retention is a congenital absence of myenteric and submucosal intramural plexuses (aganglionosis) in the caudal part of the colon. Acquired megacolon is further subdivided according to the suspected cause of the disorder, or is termed idiopathic if no cause is apparent.

Megacolon is uncommon in companion animals but has been reported in both dogs and cats (Bright *et al.*, 1986; Matthiesen *et al.*, 1991). Mechanical obstruction from various causes (pelvic trauma, colonic or rectal neoplasms, foreign bodies or extracolonic masses) and dietary changes can all cause megacolon (Figure 8.7). Megacolon is a frequent complaint in older Manx cats. The pathogenesis is not understood but it is likely to relate to interference with the defecation reflex caused by the sacral spinal cord deformities present in this breed.

Extraluminal expression	Pelvic deformity/fractures Prostatomegaly Pelvic masses Strictures
Intraluminal obstruction	Constipation Foreign bodies Neoplasia Non-neoplastic strictures
Metabolic	Hypokalaemia Hypothyroidism
Neuromuscular abnormalities	Sacral spine cord deformities (Manx cats) Ileus Dysautonomia Idiopathic Aganglionosis?

8.7 Causes of megacolon.

In most cats the cause of megacolon remains obscure. Megacolon has been reported in cats as young as 1 year and as old as 15 years, but most cases are seen in middle-aged cats. The hallmark of idiopathic megacolon is a dilated colon with no evidence of physical or functional obstruction. *In vitro* studies have shown that megacolon smooth muscle develops less isometric stress in response to neurotransmitters, membrane depolarization and electrical field stimulation than normal colonic smooth muscle (Washabau and Stalis, 1996). It is believed that there is a generalized dysfunction of longitudinal and circular smooth muscle due to a disturbance in the activation of the smooth muscle myofilaments. To date, no specific histological abnormality of the smooth muscle cells or of myenteric or submucosal plexus neurons has been recognized.

Most owners are not aware of their cat's toilet habits, and hence diagnosis and treatment are often initiated only when clinical signs (Figure 8.8) are severe and the condition is long-standing. Chronic obstipation may be associated with anaemia as well as fluid, electrolyte and acid–base abnormalities. Hypokalaemia secondary to vomiting and anorexia is also a complicating factor. It has been suggested that the systemic signs result from a

- Constipation/obstipation
- Anorexia
- Tenesmus
- Vomiting
- Weight loss
- Dehydration
- Crying, arched back, stiff gait, reluctance to move

8.8 Clinical signs of megacolon.

breakdown of the mucosal barrier and absorption of toxic luminal products such as those produced by clostridia, which are thought to multiply in the static colonic contents.

Diagnosis

A diagnosis of constipation/obstipation can usually be made from the history and physical examination findings alone. Abdominal palpation and rectal examination are usually sufficient to identify an impacted colon and to rule out certain causes, such as atresia ani and prostato-megaly (dogs). The integrity of the pelvic diaphragm should also be assessed during rectal examination. It is not uncommon for cats with megacolon to have uni- or bilateral perineal hernias (see section on Perineal hernias). Radiography and laboratory data are helpful to identify any underlying cause. Radiography is used primarily to characterize the severity of colonic impaction (Figure 8.9) and to rule out obstructive diseases such as pelvic fracture malunion, sacrocaudal spinal trauma or deformities, and intramural or mural colonic or rectoanal obstructive lesions.

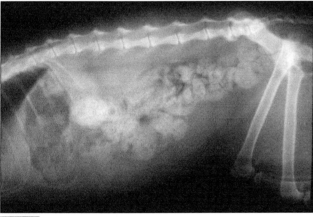

8.9 Lateral radiograph of a cat with idiopathic megacolon.

Treatment

Initial management involves correction of dehydration, and of acid–base and electrolyte abnormalities if obstipation has been prolonged. Occasionally, acquired megacolon can be successfully managed medically, but ultimately most patients undergo colectomy (see Operative Technique 8.2) or are euthanased. For some cats with megacolon secondary to pelvic canal stenosis, pelvic osteotomy without colectomy may be sufficient. In most cases, even if the cause of colonic obstruction that resulted in acquired mega-colon can be identified and readily corrected, the changes in the dilated colon are usually irreversible.

Palliative medical therapies involve manual removal of faecoliths from the colon using stool softeners and enemas. Sedation or preferably general anaesthesia is

necessary to allow adequate decompression of the colon. Perioperative antibiotics should be administered prior to manual removal of faecoliths, because some trauma to the mucosa is inevitable. Copious warm-water irrigation is best used to soften the faecoliths, with the addition of a water-soluble lubrication jelly. Post-enema radiographs should be taken to confirm removal of all impacted faecal material.

> **WARNING**
>
> Manual removal of softened faecoliths should be performed with care to minimize trauma to the mucosal barrier, thus preventing further absorption of luminal bacteria and toxins into the systemic circulation

> **WARNING**
>
> Phosphate enemas should *never* be used in cats, because they will lead to severe dehydration, hypocalcaemia, hypophosphataemia and death

Once the retained faeces have been removed, lax-atives can be used to try and prevent recurrence. Trad-itionally, long-term management has involved the use of stool softeners, high-fibre diets and periodic enemas. Some constipated cats will respond to supplementation of the diet with one of these products. Dietary fibre is preferable, because it is well tolerated, more effective and more physiological than other laxatives. Cats should be well hydrated before commencing fibre supplement-ation, to maximize the therapeutic effect and minimize the impaction of fibre in the constipated colon.

Lactulose is a useful agent for the medical manage-ment of megacolon and is better tolerated by cats than many other laxatives. It is a disaccharide that cannot be hydrolysed by mammals, but is metabolized by the colonic bacteria, resulting in the formation of low molecular weight organic acids. These acids increase the osmotic pressure, drawing water into the bowel and resulting in a laxative effect. There is no set dosage and recommendations vary from 1 ml/4.5 kg orally q8h to 5 ml/cat orally q12h and 5–25 ml/dog q8–12h.

> **PRACTICAL TIP**
>
> Owners should be instructed to monitor the consistency of the stools and adjust the dose of lactulose as necessary to achieve a soft but formed stool

> **WARNING**
>
> Use of mineral oil as a stool softener is not advised because of the danger of aspiration during administration. It also tends to flow around the faecoliths rather than softening them appreciably. Chronic administration of mineral oil can lead to malabsorption of fat-soluble vitamins

Cisapride is a prokinetic agent that works by causing the release of acetylcholine from the enteric nervous sys-tem, which stimulates colonic smooth muscle to contract. In the past it has been used alone, and in combination with lactulose, for the treatment of megacolon in cats. Cisapride tended to be more effective in stimulating colonic propulsive motility in cats affected with mild to moderate idiopathic constipation. Cats with long-standing constipation and megacolon did not always respond. Cisapride is available under special licence in the UK and from Food and Drug Administration (FDA)-approved compounding pharmacies in the USA; the recommended dose is 2.5 mg per cat q8–12h.

Colectomy: Subtotal colectomy (see Operative Technique 8.2) involves removal of 90–95% of the colon. The primary indication is the treatment of obstipation related to megacolon. Other indications include trauma, perforation, neoplasia or irreducible intussusception.

> **PRACTICAL TIP**
>
> Preserve the ileocolic valve when possible, because this shortens the postoperative recovery period and decreases the likelihood of intractable diarrhoea from small intestinal bacterial overgrowth. It can, however, be more difficult to achieve a tension-free anastomosis when the valve is preserved, and in cats the ileocolic valve can be resected with very few postoperative complications

Following total colectomy with ileorectal anastomosis, cats initially pass small volumes of watery diarrhoea. Experimental studies have shown postoperative increases in villus height, enterocyte height and enterocyte density over a 2-month period and stool consistency improves to a semi-solid formed stool as ileal adaptation occurs (Bertoy *et al.*, 1989). Dogs do not adapt as well as cats following colectomy and the ileocolic valve should be preserved if at all possible.

> **PRACTICAL TIP**
>
> Meticulous tissue handling, careful apposition and a tension-free anastomosis are vital to surgical success

Colonic torsion

Torsion of the descending colon is a rarely described condition in which the descending colon twists about its long axis (Halfacree *et al.*, 2006). It has been reported in two collie dogs (Marks, 1986). It is theorized that torsion is rare because of the short mesentery that attaches the colon to the dorsal abdominal wall, and that a defect in the descending mesocolon would be necessary to permit torsion to occur. Dogs present depressed and in shock, with abdominal pain and progressive abdominal distension. Prompt diagnosis and immediate surgical exploration are required because of the rapid build-up and absorption of toxins, necrosis of the colonic wall and peritonitis. Abdominal palpation may reveal a large painful mass in the caudal abdomen. Radiographs may show a megacolon ending abruptly at the pelvic inlet. Treatment consists of reducing the torsion as quickly as possible and assessing whether colopexy or intestinal resection is necessary

Colonic neoplasia

Dogs develop large intestinal tumours more commonly than cats, in which the small intestine is most frequently affected (see Chapter 7). Adenomas, adenocarcinomas,

lymphosarcomas, leiomyomas, leiomyosarcomas, carcinoids and plasmacytomas have all been reported. Adenocarcinoma of the large intestine often occurs in the mid to distal rectum and in several forms: nodular, pedunculated, or as an annular constriction. Metastasis can occur to the regional lymph nodes, mesentery and liver. Metastasis to the spinal meninges, testes and skin has also been reported (Phillips, 2003). In cats, the most common tumour types are adenocarcinoma, lymphoma, mast cell tumours and neuroendocrine tumours. Metastatic disease is found in between 75% and 80% of cats with colonic neoplasia.

The most common clinical signs in dogs with colonic neoplasia include tenesmus, haematochezia, dyschezia, constipation and rectal prolapse. Diarrhoea, weight loss and vomiting may also be observed. Dogs with mesenchymal caecal tumours can present with fever, collapse and septic peritonitis. In cats, clinical signs associated with colonic neoplasia include weight loss, anorexia, vomiting and diarrhoea. Haematochezia and tenesmus are seen far less commonly than in the dog.

Large intestinal tumours can sometimes be felt on abdominal palpation and distal colonic/rectal tumours may be palpated per rectum. Animals may be cachexic and dehydrated, with or without abdominal pain. A complete blood count can reveal a mild to moderate anaemia and leucocytosis. Abdominal radiography (including contrast studies), ultrasonography and colonoscopy are all useful in the diagnosis and staging of colonic tumours. Wide *en bloc* excision, with margins of 4–6 cm, is recommended for isolated malignant masses, followed by colonic anastomosis. Pelvic osteotomy may be required to achieve adequate margins in some cases.

Prognosis

The mean survival time after surgical resection of colorectal adenocarcinomas in dogs is 6–22 months, whereas in cats mean survival time following mass resection alone is 68 days *versus* 138 days in cats treated with subtotal colectomy. Chemotherapy does significantly increase survival time for cats with adenocarcinomas but does not seem to make a difference to cats with colonic lymphoma (Slawienski *et al.*, 1997).

Colonic entrapment

Colonic entrapment has been reported after ovariohysterectomy and castration, secondary to adhesion formation. In all reported cases that occurred after ovariohysterectomy, the prognosis was good after resection of the fibrous band compressing the colon. Scar tissue resection can be performed laparoscopically or via exploratory coeliotomy.

Entrapment and strangulation may occur after rupture of the duodenocolic ligament (Hassinger, 1997). The clinical findings at presentation include vomiting, collapse, marked cranial abdominal distension, and a palpable tubular viscus with large distended gas-filled bowel loops visible on plain radiographs. During surgery, the colon and small intestine are found on the right side of the abdomen because of herniation through the torn duodenocolic ligament. The colon is decompressed and any remaining remnant of the ventral band of the duodenocolic ligament is transected before the intestine is returned to its normal position. The prognosis is favourable as long as there is no significant vascular compromise of the entrapped bowel.

Colonic or rectal trauma

Traumatic perforation of the colon or rectum is very uncommon in dogs and cats. It may be caused by bites, by gunshot or knife wounds, or by bone fragments from pelvic fractures. The passage of bloody faeces after a traumatic episode should raise the index of suspicion of colonic perforation. Occasionally procedures such as endoscopy, proctoscopy or enemas can cause perforation. Bacterial peritonitis and septic shock quickly ensue. Clinical signs, diagnosis and treatment of peritonitis are covered in Chapter 18.

Colonic perforation has also been reported in dogs that have been treated with parenteral dexamethasone (Toombs *et al.*, 1980). Colonic perforation in the absence of trauma occurs most frequently in dogs with intervertebral disc disease that undergo surgery. Spinal cord injury, surgical stress and decreased colonic mucus production lead to an increased colonic transit time, erosion of the mucosa, perforation, peritonitis and death. Clinical signs often occur 3–8 days after surgery and include anorexia, depression, vomiting, pyrexia, melaena and abdominal pain.

Perforations most commonly occur on the antimesenteric side of the proximal descending colon. Changeovers between vagal and pelvic sources of parasympathetic innervation, and between coeliacomesenteric and caudal mesenteric sources of sympathetic innervation, occur at this location. It has been suggested that this creates an imbalance of autonomic innervation, resulting in decreased motility and microvascular supply of this portion of the colon, making it more susceptible to perforation.

Colorectal neoplasia

Benign leiomyoma and adenomatous polyps are commonly seen in dogs, with adenomatous polyps being the most frequently reported colorectal tumour. There is evidence that, as with familial polyposis In humans, malignant transformation can occur in approximately 25% of cases. In the dog, malignant tumours include adenocarcinoma, leiomyosarcoma and lymphosarcoma. The ratio of benign to malignant tumours is approximately 40:60. In the cat, adenocarcinoma is the most commonly reported tumour, followed by lymphoma and mast cell tumours. The median age for colorectal tumours is 6–9 years in dogs and 12 years for cats.

Patients with large intestinal and rectal tumours consistently present with dyschezia and/or haematochezia, although signs such as anal discharge, frank haemorrhage, increased faecal frequency or constipation are also seen. Occasionally owners will notice a temporary prolapse of a mass after the patient has defecated. Lower colorectal lesions are readily detected by digital rectal examination, which allows the site and extent of the lesion to be identified. Open illuminated proctoscopes are invaluable in the investigation of all colorectal lesions, and are preferred to fibreoptic endoscopes for lower colonic examination. Proctoscopes allow a direct view of the lesion so that deep representative biopsy samples can be obtained. Radiography (including survey films and contrast studies) often adds little information to that gained from rectal and proctoscopic examination. Survey films for evidence of metastatic spread to the sublumbar (iliac) lymph nodes and thorax should be carried out routinely. Positive contrast radiographs (barium enema) may reveal mural filling defects (Figure 8.10) and classically an 'apple core' appearance is seen.

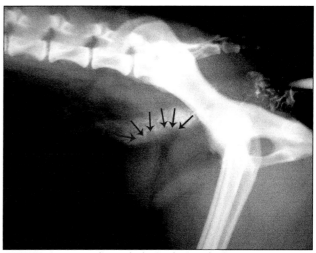

8.10 Contrast radiograph obtained using a barium enema. Arrows outline a filling defect in ventral colorectal wall.

Owing to their potential for malignant transformation, all colorectal polyps, as well as malignant lesions, should be excised as early as possible and with a wide surgical margin of 1–2 cm. Access to a significant number of colorectal masses is limited because they are intrapelvic, making it difficult to achieve adequate surgical margins. A number of techniques have been described for the management of intrapelvic colorectal tumours. The majority of these techniques involve an anal or perineal approach, which requires the patient to be placed in sternal recumbency with the tail tied upwards and forwards, with the hindlimbs hanging over the end of a table (perineal stand). To facilitate surgery, the table can be tipped at an angle, taking care not to exceed 25–30 degrees (Figure 8.11). A tilt greater than this may compromise respiration, as a result of cranial shifting of the abdominal organs.

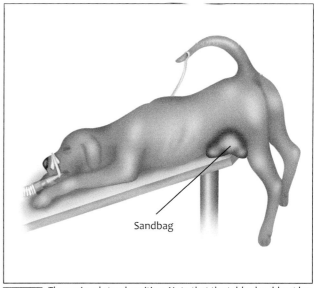

Sandbag

8.11 The perineal stand position. Note that the table should not be tilted more than 25–30 degrees.

PRACTICAL TIP

It is usually preferable for the surgeon to sit when carrying out anal or perineal surgery

Local excision and the anal 'pull-out' procedure

Eversion of small non-malignant rectal masses adjacent to the anus is a simple and practical procedure (Figure 8.12). Following eversion, stay sutures can be placed in the rectal mucosa around the lesion. The lesion is excised along with the mucosa. A full-thickness excision is usually not required. The mucosal defect is closed with simple appositional absorbable sutures.

It is also often possible to evert larger distal colorectal lesions by traction and then carry out a full-thickness resection, with adequate margins (see Operative Technique 8.5). The resulting defect is closed with simple interrupted sutures, while for distal annular lesions a standard end-to-end anastomosis is performed.

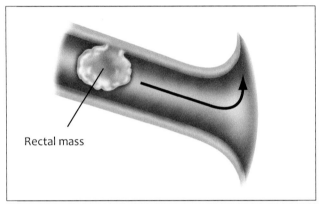

Rectal mass

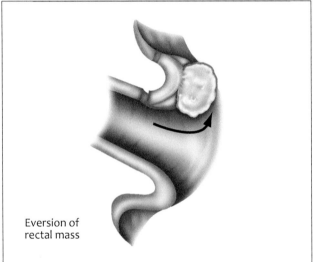

Eversion of rectal mass

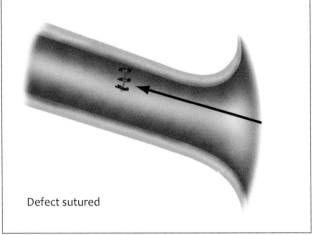

Defect sutured

8.12 Anal 'pull-out' and local excision. For small lesions, full-thickness resection is not always required.

Rectal 'pull-through' technique

The rectal 'pull-through' technique (see Operative Technique 8.6) is preferable for large or annular lesions that are located in the caudal to mid part of the pelvic canal. It involves incising the rectum circumferentially, immediately cranial to the anus. One author [JW] finds this technique preferable to anal pull-out for large lesions, because the incidence of stricture formation or dehiscence is less.

Dorsal approach

An inverted horseshoe-shaped incision between the anus and the base of the tail allows good access to the rectum (see Operative Technique 8.7). The paired rectococcygeus muscles must be transected to allow separation of the rectum from its pelvic attachments so that it may be exteriorized. In most cases a standard resection and end-to-end anastomosis is performed. Care must be taken not to resect more than 6 cm of rectum, because the risk of faecal incontinence becomes much greater if more is excised.

Perineal approach

In this modification of the dorsal approach, a unilateral incision is made from the base of the tail to the ischial tuberosity (see below). This gives limited access to the lateral aspect of the pelvic canal; separation of the levator ani and coccygeus muscles may be required for more cranial lesions. The technique is useful only for excision of small serosal lesions of the rectum and well encapsulated benign lesions (e.g. fibroleiomyoma, lipoma).

Ventral approach

In some cases, colorectal tumours may be exposed via a posterior midline laparotomy, which may be combined with a pubic symphysiotomy or osteotomy (see Operative Technique 8.8). In one author's experience [JW], this gives limited access and requires considerable postoperative analgesia. It is generally only considered when other techniques are not feasible.

Complications and prognosis

Complications that may be encountered following colorectal surgery include stenosis, persistent tenesmus, dehiscence, incontinence and pararectal abscessation. Stenosis at the surgical site is most likely when more than half the circumference of the rectum is excised. Rectal polyps have a very favourable prognosis, but with malignant lesions local recurrence and regional metastasis are common after surgery. Mean postsurgical survival time for dogs with rectal adenocarcinoma is reported as 6–9 months.

Atresia ani

Congenital abnormalities of the anal region are thought to be rare but the recorded incidence may not be a true one, because many animals are euthanased owing to the poor prognosis associated with these conditions. Atresia ani is the most commonly reported congenital anomaly in dogs and is classified into four types:

- *Type I*: Congenital stenosis of the anus
- *Type II*: Persistent anal membrane with a blind-ending rectal pouch just cranial to the anus
- *Type III*: Closed anus with the rectum ending more cranially within the pelvic canal (Figure 8.13)
- *Type IV*: Anus and distal rectum normal; proximal rectum ends as a pouch within the pelvic canal.

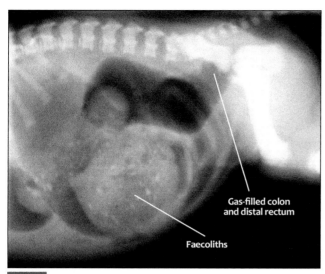

8.13 Radiograph of Boxer puppy with Type III atresia ani.

These cases usually present in the first few weeks of life with tenesmus and constipation. On examination, patients usually have an imperforate anus (Figure 8.14) (apart from Type IV) and are thin, in poor condition but very potbellied. Surgical correction may be attempted but is often unsuccessful and may require repeated procedures. Complications of surgery include rectoanal stricture formation, faecal incontinence or constipation due to irreversible megacolon. A recently described technique may reduce the risk of dehiscence (Mahler and Williams, 2005).

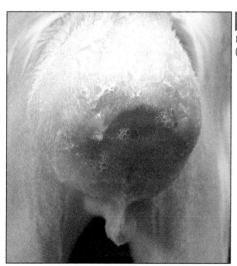

8.14 Imperforate anus (atresia ani).

Anogenital cleft

In this condition there is a failure of the embryological cloaca to separate and so there is direct communication between the anus and the vagina or urethra. In males, the condition is often associated with hypospadias (incomplete formation of the urethra ventrally); both faecal and urinary continence are usually maintained. In females, faecal incontinence is common and, more importantly, there is often severe faecal contamination of the urinary tract, which may result in pyelonephritis.

Surgical correction may be attempted in both males and females and can be successful, although wound dehiscence and infection are commonly encountered. In the male, as well as reconstruction of the ventral anus, a ventral or scrotal urethrostomy may be required. In cases of hypospadias there is often insufficient tissue present to allow reconstruction.

Pseudocoprostasis

Pseudocoprostasis is a condition (usually of long-haired animals) where perineal hair and faeces are matted over the anus, resulting in a physical obstruction of the anus. The condition tends to occur either in poorly groomed individuals or following diarrhoea. Treatment simply involves clipping the hair away and removing any anorectal faecoliths.

Anal sac disease

Anal sac problems account for approximately 12% of canine clinical presentations, but cats are less commonly presented (Van Duijkeren, 1995). The classical presenting signs for any anal sac problem are summarized in Figure 8.15.

- Chewing or licking excessively over tail base or anus
- Reluctance/discomfort on sitting
- 'Scooting' (dragging anus along the ground with hindlimbs extended)
- Dyschezia (may be noted in extreme cases)
- Draining tracts in ruptured abscesses

8.15 Anal sac presenting signs.

It is thought that most anal sac disease is related to some degree of obstruction of the anal sac duct, though the precise aetiology is not fully understood. Factors that are believed to initiate or perpetuate anal sac problems are listed in Figure 8.16.

- Stool consistency
- Diet
- Lack of anal sphincter muscle tone
- Inactivity
- Obesity
- Generalized seborrhoea
- Recent oestrus
- Anal furunculosis/perianal fistulae
- Breed predisposition

8.16 Factors initiating anal sac problems.

Anal sac impaction

Anal sac impaction is the most common presentation and is straightforward to treat by digital expression of the anal sacs, situated at 4 and 8 o'clock. Internal (per rectum) compression is preferable and more effective than external compression. External compression is reserved for only the smallest of dogs or cats where digital rectal examination is not feasible. The anal sac secretion is viscous, often grey in colour and has a putty-like consistency. In some cases digital expression may be required at regular intervals and in chronic cases anal sacculectomy may be considered (see below).

Anal sacculitis

In cases of anal sacculitis, the anal sacs are often very painful and either sedation or a general anaesthetic may be required in order to express them. Following expression of the infected anal sacs, they should be cannulated and flushed. The sacs can either be flushed with a sterile isotonic solution, such as lactated Ringer's, or a mild antiseptic solution (0.05% chlorhexidine). There is some debate as to the effectiveness of instilling an antibiotic, an antibiotic plus corticosteroid, or a corticosteroid alone into the sacs after flushing. If there is an infection present a suitable systemic antibiotic is likely to prove more effective, because the tissue concentration of the anti-biotic can be maintained for longer than with a single application of a topical antibiotic. The effectiveness or otherwise of instilling corticosteroids has not been proven. Anal sac flushing may be required at intervals of 10–14 days until the problem resolves. In refractory cases, anal sacculectomy can be considered (see below).

Anal sac abscessation

As with all abscesses, it is essential to incise and drain the infected sacs. It is also beneficial to lavage with an isotonic solution or dilute chlorhexidine (dilute povidone–iodine is of little value, as it is inactivated by organic matter). The incised sacs should be left open and the animal given a systemic broad-spectrum antibiotic, pending the results of culture and sensitivity. The most frequently cultured organisms are *Escherichia coli*, *Streptococcus faecalis* and *Proteus* spp. Recurrent anal sac abscessation is best managed by anal sacculectomy (see below).

Anal sacculectomy: The procedure of choice for removing the infected tissue is open excision (see Operative Technique 8.10). This procedure can also be used when dealing with anal sac adenocarcinoma or when anal sac excision is required in the management of anal furunculo-sis. The use of resins and other materials to pack the anal sac is to be avoided as they may leak into the surrounding tissues, producing a chronic focus for infection.

Anal sac gland adenocarcinoma

Anal sac (apocrine) gland adenocarcinoma predominantly affects older bitches (>90% of cases) and is highly malignant, tending to metastasize readily to the medial iliac lymph nodes. The presenting clinical signs are those typically seen with anal disease and include dyschezia, tenesmus, flattened (ribbon-like) stools and a perineal swelling. Very occasionally a perianal mass is noted during a routine clinical examination. This condition is extremely rare in cats and the prognosis is poor.

Anal sac adenocarcinoma may also present initially with polydipsia/polyuria. This is due to the paraneoplastic effects caused by a parathyroid hormone-related protein (PTHrP) that is produced by the tumour. Release of PTHrP results in hypercalcaemia and hypophosphataemia. Excess circulating calcium has a toxic effect on the renal tubular epithelial cells that leads to the polydipsia.

> **PRACTICAL TIP**
>
> In all cases of a suspected anal sac mass, it is important to obtain a full biochemistry profile to assess the levels of calcium and phosphate. It is also essential to assess renal function

In cases with hypercalcaemia, normal (0.9%) saline should be administered at rates in excess of maintenance to diurese the calcium. Once the patient is normocal-caemic, furosemide may be administered (2 mg/kg i.v.) to prevent calcium resorption.

Given that metastasis is reportedly seen in >50% of cases at presentation (Aronson, 2003), it is essential to assess the draining lymph nodes and to check for thoracic metastases. Although the medial iliac lymph nodes are occasionally palpable per rectum in small dogs, if the node is massive, it is better to take caudal abdominal radiographs (Figure 8.17) or to use trans-abdominal ultrasonography for assessment.

If there are no detectable metastases and the patient is normocalcaemic, the treatment of choice is surgical excision of the mass. The success in removal will depend on the size of the tumour, which has been reported to be between 1 and 10 cm. Potential postoperative sequelae include wound dehiscence, infection, faecal incontinence and local recurrence (25% of cases). Recurrence of hyper-calcaemia without local tumour recurrence is reported in 35–50% of cases as a consequence of paraneoplastic effects from metastatic tumour deposits. It is therefore important to assess blood calcium levels regularly as well as check for local regrowth in these patients. Postsurgical survival ranges from 2 to 39 months, with average survival being around 8 months for patients undergoing surgery alone. It is reasonable to expect average survival rates of around 18 months if surgery is followed with either chemotherapy or radiation therapy.

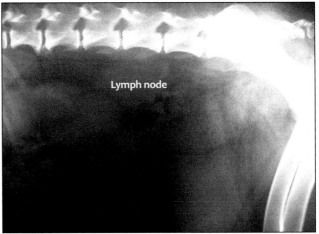

8.17 Radiograph showing an enlarged iliac lymph node. (Reproduced from the BSAVA *Manual of Canine and Feline Gastroenterology*)

Anal furunculosis/perianal fistula

Anal furunculosis/perianal fistulae are extremely frustra-ting diseases characterized by chronic infection and ulceration of the tissues around the anus (see BSAVA *Manual of Canine and Feline Gastroenterology* and BSAVA *Manual of Canine and Feline Wound Management and Reconstruction*). There are often deeply infiltrating sinus tracts, which can form true fistulae with the rectum. The underlying cause of this disease remains elusive. Successful long-term management is also elusive but use of immunosuppressive agents, such as oral prednisone in combination with a novel protein diet, oral ciclosporin (cyclosporine) or topical tacrolimus ointment (Misseghers *et al.*, 2000), holds out the best hope. Ciclosporin shows marked variation in absorption and metabolism between animals and regular blood level monitoring is recom-mended to ensure that the dose is maintained within an appropriate therapeutic range. Doses of 2–15 mg/kg orally q12–24h have been suggested. It is generally well tolerated but is very expensive. Side effects can include vomiting, diarrhoea, anorexia and increased susceptibility to infection.

Ketoconazole has been used in conjunction with ciclosporin. It inhibits cytochrome P450 oxidase activity in the liver and intestines and results in increased blood ciclosporin levels, which can decrease the cost of therapy. Where there is recurrence after immunosuppression, or if the lesions are reduced but not resolved with drug therapy, surgical excision of the lesions can be considered (Patterson and Campbell, 2005; Milner, 2006). Ketoconazole is not available in the UK at the time of publication.

Anal stricture

Strictures occur secondary to trauma, anal furunculosis, neoplasia or surgery. The clinical signs are faecal tenesmus, dyschezia and haematochezia with flattened stools. Confirmatory diagnosis is by digital rectal examination but many patients require anaesthesia for this to be carried out owing to the painful nature of the condition. Megacolon may develop secondarily to constipation caused by severe rectal strictures.

Treatment consists of bougienage to dilate the stricture ± intralesional injection of a steroid such as triamcinolone. This may need to be carried out at regular intervals (once or twice weekly for several weeks) but strictures can recur. In severe cases surgical excision can be attempted, but stricture may recur at the surgical site. In extreme cases anal resection (anoplasty) and a rectal pull-through procedure can be considered (see Operative Technique 8.11). Although a radical procedure, this can greatly improve the patient's quality of life, and the degree of faecal incontinence is usually mild.

Anal prolapse

This is a prolapse that presents with oedematous red anal mucosa protruding through the anal orifice at the end of defecation. The cause is usually associated with faecal tenesmus and it is essential to determine and treat the underlying cause of the tenesmus as well as managing the prolapse.

In most cases the prolapse can be reduced digitally, following lubrication. For recurrent cases a temporary purse-string suture can be placed in the anus for 48–96 hours; some authors suggest that the purse-string suture is tied loosely to allow faecal passage but prevent mucosal prolapse. While the suture is in place the animal should be fed a low-residue diet and placed on a stool softener such as lactulose. In severe cases, where the mucosa appears devitalized, mucosal resection should be carried out. In cases with recurrent prolapse in which the mucosa is viable, an incisional colopexy (see Operative Technique 8.4) should be carried out.

Anal trauma

Perianal and perineal trauma may be the result of projectile injuries, bite wounds or severe road traffic accidents. The management of such wounds may be problematic, as either faecal incontinence or stricture formation may result. For further discussion see the *BSAVA Manual of Canine and Feline Wound Management and Reconstruction.*

Circumanal gland adenoma

The circumanal gland (hepatoid or perianal gland) adenoma is the commonest anal tumour of the dog, with some 85% being reported in the older intact male; it is rarely reported in cats. Circumanal gland adenocarcinomas are very rare. Anatomically the adenomas are found in the external region of the outer cutaneous zone; they may be single or multiple.

They may be seen and palpated as discrete swellings; they often have a bluish coloration and may be large and ulcerated. Many owners do not realize that there is a problem until there is either fresh blood seen on the stools or frank haemorrhage from the ulcerated tumour.

As these tumours are known to respond to androgenic stimulation, castration of the intact male is the treatment of choice. Once the animal has been castrated, the tumour (even if ulcerated) will regress. If the tumour is large, surgical excision can be carried out in addition to castration.

The perineum
Anatomy

The perineum comprises the structures that make up the boundary of the pelvic outlet. It extends externally from the dorsal aspect of the scrotum/vulva to the base of the tail; its lateral margins extend to the skin covering the tubers ischii and superficial gluteal muscles. The deep portion is delineated by the ischial arch ventrally, the third coccygeal vertebra dorsally and, in the dog, by the sacrotuberous ligament laterally. In the cat the lateral margins are less well defined, owing to the absence of a sacrotuberous ligament. The perineum essentially surrounds the anal and urogenital canals.

Within the perineum the most important structures are those that make up the pelvic diaphragm: the levator ani and coccygeal muscles. These muscles act as a division between the pelvic canal and the wedge-shaped ischiorectal fossa, which is bounded laterally by the caudal portion of the superficial gluteal muscle, medially by the external anal sphincter, levator ani and coccygeus muscles, and ventrally by the internal obturator muscle (Figures 8.18 and 8.19). The muscles of the pelvic diaphragm are essential in supporting the rectum and not only act as a physical partition but are essential in counteracting the effects of raised intra-abdominal pressure. Failure of these muscles has the potential to allow abdominal viscera to herniate through the pelvic canal, as happens in a perineal hernia (see below).

Within the ischiorectal fossa lie the internal pudendal artery and vein and the pudendal nerve, together with fat. The pudendal nerve gives rise to the caudal rectal nerves that supply the external anal sphincter and are responsible for maintaining faecal continence. The neurovascular structures course caudomedially from the ventrolateral aspect of the coccygeus, over the internal obturator muscle, towards the clitoris or the root of the penis. Lymphatic drainage of the perineum is via the internal (medial) iliac lymph nodes, while the cutaneous anal area drains via the superficial inguinal lymph nodes.

Perineal hernia

Perineal hernias or ruptures are mostly seen in middle-aged to older intact male dogs, though they are also reported in bitches and in the cat, and one case was recently reported in a 4-month-old puppy (Vyacheslav and Ranen, 2009). The aetiology remains unclear but is associated with degenerative changes in the muscles of the pelvic diaphragm. Many factors have been implicated in the aetiopathogenesis but none has been fully substantiated. They include prostatomegaly, reduced numbers of androgen receptors in the levator ani and coccygeus muscles, rectal sacculation (most likely to be secondary to herniation), colitis and docking.

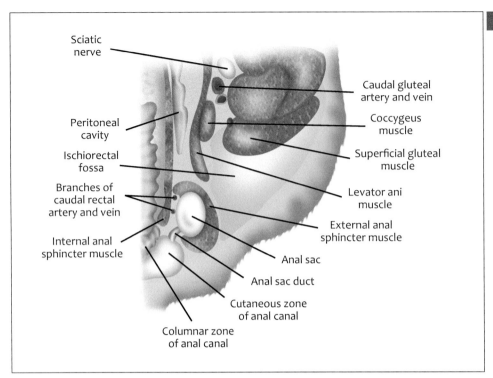

8.18 Horizontal section through perineal area.

Labels:
Sciatic nerve
Caudal gluteal artery and vein
Peritoneal cavity
Coccygeus muscle
Ischiorectal fossa
Superficial gluteal muscle
Branches of caudal rectal artery and vein
Levator ani muscle
Internal anal sphincter muscle
External anal sphincter muscle
Anal sac
Anal sac duct
Cutaneous zone of anal canal
Columnar zone of anal canal

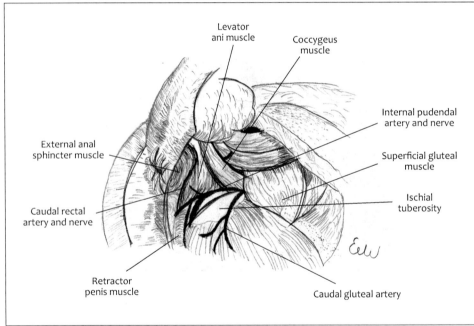

8.19 Schematic drawing of perineal anatomy.
(Reproduced from the *BSAVA Manual of Canine and Feline Gastroenterology*)

Labels:
Levator ani muscle
Coccygeus muscle
Internal pudendal artery and nerve
External anal sphincter muscle
Superficial gluteal muscle
Ischial tuberosity
Caudal rectal artery and nerve
Retractor penis muscle
Caudal gluteal artery

Four types of perineal hernia have been reported in dogs, but the hernia is usually caudal and located between the levator ani and coccygeus muscles and the external anal sphincter muscle (see Figures 8.19, 8.20 and 8.21). With the loss of lateral support there is progressive rectal deviation, which leads to enlargement. Unilaterally this is termed *sacculation*, whilst bilateral disease is termed *dilatation*. True rectal diverticula with rectal mucosa protruding through the rectal musculature are extremely rare (Figure 8.22). Hernias may be complicated by the inclusion of pelvic and peritoneal fat, loops of small intestine, prostate gland, paraprostatic or prostatic cysts and, in severe cases, by retroflexion of the bladder (Figure 8.23).

Type of perineal hernia	Location	Incidence
Sciatic	Between sacrotuberous ligament and coccygeus muscle	Rare
Ventral	Between bulbocavernosus and ischiocavernosus muscles	Rare
Dorsal	Between coccygeus and levator ani muscles	Uncommon
Caudal	Between external anal sphincter, levator ani and internal obturator muscles	Most common

8.20 The four types of perineal hernia.

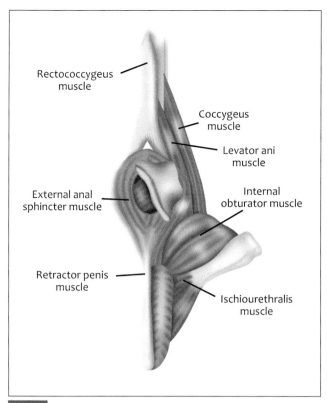

Rectococcygeus muscle
Coccygeus muscle
Levator ani muscle
External anal sphincter muscle
Internal obturator muscle
Retractor penis muscle
Ischiourethralis muscle

8.21 Perineal musculature.

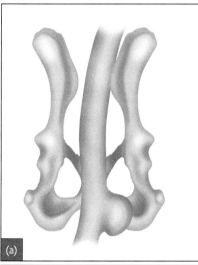

(a)

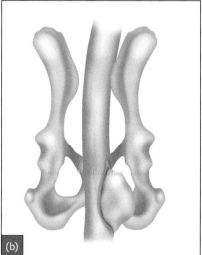

(b)

8.22 (a) Rectal sacculation. (b) Rectal diverticulum (rare; note the mucosa protruding through the muscularis and serosal layers of rectum).

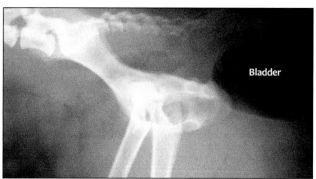

Bladder

8.23 Pneumocystogram of a Cocker Spaniel bitch with perineal hernia and retroflexed bladder.

The clinical signs and main differential diagnoses are summarized in Figures 8.24 and 8.25. Diagnosis of perineal hernias is confirmed by rectal examination, where sacculation and lack of lateral rectal wall support are noted (Figure 8.26). Contrast radiography or ultrasonography is of use to confirm a retroflexed bladder (see Figure 8.23) and aid in the diagnosis of concurrent prostatic disease. Megacolon, perineal masses, trauma, fibrosing colitis and previously performed perineal urethrostomy have all been reportedly associated with perineal hernias in cats. Signs include tenesmus and constipation but, unlike dogs, cats rarely show perineal swelling. Cats with mild clinical signs may be able to be managed medically. Those with more severe clinical signs require surgical repair using internal obturator muscle transposition.

Owing to the risk of bladder involvement, all perineal hernias in dogs should be managed surgically by reconstruction of the pelvic diaphragm. In those cases that have bladder retroflexion, renal and electrolyte status should be assessed and corrected by fluid therapy before undertaking surgery. If urinary catheterization is not possible, relief can be provided by perineal cystocentesis. Where there is preoperative bladder retroflexion, replacement into the abdomen whilst carrying out a perineal approach together with herniorrhaphy can be performed and is, in the opinion of the authors, usually adequate; this precludes the need for cystopexy or vas deferensopexy. Alternatively, cystopexy or vas deferensopexy (see Operative Technique 15.4) can be performed via an abdominal approach prior to definitive herniorrhaphy.

Perineal swelling	Unilateral (more commonly reported on the right) Bilateral
Defecatory tenesmus	75–80% of cases
Dysuria and stranguria if there is bladder herniation	Reportedly in up to 20% of cases, though likely to be less common
Bloody stool	4% of cases
Vomiting	3% of cases
Urinary incontinence	3% of cases

8.24 Clinical signs of perineal hernia.

- Perineal hernia
- Perineal/intrapelvic mass
- Paraprostatic cysts
- Perineal trauma
- Neoplasia

8.25 Differential diagnoses for perineal swelling.

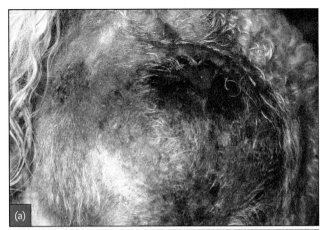

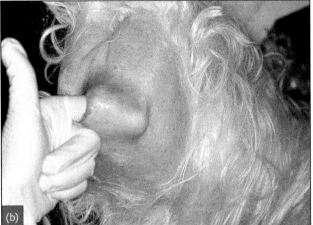

8.26   (a) Large perineal swelling, suggestive of a perineal hernia.
(b) Perineal hernia being confirmed by rectal examination;
note the lack of lateral rectal wall support.
(Reproduced from the BSAVA Manual of Canine and Feline Gastroenterology)

Surgery

Castration is carried out routinely in the management of perineal hernia, as there is evidence of a reduced incidence of recurrence. The authors prefer to carry out castration in the dorsally recumbent patient prior to undertaking herniorrhaphy. There is no indication for multiple anaesthetic episodes in these cases; castration and bilateral herniorrhaphy (where indicated) should be performed at the same time (see Operative Techniques 8.9 and 15.4).

A number of techniques have been described for the repair of perineal hernias, but the technique with the highest success rate (80–90%) is a combination of the 'conventional' or dorsal repair with transposition of the internal obturator muscle.

Ventral herniation and/or sacculation of the rectum:
The presence of significant ventral herniation and/or sacculation (see Figure 8.26) presents a considerable challenge to the surgeon. If the degree of sacculation is small, suturing the elevated obturator muscle flaps as far medially as possible is often satisfactory, taking care to identify and avoid the urethra.

PRACTICAL TIP

Place a urethral catheter preoperatively to help identify the urethra

With larger defects the surgeon should consider either a colopexy procedure (see Operative Technique 8.4) or transposition of the semitendinosus muscle (Figure 8.27). (For further description of the use of this muscle flap, see the *BSAVA Manual of Canine and Feline Wound Management and Reconstruction*.) There are a number of case reports indicating that colopexy with cystopexy can be successful when combined with perineal hernia repair. Whether these additional procedures are performed at the time as perineal herniorrhaphy or not is based on the surgeon's preference; however, in dogs with retroflexed bladders or large rectal dilatations, performing the abdominal procedures a few days before the perineal approach often facilitates the herniorrhaphy. One report of 32 cases suggested successful treatment of perineal hernias by colopexy, cystopexy and vasopexy without definitive herniorrhaphy (Maute *et al.*, 2001). The reported recurrence rate was 22%, which compares favourably with other reports.

Use of prosthetic materials: Prosthetic materials that may be used include porcine dermal collagen sheets, polyester mesh and porcine small intestine submucosa (SIS). It must be remembered that biomaterials increase the risk of infection. In one series of 59 dogs in which polypropylene mesh was used, the reported infection rate was 5.6% and the recurrence rate was 12.5% (Szabo *et al.*,

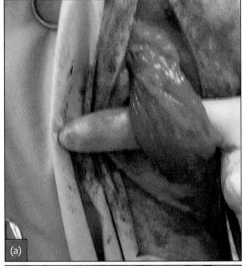

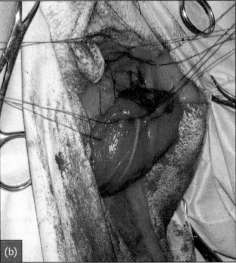

8.27   (a) Semitendinosus muscle being dissected prior to distal transection and used to repair a ventral perineal hernia.
(b) Semitendinosus muscle being sutured in ventral portion of hernia.

2007). In a study where porcine dermal collagen was used to treat perineal hernias in 21 dogs the success rate was only 59.3%, and 33% of dogs developed a serosanguineous discharge from the wound (Frankland, 1986). Porcine SIS may offer advantages over polypropylene mesh in that it promotes vascular ingrowth, is more resistant to infection and induces a regenerative response from the tissues in which it is implanted. Overall, there is a paucity of long-term follow-up in cases where prosthetic materials have been used, and thus their routine use is not currently advocated. Autogenous fascia lata grafts and the use of tunica vaginalis have also recently been reported in very small numbers of dogs.

Complications and prognosis

The most common complication is wound dehiscence or infection at the surgical site, with a reported incidence of 6–26%. Drainage, lavage and appropriate antimicrobial therapy are usually curative.

* *Faecal incontinence* due to loss of external anal sphincter function may occur if the caudal rectal or internal pudendal nerves are damaged during herniorrhaphy. Function may return in cases of unilateral nerve damage due to re-innervation from the contralateral side. Bilateral nerve damage can result in permanent faecal incontinence.
* *Rectal eversion/prolapse* may occur immediately after surgery. Lubrication with local anaesthetic gel and gentle reduction, combined with a temporary purse-string suture (24–96 hours), are usually all that is necessary. In cases where there is prolonged tenesmus, epidural anaesthesia should be considered. Where rectal prolapse recurs, incisional colopexy (see Operative Technique 8.4) should be performed to prevent further prolapse. It is also necessary to establish a cause for the tenesmus and to treat it.
* *Sciatic paralysis* is very rare but may occur where sutures are inadvertently placed lateral to the sacrotuberous ligament. Its presence is characterized by pain and lameness on the affected side. If it is noted, the sutures must be removed immediately and this can be achieved either by revision of the original repair or via a caudolateral approach to the sciatic nerve.
* *Rectocutaneous fistulae* are a rare complication but may occur if the suture material inadvertently penetrates the rectal mucosa. Digital rectal examination should be carried out immediately after removing the purse-string suture. Any offending suture material should be cut per rectum.

Recurrence is uncommon when internal obturator muscle transposition has been properly performed, and is reported at between 10% and 20%. Studies have shown a significantly higher recurrence rate when herniorrhaphy is performed by an inexperienced surgeon. The most common reason for recurrence is a failure to accurately identify the anatomy of the pelvic diaphragm.

Rectocutaneous fistulae: These are a rare but potentially serious complication of any perianal surgery where there may be inadvertent penetration of the rectal lumen with a scalpel or suture materials. The clinical signs are those of dyschezia, initially with a perineal swelling. Ultimately faeces will be seen to leak from a cutaneous wound (Figure 8.28). The options for management include primary repair,

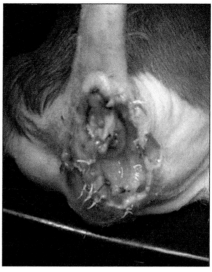

8.28 Rectocutaneous fistula.

a rectal 'pull-through' procedure, anoplasty (see Operative Technique 8.11, below) or primary repair with omental reinforcement. One author [JW] has had some success in using the latter technique.

1. The patient initially undergoes a laparotomy, and the omentum is lengthened as described by Ross and Pardo (1993) (see *BSAVA Manual of Canine and Feline Wound Management and Reconstruction*).
2. The omentum is placed within the pelvic canal lateral to the rectum.
3. The laparotomy wound is closed routinely and the patient is placed in the perineal stand position.
4. The perineal area is cleaned and the edges of the rectum are debrided as necessary.
5. Closure of the rectal defect is achieved with simple interrupted sutures of 2 or 3 metric (3/0 or 2/0 USP) monofilament absorbable suture material.
6. If the pelvic diaphragm is intact, it is necessary to break down the attachment between the levator ani and the coccygeus muscles to allow access to the omentum. This is then drawn caudally into the perineal space and sutured over the rectal closure.

It is essential to close the perineal diaphragm as described above, taking care not to damage the omental vasculature (Figure 8.29).

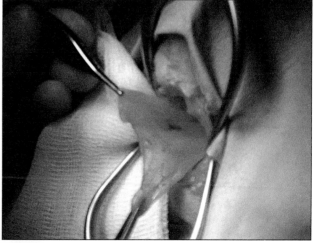

8.29 Omentalization of the perineal wound in Figure 8.28.

References and further reading

Aronson L (2003) Rectum and anus. In: *Textbook of Small Animal Surgery, 3rd edn*, ed. D Slatter, pp.665–682. WB Saunders, Philadelphia

Bellenger CR and Canfield RB (2003) Perineal hernia. In: *Textbook of Small Animal Surgery, 3rd edn*, ed. D Slatter, pp.487–498. WB Saunders, Philadelphia

Bertoy RW, MacCoy DM, Wheaton LG and Gelberg HB (1989) Total colectomy with ileorectal anastomosis in the cat. *Veterinary Surgery* **18**, 204–210

Bongartz A, Carofiglio F, Balligand M, Heimann M and Hamaide A (2005) Use of autogenous fascia lata graft for perineal herniorrhaphy in dogs. *Veterinary Surgery* **34**, 405–413

Bright RM, Burrows CF, Goring R, Fox S and Tilmant L (1986) Subtotal colectomy for treatment of acquired megacolon in the dog and cat. *Journal of the American Veterinary Medical Association* **188**, 1412–1416

Carberry CA and Flanders JA (1993) Caecal-colic volvulus in two dogs. *Veterinary Surgery* **22**, 225–228

De Novo RC and Bright RM (2000) Rectoanal disease. In: *Textbook of Veterinary Internal Medicine, 5th edn*, ed. SJ Ettinger and EC Feldman, pp.1257–1271. WB Saunders, Philadelphia

Drobatz KJ (1996) Volvulus of the colon in a cat. *Journal of Veterinary Emergency and Critical Care* **6**, 99

Eggertsdottir AV, Stigen y Ø, Lonaas L *et al.* (2001) Comparison of the recurrence rate of gastric dilatation with or without volvulus in dogs after circumcostal gastropexy versus gastrocolopexy. *Veterinary Surgery* **30**, 546–551

Frankland AL (1986) Use of porcine dermal collagen in the repair of perineal hernia in dogs – a preliminary report. *Veterinary Record* **119**, 13–14

Gibbons GC and Murtaugh RJ (1989) Caecal smooth muscle neoplasia in the dog: report of 11 cases and literature review. *Journal of the American Animal Hospital Association* **25**, 191–197

Halfacree ZJ, Beck AL, Lee KC *et al.* (2006) Torsion and volvulus of the transverse and descending colon in a German shepherd dog. *Journal of Small Animal Practice* **47**, 468–470

Hall EJ, Simpson JW and Williams DA (2005) *BSAVA Manual of Canine and Feline Gastroenterology, 2nd edn*. BSAVA Publications, Gloucester

Harkin KR, Walshaw R and Mullaney TP (1996) Association of perineal fistula and colitis in German Shepherd Dogs: response to high dose prednisone and dietary therapy. *Journal of the American Animal Hospital Association* **32**, 515–520

Hassinger KA (1997) Intestinal entrapment and strangulation caused by rupture of the duodenocolic ligament in four dogs. *Veterinary Surgery* **26**, 275–280

Kapatkin AS, Mullen HS, Matthiesen DT and Patnaik AK (1992) Leiomyosarcoma in dogs: 44 cases (1983–1988). *Journal of the American Veterinary Medical Association* **201**, 1077–1079

Kudisch M and Pavletic MM (1993) Subtotal colectomy with surgical stapling instruments via a trans-caecal approach for treatment of acquired megacolon in cats. *Veterinary Surgery* **22**, 457–463

Mahler S and Williams G (2005) Preservation of the fistula for reconstruction of the anal canal and the anus in atresia ani and rectovestibular fistula in two dogs. *Veterinary Surgery* **34**(2), 148–152

Marks A (1986) Torsion of the colon in a Rough Collie. *Veterinary Record* **118**, 400

Mathews KA, Ayres SA, Tano CA *et al.* (1997) Cyclosporin treatment of perianal fistulas in dogs. *Canadian Veterinary Journal* **38**, 39–41

Matthiesen DT, Scavelli TD and Whitney WO (1991) Subtotal colectomy for the treatment of obstipation secondary to pelvic fracture malunion in cats. *Veterinary Surgery* **20**, 113–117

Maute AM, Kock DA and Montovon PM (2001) Perineal hernia in dogs – colopexy, vasopexy, cystopexy and castration as elective therapies in 32 dogs. *Schweizer Archiv für Tierheilkunde* **143**, 360–367

Milner HR (2006) The role of surgery in the management of canine anal furunculosis. A review of the literature and a retrospective evaluation of treatment by surgical resection in 51 dogs. *New Zealand Veterinary Journal* **54**(1), 1–9

Misseghers BS, Binnington AG and Mathews KA (2000) Clinical observations of the treatment of canine perianal fistulas with topical tacrolimus in 10 dogs. *Canadian Veterinary Journal* **41**, 623–627

Patterson AP and Campbell KL (2005) Managing anal furunculosis in dogs. *Compendium on Continuing Education for the Practicing Veterinarian* **27**(5), 339–355

Phillips BS (2003) Tumors of the intestinal tract. In: *Textbook of Small Animal Clinical Oncology, 2nd edn*, ed. SJ Withrow and EG McEwan, pp.335–346. WB Saunders, Philadelphia

Pratummintra K, Chuthatep S, Banlunara W and Kalpravidh M (2013) Perineal hernia repair using an autologous tunica vaginalis communis in nine intact male dogs. *Journal of Veterinary Medicine and Science* **75**, 337–341

Ross WE and Pardo AD (1993) Evaluation of an omental pedicle extension technique in a dog. *Veterinary Surgery* **22**, 37–43

Slawienski MJ, Mauldin GE and Mauldin GN (1997) Malignant colonic neoplasia in cats: 46 cases (1990–1996). *Journal of the American Veterinary Medical Association* **211**, 878–881

Szabo S, Wilkens B and Radasch RM (2007) Use of polypropylene mesh in addition to internal obturator transposition: a review of 59 cases (2000–2004). *Journal of the American Animal Hospital Association* **43**, 136–142

Toombs JP, Caywood DD, Lipowitz AJ and Stevens JB (1980) Colonic perforation following neurosurgical procedures and corticosteroid therapy in 4 dogs. *Journal of the American Veterinary Medical Association* **177**, 68–72

Van Duijkeren E (1995) Disease conditions of canine anal sacs. *Journal of Small Animal Practice* **36**, 12–16

Vyacheslav H and Ranen E (2009) Perineal hernia with retroflexion of the urinary bladder in a 4 month old puppy. *Journal of Small Animal Practice* **50**, 625

Washabau RJ and Stalis IH (1996) Alterations in colonic smooth muscle function in cats with idiopathic megacolon. *American Journal of Veterinary Research* **57**, 580–587

Wells KL, Bright RM and Wright KN (1995) Caecal impaction in a dog. *Journal of Small Animal Practice* **36**, 455–457

Westermarch E and Rimaila-Parnanen E (1989) Mesenteric torsion in dogs with exocrine pancreatic insufficiency: 21 cases (1978–1987). *Journal of the American Veterinary Medical Association* **195**, 1404–1406

White RN (1997) Chronic caecal faecolithiasis in a dog. *Journal of Small Animal Practice* **38**, 459–461

Williams JM (2012) Colon. In: *Veterinary Surgery: Small Animal*, ed. KM Tobias and SA Johnston, pp.1542–1563. Elsevier, St Louis

Williams JM and Moores A (2009) *BSAVA Manual of Canine and Feline Wound Management and Reconstruction, 2nd edn*. BSAVA Publications, Gloucester

---

OPERATIVE TECHNIQUE 8.1

Colotomy

PREOPERATIVE PLANNING

- Correct any electrolyte and acid–base abnormalities and ensure adequate hydration status.
- Administer prophylactic antibiotics intravenously at anaesthetic induction and then every 2 hours during surgery.
- Preoperative enemas should be avoided, to prevent potential leakage of fluid from the colon.

POSITIONING

Dorsal recumbency.

→ **OPERATIVE TECHNIQUE 8.1 CONTINUED**

ASSISTANT

Not required.

EQUIPMENT EXTRAS

Balfour abdominal retractor; large abdominal swabs; suction; two Doyen non-crushing bowel clamps.

SURGICAL TECHNIQUE

Approach

Routine midline abdominal incision.

Surgical manipulations

1 Isolate the colon and pack it off well with large abdominal swabs.

2 'Milk' colonic contents away from the proposed incision site. Reflux into the surgical site is prevented either by an assistant's fingers or by the use of Doyen bowel clamps.

3 Make a longitudinal incision in the antimesenteric border over the foreign body.

4 For colonic biopsy, a stay suture can be placed through one side of the incision to minimize crushing of the biopsy sample with forceps, and a second incision is made with fine Metzenbaum scissors to form an ellipse around the stay suture.

5 Clean the incision edges and close with simple interrupted or continuous sutures of a monofilament absorbable, (polydioxanone) or non-absorbable (polypropylene) suture material.

6 Before removing the abdominal swabs, gently lavage the area of bowel adjacent to the colotomy with warm saline. Lavage fluid should not be allowed to spill into the peritoneal cavity.

7 Cover the colotomy incision line with omentum.

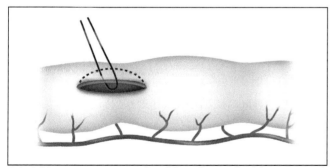

Colonic biopsy. A stay suture is placed through one side of the incision and a second incision is made with fine Metzenbaum scissors to form an ellipse around the stay suture.

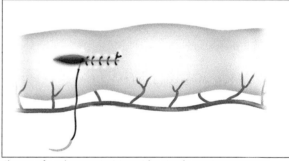

Closure of a colostomy incision with a simple continuous suture pattern. Note: all sutures penetrate the submucosa.

Wound closure

Abdominal closure is routine.

POSTOPERATIVE MANAGEMENT AND COMPLICATIONS

Intravenous fluids are continued until the animal is eating and drinking normally. The animal is monitored closely for signs of peritonitis.

Colectomy

PREOPERATIVE PLANNING

- Correct any electrolyte and acid–base abnormalities and ensure adequate hydration status.
- Administer prophylactic antibiotics intravenously at anaesthetic induction and then every 2 hours during surgery.
- Preoperative enemas should be avoided, to prevent potential leakage of fluid from the colon.

POSITIONING

Dorsal recumbency.

ASSISTANT

Ideally.

EQUIPMENT EXTRAS

Balfour abdominal retractor; large abdominal swabs; suction; two Doyen non-crushing bowel clamps; two Carmalt crushing forceps. Optional: end-to-end anastomosis stapling device.

SURGICAL TECHNIQUE

Approach

Routine ventral midline abdominal incision, starting from a point midway between the xiphoid process and umbilicus and extending caudally to the brim of the pubis.

Surgical manipulations

1 Exteriorize the colon, caecum and distal ileum and pack off from the rest of the abdominal cavity using large moistened abdominal swabs.

2 Identify the cranial resection site either just distal to the ileocolic valve (A), or into the ileum if the ileocolic valve is to be resected (B). Identify the resection site in the distal colon (C).

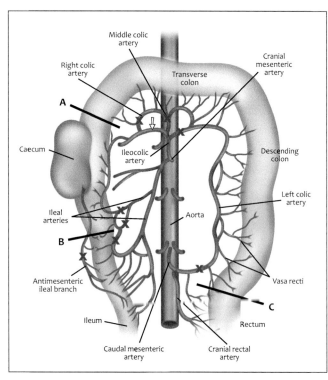

Subtotal colectomy is performed after identifying the proximal (A or B) and distal (C) resection sites and ligating the appropriate blood vessels (blue crosses). If the ileocolic valve is to be removed, the ileocolic artery and vein need to be ligated (arrowed).

→ **OPERATIVE TECHNIQUE 8.2 CONTINUED**

3 Isolate, double ligate and divide the appropriate colic vessels 1–2 cm from the mesenteric side of the colon. To preserve as much of the blood supply as possible to the distal colon, the vasa recta of the left colic and caudal mesenteric arteries can be ligated rather than the main vessels. If the ileocolic valve is being removed, the ileocolic artery and vein also need to be ligated.

4 'Milk' the faecal contents towards the centre of the colon and place non-crushing Doyen clamps to the brim of the pubis.

> **PRACTICAL TIP**
>
> Remember to leave 1.5–2 cm of colon cranial to the brim of the pubis to facilitate anastomosis

5 If the ileocolic valve is being preserved, place a second set of non-crushing forceps across the proximal colon, 1 cm distal to the valve. If the valve is being resected, place the non-crushing forceps across the ileum, just proximal to the valve. Place the crushing (Carmalt) forceps inside each of the previously placed non-crushing forceps.

6 Transect the colon next to the crushing forceps and remove. The crushing forceps prevent leakage from the resected section of bowel. The non-crushing forceps prevent leakage from the retained bowel, without damaging the blood supply to the tissue.

7 Any luminal disparity is corrected prior to anastomosis if necessary (see Chapter 7).

8 Perform an end-to-end anastomosis using a monofilament suture material such as polydioxanone or polypropylene. Use a simple interrupted full-thickness appositional suture pattern or continuous suture pattern. Simple interrupted sutures should be placed at 2–3 mm intervals.

9 Irrigate the anastomosis site, without allowing any fluid to enter the abdominal cavity. Remove the swabs and omentalize the anastomosis site.

Subtotal colectomy with surgical stapling instruments via a transcaecal approach has also been described for the treatment of acquired megacolon in cats (Kudisch and Pavletic, 1993).

Wound closure

New gloves and a new set of sterile instruments are used to close the abdomen. Routine abdominal closure is performed.

POSTOPERATIVE MANAGEMENT AND COMPLICATIONS

- The patient is kept on intravenous fluids for 48–72 hours.
- Monitor for signs of peritonitis for 3–5 days.
- Tenesmus and loose stools are commonly seen after colectomy. The character of the faeces should gradually change from diarrhoea to formed stool over 6–8 weeks. The frequency of defecation usually increases by 30–50%.
- Potential complications following colectomy include leakage, dehiscence, peritonitis, ischaemic necrosis, stricture and abscess formation. Persistent diarrhoea may be the result of small intestinal bacterial overgrowth or hypersecretion. Constipation following subtotal colectomy is managed by dietary modification and stool softeners.

OPERATIVE TECHNIQUE 8.3

Typhlectomy (caecal resection)

PREOPERATIVE PLANNING

- Correct any electrolyte and acid–base abnormalities and ensure adequate hydration status.
- Administer prophylactic antibiotics intravenously at anaesthetic induction and then every 2 hours during surgery.

POSITIONING

Dorsal recumbency.

ASSISTANT

Not necessary.

EQUIPMENT EXTRAS

Balfour abdominal retractor; large abdominal swabs; suction; two Doyen non-crushing bowel clamps. Optional: TA stapler.

SURGICAL TECHNIQUE

Approach

Routine ventral midline abdominal incision, starting from a point midway between the xiphoid process and umbilicus and extending caudally to the brim of the pubis.

Surgical manipulations

If possible, the caecum is everted prior to resection. Reduction may need to be performed via an antimesenteric colotomy incision if manual reduction is not possible.

1 Dissect the ileocaecal fold to free the caecum from the distal ileum.

2 Ligate the branches of the ileocaecal artery supplying the caecum.

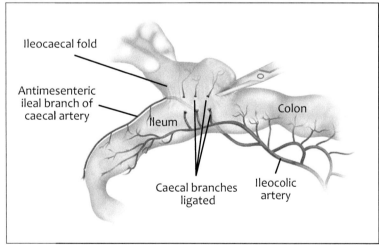

The ileocaecal fold is dissected and branches of the ileocaecal artery supplying the caecum are ligated.

3 Once the caecum is isolated from its attachments and blood supply, place two non-crushing Doyen clamps across its base and amputate the caecum between the two forceps.

4 Oversew the base of the caecum with synthetic absorbable suture material using a Parker–Kerr suture pattern. A continuous Lembert inverting suture pattern can be placed as a second layer. Alternatively, a linear stapling device (TA stapler; see Chapter 2) can be placed across the base of the caecum and the distal portion is then amputated. →

→ **OPERATIVE TECHNIQUE 8.3 CONTINUED**

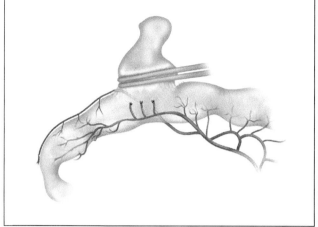

Two non-crushing intestinal clamps are placed across the base of the caecum and it is amputated between the two forceps.

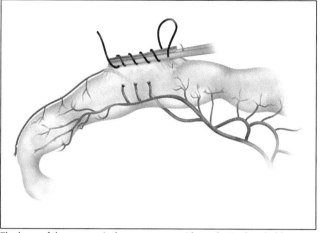

The base of the caecum is then oversewn with synthetic absorbable suture material using a Parker–Kerr suture pattern.

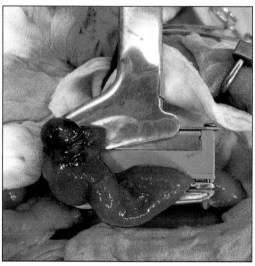

TA stapling device being used to resect a perforated caecal mass in a 10-year-old Greyhound bitch. Histopathology revealed the mass to be a leiomyosarcoma.

Wound closure

A new set of sterile instruments is used for routine abdominal closure.

POSTOPERATIVE MANAGEMENT AND COMPLICATIONS

- The patient is kept on intravenous fluids for 48–72 hours.
- Monitor for signs of peritonitis for 3–5 days.

OPERATIVE TECHNIQUE 8.4

Incisional colopexy

PREOPERATIVE PLANNING

- Identify and treat underlying causes of tenesmus predisposing to recurrent rectal prolapse.
- Administer prophylactic antibiotics intravenously at anaesthetic induction and then every 2 hours during surgery.

POSITIONING

Dorsal recumbency.

ASSISTANT

Ideally.

EQUIPMENT EXTRAS

Balfour abdominal retractor; large abdominal swabs.

SURGICAL TECHNIQUE

Approach

Routine ventral midline abdominal incision, starting from a point midway between the xiphoid process and umbilicus and extending caudally to the brim of the pubis.

Surgical manipulations

1   Via a midline laparotomy incision, reduce the rectal prolapse by placing gentle cranial traction on the descending colon. Gentle cranial traction is applied similarly when attempting to decrease rectal sacculation associated with perineal herniation.

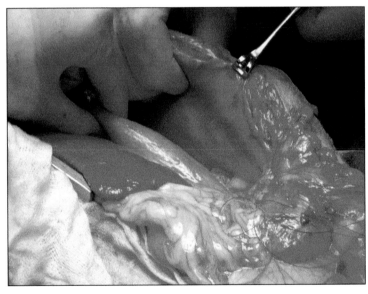

Incisional colopexy. Gentle cranial traction is applied to the descending colon.

2   Make a longitudinal seromuscular incision using a scalpel along the antimesenteric border of the colon. The incision should be approximately 3–4 cm long. The lumen of the colon should not be penetrated.

3   Make an incision of similar length into the peritoneum and underlying musculature of the left abdominal wall, located cranially enough so that when the two incisions are brought together the colon is tractioned sufficiently cranially.

→ **OPERATIVE TECHNIQUE 8.4 CONTINUED**

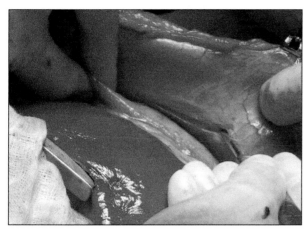

Incisions of similar length are made in the peritoneum of the left abdominal wall and through the seromuscular layer of the descending colon.

4 Starting with the deepest side of the incision, suture the colon to the abdominal wall using a simple continuous suture pattern with either polypropylene or polydioxanone suture material of an appropriate size.

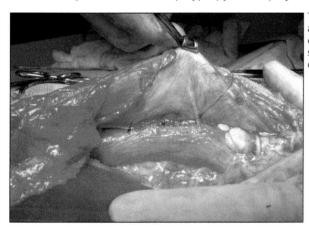

The colon is sutured to the abdominal wall using a simple continuous suture pattern, starting with the deepest side of the incision.

5 Suture the superficial side of the incision similarly so that the bleeding surfaces of the colon and abdominal wall are directly apposed.

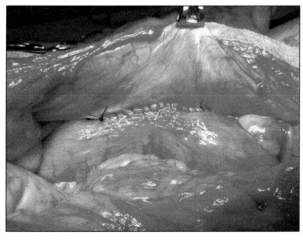

The superficial side of the incision is sutured similarly to complete the colopexy.

Wound closure

Routine abdominal closure is performed.

POSTOPERATIVE MANAGEMENT AND COMPLICATIONS

The use of stool softeners to prevent excessive straining in the postoperative period should be considered. Recurrence of rectal prolapse following colopexy suggests breakdown of the pexy site.

OPERATIVE TECHNIQUE 8.5

Anal 'pull-out' procedure for lesions requiring full-thickness resection

PREOPERATIVE PLANNING

- Assess preoperative biopsy results; use thoracic and abdominal radiography to assess for any possible metastases.
- Administer prophylactic antibiotics intravenously at anaesthetic induction.
- Clip the perineal area and prepare aseptically. Insert a swab soaked in an alcohol-free antiseptic solution per rectum.

> **WARNING**
>
> Do not administer preoperative enemas or purgatives

POSITIONING

Perineal stand (see Figure 8.11).

ASSISTANT

Not essential.

EQUIPMENT EXTRAS

Polypropylene suture material (3 metric; 2/0 USP) to use as stay sutures; Babcock tissue forceps.

SURGICAL TECHNIQUE

Approach

Per anus.

Surgical manipulations

1 Large or annular colorectal lesions are prolapsed or everted by careful and gentle traction, using stay sutures and/or Babcock forceps placed proximal and distal to the lesion.

2 Incise the rectum distal to the mass, thus allowing dissection of the mesorectum to free up the proximal portion.

3 Resect larger or annular masses, full-thickness and intact, with adequate margins.

4 Perform an 'end-to-end' anastomosis.

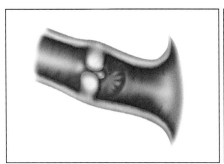
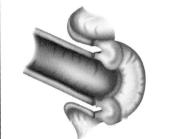
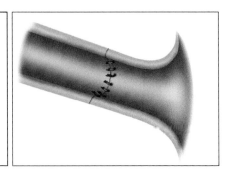

Anal 'pull-out' procedure for annular lesions.

➜ **OPERATIVE TECHNIQUE 8.5 CONTINUED**

5   Close the defect with simple interrupted sutures of an absorbable 2 or 3 metric (3/0 or 2/0 USP) monofilament suture material (polydioxanone or glycomer 610), with the knots in the rectal lumen.

> **PRACTICAL TIP**
>
> It is helpful initially to place four sutures at 90 degrees to each other at the four points of the compass, and then to fill in the gaps

POSTOPERATIVE MANAGEMENT AND COMPLICATIONS

- Mild postoperative tenesmus and haemorrhage are not uncommon for 24–48 hours.
- Prolonged tenesmus or dyschezia suggests possible stricture formation.
- Excessive discomfort or any perineal swelling would suggest wound dehiscence with perineal abscessation and/or rectal fistula formation.

It is essential that any dehiscence or stricture formation is diagnosed and dealt with promptly. Conservative management is rarely helpful and the patient is more likely to benefit from aggressive surgical intervention. One of the authors [JW] prefers to carry out a rectal 'pull-through' procedure in the event of such complications occurring (see Operative Technique 8.6).

OPERATIVE TECHNIQUE 8.6

Rectal 'pull-through' procedure

PREOPERATIVE PLANNING

- Assess preoperative biopsy results; take thoracic and abdominal radiographs to assess for any possible metastases.
- Administer prophylactic antibiotics intravenously at anaesthetic induction.
- Clip the perineal area and prepare aseptically. Insert a swab soaked in an alcohol-free antiseptic solution per rectum.

> **WARNING**
>
> Do not administer preoperative enemas or purgatives

POSITIONING

Perineal stand (see Figure 8.11).

ASSISTANT

Not essential but useful.

EQUIPMENT EXTRAS

Polypropylene suture material (3 metric; 2/0 USP) to use as stay sutures; Babcock tissue forceps.

SURGICAL TECHNIQUE

Approach

Per anus.

→ **OPERATIVE TECHNIQUE 8.6 CONTINUED**

Surgical manipulations

1 Incise the rectum circumferentially at the mucocutaneous junction, keeping medial to the external anal sphincter muscle.

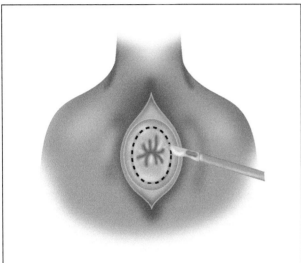

The skin incision is made with care to avoid the anal sacs and their ducts.

WARNING

Avoid damaging the openings of the anal sacs

2 Dissect the rectum free from the external anal sphincter and surrounding tissues, using a combination of blunt and sharp dissection, to a point 2 cm cranial to the mass. Care must be taken to deal with haemorrhage from the caudal rectal artery and vein, and branches of the caudal gluteal artery and vein that run dorsal to the rectum.

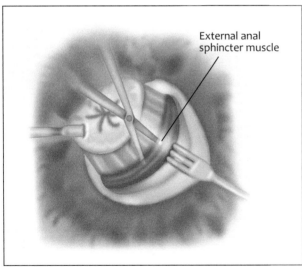

External anal sphincter muscle

A combination of sharp and blunt dissection is carried out to free the rectum from the external anal sphincter muscle.

PRACTICAL TIP

The rectum can be opened longitudinally to ensure that an adequate cranial margin of disease-free tissue has been obtained prior to resection

3 Place stay sutures proximal to the mass and amputate the rectocolon. A cut-and-sew technique is recommended.

→ **OPERATIVE TECHNIQUE 8.6 CONTINUED**

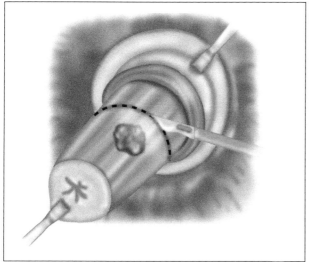

The rectum is excised 1–2 cm proximal to the lesion.

4 Resect one-quarter of the circumference of the rectum and anastomose the normal rectal tissue to form a new mucocutaneous junction. This prevents cranial retraction of the rectum.

5 Cut and sew each additional quarter circumference in the same fashion.

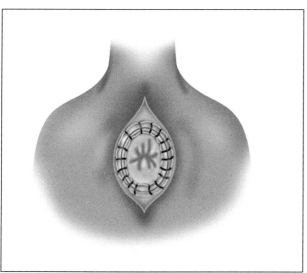

The rectum is sutured to the skin using absorbable suture material in a simple interrupted pattern.

POSTOPERATIVE MANAGEMENT AND COMPLICATIONS

- Mild postoperative tenesmus and haemorrhage are not uncommon for 24–48 hours.
- Prolonged tenesmus or dyschezia would suggest possible stricture formation.
- Excessive discomfort or any perineal swelling suggests wound dehiscence with perineal abscessation and/or rectal fistula formation.

OPERATIVE TECHNIQUE 8.7

Dorsal rectal approach

PREOPERATIVE PLANNING

- Assess preoperative biopsy results; take thoracic and abdominal radiographs to assess for any possible metastases.
- Administer prophylactic antibiotics intravenously at anaesthetic induction.
- Clip the perineal area and prepare aseptically. Insert a swab soaked in an alcohol-free antiseptic per rectum.

> ### WARNING
>
> Do not administer preoperative enemas or purgatives

POSITIONING

Perineal stand (see Figure 8.11).

ASSISTANT

Not essential but useful.

EQUIPMENT EXTRAS

Polypropylene suture material (3 metric; 2/0 USP) to use as stay sutures; Babcock tissue forceps; Doyen bowel clamps; Gelpi retractors.

SURGICAL TECHNIQUE

Approach

Dorsal perineal.

Surgical manipulations

1   Make an inverted horseshoe-shaped incision dorsal to the anus.

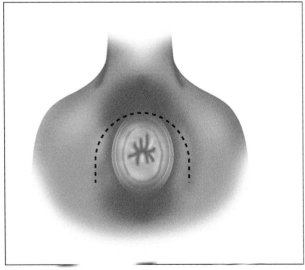

A horseshoe-shaped incision is made dorsal to the anus.

2   Transect the fused (paired) rectococcygeus muscle to allow access to the pelvic canal. Separation of the rectum from its pelvic attachments is required so that it may be exteriorized. In some cases it may be necessary to transect the levator ani muscles either unilaterally or bilaterally to improve access.

→ **OPERATIVE TECHNIQUE 8.7 CONTINUED**

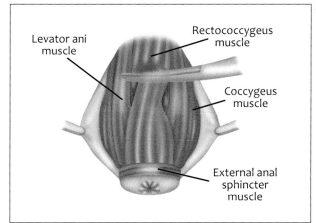

Muscles exposed via the dorsal approach.

Levator ani muscle
Rectococcygeus muscle
Coccygeus muscle
External anal sphincter muscle

WARNING

Care should be taken to avoid damaging the pelvic nerve plexus that runs along the lateral aspect of the rectum in the peritoneal reflection

3 Once exteriorized, isolate the mass with 2 cm margins by means of Doyen bowel clamps. Care must be taken not to resect more than 6 cm of rectum, as the risk of faecal incontinence becomes much greater.

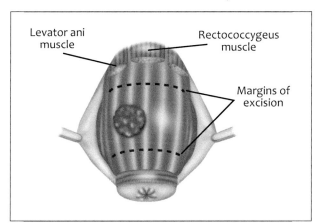

Levator ani muscle
Rectococcygeus muscle
Margins of excision

The rectum and lesion are identified and the area to be excised planned.

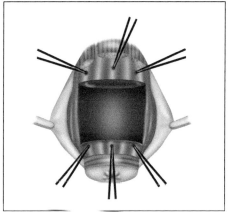

Stay sutures are used to reduce the risk of retraction of the severed ends of the rectum.

4 After resection, perform an end-to-end anastomosis using 2 or 3 metric (3/0 or 2/0 USP) absorbable monofilament suture material (polydioxanone or glycomer 631).

5 Reappose the transected muscles using 3 metric (2/0 USP) absorbable monofilament suture material (polydioxanone or glycomer 631).

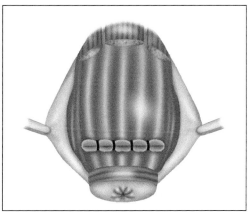

The rectum is anastomosed using monofilament absorbable suture material.

→ **OPERATIVE TECHNIQUE 8.7 CONTINUED**

Wound closure

Subcutaneous and skin closure is routine.

- Mild postoperative tenesmus and haemorrhage are not uncommon for 24–48 hours.
- Prolonged tenesmus or dyschezia would suggest possible stricture formation.
- Excessive discomfort or any perineal swelling suggests wound dehiscence with perineal abscessation and/or rectal fistula formation.

It is essential that any dehiscence or stricture formation is diagnosed and dealt with promptly. Conservative management is rarely helpful and the patient is more likely to benefit from aggressive surgical intervention. One of the authors [JW] prefers to carry out a rectal 'pull-through' procedure in the event of such complications occurring (see Operative Technique 8.6).

- Postsurgical faecal incontinence suggests that more than 6 cm of rectum has been excised.
- Cutaneous wound dehiscence is not uncommon.

OPERATIVE TECHNIQUE 8.8

Ventral approach to the rectum

PREOPERATIVE PLANNING

- Assess preoperative biopsy results; take thoracic and abdominal radiographs to assess for any possible metastases.
- Administer prophylactic antibiotics intravenously at anaesthetic induction.
- Clip the ventral abdomen and prepare aseptically from the xiphoid to the vulvar or scrotal area.

WARNING

Do not administer preoperative enemas or purgatives

POSITIONING

Dorsal recumbency.

ASSISTANT

Ideally.

EQUIPMENT EXTRAS

Finochietto rib retractor; oscillating saw (or orthopaedic mallet and osteotome); sterile drill and drill bits; orthopaedic wire; rongeurs; Babcock tissue forceps; Doyen bowel clamps; Gelpi retractors.

SURGICAL TECHNIQUE

Approach

Caudal ventral laparotomy with extension over the pelvis.

Surgical manipulations

1 Make an incision from cranial to the umbilicus to the caudal pelvic brim (in the male dog this will necessitate a parapreputial skin incision; see Chapter 4). The incision is made through the linea alba to the cranial pelvic brim.

➜ **OPERATIVE TECHNIQUE 8.8 CONTINUED**

2 The degree of osteotomy/ostectomy required for access depends on the size and location of the lesion.

- For small masses it may be sufficient to remove a window of pubic bone using a small oscillating saw or rongeurs.
- For larger or mid-pelvic lesions in young dogs, a pubic symphysiotomy should be carried out using either an oscillating saw or a mallet and osteotome. Holes should be pre-drilled on either side of the pubic symphysis to allow placement of orthopaedic wire. The symphysiotomy site is distracted and maintained using Finochietto rib retractors.
- For larger or mid-pelvic lesions in older dogs, it is necessary to create a pubic–ischial flap following osteotomies of the pubic and ischial bones. Holes should be pre-drilled on either side of each osteotomy site to allow reattachment with orthopaedic wire.

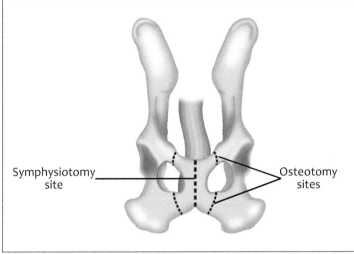

Pelvic symphysiotomy. Symphysiotomy/osteotomy sites.

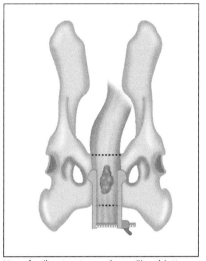

Use of a rib retractor, such as a Finochietto retractor, helps to improve exposure.

> **WARNING**
>
> In old dogs, it is difficult to gain sufficient access by pelvic symphysiotomy alone

3 Exteriorize the rectum and isolate the mass with 2 cm margins by means of Doyen bowel clamps. Care must be taken not to resect more than 6 cm of rectum as the risk of faecal incontinence becomes much greater.

4 Once resected, perform an end-to-end anastomosis using 2 or 3 metric (3/0 or 2/0 USP) absorbable monofilament suture material (polydioxanone or glycomer 631).

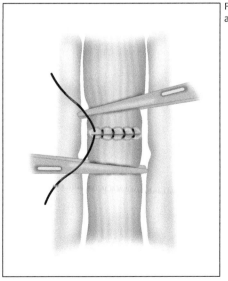

Following resection of the rectal lesion, a routine anastomosis is carried out.

→ **OPERATIVE TECHNIQUE 8.8 CONTINUED**

Wound closure

Reappose osteotomy or symphysiotomy sites using orthopaedic wire sutures, through pre-drilled holes. Soft tissue closure is routine.

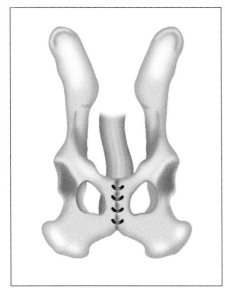

The symphysis or osteotomy is repaired with orthopaedic wire passed through pre-drilled holes.

POSTOPERATIVE MANAGEMENT AND COMPLICATIONS

- There may be severe postoperative discomfort, requiring opioid or epidural analgesia.
- Mild postoperative tenesmus and haemorrhage are not uncommon for 24–48 hours.
- Prolonged tenesmus or dyschezia suggests possible stricture formation.
- Excessive discomfort, perineal swelling or abdominal guarding would suggest wound dehiscence with perineal abscessation, rectal fistula formation or peritonitis (see Chapter 18).
- There may be avascular necrosis or sequestrum formation of the pubic–ischial bone flap.

In some cases, colorectal tumours may be exposed via a posterior midline laparotomy, which may be combined with a pubic symphysiotomy or osteotomy. In one author's experience [JW], this gives limited access and requires considerable postoperative analgesia. It is generally only considered when other techniques are not feasible.

OPERATIVE TECHNIQUE 8.9

Perineal herniorrhaphy in a male dog

PREOPERATIVE PLANNING

- Preparation for surgery should include suitable perioperative analgesia; epidural analgesia can be considered.
- Carry out a wide bilateral perineal clip, followed by manual evacuation of the faeces from the rectum, and purse-string suture closure of the anus (some surgeons favour placing a swab as a tampon within the rectal lumen prior to placing a purse-string suture). If faeces persist in leaking from the rectum, a sterile adhesive drape can be applied.
- Administer perioperative broad-spectrum antibiotics and prepare the perineal area aseptically.

WARNING

Enemas should not be given preoperatively because they will create a liquid slurry that will leak from the anus on to the surgical field

POSITIONING

Perineal stand (see Figure 8.11). If the patient has not been castrated, he should be placed in dorsal recumbency and a routine castration carried out prior to herniorrhaphy.

ASSISTANT

Not essential.

EQUIPMENT EXTRAS

Gelpi retractors; extra mosquito forceps (useful); polypropylene suture material swaged on a 'J'-shaped needle.

SURGICAL TECHNIQUE

Approach

Lateral perineal.

Surgical manipulations

1 Make a straight incision from the base of the tail to the ischial tuberosity.

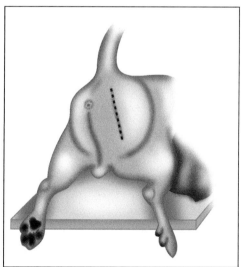

Incision from the base of the tail to the ischial tuberosity.

WARNING

Do not be tempted to incise over the most prominent part of the perineal swelling. This will place the incision either too far laterally or too far medially to allow accurate identification of the perineal structures

→ **OPERATIVE TECHNIQUE 8.9 CONTINUED**

2   Once the skin has been incised, it is common to find the perineal space filled with pelvic and peritoneal fat together with variable quantities of serosanguineous fluid. The fat can usually be replaced into the peritoneal cavity, gently repelling with a moist swab; occasionally it may be necessary to excise it. Other structures that may be encountered within the hernia are the bladder, prostate gland, or paraprostatic and prostatic cysts. *The surgeon should ensure that any structure to be excised is not the bladder or prostate gland.*

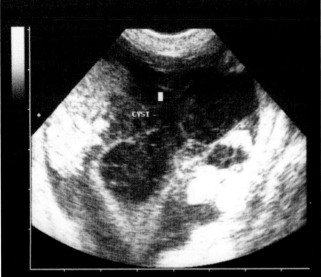

Ultrasound scan of a perineal prostatic cyst.

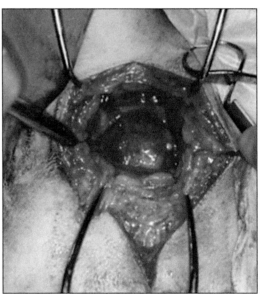

Perineal prostatic cyst at surgery.

3   Identify the structures of the perineum, taking care to identify the internal pudendal nerves and vessels. Identify the coccygeus and levator ani muscles together with the external anal sphincter muscle. If the lateral muscles are deficient, the sacrotuberous ligament may be used (with care taken to avoid the sciatic nerve that courses cranial to it) to anchor the sutures. It is preferable to pass the suture material through the ligament rather than around it.

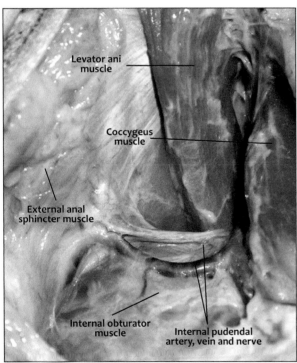

Perineal anatomy in a dog without a perineal hernia.
(Courtesy of M McLoughlin)

4   Elevate the internal obturator muscle from its ventral position using fine Metzenbaum scissors or a periosteal elevator. There is some debate as to whether to perform a tenotomy on the internal obturator muscle, but most surgeons perform either a partial or complete tenotomy.

→ OPERATIVE TECHNIQUE 8.9 CONTINUED

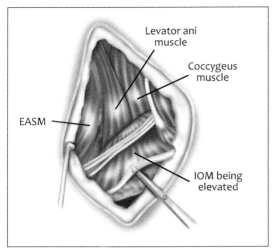

Elevation of the internal obturator muscle (IOM). EASM = external anal sphincter muscle.

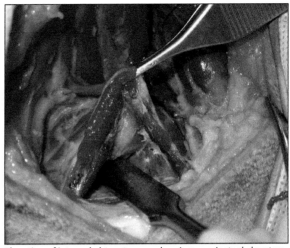

Elevation of internal obturator muscle using a periosteal elevator.
(Courtesy of M McLoughlin)

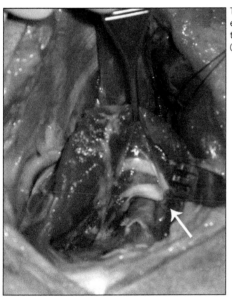

The internal obturator muscle has been elevated. Note that the internal obturator tendon has been transected (arrowed).
(Courtesy of M McLoughlin)

5 Pre-place permanent suture material (3.5 metric (0 USP), polypropylene) in a simple interrupted pattern, passing from the coccygeus, levator ani and internal obturator muscles to the external anal sphincter muscles before tying.

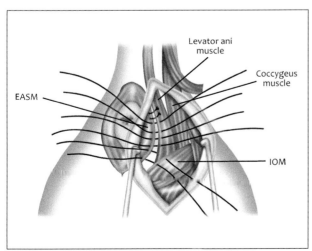

Surgical anatomy of a perineal hernia; note suture placement. EASM = external anal sphincter muscle; IOM = internal obturator muscle.

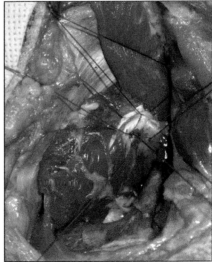

Polypropylene sutures have been pre-placed between: the levator ani/coccygeus and the external anal sphincter muscles; the levator ani/coccygeus and the internal obturator muscles; and the internal obturator and external anal sphincter muscles.
(Courtesy of M McLoughlin)

→ **OPERATIVE TECHNIQUE 8.9 CONTINUED**

PRACTICAL TIP

Using a 'J'-shaped needle swaged on to the suture material makes it easier to pass through the muscles/sacrotuberous ligament, which are deep within the perineum

PRACTICAL TIP

It is recommended to tie the sutures from dorsal to ventral

WARNING

Chromic catgut does not stimulate the formation of strong fibrous adhesions and its use should be avoided

Wound closure

After routine closure of the subcutaneous tissues and skin, the purse-string suture must be removed from the anus.

POSTOPERATIVE MANAGEMENT AND COMPLICATIONS

- Postoperative analgesia should be provided. If the animal strains excessively in the immediate postoperative period, an epidural is beneficial.
- Stool softeners should be used and defecatory function should be monitored for the first 1–2 days.

Complications

See main text.

OPERATIVE TECHNIQUE 8.10

Anal sacculectomy

PREOPERATIVE PLANNING

- Administer prophylactic antibiotics intravenously at anaesthetic induction.
- Clip the perineal area and prepare aseptically. Insert a swab soaked in an alcohol-free antiseptic solution per rectum.

WARNING

Do not administer preoperative enemas or purgatives

POSITIONING

Perineal stand (see Figure 8.11).

ASSISTANT

Not essential.

EQUIPMENT EXTRAS

Sterile surgical probe.

SURGICAL TECHNIQUE

Approach

Perianal.

→ **OPERATIVE TECHNIQUE 8.10 CONTINUED**

Surgical manipulations

1 Insert a sterile probe or straight mosquito forceps into the anal sac via the opening.

2 Incise through the skin and anal sac lining on to the probe.

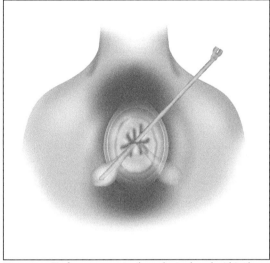

Fine mosquito forceps or a sterile probe is placed within the duct of the anal sac.

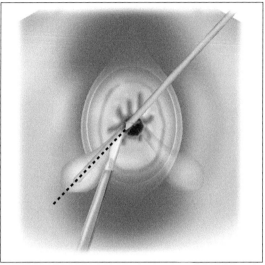

Incise on to the probe with a No. 15 scalpel blade; the incision is extended into the anal sac.

3 Once the sac is opened, dissect it free from the surrounding tissues using fine Metzenbaum scissors and amputate it at the anal sac opening.

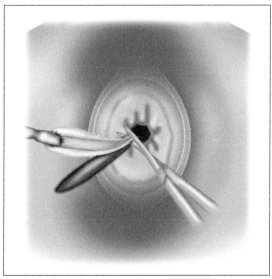

The anal sac is dissected free and amputated at the level of the duct opening.

PRACTICAL TIP

Placing one or two stay sutures into the incised edges of the anal sac can facilitate dissection

PRACTICAL TIP

The anal sac is invested in fibres of the external anal sphincter muscle. Stay close to the anal sac wall during dissection to minimize damage to this muscle

→ **OPERATIVE TECHNIQUE 8.10 CONTINUED**

Wound closure

Suture the deep tissues with 2 metric (3/0 USP) absorbable monofilament suture material and close the skin with simple interrupted sutures of a 2 metric (3/0 USP) monofilament nylon suture material.

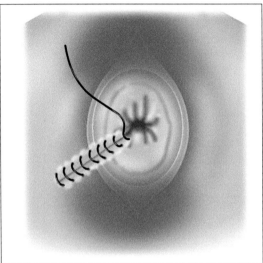

The defect is closed routinely with absorbable sutures subcutaneously and monofilament nylon in the skin.

POSTOPERATIVE MANAGEMENT AND COMPLICATIONS

• Use stool softeners.
• Wound dehiscence may occur; this will require resuturing.

OPERATIVE TECHNIQUE 8.11

Anoplasty

PREOPERATIVE PLANNING

• Administer prophylactic antibiotics intravenously at anaesthetic induction.
• Clip the perineal area and prepare aseptically. Insert a swab soaked in an alcohol-free antiseptic solution per rectum.

WARNING

Do not administer preoperative enemas or purgatives

POSITIONING

Perineal stand (see Figure 8.11).

ASSISTANT

Not essential.

EQUIPMENT EXTRAS

Polypropylene suture material (3 metric; 2/0 USP) to use as stay sutures; Babcock tissue forceps.

→ **OPERATIVE TECHNIQUE 8.11 CONTINUED**

Approach

Perianal.

Surgical manipulations

1 Make a 360-degree incision around the anus; include any perianal fistulae, trying to keep medial to the external anal sphincter muscle. This may not be possible owing to the extent of the disease process and involvement of the external anal sphincter. Any areas of fibrosis should be resected.

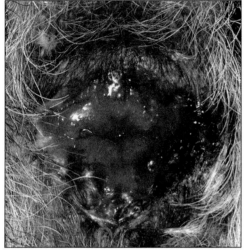
A 9-year-old male crossbreed dog with mild perianal fistulae.

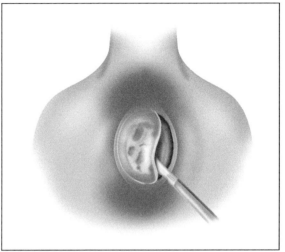
A 360-degree incision is made around the anus, incorporating all fistulous tracts.

PRACTICAL TIP

Bilateral anal sacculectomy is usually required with this procedure

---

2 If necessary, dissect the rectum and mesorectum free.

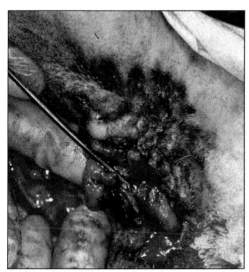
Anal sacculectomy being performed owing to secondary involvement of the anal sacs in a German Shepherd Dog with severe perianal fistulae. Note that a surgical probe has been placed into the anal sac.

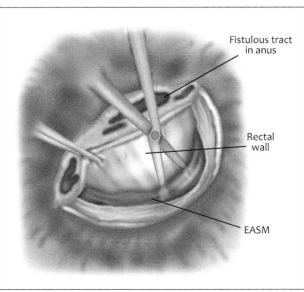
The diseased tissue (including the anus) is dissected free. The external anal sphincter muscle (EASM) should be preserved if possible.

Fistulous tract in anus

Rectal wall

EASM

→ **OPERATIVE TECHNIQUE 8.11 CONTINUED**

3   Amputate the distal portion of the rectum at an appropriate level. Care must be taken to deal with haemorrhage from the caudal rectal artery and vein, and branches of the caudal gluteal artery and vein, which run dorsal to the rectum.

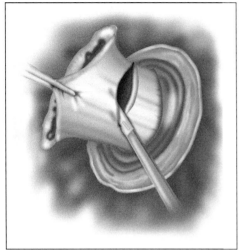

The rectum and anus are amputated.

Wound closure

Suture the rectal mucosa to the skin with 2 or 3 metric (3/0 or 2/0 USP) polydioxanone or glycomer 361 suture material.

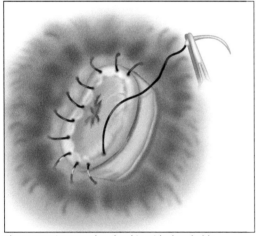

The rectum is sutured to the skin with absorbable monofilament suture material.

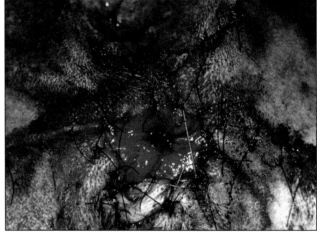

Following excision of all diseased tissue the anus has been reconstructed by closing the skin defect and suturing the rectal mucosa to the skin.

POSTOPERATIVE MANAGEMENT AND COMPLICATIONS

- Stool softeners should be used.
- Mild postoperative tenesmus and haemorrhage are not uncommon for 24–48 hours.
- If the external anal sphincter muscle is preserved faecal incontinence is rare, although faecal urgency is common.
- Wound dehiscence is not uncommon and will require resuturing.

Chapter 9

The liver and biliary tract

Jacqui D. Niles

Small animal patients commonly present with conditions of the liver and biliary tract that require surgical intervention. Techniques such as liver biopsy, partial hepatectomy and simple exploration of the biliary tract can be performed in general veterinary practice, but it is important to remember that the liver has many diverse functions. It is the primary site of protein, carbohydrate and fat metabolism; it detoxifies and excretes many drugs and toxins; and it is responsible for the formation of bile and coagulation factors. Owing to the large functional reserve, clinical signs of hepatic disease may not be apparent until the disease is advanced and by that time many metabolic abnormalities may be present. In addition to adequate patient preparation, it is extremely important to understand the pathophysiology of the underlying disease processes and to review the anatomy and specific surgical techniques preoperatively.

The liver

Anatomy

The liver is divided into six lobes: the right lateral, right medial, caudate, quadrate, left medial and left lateral. In addition the caudate lobe is divided into the caudate process and the papillary process (Figure 9.1a). The liver lobes are clearly separate near the periphery, but at the hilus the parenchyma becomes confluent. The right medial, right lateral and caudate lobes envelope the caudal vena cava as it passes the liver and these lobes are joined to the rest of the liver over a broad area.

The triangular, hepatogastric and hepatoduodenal ligaments form the major attachments from the liver to the body wall and other organs. The right and left triangular ligaments tether the more central parts of the right and left lobes to the diaphragm. The hepatorenal ligament is a thin fold of peritoneum that extends from the renal fossa of the caudate lobe to the ventral surface of the right kidney (Figure 9.1b). The hepatogastric and hepatoduodenal ligaments are components of the lesser omentum. The falciform ligament extends on the midline from the liver to the diaphragm and ventral abdominal wall. In some dogs this mesenteric remnant is large and fat-filled.

The portal vein supplies 80% of the total blood flow to the liver, the remaining 20% coming from the hepatic artery. The portal system is a low pressure system (6–12 mmHg) and is derived from the confluence of splanchnic veins bringing blood to the liver from the intestines, pancreas and spleen. It can be seen ventral to the caudal vena cava, in the root of the mesoduodenum. In

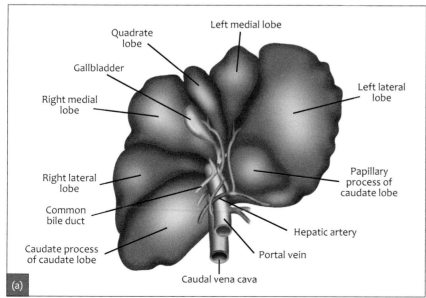

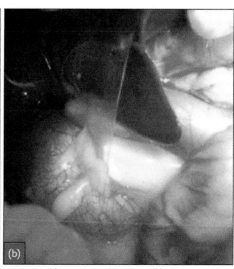

(a) Anatomy of the liver. (b) The
9.1 hepatorenal ligament extending from the caudate lobe to the right kidney.

Labels in figure (a): Quadrate lobe; Left medial lobe; Gallbladder; Left lateral lobe; Right medial lobe; Papillary process of caudate lobe; Right lateral lobe; Hepatic artery; Common bile duct; Portal vein; Caudate process of caudate lobe; Caudal vena cava

conjunction with the hepatic artery, the portal vein forms the ventral boundary of the epiploic foramen (Figure 9.2). At the hepatic hilus the portal vein splits consistently into three major branches – right lateral, right medial and left lateral – before intrahepatic branching occurs (Figure 9.3). Pancreatic hormones (insulin and glucagon) are present in the portal blood and have important hepatotrophic properties. The hepatic artery is a branch of the coeliac artery and gives off numerous branches (three to five) to supply the liver lobes. The hepatic veins drain the liver and flow directly into the caudal vena cava at the level of the diaphragm. They tend to be short and broad and are often obscured from view by the liver parenchyma.

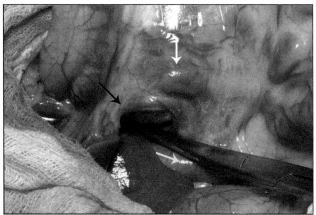

9.2 The epiploic foramen bounded by the hepatic artery (black arrow), portal vein (white arrow) and caudal vena cava (yellow arrow).

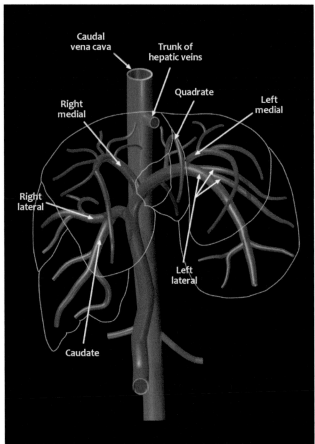

9.3 Intrahepatic portal vein anatomy.
(Illustration by T Vojt, courtesy of S Birchard)

Evaluation of the patient: imaging techniques

The liver can be assessed non-invasively using a variety of imaging modalities. Radiographic lesions of the liver are frequently non-specific but abdominal radiographs may support diagnoses indicated by other data. The most common radiographic change in the liver is an increase in its size (Figure 9.4), but generalized hepatomegaly is a non-specific finding and differential diagnoses include hepatitis, fatty infiltration, hyperadrenocorticism, passive congestion, primary neoplasia (e.g. hepatocellular carcinoma, mast cell tumour, lymphosarcoma) and metastatic neoplasia (e.g. haemangiosarcoma).

Lateral view
• Increased angulation of the gastric shadow
• Extension of the central hepatic border beyond the 13th rib and chondral cartilages
• Rounding of the hepatic borders

Ventrodorsal view
• Displacement of the pylorus towards the midline by the right liver lobes
• Displacement of the cardia towards the midline by the left liver lobes
• Caudal displacement of the stomach, small intestines and right kidney

9.4 Radiographic signs of hepatomegaly.

Occasionally the liver may appear smaller, with the stomach closer to the diaphragm than normal. Differential diagnoses for microhepatica include portosystemic shunts, arteriovenous (AV) fistulae and cirrhosis. Cirrhosis may be due to portosystemic shunts, as well as toxic, metabolic, inflammatory or idiopathic causes. Irregular lumpy liver margins may be caused by neoplasia, abscesses, cysts, cirrhosis or nodular hyperplasia. Ascites may be seen with any chronic hepatic disease, particularly cirrhosis or neoplasia.

Ultrasonography is excellent for demonstrating the anatomy of the liver, detecting focal changes and allowing fine-needle aspiration or core biopsy to be performed. It should be remembered that the correlation between ultrasonographic appearance and histopathology is poor (Warren-Smith et al., 2012). Fine-needle aspiration is the least invasive technique available to obtain samples for cytological evaluation and can be performed in debilitated patients with minimal risk; however, given the small sample of cells obtained the diagnostic accuracy is poor. Ultrasonography is superior to radiography for evaluation of the gallbladder and bile ducts. (For a more detailed discussion of radiography and ultrasonography, see the BSAVA Manual of Canine and Feline Radiography and Radiology and the BSAVA Manual of Canine and Feline Ultrasonography.)

Computed tomography (CT) and magnetic resonance imaging (MRI) are increasingly available in veterinary medicine to achieve non-invasive diagnosis and help with preoperative planning. Minimally invasive laparoscopic techniques are also being increasingly used, and laparoscopic liver biopsy is considered by many to be the preferred method of obtaining a liver sample, as it allows direct visualization of >85% of the hepatic surface and evaluation of the extrahepatic biliary system. Additional advantages include the ability to take directed tissue biopsy samples and to monitor for excessive bleeding immediately after biopsy. Multiple samples should be taken to maximize the chances of obtaining an accurate histopathological diagnosis (Petre et al., 2012).

In humans, endoscopic retrograde cholangiopancreatography is used extensively to achieve a diagnosis. The technique involves retrograde injection of an iodinated contrast material through the duodenal papilla. Therapeutic applications include cholelith removal and stent placement, and, although this minimally invasive technique has not yet been described in clinical veterinary cases, it may hold promise for the future.

Preoperative considerations

> **PRACTICAL TIP**
>
> Liver disease can cause a variety of significant metabolic and haematological disorders and is not a static situation. Current preoperative bloodwork should be performed. In particular, packed cell volume (PCV), serum albumin, glucose and electrolytes should be monitored closely. In addition, measurements of liver function such as pre- and postprandial bile acids and blood ammonia concentrations will provide further information prior to anaesthesia and surgery

Hypoglycaemia

The liver maintains plasma glucose concentrations through gluconeogenesis and glycogenolysis. Hypoglycaemia can result from severe liver disease. If the animal is hypoglycaemic, intravenous fluids supplemented with glucose should be given before and during surgery (e.g. 5% dextrose in lactated Ringer's solution).

Anaemia

Mild to moderate anaemia can occur secondary to liver disease because of blood loss (coagulopathy or gastrointestinal ulceration), or may be associated with anaemia of chronic disease. Animals with a PCV <20% should be given a preoperative blood transfusion, and blood loss during and after surgery should be monitored closely.

Coagulopathy

> **WARNING**
>
> Animals with severe or chronic liver disease may bleed excessively. A coagulation profile should be performed in any animal with hepatobiliary disease that will be undergoing an invasive procedure

The liver is responsible for synthesis of all coagulation factors except factor VIII. In addition, activated clotting factors and fibrinolytic enzymes are cleared by the liver. Mechanisms of excessive bleeding associated with hepatobiliary disease include decreased synthesis of clotting factors, disseminated intravascular coagulation (DIC) and vitamin K deficiency (deficiency of factors II, VII, IX and X). Vitamin K deficiency is usually caused by malabsorption of vitamin K secondary to complete bile duct obstruction, but can also occur in association with severe hepatic insufficiency. Treatment with subcutaneous injections of vitamin K1 usually results in normalization of coagulation within a few hours. If coagulation is abnormal at the time of surgery, fresh whole blood or fresh frozen plasma can be administered.

Hypoalbuminaemia and ascites

Albumin is synthesized exclusively by the liver. The liver has a large reserve capacity for production, and hypoalbuminaemia typically does not occur until the functional hepatic mass is reduced by 70–80%. In end-stage liver disease there is both decreased albumin synthesis and dilution of serum albumin due to sodium and water retention. Ascitic fluid that accumulates secondary to liver disease and hypoalbuminaemia (serum albumin <15 g/l) is usually a transudate. Administration of plasma should be considered if albumin levels are significantly low.

> **WARNING**
>
> A large accumulation of ascitic fluid can displace the diaphragm and restrict lung expansion. Removal of some of the fluid immediately prior to anaesthetic induction may help to prevent hypoventilation

Hepatic encephalopathy

Dementia, disorientation, circling, head pressing, hypersalivation, seizures or coma may all be signs of hepatic encephalopathy, a metabolic encephalopathy that occurs secondary to severe liver disease or portosystemic shunting of blood (see Chapter 10). These signs should be stabilized prior to surgery using dietary and medical management. (For a more detailed discussion see Chapter 10 and the *BSAVA Manual of Canine and Feline Gastroenterology*.)

Anaesthetic considerations

Animals with hepatic disease may have impaired ability to metabolize and inactivate some drugs, resulting in a prolonged duration of action or altered function of drugs (see Chapter 1 and the *BSAVA Manual of Canine and Feline Anaesthesia and Analgesia*).

Antibiotics

Prophylactic antibiotics are warranted in almost all patients undergoing hepatic surgery. There is evidence to suggest that the canine liver is colonized by anaerobes (*Clostridium* spp.) and that these bacteria may proliferate if there is hepatic ischaemia or hypoxia. In addition, bacteria can migrate to the liver via portal venous blood. The reticuloendothelial system of the liver normally clears these bacteria but this mechanism is compromised in an animal with severe liver disease, obstructive jaundice or portosystemic shunting of blood.

Cephalosporins provide broad-spectrum activity and high tissue concentrations when given intravenously immediately prior to surgery. Penicillin derivatives, metronidazole and clindamycin may also be used, although high doses of metronidazole may cause neurological signs in some dogs. Continuation of the antibiotics is determined by the findings at surgery and the results of bacterial culture and sensitivity testing.

Surgical management of hepatic disease

A large laparotomy incision is essential for thorough examination and surgical manipulation of the liver and biliary tract. A ventral midline laparotomy incision should be made from the xiphoid cartilage to the pubis, and the falciform ligament should be removed.

Using either Mayo scissors or electrocautery, incise the falciform ligament along its attachment to the ventral body wall (Figure 9.5). Once free from these attachments, place a circumferential ligature around the base and transect the falciform ligament distal to the ligature. Removal of the falciform ligament and fat will greatly improve visibility of the cranial abdomen

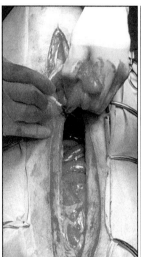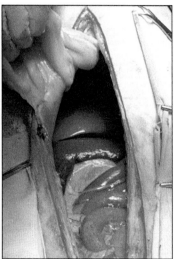

9.5 Removal of the falciform ligament to improve visualization of the cranial abdomen.

In the majority of dogs, incising up to or through the cartilaginous portion of the xiphoid process provides adequate exposure of the liver and biliary tract. In some cases a caudal sternotomy or a transverse paracostal incision can be made after the abdomen is open if further access is required. Manipulation and examination of the liver can be facilitated by taking down the peritoneal folds that suspend the liver from the abdominal wall and diaphragm. By placing a hand over the ventral surface of the liver and gently retracting it caudally, the coronary and triangular ligaments can be seen and carefully transected. Extreme care needs to be taken not to cut the wall of the vena cava as it courses through the caval foramen of the diaphragm or the wall of the left hepatic vein, which empties into the vena cava just before the caval foramen. Additionally, a ventrodorsal incision into the diaphragm from the xiphoid towards the caval foramen (taking care not to incise the vena cava) allows further caudal retraction of the liver.

Balfour abdominal retractors (see Chapter 2) should be placed into the incision and the abdomen should be thoroughly explored. Each lobe of the liver should be visually inspected and carefully palpated.

An assistant can retract caudally using stay sutures placed in the greater curvature of the stomach to facilitate manipulation of the liver

The gallbladder should be visualized and palpated and the cystic duct and common bile duct identified.

Identification and retraction of the descending duodenum aids in locating the common bile duct

Hepatic biopsy techniques and partial lobectomy

Liver biopsy samples (see Operative Technique 9.1) should be routinely obtained during abdominal exploratory surgery in animals with known or suspected hepatobiliary disease. Surgical biopsy has the advantage of allowing the whole liver to be examined, ensuring appropriate lesion localization and that representative biopsy samples are taken. In addition, haemorrhage from the biopsy site can be easily identified and controlled. For diffuse hepatic disease the biopsy sample should be obtained from the most accessible site (marginal biopsy). For focal disease the entire liver should be palpated to determine whether intraparenchymal nodules or cavitary lesions are present and representative samples should be obtained. Regardless of the technique used, it is important to handle the biopsy sample gently to avoid causing artefactual changes. Samples for microbial culture should be taken as soon as possible after opening the abdomen. Partial lobectomy (see Operative Technique 9.1) may be indicated in some conditions where disease only involves a portion of a liver lobe (e.g. peripheral hepatic AV fistula, focal neoplasia, hepatic abscess or trauma).

Techniques for excision of complete or partial liver lobes are similar. Hepatic parenchyma can be bluntly dissected using the flat end of a scalpel handle or the inner cannula of a Poole suction tip. Smaller vessels can be cauterized. Large vessels should be tied off or sealed with metal clips, surgical stapling devices or a vessel sealant device. Several devices developed for laparoscopic surgery can be used in open liver surgery. These include vessel sealant devices that use high-current low-voltage radiofrequency energy (e.g. LigaSure™ or Enseal®), ultrasonic scalpels (e.g. Harmonic® scalpel) and encircling suturing devices (a pre-tied suture loop, e.g. Surgitie™). One study (Risselada et al., 2010) compared five different surgical techniques for partial liver lobectomy in the dog, including use of a Harmonic® scalpel, vessel sealant device and a linear thoracoabdominal (TA) stapler. The encircling suturing devices had not been described previously for use in dogs or in partial liver lobectomy. There were no significant differences in surgical times between the techniques but the suction and clip method led to significantly more blood loss than the other techniques.

The Harmonic® scalpel is increasingly being used in both human and veterinary surgical laparoscopic procedures as an alternative to electrical energy sources such as mono- or bipolar electrocautery or even traditional surgical techniques such as suturing or sharp scissor dissection. The scalpel is ultrasonically activated and controls bleeding by protein denaturation, in contrast with electrosurgery and lasers that deliver localized intense heat to destroy tissue. The blade tip of the Harmonic® scalpel vibrates approximately 55,000 times per second and will seal blood vessels up to 5 mm in diameter without charring or desiccating the tissue.

Complete lobectomy

Complete lobectomy (see Operative Technique 9.2) may be necessary for some focal lesions (e.g. traumatic laceration, AV fistula, neoplasia). The standard exploratory laparotomy incision may need to be extended to improve access to the entire liver, either by splitting the xiphoid and caudal two to three sternebrae, or by extending paracostally; incising the diaphragm ventrodorsally (see above) will also improve access. The gallbladder must be mobilized from its fossa when either the right medial or the quadrate lobe is removed (see below).

Partial hepatectomy

Multiple lobes of the liver can be removed if necessary and this may sometimes be indicated for treatment of abscesses, neoplasia or trauma. The use of surgical stapling devices is recommended. Removal of large portions of the liver in dogs does not usually lead to the bleeding diathesis commonly reported after hepatic resection in humans. Intra-abdominal haemorrhage during and after partial hepatectomy in dogs and cats is most commonly due to failure of the ligatures.

After massive hepatic resection, liver function should be monitored closely. The normal liver has an incredible regenerative capacity. Liver function reportedly remains normal after resection of up to 70% of the normal canine liver. Liver regeneration begins within hours and peaks within 3 days with nearly complete compensatory hypertrophy and hyperplasia reached by 6 days, although it can take up to 6–10 weeks. It is important to remember that the patient's general health and the condition of the remaining liver have a profound effect on survival when a large amount of liver is removed. Mild increases in alkaline phosphatase (ALP) and alanine aminotransferase (ALT) can persist for up to 6 weeks after partial hepatectomy in dogs. High levels of ALT after the first week postoperatively may be indicative of continued hepatic necrosis. It has been shown that, when serum albumin is <20 g/l, dogs with obstructive jaundice do not survive a 70% hepatectomy (Mizumoto *et al.*, 1979) and that dogs with experimentally produced liver cirrhosis can tolerate removal of no more than 40% of the liver (Kohno *et al.*, 1977).

Hepatic cysts and abscesses

Hepatic cysts are closed fluid-filled sacs lined with secretory epithelium. They may be congenital or acquired, single or multiple, and can affect one or several lobes of the liver. Congenital cysts are often multiple and have been reported in association with polycystic kidney disease in cats and in Cairn (McKenna and Carpenter, 1980) and West Highland White Terriers (McAloose *et al.*, 1998). Acquired cysts are usually solitary and can occur secondary to trauma. They may also be caused by benign bile duct adenomas or biliary cystadenomas.

Hepatic cysts are usually an incidental finding but occasionally animals present with abdominal enlargement secondary to an enlarged cyst or abdominal fluid accumulation. If hepatic cysts are found in an animal with clinical evidence of hepatic dysfunction, biopsy samples should be obtained. Large solitary cysts may be excised via partial lobectomy or they may be 'de-roofed' and omentalized.

Hepatic abscesses are rare in cats and dogs but the clinical signs and clinicopathological findings are similar to those for other types of inflammatory hepatic disease. Anorexia and lethargy are the most common historical complaints, followed by vomiting and diarrhoea. Rupture of a hepatic abscess rapidly leads to peritonitis, septic shock and death.

Physical abnormalities are vague and include fever, dehydration, signs of abdominal pain, abdominal distension, hepatomegaly and mucosal bleeding. Haematological abnormalities include leucocytosis with neutrophilia, mild to moderate thrombocytopenia and mild anaemia. Serum biochemical abnormalities include high ALP and ALT activities and a high bilirubin concentration; hypoalbuminaemia and prolonged coagulation values have also been reported.

Abdominal radiography may reveal hepatomegaly, poor abdominal detail, a hepatic mass or splenomegaly. Masses may be identified by ultrasonography. On abdominal ultrasonography, abscesses can be hypoechoic or hyperechoic, round, oval or irregular lesions, often with central cavitation. Enhancement artefacts, abdominal effusion, regional lymphadenopathy and hyperechoic perihepatic fat may also be identified. Ultrasound-guided fine-needle aspiration for cytology and culture may be diagnostic.

Abscesses are usually due to polymicrobial infections. *Escherichia coli*, *Clostridium* spp., *Klebsiella pneumoniae*, *Enterococcus* spp., *Staphylococcus epidermidis* and *S. intermedius* are the most common bacteria isolated. Potential sources of bacteria include ascension via the bile ducts, haematogenous spread, direct extension from local suppurative diseases and penetrating abdominal wounds. Concurrent infections are often identified in humans and may be detected in the biliary tract, spleen, blood, endocardium, lung, prostate gland, peritoneum, lymph nodes, salivary gland or brain. Umbilical infections are the most common cause of hepatic abscesses in young animals.

Treatment of hepatic abscesses can be medical or surgical. Ultrasound-guided percutaneous abscess drainage has been advocated for the treatment of single abscesses, in conjunction with fluid and antibiotic therapy, but there is a risk that the abscess will rupture into the abdomen, causing diffuse peritonitis. Surgical treatment involves partial or complete lobectomy for single or multiple abscesses confined to one liver lobe, followed by long-term antibiotic therapy based on the results of bacterial culture and sensitivity testing.

Liver lobe torsion

Liver lobe torsion is rare in both dogs and cats. Twisting of a liver lobe around its vascular pedicle results initially in venous obstruction, increased hydrostatic pressure, ascites and arterial and venous thrombosis and, eventually, in tissue necrosis.

Clinical signs may be vague and non-specific and include lethargy, anorexia, polyuria/polydipsia or signs indicative of a severe intra-abdominal problem, with acute onset of weakness, abdominal pain, vomiting, collapse and shock. In most cases an underlying cause is never identified. Bloodwork abnormalities are non-specific but generally reveal elevated liver enzymes. A cranial abdominal mass may be identified on abdominal radiographs or ultrasound examination.

The diagnosis is confirmed by abdominal exploratory surgery (Figure 9.6). Torsion of the left lateral liver lobe is most commonly reported and has been suggested to be due to its mobility, large size and relative separation from the other lobes (Swann and Cimino Brown, 2001). A complete lobectomy should always be performed (see Operative Technique 9.2) without derotating the twisted lobe. Derotation can result in the release of bacterial toxins, reperfusion injury and death. Torsion of the gallbladder has also been reported in association with torsion of the right middle and quadrate liver lobes (Massari *et al.*, 2012).

Hepatic arteriovenous fistulae

Hepatic AV fistulae have been reported in both dogs and cats but they occur rarely. Most are diagnosed in animals less than 1 year of age and are believed to be congenital, the result of a failure of the common embryological capillary plexus to differentiate into an artery or vein. AV fistulae may also be acquired, as a result of abdominal

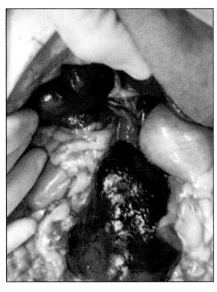

9.6 Torsion of the left medial liver lobe in a 7-year-old Cocker Spaniel bitch.

trauma, hepatic surgery, hepatic neoplasia, cirrhosis or rupture of a hepatic arterial aneurysm. Any liver lobe may be affected but the right medial lobe is the most frequently reported (Whiting *et al.*, 1986). Affected animals usually develop portal hypertension and multiple collateral shunting vessels, and often have ascites. With excessive AV shunting, diastolic arterial pressure decreases, resulting in increased cardiac output and heart rate and possibly ventricular failure. History and clinical findings are similar to those for congenital portosystemic shunts. On physical examination a systolic cardiac murmur may be noted and auscultation of the abdomen over the area of the liver reveals a continuous machinery murmur (bruit) caused by runoff of arterial blood into the portal system.

Tortuous anechoic tubular structures may be seen on ultrasound examination of the liver. Colour-flow Doppler can be used to differentiate AV fistulae from congenital portosystemic shunts and to determine the direction of blood flow. The diagnosis is confirmed by coeliac arteriography, which demonstrates communication between the hepatic artery and portal vein. At exploratory laparotomy, AV fistulae appear as thin-walled tortuous pulsating vascular channels that distort the hepatic parenchyma and elevate the overlying hepatic capsule.

Treatment involves surgical ligation of the AV fistula or resection of the affected liver lobe. With closure of the fistula, reflex bradycardia can occur (Branham's reflex), and animals should be premedicated with glycopyrrolate or atropine to help prevent this. Dearterialization is required if multiple lobes are involved. Following surgery, clinical signs are decreased in 57% of cases but often hepatic function does not return to normal, owing to persistent shunting through acquired portosystemic shunt vessels.

Hepatobiliary neoplasia

Tumours involving the liver are categorized according to the tissue they arise from (see *BSAVA Manual of Canine and Feline Oncology*). Primary hepatic tumours are rare and arise either from the hepatocytes (e.g. hepatocellular adenoma (hepatoma) or carcinoma) or the bile duct epithelium (e.g. biliary adenoma or carcinoma; Figure 9.7ab). Metastatic tumours are most common in dogs, especially haemangiosarcoma, pancreatic adenocarcinoma, insulinoma and other tumours of the gastrointestinal and urinary tracts. In cats, haemolymphatic tumours are most commonly diagnosed (e.g. lymphosarcoma, mast cell tumour).

Hepatocellular carcinomas and bile duct carcinomas can occur in one of three distinct pathological forms:

- Solitary or massive form (single large mass in one liver lobe)
- Multifocal nodules (discrete nodules of different sizes in various lobes) (Figure 9.7c)
- Diffuse infiltration of large portions of the liver (Figure 9.7d).

These tumours have a high metastatic rate, which is variable depending on the tumour subtype. For hepatocellular carcinomas, metastasis at the time of diagnosis has been reported as 100% for the diffuse, 93% for the nodular and 36.6% for the solitary type (Patnaik *et al.*, 1980). The reported metastatic rate for bile duct carcinomas is 87.5% (Patnaik *et al.*, 1981). Common metastatic sites for both tumour types include the hepatic lymph nodes, lung and peritoneum.

Older dogs and cats (>10 years) are usually affected and show vague non-specific signs of hepatic dysfunction that often do not appear until late in the course of

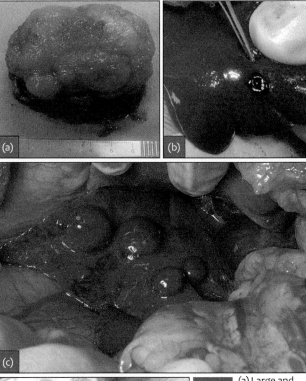

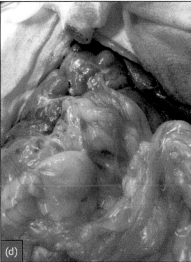

9.7 (a) Large and (b) small biliary cystadenomas in the liver of a cat. (c) Multifocal hepatocellular carcinoma. (d) Diffuse form of hepatocellular carcinoma, which is not amenable to surgical resection.

the disease. Clinical signs include lethargy, anorexia, weight loss, vomiting and polyuria/polydipsia. Other signs may include jaundice, ascites and signs of hepatic encephalopathy due to liver dysfunction or central nervous system metastasis.

Diagnosis

Physical examination findings in animals with hepatobiliary neoplasia include:

- Cranial abdominal mass or marked hepatomegaly
- Ascites
- Haemoperitoneum (most likely with rupture of hepatocellular adenoma, hepatocellular carcinoma or haemangiosarcoma)
- Jaundice
- Anaemia
- Marked weight loss.

Bloodwork changes may reveal anaemia and mild to marked increases in ALT and ALP, but these changes are present inconsistently. Serum bilirubin concentrations may be elevated, particularly if an extrahepatic biliary tract obstruction occurs. Hypoglycaemia is occasionally detected and coagulation times may be prolonged. Abdominal radiography and ultrasonography provide the mainstay of diagnosis. Thoracic radiographs should be taken to look for evidence of metastatic disease.

Treatment

Surgical excision is the treatment of choice but only solitary masses are amenable to surgical resection via hepatic lobectomy. The entire abdomen should be thoroughly explored and biopsy samples of the hepatic lymph nodes should be taken.

Prognosis

Little information exists regarding prognosis following resection of hepatobiliary tumours in dogs and cats. Prognosis following excision for benign tumours is good. Diffuse hepatic neoplasia carries a very poor prognosis, but patients with localized tumours that can be resected may survive more than 1 year. In one study 50% of dogs were alive, without evidence of disease, a median of 377 days following excision of hepatocellular carcinoma and the cause of death was rarely tumour related.

The biliary tract

> *Every biliary operation is, in essence, an exploratory one, and the type of procedure to be performed should be dictated by the operative findings*
> WS Halsted (1899)

Extrahepatic bile duct obstruction and trauma are the two most common indications for biliary tract surgery.

Anatomy

The gallbladder is a pear-shaped sac that lies in a fossa between the right medial and quadrate lobes of the liver and is connected to the common bile duct by the cystic duct. It is divided anatomically into the fundus, body and neck and receives its blood supply from the cystic artery, a branch of the hepatic artery. The wall consists of a mucosal lining, smooth muscle fibres, submucosa and an outer serosal covering. It has a capacity of approximately 1 ml/kg bodyweight.

The extrahepatic portion of the biliary system consists of a variable number of hepatic ducts that enter the common bile duct at several locations (Figure 9.8). The free portion of the bile duct (Figure 9.9a) runs through the lesser omentum within the hepatoduodenal ligament and is about 5 cm long and 2.5 mm in diameter. In dogs, the distal portion of the bile duct (intramural portion) enters the dorsal mesenteric wall of the duodenum, courses obliquely through the duodenal wall for 1.5–2 cm and terminates alongside but separate from the pancreatic duct at the major duodenal papilla (Figure 9.9b). In cats, the terminal portion of the bile duct merges with the major pancreatic duct just before it empties into the cranial duodenum through a common ampulla.

Bile

Bile is a slightly alkaline isotonic solution that consists of water, inorganic electrolytes and organic solutes, such as bile acids, cholesterol, phospholipid and bilirubin. Efficient digestion and absorption of dietary lipids depends on adequate secretion of bile. Fat maldigestion results in malabsorption of fat-soluble vitamins, most importantly vitamin K. The production of activated prothrombin complex factors II, VII, IX and X depends on vitamin K. Deficiencies can develop with fat malabsorption leading to coagulopathies. Absence of bile from the duodenum (obstruction or surgical diversion) leads to an increase in gastric acid secretion and a decrease in gastric acid neutralization in the duodenum. Duodenal ulceration may develop as a sequela.

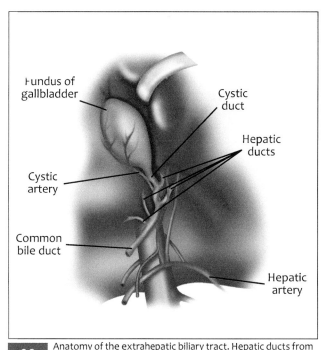

9.8 Anatomy of the extrahepatic biliary tract. Hepatic ducts from the quadrate and right medial lobes (central division of the liver) enter the bile duct at its origin, along with the cystic duct from the gallbladder. Hepatic ducts from the right lateral and caudate lobes, left lateral and medial lobes and the papillary process of the caudate lobe enter the free portion of the bile duct more distally.

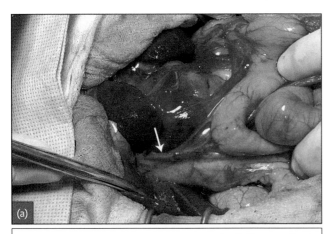

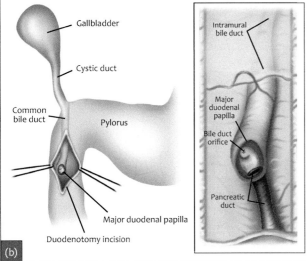

(a) Common bile duct (arrowed) entering the dudonenum.
(b) The distal portion of the bile duct in the dog is intramural.
It courses obliquely through the duodenal wall and terminates alongside
but separate from the pancreatic duct at the major duodenal papilla.

9.9

Congenital
• Biliary atresia
• Choledochal cysts

Acquired

• Luminal:
  – Inspissated bile
  – Gallbladder mucocele
  – Stones
  – Blood clots
  – Parasites (flukes)
• Mural:
  – Cholangitis (infectious, sclerosing)
  – Biliary carcinoma
  – Cholecystitis
  – Stricture
• Extraluminal:
  – Pancreatitis (chronic fibrosing, acute)
  – Pancreatic abscess
  – Neoplasia (biliary, hepatic, pancreatic, gastrointestinal, lymph node)
  – Duodenal foreign body
  – Diaphragmatic hernia with gallbladder entrapment

9.10   Causes of extrahepatic biliary obstruction.

Bile duct obstruction

Obstruction of the biliary system is the most common cause of hyperbilirubinaemia. Obstruction can be intra- or extrahepatic. Hyperbilirubinaemia can also be seen with biliary tract rupture, since bile drains into the abdominal cavity and is absorbed. In animals with extrahepatic biliary obstruction, hyperbilirubinaemia is evident within several hours and jaundice may be detectable as early as 48 hours. Causes of extrahepatic biliary obstruction are shown in Figure 9.10.

Gallbladder mucocele

Gallbladder mucoceles are being recognized with increasing frequency in dogs but have not been reported in cats. Older small-breed dogs tend to be affected, with Cocker Spaniels, Shetland Sheepdogs and Miniature Schnauzers being over-represented in the literature, and Border Terriers in the UK. Hyperplasia of the mucus-secreting glands within the mucosa of the gallbladder leads to an abnormal accumulation of mucus within the gallbladder lumen. Accumulation of bile-laden mucus within the hepatic, cystic and common bile ducts results in extrahepatic biliary obstruction and can ultimately lead to rupture of the gallbladder. The aetiology is uncertain but biliary stasis, cholecystitis and liver disease have all been suggested to predispose to mucocele formation.

Genetic predisposition may also play a role; for example, Shetland Sheepdogs are predisposed to gallbladder disorders, with mucoceles and concurrent dyslipidaemia or dysmotility occurring in many affected dogs (Aguirre et al., 2007). Recently it has been suggested that dogs with hyperadrenocorticism are at a 29 times greater risk of developing biliary mucoceles than dogs without hyper-adrenocorticism (Mesich et al., 2009).

Dogs usually present with non-specific signs such as vomiting, lethargy and anorexia, but some dogs have no clinical signs at all. Diagnosis therefore relies on a combination of clinical signs, bloodwork abnormalities and the results of diagnostic imaging studies. Common examination findings include abdominal pain, fever and jaundice. Total bilirubin, ALT, ALP and total white blood cell count are usually elevated; however, bilirubin can be normal in early cases. Abdominal radiographs are usually non-specific. Ultrasonographically, biliary mucoceles are characterized by the appearance of stellate or finely striated bile patterns ('kiwi fruit-like' pattern) and differ from biliary sludge by the absence of gravity-dependent bile movement. The wall of the gallbladder is variably thickened (Besso et al., 2000). Gallbladder wall discontinuity is suggestive of gallbladder rupture, as is the presence of pericholecystic hyperechoic fat or the accumulation of fluid within the abdomen.

> **WARNING**
>
> Gallbladder rupture secondary to ischaemic necrosis of the gallbladder wall is present in up to 60% of dogs with gallbladder mucocele. Emergency cholecystectomy should be performed

Cholecystectomy (see Operative Technique 9.4) is the treatment of choice because it is the gallbladder wall that is considered to be the source of the abnormal mucus production. The gallbladder should always be submitted for histopathology, and a sample of bile and gallbladder wall should be submitted for culture. Enterococcus spp. and Eschericia coli are reported as being most commonly isolated; however, in the author's experience, bacterial cultures are most frequently negative. Liver biopsy should be performed routinely at the time of cholecystectomy. The most common histopathological findings are cholangiohepatitis, biliary hyperplasia and cholestasis.

Potential complications include leakage of bile, pancreatitis and re-obstruction of the common bile duct with gelatinous bile. Reported perioperative mortality rates range from 21.7% to 40% and, in a recent study (Malek *et al.*, 2013), elevations in serum lactate concentrations and immediate postoperative hypotension in dogs were associated with poor clinical outcomes. Despite this, if treated early, before the gallbladder has ruptured, the prognosis is generally good if the dog survives the immediate postoperative period (Besso *et al.*, 2000; Mehler, 2004; Amsellem *et al.*, 2006).

Ursodiol

The use of agents such as ursodiol is controversial in cases of hepatobiliary disease. Ursodiol is known to have choleretic activity, as well as anti-apoptotic and immunomodulatory properties (Webster and Cooper, 2009). However, because of lack of published clinical trials, the true therapeutic potential of ursodiol in companion animals with hepatobiliary disease is largely unknown.

Pancreatitis

Animals with pancreatitis should initially be managed medically. If clinical or laboratory evidence of improvement is not seen within 10 days, or if deterioration occurs despite appropriate medical therapy, biliary decompression procedures can be considered. Obstruction from fibrosis secondary to pancreatic inflammation is most often seen 10–14 days after an acute vomiting crisis, though it can occur at any time after multiple episodes of low-grade pancreatitis.

> **WARNING**
>
> At surgery a pancreatic granuloma or fibrotic tissue can easily be confused with a neoplastic process. Unless numerous metastatic nodules are seen in other organs and confirmed cytologically, biopsy samples should be taken

Cholelithiasis

Cholelithiasis is rare in dogs and cats and many animals with choleliths are asymptomatic. In humans, gallstones are classified into two categories: cholesterol stones and pigment stones. Cholesterol stones are the most frequently formed in humans, whereas in dogs and cats bile pigment (calcium bilirubinate) stones predominate. Pigment stones rarely result in clinical signs unless obstruction or infection of the biliary system occurs. The gallbladder is the site of formation of most choleliths but stones can form primarily in the duct. This usually requires an abnormality that produces bile stasis, such as partial obstruction or marked dilatation.

Older small-breed bitches appear to be at an increased risk of developing choleliths. Clinical signs range from mild and intermittent to severe, with fever, vomiting, abdominal pain and jaundice. Choleliths may be a factor predisposing to cholecystitis and they should be removed in any patient presenting with signs of biliary tract disease.

Bile duct carcinoma (cholangiocellular carcinoma)

Bile duct carcinomas are the second most common primary hepatobiliary tumour of dogs, occurring more frequently in bitches. These tumours arise from the intrahepatic bile duct epithelium, though in rare instances they may arise from the extrahepatic bile ducts or gallbladder. They are highly metastatic, commonly metastasizing to the hepatic lymph nodes, lung and peritoneum. Clinical signs include weight loss, anorexia, depression, vomiting and an enlarged abdomen. Jaundice may occur and hepatomegaly is noted on abdominal palpation.

Evaluation of the patient: imaging techniques

Common imaging techniques used to evaluate the biliary tract include abdominal radiography and ultrasonography. Radiographic findings depend on the underlying disease but images may show radiopaque densities in the area of the gallbladder if choleliths containing calcium are present. Occasionally, a large fluid-filled gallbladder can be seen superimposed over the liver. Other findings may include evidence of pancreatitis, emphysematous cholecystitis and hepatomegaly, but radiographs are frequently non-diagnostic. Ultrasonography may help in identifying underlying causes of biliary obstruction, such as pancreatitis, neoplasia, cholelithiasis or gallbladder mucocele. Ultrasound examination can detect both radiolucent and radiopaque choleliths and reveal distension of the gallbladder and intra- and extrahepatic bile ducts (Figure 9.11). In cases of gallbladder rupture, intra-abdominal fluid will be detected and no gallbladder will be observed.

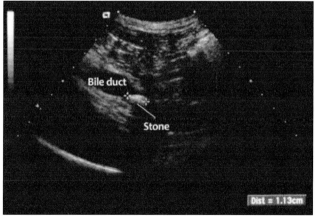

9.11 Ultrasonogram showing a choledocholith with distension of the common bile duct proximal to it.

A combination of findings from the physical examination, bloodwork abnormalities and ultrasound examination often indicates a problem with the biliary tract. If a diagnosis is not confirmed, CT, hepatobiliary scintigraphy or laparoscopy can aid diagnosis. These techniques are usually only available at referral centres and often an exploratory laparotomy is required for definitive diagnosis and treatment.

Preoperative considerations

Animals with biliary tract disease are usually very ill and are poor candidates for immediate surgery. Biliary obstruction causes icterus, elevation of liver enzymes and coagulopathy. Vomiting and anorexia are frequent problems in these patients and intravenous fluids are indicated preoperatively. Preoperative and intraoperative considerations for animals with biliary tract disease are summarized in Figure 9.12.

Preoperative considerations

- Correct fluid, electrolyte and acid–base deficiencies preoperatively
- Check blood glucose and albumin levels
- Determine whether vitamin K deficiency is present: check one-stage prothrombin time (OSPT) or proteins induced by vitamin K absence (PIVKA) and if either are increased begin vitamin K therapy (1–2 mg/kg bodyweight q8h). In most cases coagulation times normalize within 3 hours
- Intravenous antibiotics, which reach high levels in bile, should be given perioperatively: acute *versus* enteric organisms (*Escherichia coli*, *Klebsiella* spp., *Proteus* spp., *Streptococcus* spp., *Pseudomonas* spp., *Clostridium* spp.,) i.e. cephalosporins
- Plasma or whole blood may be required before, during or after the surgery
- Severely compromised animals will not survive prolonged surgical procedures (i.e. cholecystoduodenostomy/cholecystojejunostomy) and consideration should be given to performing palliative procedures (i.e. tube drainage of the biliary tract) to allow the patient's physiological condition to improve prior to a definitive surgical correction

Intraoperative considerations

- Routine liver biopsy will provide information on severity and progression of structural liver alterations and help with diagnosis, prognosis and long-term management
- Cholecystectomy (see Operative Technique 9.4) is preferred over cholecystotomy (see Operative Technique 9.3) for stone removal. Secondary changes of the gallbladder that result from the presence of stones include hyperplasia, inflammation and necrosis. Removing the gallbladder removes the reservoir for subsequent stone formation and may have a lower rate of surgical morbidity than cholecystotomy
- Always determine patency of the lower biliary tract. If patency cannot be determined by passing a catheter via cholecystectomy and cannulation of the cystic duct, a duodenotomy incision should be made over the major duodenal papilla and the common bile duct cannulated (see Figure 9.13)
- If biliary obstruction cannot be relieved in cases other than those with stones, a biliary diversion procedure will be necessary. Cholecystoduodenostomy (see Operative Technique 9.5) is the procedure of choice
- In very ill patients temporary biliary decompression using a cholecystostomy tube should be considered to minimize surgical time
- Culture bile. Biliary sepsis is not uncommon in patients with chronic hepatobiliary disease

9.12 Pre- and intraoperative considerations for animals with biliary tract disease.

Surgical management of biliary tract disease

Tube drainage of the biliary tract

A soft tube to provide temporary drainage of the biliary tract can be inserted directly into the gallbladder (tube cholecystostomy), or via the major duodenal papilla (transpapillary biliary endoprosthesis) (Figure 9.13) and into the common bile duct.

Whenever a transpapillary biliary endoprosthesis is used, the local effects on the extrahepatic bile ducts and the possibility of subsequent bacterial contamination should be considered. Experimental studies have shown that 4 weeks of stenting of normal or obstructed canine common bile ducts resulted in fibrosed bile ducts, with chronic inflammation and papillary hyperplasia of the epithelium, and that in all cases bile cultures grew faecal bacteria (Karsten *et al.*, 1994).

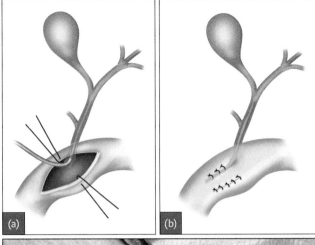

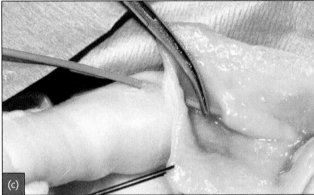

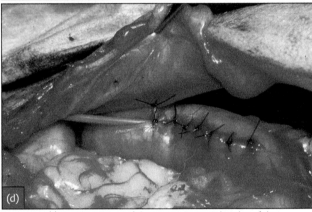

9.13 (a) Duodenotomy of the antimesenteric border of the proximal duodenum allowing visualization of the major duodenal papilla and cannulation of the common bile duct. (b) From the duodenal approach the tube may be ended within the lumen of the duodenum and held in place with absorbable sutures. This allows bile to flow into the duodenal lumen. The tube migrates into the duodenum postoperatively and passes from the body with the faeces.
(c–d) Alternatively the tube can be placed through the abdominal wall on the right side, then tunnelled through the duodenum, similar to a jejunostomy tube. This has the advantage that cholangiography can be performed and the tube can be easily removed.
(Photographs courtesy of S Birchard)

Tube cholecystostomy

Tube cholecystostomy is used for biliary diversion either when the bile duct is temporarily obstructed (acute pancreatitis) or in severely ill patients requiring biliary decompression prior to definitive treatment of the bile duct obstruction. An advantage of this technique is that it allows positive contrast cholangiography to be performed to determine bile duct patency prior to tube removal. A Foley catheter is introduced through the right ventrolateral body wall (Figure 9.14) just caudal to the costal arch and passed through a layer of omentum. The gallbladder is packed off and a purse-string suture is made in the fundus of the gallbladder using 2 metric (3/0 USP) monofilament absorbable suture material. A stab incision is made into the fundus within the limits of the purse-string suture and the end of the tube is passed into the gallbladder. The purse-string suture is tied and the bulb of the Foley catheter is inflated. Mobilization of the gallbladder is not generally required, as the omentum forms a fibrous tract

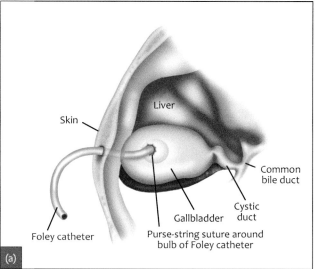

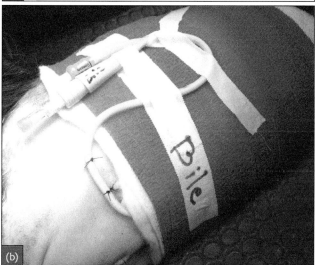

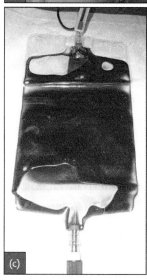

9.14 (a) Tube cholecystotomy. (b–c) The Foley catheter should be connected to a closed connecting system and the amount of bile produced should be monitored.

around the tube that collapses and seals off the gallbladder stoma after the tube has been removed.

The tube can be removed as early as 5 days later or left in place until resolution of the problem. The temporary exclusion of bile from the gastrointestinal tract does not usually alter digestion or haemostasis beyond those changes already occurring as a result of the disease process. If the tube is to remain in place for longer than 10 days, it is possible to collect the diverted bile and place it into gelatin capsules to be administered orally at the time of feeding. However, this is often an impractical suggestion: a large number of capsules are usually required (owing to the volume of bile collected); these patients may be on *nil per os* regimes as a consequence of pancreatitis; and even if they are being offered food, patients often remain anorexic for prolonged periods.

Cholecystotomy

Cholecystotomy, or incision into the gallbladder (see Operative Technique 9.3), is performed to allow removal of gallbladder contents (stones or inspissated bile) and to allow tube exploration and flushing of the extrahepatic biliary tract. If the gallbladder appears normal, moderately increasing pressure can be applied to it prior to cholecystotomy to determine whether the extrahepatic biliary tract is patent. This should be performed carefully so as not to damage or rupture the gallbladder wall.

Cholecystectomy

The decision to remove the gallbladder rather than save it is based upon the apparent viability of the tissue and severity of the trauma or disease. Cholecystectomy (see Operative Technique 9.4) is indicated when the gallbladder is the primary source of the disease process, when it is secondarily involved but has undergone severe structural changes, or when leaving it is likely to cause recurrence of disease. Cholecystectomy is performed for diseases such as severe cholecystitis, cholelithiasis, neoplasia and traumatic rupture. Surgical objectives include removing the gallbladder while minimizing trauma to the surrounding hepatic parenchyma, preventing leakage of bile into the peritoneal cavity and avoiding damage to the rest of the biliary tract.

> **WARNING**
>
> It is important to realize that removal of the gallbladder removes the option to perform a cholecystoduodenostomy or cholecystojejunostomy to improve bile drainage

Choledochotomy

Choledochotomy involves an incision into the common bile duct for exploration or for the removal of a calculus (Figure 9.15). It is usually only possible in animals with marked dilatation secondary to chronic obstruction. Prior to choledochotomy, attempts should first be made to remove the obstruction by flushing the common bile duct, via either a cholecystotomy or duodenotomy incision.

Once the duct has been opened and drained, sequential flushing and probing should be carried out to ensure that the lumen is completely free of obstruction. If luminal or mural obstructive lesions are not removable, a biliary

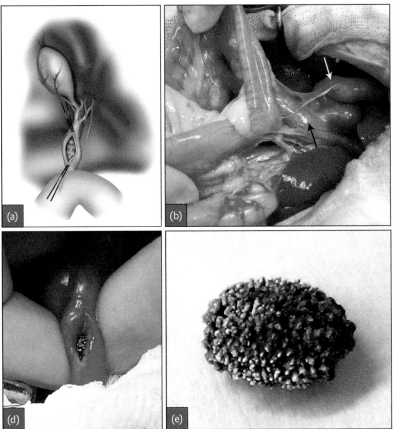

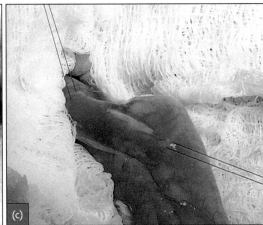

9.15 Choledochotomy. (a) Fine stay sutures of polypropylene should be placed to allow traction on the duct and the area should be well packed off. A small incision should be made using a No. 15 scalpel blade. (b) Markedly dilated common (black arrow) and cystic (white arrow) ducts in a cat with a choledocholith. (c) Stay sutures are placed through the wall of the common bile duct. (d) An incision is made into the duct directly over the choledocholith. (e) The choledocholith.

diversion procedure (see Operative Technique 9.5) should be performed. Extraluminal obstruction or stricture should be treated using a biliary diversion technique. The chole-dochotomy incision can be closed with 1.0 or 1.1 metric (5/0 or 4/0 USP) monofilament absorbable suture material in a simple interrupted or simple continuous pattern.

Definitive biliary diversion techniques

There are numerous biliary–intestinal diversion techniques that can be performed, including anastomosis of the gall-bladder to the stomach (cholecystogastrostomy) or the small intestine (cholecystoenterostomy), or anastomosis of the common bile duct to the small intestine (choledocho-enterostomy). In small animal surgery, anastomosis of the common bile duct to the intestine is difficult, owing to the small size of the common bile duct (1–2 mm in cats and 2–3 mm in dogs). The two most commonly performed pro-cedures are cholecystoduodenostomy and cholecysto-jejunostomy (see Operative Technique 9.5), which involve anastomosis of the gallbladder to the duodenum and jeju-num, respectively. These techniques are indicated when the common bile duct is irreversibly obstructed or trauma-tized. The anastomosis is usually performed by suturing the gallbladder to the intestinal wall in a single layer. Double-layer closures are unnecessary and likely to cause more narrowing at the stoma site. Performing the anasto-mosis with a 30 mm endo-gastrointestinal anastomosis (GIA) stapler has also been reported (Morrison et al., 2008).

Of the two options, cholecystoduodenostomy is the procedure of choice. It is more physiological than chole-cystojejunostomy because bile enters the intestine closer to its normal position and it is the presence of bile in the duodenum that inhibits gastric acid secretion. However, in some cases excessive tension can be encountered when trying to anastomose the gallbladder to the duodenum, mandating the use of the jejunum. If a cholecystojejuno-stomy is performed, the proximal jejunum should be used to decrease postoperative maldigestion of lipids and con-sequent weight loss. In addition, diversion of bile into the jejunum results in a physiological increase in gastric acid secretion and a decrease in neutralization of gastric secretions in the duodenum. This leads to an increased incidence of duodenal ulceration.

Rupture of the biliary tract

Biliary tract rupture secondary to necrotizing cholecystitis, cholelithiasis or trauma causes a severe chemical perito-nitis, which may or may not be associated with sepsis (see Chapter 18). Identification and repair of the leak should be performed as soon as possible, because the metabolic alterations are serious and can rapidly become life-threatening. When leakage of bile occurs following trauma it is rarely from the gallbladder and much more commonly from the common bile duct or hepatic ducts. The common bile duct can also become avulsed from the duodenum or the hepatic ducts can become avulsed from their entrance into the common bile duct. There is usually a prolonged delay (days to weeks) before the clinical signs of biliary leakage are evident.

Primary repair of biliary trauma

Rupture of the gallbladder is easily recognized at surgery and is treated by cholecystectomy. Recognition of trau-matic rupture of the bile ducts is usually delayed, owing to their small diameter, and identifying the area of leakage can be difficult. The most frequent area of rupture is the common bile duct distal to the last hepatic duct, followed by the junction of the common bile duct with the duodenum (Parchman and Flanders, 1990). Primary repair has a high morbidity associated with surgical complications and is reserved for selected cases in which ductal tissue appears healthy, wound tension is minimal and biliary diversion is not an option (i.e. patients with proximal ductal lacerations or avulsions of the cystic duct from the bile duct).

The simplest method of repair involves ligating a hepatic duct when there has been avulsion of a hepatic duct from the bile duct; this will resolve the leakage. Ligation of a hepatic duct can be performed safely, because dogs have an auxiliary network of small ducts that may permit drainage of hepatic bile from one lobe to another when the hepatic duct is obstructed. Alternatively, the portion of liver drained by the dilated duct may undergo atrophy whilst the unaffected liver hypertrophies in compensation and assumes the function of excreting all the bile (Martin *et al.*, 2003).

Avulsion of the bile duct at its junction with the duodenum is not usually amenable to primary repair and requires biliary diversion (cholecystoduodenostomy). The bile duct should be ligated proximal to the site of injury to prevent further leakage of bile. Proximal lacerations of the free portion of the bile duct can be sutured primarily with absorbable suture material but leakage is common. Lacerations of the bile duct not amenable to suturing can be managed with stent tubing (see above), although its use is controversial. No consensus exists as to how long the stent should remain in place. The stent may interfere with normal bile flow, promote stricture formation and cause cholangitis. The use of vascular grafts and autologous vein grafts in conjunction with stenting has also been reported for the treatment of experimental biliary tract injuries in dogs (Karaayvaz *et al.*, 1998; Gomez *et al.*, 2002).

References and further reading

Aguirre AL, Center SA, Randolph JF, *et al.* (2007) Gallbladder disease in Shetland sheepdogs: 38 cases (1995–2005). *Journal of the American Veterinary Medical Association* **231**, 79–88

Amsellem PM, Seim HB and MacPhail CM (2006) Long-term survival and risk factors associated with biliary surgery in dogs: 34 cases (1994–2004). *Journal of the American Veterinary Medical Association* **229**, 1451–1457

Barr F and Gaschen L (2011) *BSAVA Manual of Canine and Feline Ultrasonography*. BSAVA Publications, Gloucester

Besso JG, Wrigley RH, Gliatto JM and Webster CRL (2000) Ultrasonographic appearance and clinical findings in 14 dogs with gallbladder mucocele. *Veterinary Radiology and Ultrasound* **41**, 261–271

Bjorling DE, Prasse KW and Holmes RA (1985) Partial hepatectomy in dogs. *The Compendium for Continuing Education (Small Animal)* **7**, 257–264

Dobson J and Lascelles D (2011) *BSAVA Manual of Canine and Feline Oncology, 3rd edn*. BSAVA Publications, Gloucester

Downs MO, Miller MA, Cross AR *et al.* (1998) Liver lobe torsion and liver lobe abscess in a dog. *Journal of the American Veterinary Medical Association* **212**, 678–680

Farrar ET, Washabau RJ and Saunders HM (1996) Hepatic abscesses in dogs: 14 cases (1982–1994). *Journal of the American Veterinary Medical Association* **208**, 243–247

Francavilla A, Porter KA and Benichou J (1978) Liver regeneration in dogs: morphologic and chemical changes. *Journal of Surgical Research* **25**, 409–419

Gomez NA, Alvarez LR, Mite A, *et al.* (2002) Repair of bile duct injuries with Gore-Tex vascular grafts: experimental study in dogs. *Journal of Gastrointestinal Surgery* **6**, 116–120

Grooters AM, Sherding RG, Biller DS and Johnson SE (1994) Hepatic abscesses associated with diabetes mellitus in two dogs. *Journal of Veterinary Internal Medicine* **8**, 203–206

Hall E, Simpson J and Williams D (2005) *BSAVA Manual of Canine and Feline Gastroenterology, 2nd edn*. BSAVA Publications, Gloucester

Holloway A and McConnell F (2013) *BSAVA Manual of Canine and Feline Radiography and Radiology*. BSAVA Publications, Gloucester

Karaayvaz M, Ugras S, Guler O *et al.* (1998) Use of an autologous vein graft and stent in the repair of common bile defects: an experimental study. *Surgery Today* **28**, 830–833

Karsten TM, Davids PH, van Gulik TM *et al.* (1994) Effects of biliary endoprosthesis on the extrahepatic bile ducts in relation to subsequent operation of the biliary tract. *Journal of the American College of Surgeons* **178**, 343–352

Kirpensteijn J, Fingland RB, Ulrich T, Sikkema DA and Allen SW (1993) Cholelithiasis in dogs: 29 cases (1980–1990). *Journal of the American Veterinary Medical Association* **202**, 1137–1142

Kohno A, Mizumoto R and Honjo I (1977) Changes after major resection of experimental cirrhotic liver. *American Journal of Surgery* **134**, 248–252

Kosovsky JE, Mafia-Marretta S, Matthiesen DT and Patnaik AK (1989) Results of partial hepatectomy in 18 dogs with hepatocellular carcinoma. *Journal of the American Animal Hospital Association* **25**, 203–206

Ludwig LL, McLoughlin MA, Graves TK and Crisp MS (1997) Surgical treatment of bile peritonitis in 24 dogs and 2 cats: a retrospective study (1987–1994). *Veterinary Surgery* **26**, 90–98

Malek S, Sinclair E, Hosgood G *et al.* (2013) Clinical findings and prognostic factors for dogs undergoing cholecystectomy for gall bladder mucocele. *Veterinary Surgery* **42**(4), 418–426

Martin RA, Lanz OI and Tobias KM (2003) Liver and biliary system. In: *Textbook of Small Animal Surgery, 3rd edn*, ed. D Slatter, pp.708–725. WB Saunders, Philadelphia

Massari F, Verganti S, Secchiero B *et al.* (2012) Torsion of quadrate and right middle liver lobes and gallbladder in a German Shepherd Dog. *Australian Veterinary Journal* **90**, 44–47

McAloose D, Casal M, Patterson DF and Dambach DM (1998) Polycystic kidney and liver disease in two related West Highland White Terrier litters. *Veterinary Pathology* **35**, 77–81

McConkey S, Briggs C, Solano M and Illanes O (1997) Liver torsion and associated bacterial peritonitis in a dog. *Canadian Veterinary Journal* **38**, 438–439

McKenna SC and Carpenter JL (1980) Polycystic disease of the kidney and liver in the Cairn Terrier. *Veterinary Pathology* **17**, 436–442

Mehler SJ, Mayhew PD, Drobatz KJ and Holt DE (2004) Variables associated with outcome in dogs undergoing extrahepatic biliary surgery: 60 cases (1988–2002). *Veterinary Surgery* **33**(6), 644–649

Mesich ML, Mayhew PD, Paek M, Holt DE and Brown DC (2009) Gall bladder mucoceles and their association with endocrinopathies in dogs: a retrospective case-control study. *Journal of Small Animal Practice* **12**, 630–635

Mizumoto R, Kawarada Y, Yamawaki T, Noguchi T and Nishida S (1979) Resectability and functional reserve of the liver with obstructive jaundice in dogs. *American Journal of Surgery* **137**, 768–772

Morrison S, Prostredny J and Roa D (2008) Retrospective study of 28 cases of cholecytoduodenostomy performed using endoscopic gastrointestinal anastomosis stapling equipment. *Journal of the American Animal Hospital Association* **44**, 10–18

Ogata A, Miyazaki M, Ohtawa S, Ohtsuka M and Nakajima N (1997) Short term effect of portal arterialization on hepatic protein synthesis and endotoxaemia after extended hepatectomy in dogs. *Journal of Gastroenterology and Hepatology* **12**, 633–638

Parchman MB and Flanders JA (1990) Extrahepatic biliary tract rupture: evaluation of the relationship between the site of rupture and the cause of rupture in 15 dogs. *Cornell Veterinarian* **80**, 267–272

Patnaik AK, Hurvitz AI and Lieberman PH (1980) Canine hepatic neoplasms: a clinicopathologic study. *Veterinary Pathology* **17**, 553–563

Patnaik AK, Hurvitz AI, Lieberman PH and Johnson GF (1981) Canine bile duct carcinoma. *Veterinary Pathology* **18**, 439–444

Petre SL, McClaran JK, Bergman PJ and Monette S (2012) Safety and efficacy of laparoscopic hepatic biopsy in dogs: 80 cases (2004–2009). *Journal of the American Veterinary Association* **240**, 181–185

Risselada M, Ellison GW, Bacon NJ *et al.* (2010) Comparison of 5 surgical techniques for partial liver lobectomy in the dog for intraoperative blood loss and surgical time. *Veterinary Surgery* **7**, 856–862

Schwarz LA, Penninck DG and Leveille-Webster C (1998) Hepatic abscesses in 13 dogs: a review of the ultrasonographic findings, clinical data and therapeutic options. *Veterinary Radiology and Ultrasound* **39**, 357–365

Seymour C and Duke-Novakovski T (2007) *BSAVA Manual of Canine and Feline Anaesthesia and Analgesia, 2nd edn*. BSAVA Publications, Gloucester

Stebbins KE (1989) Polycystic disease of the kidney and liver in an adult Persian cat. *Journal of Comparative Pathology* **100**, 327–330

Swann HM and Cimino Brown D (2001) Hepatic lobe torsion in 3 dogs and a cat. *Veterinary Surgery* **30**, 482–486

Szawlowski AW, Saint-Aubert B and Gouttebel MC (1987) Experimental model of extended repeated partial hepatectomy in the dog. *European Surgical Research* **19**, 375–380

Warren-Smith CM, Andrew S, Mantis P and Lamb CR (2012) Lack of associations between ultrasonographic appearance of parenchymal lesions of the canine liver and histological diagnosis. *Journal of Small Animal Practice* **53**, 168–173

Webster CRL and Cooper J (2009) Therapeutic use of cytoprotective agents in canine and feline hepatobiliary disease. *Veterinary Clinics of North America Small Animal Practice* **39**, 631–652

Whiting PG, Breznock EM, Moore P *et al.* (1986) Partial hepatectomy with temporary hepatic vascular occlusion in dogs with hepatic arteriovenous fistulae. *Veterinary Surgery* **15**, 171–180

OPERATIVE TECHNIQUE 9.1

Hepatic biopsy techniques and partial lobectomy

PREOPERATIVE PLANNING

- Measure PCV and coagulation status preoperatively (measuring coagulation status is not essential prior to routine liver biopsy but is ideal prior to partial lobectomy).
- Administer intravenous antibiotic at anaesthetic induction.
- Prepare the entire ventral abdomen and caudal one-third of the sternum for surgery.

POSITIONING

Dorsal recumbency.

ASSISTANT

Optional.

EQUIPMENT EXTRAS

Balfour retractor; gelatin or collagen haemostatic swab (see Chapter 2); skin biopsy punch; core biopsy needle; thoracoabdominal (TA) stapling device; large crushing forceps for partial lobectomy; Harmonic® scalpel.

SURGICAL TECHNIQUE

Approach

Use a ventral midline laparotomy, ensuring that the incision extends all the way to the xiphoid process. Following resection of the falciform ligament, Balfour retractors are used to improve exposure of the liver. Each lobe of the liver is visually inspected and palpated to identify nodules or cavities, and the areas to be sampled or removed are identified. If necessary, the triangular ligaments are incised to mobilize the liver lobes.

Surgical manipulations: hepatic biopsy

Liver biopsy can be achieved by a variety of techniques. If generalized hepatic disease is present the biopsy sample can be taken from the most accessible site (marginal or peripheral biopsy).

Guillotine technique for peripheral lesions

1 Place a loop of absorbable suture material around a small portion of the tip of a liver lobe.

2 Tie the suture tight to cut through the parenchyma and occlude the blood vessels and bile ducts.

3 Using a sharp scalpel blade, cut the hepatic tissue approximately 3–5 cm distal to the ligature. To avoid crushing, the sample should not be handled with tissue forceps.

PRACTICAL TIP

Place a suture packet below the liver tip to be resected and use that as a 'cutting board' when excising the biopsy sample. The suture packet plus sample can then be handed to an assistant to place into formalin for histopathology

---

→ **OPERATIVE TECHNIQUE 9.1 CONTINUED**

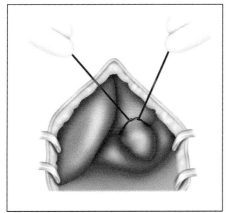

A loop of absorbable suture material is placed around the tip of a liver lobe.

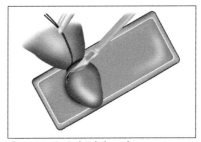

The suture is tied tightly and an empty suture packet is placed below the tip of the liver to act as a 'cutting board'. The hepatic tissue is cut approximately 5 mm from the ligature.

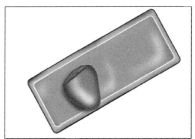

The biopsy sample and suture packet can then be handed to a non-sterile assistant to be put into formalin.

4 Check the biopsy site for bleeding and, if necessary, place a small piece of gelatin or collagen haemostatic swab over the cut surface to aid haemostasis.

Needle/punch biopsy

A core biopsy needle or skin biopsy punch can be used to obtain small pieces of liver tissue. This technique is useful for hepatic lesions located away from the periphery of the lobe.

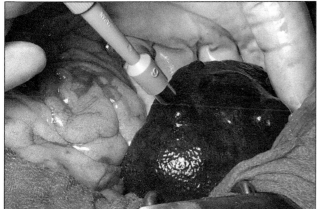

The focal lesion is identified.

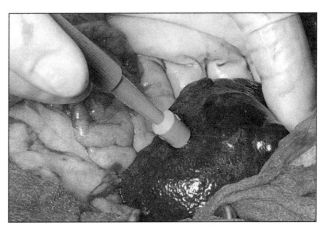

The skin biopsy punch is pushed into the parenchyma to cut a core sample.

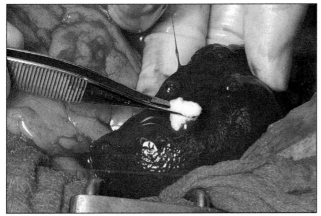

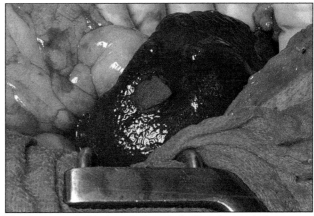

The biopsy site can be packed with a small piece of Gelfoam® or omentum following removal of the hepatic tissue to facilitate haemostasis.

→ OPERATIVE TECHNIQUE 9.1 CONTINUED

Overlapping guillotine suture technique for focal lesions

Resection of larger lesions can be achieved using the overlapping guillotine suture technique. Several overlapping simple interrupted (full-thickness) sutures are placed through the liver along the margins of the liver to be resected. As the sutures are tightened they crush through the parenchyma and ligate vascular elements. It is important to ensure that the entire thickness of the hepatic parenchyma is included in the sutures. After the sutures have been tightened, a sharp scalpel blade is used to remove the hepatic tissue distal to the ligature, allowing a stump of crushed tissue to remain.

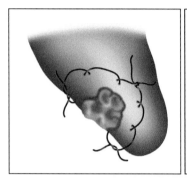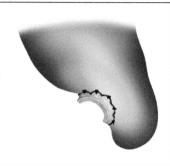

Overlapping guillotine suture technique.

Surgical manipulations: partial lobectomy

Finger fracture technique

1 Determine the line of separation between normal hepatic parenchyma and that to be removed and sharply incise the liver capsule along the selected site.

2 Bluntly fracture the liver with fingers or the blunt end of a scalpel handle and expose the parenchymal vessels. Large vessels that are encountered during the dissection are ligated; small vessels may be occluded by electrocoagulation.

> **PRACTICAL TIP**
>
> The larger vessels (>2 mm diameter) are located deeper in the hepatic parenchyma where the hepatic veins coalesce near the concave surface of the liver

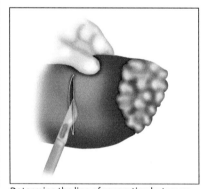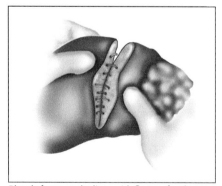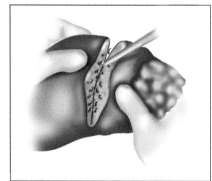

Determine the line of separation between the normal parenchyma and that to be removed.

Bluntly fracture the liver with fingers (or the blunt end of a scalpel handle) to expose parenchymal vessels.

Large vessels encountered during the dissection are ligated.

Parenchymal crushing (overlapping mattress suture) technique

1 Place a single large crushing clamp or two smaller clamps across the lobe, proximal to the lesion.

2 Similar to the overlapping guillotine suture technique above, place several overlapping guillotine sutures through the liver just proximal to the site of the proposed lobectomy incision. It is important to ensure that the entire width of the hepatic parenchyma is included in the suture and that a stump of crushed tissue is left distal to the ligatures.

3 After tightening the sutures, use a sharp scalpel blade to remove the hepatic tissue distal to the ligatures, allowing a stump of crushed tissue to remain.

→ OPERATIVE TECHNIQUE 9.1 CONTINUED

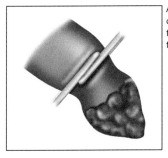
A large crushing clamp can be placed across the lobe proximal to the lesion.

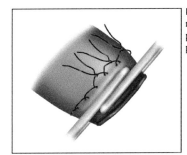
Large overlapping mattress sutures are placed through the parenchyma of the liver.

Stapling

Surgical stapling devices (see Chapter 2) crush the hepatic tissue and ligate the vessels in one step and may be used for partial lobectomy. Care should be taken with these instruments, because haemorrhage may occur if the staples do not adequately compress the hepatic tissue.

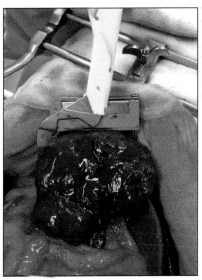
TA55 stapler being used to perform a partial hepatic lobectomy. The stapler is placed around the portion of the lobe to be resected, the appropriate lever is pulled and the staples are fired.

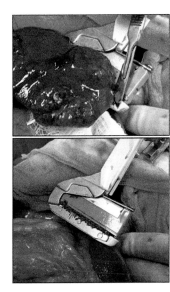
Once the staples have been fired, the lobe is amputated by cutting along the edge of the staple cartridge with a scalpel. The lobe is then released and the stump is checked for bleeding.

PRACTICAL TIP

TA55 or TA90 staplers place two overlapping rows of staples. The 3.5 mm staples (blue cartridge) close to 1.5 mm and can result in minor arterial haemorrhage from small vessels that are not completely sealed by the staples. To obtain the best vascular closure use a TA30 V3 stapler with staples that close to 1 mm and have three staggered rows. If a lobe is too thick for a TA stapler, or too wide to use a TA30 stapler, skeletonization of the vessels within the parenchyma (using the blunt end of a scalpel handle or the inner cannula of a Poole suction tip) before applying the TA stapler improves haemostasis

On completion of a partial lobectomy, the raw liver surface should be dry and free from haemorrhage. A gelatin or cellulose haemostatic swab or omentum can be placed over the cut surface. If there is any significant bleeding, full-thickness mattress sutures should be placed through the parenchyma and tied tightly.

Wound closure

Routine ventral midline closure should be used. Additional samples should be taken if cultures or special tests (e.g. copper analysis) are required. Biopsy sites should be checked for haemorrhage, and a haemostatic swab or omentum applied as required.

POSTOPERATIVE MANAGEMENT AND COMPLICATIONS

- Signs of internal haemorrhage are monitored by checking mucous membrane colour, pulse and capillary refill time regularly during the 12–24 hour post-biopsy period. If the PCV drops below 20%, whole blood should be administered.
- Supportive therapy with intravenous fluids and glucose is continued until oral intake of food and water resumes.
- The patient should be monitored for evidence of pancreatitis.

OPERATIVE TECHNIQUE 9.2

Complete hepatic lobectomy

PREOPERATIVE PLANNING

- Check PCV, blood glucose, electrolytes, albumin levels and coagulation status before surgery. If possible, perform a cross-match and have whole blood available. Animals with a PCV of 20% or less should have a preoperative blood transfusion.
- In addition to routine abdominal preparation, clip and aseptically prepare the caudal one-third of the sternum in case a caudal sternotomy is required.
- Administer intravenous antibiotics at anaesthetic induction.

POSITIONING

Dorsal recumbency.

ASSISTANT

Essential.

EQUIPMENT EXTRAS

Balfour abdominal retractor; malleable retractor; assortment of right-angled dissecting forceps; TA stapling device of appropriate size (30 mm, 55 mm, 90 mm) with appropriate staples (V3, 3.5 mm or 4.8 mm); topical haemostatic agents (see Chapter 2); Doyen bowel clamps.

SURGICAL TECHNIQUE

Approach

Ventral midline; make a large incision from the xiphoid process to the pubis. If necessary, a paracostal incision can be performed in addition, to facilitate access and positioning of a stapling device (particularly for the right side of the liver).

Surgical manipulations

1   Free any hepatic lobe to be excised from its attachments to adjacent structures (diaphragm, kidney, gallbladder). The left lobes (left lateral and left medial lobes) of the liver maintain their separation near the hilus more than do the other lobes and this makes them easier to remove.

2   Take precautionary measures to control haemorrhage if necessary by pre-placing umbilical tape around the pre- and posthepatic vena cava, the hepatic artery and portal vein. This will ensure that massive haemorrhage is under sufficient control to allow repair of the appropriate vessel.

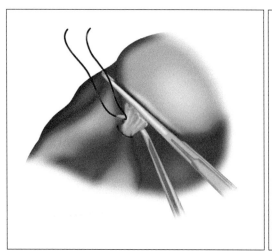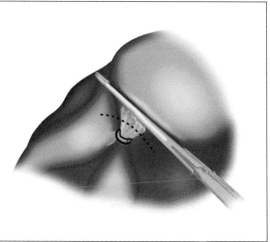

In small dogs and cats, either of the left liver lobes can be removed after placing encircling ligatures around the base of the lobe in an area that has been crushed by forceps.

→ **OPERATIVE TECHNIQUE 9.2 CONTINUED**

3   To remove central or right divisional lobes in small dogs or any lobe in large dogs, carefully dissect the hepatic parenchyma from the caudal vena cava using blunt-tipped right-angled forceps.

4   Isolate and ligate the blood vessels and biliary ducts near the hilus; double ligate large vessels. Ensure that the second suture transfixes the vessels, or oversew the end of the vessel to prevent the ligatures from slipping.

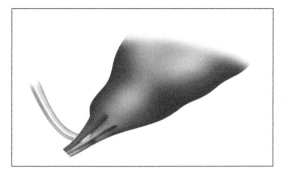 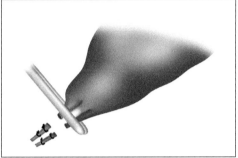

5   Alternatively, use a stapling device (this may be limited by the thickness of the lobe). The appropriate size of instrument (TA stapler; 30 mm, 55 mm, 90 mm) is based upon the width of the lobe to be resected; 3.5 mm staples close to 1.5 mm, and 4.8 mm staples close to 2 mm. The diameter and thickness of the lobe to be resected can be diminished with digital compression or pre-placement of Doyen bowel clamps. Be aware that application of stapling instruments to the central and right divisions of the liver also requires reflection of the hepatic parenchyma from the caudal vena cava; however, specific identification of the lobar vessels and biliary duct is not necessary.

- Place the stapling instrument around the base of the lobe at the hilus.
- Press the approximating lever, compressing the parenchyma between the anvil and staple cartridge, and discharge the staples.
- Use the edge of the instrument as a guide for incising the parenchyma before release.

Wound closure

Routine ventral midline closure should be used. Lobectomy sites should be checked for haemorrhage, and a topical haemostatic agent or omentum applied as required.

POSTOPERATIVE MANAGEMENT AND COMPLICATIONS

- Haemorrhage is the most common complication following hepatic resection. The animal should be monitored closely for signs of internal haemorrhage by checking mucous membrane colour, pulse and capillary refill time regularly during the 24–48 hours after lobectomy.
- Monitor blood glucose levels and continue supportive therapy with intravenous fluids and glucose until oral intake of food and water resumes.
- Monitor serum albumin levels if they are significantly low preoperatively. These are best maintained by supplemental enteral feeding or early resumption of a normal diet. Low postoperative values usually return to normal within 2–3 weeks.
- Continue antibiotics in the postoperative period based on results of bacterial culture and sensitivity testing.

Persistently high elevations in ALP or bilirubin suggest biliary obstruction. High ALT concentration, leucocytosis and fever are associated with ongoing hepatic necrosis and possibly abscess formation.

OPERATIVE TECHNIQUE 9.3

Cholecystotomy

PREOPERATIVE PLANNING

- Check PCV, blood glucose, electrolytes, albumin levels and coagulation status before surgery.
- Administer intravenous antibiotics at anaesthetic induction.

POSITIONING

Dorsal recumbency.

ASSISTANT

Optional.

EQUIPMENT EXTRAS

Balfour abdominal retractor; malleable retractor; assortment of right-angled dissecting forceps; suction.

SURGICAL TECHNIQUE

Approach

Ventral midline, make a large incision from the xiphoid to the pubis.

Surgical manipulations

1. Pack off the area around the gallbladder thoroughly and place two stay sutures in the gallbladder to facilitate manipulation and decrease the likelihood of spillage. Suction should be available.

2. Following incision into the fundus, place additional stay sutures on the sides of the incision if required.

3. Remove the gallbladder contents and send for culture.

4. Lavage the gallbladder with warmed sterile saline and use a soft latex or polyvinyl catheter (3.5–5 Fr in small dogs and cats; 8 Fr in large dogs) to catheterize the common bile duct via the cystic duct to ensure patency before the cholecystotomy is closed.

5. Collect biopsy samples from the gallbladder wall before closure and send for histopathological examination and culture.

WARNING

It can be extremely difficult to cannulate the common bile duct from the gallbladder, owing to the acute angle between the cystic and common bile ducts. If there is doubt about the patency of the common bile duct, duodenotomy and cannulation via the major papilla should be performed

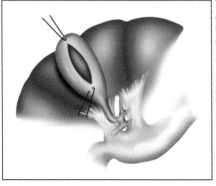

Two stay sutures are placed: one in the fundus and one in the infundibulum. These help to immobilize the gallbladder during surgical manipulation.

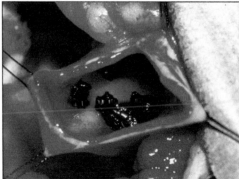

A large incision is made in the gallbladder so that all contents may be easily removed. Additional stay sutures can be placed on either side of the incision to facilitate access to the gallbladder lumen.
(Courtesy of S Birchard)

→ **OPERATIVE TECHNIQUE 9.3 CONTINUED**

Wound closure

Closure of the gallbladder is performed using 1.5 metric (4/0 USP) or 2 metric (3/0 USP) (in small dogs and cats) absorbable monofilament suture material in a one-layer inverting pattern (Lembert or Cushing). Ventral abdominal closure is routine.

POSTOPERATIVE MANAGEMENT AND COMPLICATIONS

Recovery should be uneventful. Monitor for signs of leakage from the cholecystotomy site. If there is recurrence of original signs of disease, cholecystectomy is indicated.

OPERATIVE TECHNIQUE 9.4

Cholecystectomy

PREOPERATIVE PLANNING

- Check PCV, blood glucose, electrolytes, albumin levels and coagulation status before surgery.
- Correct dehydration and electrolyte imbalances prior to surgery.
- Detect and correct any underlying coagulopathy.
- Administer intravenous antibiotics effective against Gram-negative and anaerobic bacteria at anaesthetic induction.

POSITIONING

Dorsal recumbency.

ASSISTANT

Ideal but not essential.

EQUIPMENT EXTRAS

Balfour abdominal retractor; malleable retractors; assortment of right-angled dissecting forceps, including bile duct forceps; sterile cotton-tipped applicators; topical haemostatic agent (see Chapter 2); Doyen bowel clamps; suction; haemostatic stainless steel clips can be helpful if available.

SURGICAL TECHNIQUE

Approach

A ventral midline abdominal approach is the most versatile, starting at the xiphoid cartilage and extending well beyond the umbilicus.

Surgical manipulations

1 Place stay sutures in the stomach to help traction the stomach, liver and gallbladder caudally prior to dissection.

2 Gently dissect the gallbladder away from the parenchyma of the hepatic fossa by blunt and, if necessary, sharp dissection. A selection of curved forceps and cotton-tipped applicators is helpful.

3 Control haemorrhage from the hepatic fossa by packing it with a moistened abdominal swab.

➔ **OPERATIVE TECHNIQUE 9.4 CONTINUED**

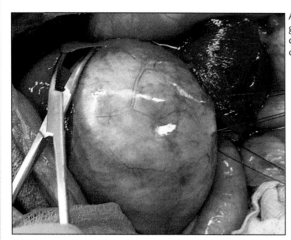

A stay suture is placed in the fundus of the gallbladder. The gallbladder is then bluntly dissected from the hepatic fossa using curved Halsted mosquito forceps.

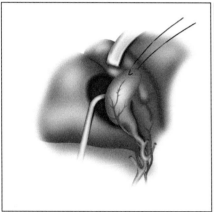
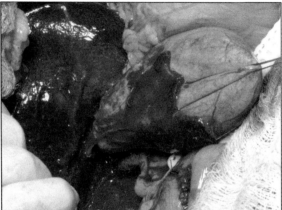

The gallbladder is dissected away from the hepatic fossa using blunt and sharp dissection.

PRACTICAL TIP

Surgery may be facilitated by aspirating some bile prior to dissection, if the gallbladder is overly distended; however, complete decompression of the gallbladder limits visualization of the cleavage plane between the gallbladder wall and hepatic fossa

---

4 Identify the cystic artery and ligate near the gallbladder.

5 Dissect the cystic duct from surrounding tissues down to its junction with the common bile duct; cross-clamp and sever.

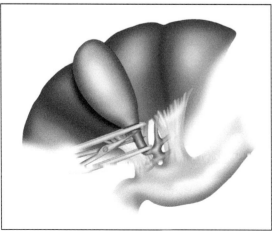

The cystic duct is dissected down to the junction with the common bile duct, clamped and severed.

→ **OPERATIVE TECHNIQUE 9.4 CONTINUED**

6 Remove the remaining clamp on the cystic duct stump and pass an orange rubber urinary catheter via the stump and down the common bile duct to ensure its patency (3.5–5 Fr in cats and small dogs; up to an 8 Fr in large dogs). Gently lavage the duct with sterile saline to remove inspissated bile.

PRACTICAL TIP

Tractioning the stump of the cystic duct to straighten the junction with the common bile duct may make it easier to pass the catheter

---

7 Once patency of the common bile duct has been determined, double ligate the stump of the cystic duct. Absorbable suture material or haemostatic clips can be used for this.

WARNING

Ensure that the common bile duct is identified and avoid damaging it during the procedure. In addition, sufficient cystic duct stump length should be left to prevent the ligatures encroaching on the hepatic ducts from the central division of the liver

---

8 If it is not possible to cannulate the common bile duct via the stump of the cystic duct, make a duodenotomy just distal to the pylorus and catheterize the duct via the major duodenal papilla.

9 Perform a biopsy of the liver.

10 Prior to closure, check the hepatic fossa for haemorrhage. It can be packed with a topical haemostatic agent (see Chapter 2) or omentum if required.

11 Submit a portion of the gallbladder wall and some bile for culture; submit the remainder of the gallbladder for histopathology.

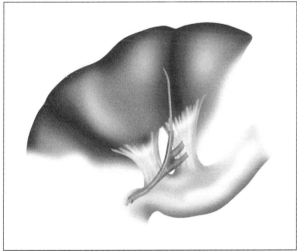
The common bile duct is cannulated via the stump of the cystic duct and flushed to ensure patency.

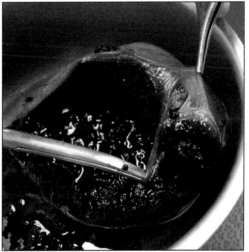
Gallbladder mucocele.

Wound closure

The duodenotomy incision is closed with a simple interrupted or a simple continuous suture pattern, using monofilament absorbable suture material. Abdominal closure is routine.

POSTOPERATIVE MANAGEMENT

- Monitor the PCV for the first 24 hours postoperatively.
- Continue supportive therapy with intravenous fluids and glucose until oral intake of food and water resumes.
- Monitor for evidence of pancreatitis and withhold food and water if it occurs.
- Continue antibiotics in the postoperative period based on results of bacterial culture and sensitivity testing.

OPERATIVE TECHNIQUE 9.5

Biliary diversion: cholecystoduodenostomy or cholecystojejunostomy

PREOPERATIVE PLANNING

- Check PCV, blood glucose, electrolytes, albumin levels and coagulation status before surgery. If possible, perform a cross-match and have whole blood available. Animals with a PCV of 20% or less should have a preoperative blood transfusion.
- Administer intravenous antibiotics at anaesthetic induction.

POSITIONING

Dorsal recumbency.

ASSISTANT

Ideal or essential to facilitate exposure and minimize the risk of contamination from the gastrointestinal or biliary tract.

EQUIPMENT EXTRAS

Balfour abdominal retractor; malleable retractors; assortment of right-angled dissecting forceps; sterile cotton-tipped applicators; suction; large abdominal swabs; topical haemostatic agent (see Chapter 2); Doyen bowel clamps.

SURGICAL TECHNIQUE

Approach

Ventral midline laparotomy with incision from the xiphoid process to the pubis.

Surgical manipulations

1   Mobilize the gallbladder from its fossa to relieve tension at the stoma site (see Operative Technique 9.4). Care must be taken to avoid trauma to the cystic artery.

> **WARNING**
>
> Tension at the stoma site predisposes to dehiscence of the anastomosis, leakage of luminal contents and stricture

2   Use stay sutures to mobilize the gallbladder and bring it into apposition with the descending duodenum (or proximal jejunum). Take care to ensure that the cystic duct is not twisted as it is advanced to the antimesenteric border of the duodenum.

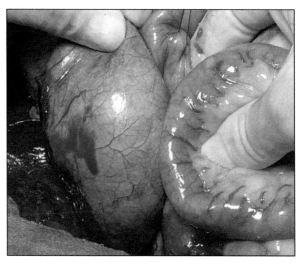

➜ **OPERATIVE TECHNIQUE 9.5 CONTINUED**

3   Pack the area with laparotomy swabs, drain the gallbladder and make an appropriate cholecystostomy.

PRACTICAL TIP

Contraction will decrease the size of the original stoma by 50%. Gallbladders vary in size: an anastomosis that corresponds to the length of an incision from the gallbladder fundus to the infundibulum should be made

---

4   Make a corresponding duodenostomy in the antimesenteric border of the duodenum (or jejunum) and aspirate the duodenal contents. Stay sutures on the duodenum permit traction on the duodenostomy site.

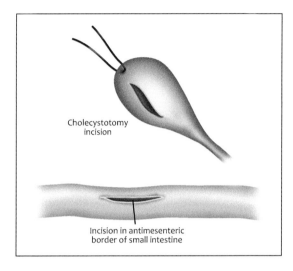

Cholecystotomy incision

Incision in antimesenteric border of small intestine

5   Perform anastomosis of the gallbladder to the intestinal wall using absorbable monofilament suture material.

6   Ensure that there is no tension on the suture line.

7   A simple interrupted pattern can be used but is more time-consuming than a continuous pattern.

8   A single-layer closure is adequate; two-layer closures are time-consuming and reduce the stoma size more.

9   Intestinal mucosa may evert after incision; trimming everted mucosa with fine Metzenbaum scissors improves the accuracy of anastomosis with the gallbladder.

10   Ensure that each suture penetrates the complete thickness of the intestinal wall as well as that of the gallbladder.

11   Place a deep row of sutures (on the far or dorsal side of the duodenostomy) first, beginning at either end of the incision. Once the deep row is completed, finish the superficial layer. Place an additional suture at the cranial and caudal ends of the anastomosis to help to relieve tension.

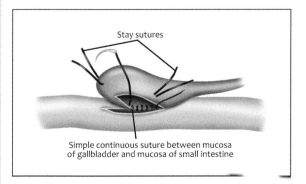

Stay sutures

Simple continuous suture between mucosa of gallbladder and mucosa of small intestine

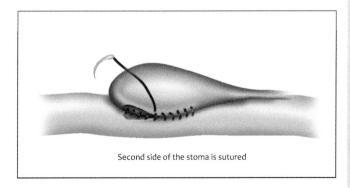

Second side of the stoma is sutured

→ **OPERATIVE TECHNIQUE 9.5 CONTINUED**

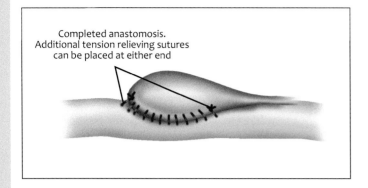

Completed anastomosis.
Additional tension relieving sutures
can be placed at either end

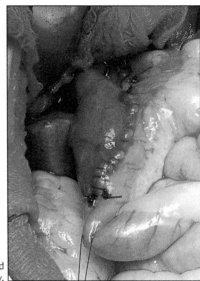

Completed
cholecystoenterostomy.

Wound closure

Routine midline abdominal closure.

POSTOPERATIVE MANAGEMENT AND COMPLICATIONS

- Closely monitor for signs of internal haemorrhage by checking mucous membrane colour, pulse and capillary refill time regularly during the 24–48 hours after biliary diversion. If the haematocrit drops below 20%, whole blood should be administered.
- Also monitor serum albumin levels.
- Monitor blood glucose levels and continue supportive therapy with intravenous fluids and glucose until oral intake of food and water resumes.
- Monitor for evidence of pancreatitis and withhold food and water if it occurs.
- Continue antibiotics in the postoperative period based on results of bacterial culture and sensitivity testing.
- Re-evaluate the patient every 3–6 months for recurrence of biliary obstruction or evidence of cholangitis. Pain, vomiting, lethargy and fever may indicate ascending biliary tract infection or can occur with stomas that are initially too small or that have developed a stricture postoperatively.

Chapter 10

Portosystemic shunts

Geraldine Hunt

Portosystemic shunts (PSS) are abnormal vascular communications between the portal venous system and the systemic venous circulation. These vascular abnormalities divert blood from the abdominal organs (especially intestinal absorption products) to the heart and systemic circulation, bypassing the liver. Portosystemic shunting of blood leads to abnormal hepatic development, decreased protein metabolism, decreased clearance of endogenous and exogenous toxins (e.g. drugs) and dysfunction of the reticuloendothelial system. Ultimately, these changes can result in liver failure. The terms microvascular dysplasia or portal vein hypoplasia refer to a condition in which portal vessels are underdeveloped or absent, in patients that do not have a macroscopic PSS.

Anatomy

The anatomical location of shunts may be very variable (Figure 10.1), with macroscopic shunts reported between almost all branches of the hepatic portal vasculature and the intra-abdominal or periabdominal systemic venous system. Microscopic intrahepatic shunts (microvascular dysplasia) may also be encountered and may be indistinguishable from macroscopic shunts on the basis of preoperative clinical and pathological criteria.

Extrahepatic shunts in dogs and cats are most likely to occur between a branch of the portal vein and the caudal vena cava. The most commonly affected sections of the portal circulation are the left gastric vein, gastrosplenic

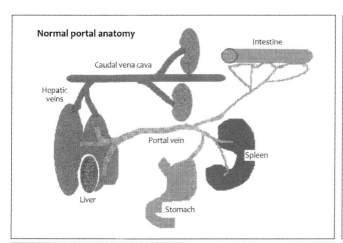

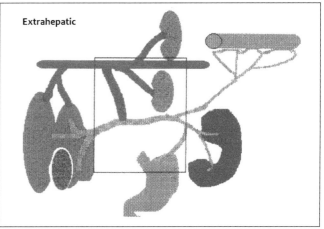

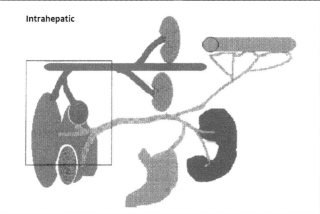

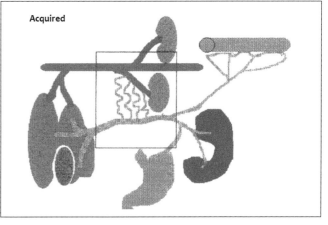

10.1 Anatomical location of different types of portosystemic shunt.

vein, pancreaticoduodenal vein and portal vein (Figure 10.2). With more widespread use of computed tomography (CT) variations in shunt anatomy are being identified more frequently in dogs; in particular, extrahepatic shunts that insert into a phrenic vein near its confluence with the left or right hepatic veins. Rarely, shunts may be found between the caudal mesenteric, ileocolic or ovarian vein and the caudal vena cava. Portoazygous shunts occur in approximately 15% of cases and travel from a branch of the portal venous system, between the crura of the diaphragm, through the caudal mediastinum to join the azygous vein in the caudal thorax (Figure 10.3).

Intrahepatic shunts are those communications arising cranial to the point of origin of the first hepatic lobar branches of the portal vein. Intrahepatic shunts may exist within the hepatic parenchyma, or travel between liver lobes. They may open into the caudal vena cava or any hepatic vein branch. Intrahepatic shunts are classified as right-divisional, central-divisional or left-divisional (Lamb and White, 1998). The anatomical form and difficulty of attenuation vary between these shunt types. In general,

right-divisional shunts take the form of discrete vessels connecting a branch of the portal vein to a lobar hepatic vein, often describing a loop within or between liver lobes (Figure 10.4a). Central-divisional shunts are more likely to be window-like communications between a dilated branch of the portal vein and the caudal vena cava (Figure 10.4b). Left-divisional shunts can arise from any portion of the left branch of the portal vein and usually insert into the left hepatic vein. The patent ductus venosus arises from the termination of the left branch of the portal vein and the left hepatic vein (Figure 10.4c).

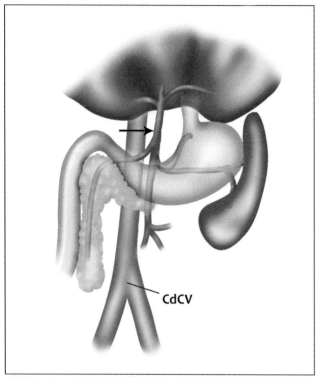

10.2 Common origins of extrahepatic shunts. The majority of extrahepatic shunts insert into the caudal vena cava (CdVC) between the right renal vein and the liver at the level of the epiploic foramen (arrowed).

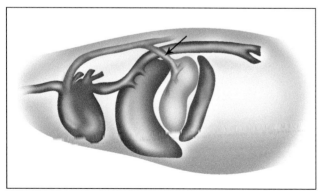

10.3 Congenital portoazygous shunt (arrowed) arising from the left gastric vein.

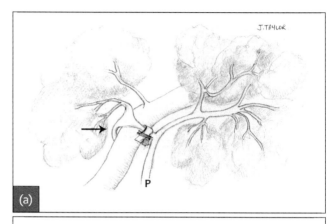

(a)

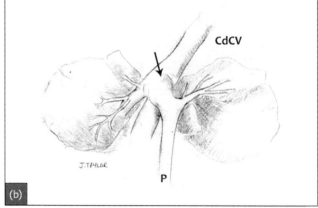

(b)

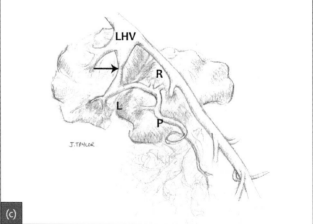

(c)

10.4 Anatomy of intrahepatic shunts. (a) Right-divisional shunt. The portal vein (P) divides into a right and left branch. The right branch gives rise to a shunt that describes a loop (arrowed) before entering the right hepatic vein. (b) Central-divisional shunt. The portal vein (P) dilates before communicating with the caudal vena cava (CdVC) via a window-like ostium (arrowed). (c) Patent ductus venosus (left dorsolateral view). The portal vein (P) divides into a right (R) and left (L) branch. The ductus venosus (arrowed) arises from the terminal portion of the left branch and enters an ampulla before joining the left hepatic vein (LHV).

Breed predisposition

Study of breed predispositions and their effect on PSS anatomy and behaviour has yielded interesting observations. It has been accepted for some time that large-breed dogs are more prone to intrahepatic shunts, whereas small-breed dogs are most likely to have extrahepatic shunts. A study of cases from Australia showed that dogs of breeds that were over-represented were significantly more likely to have characteristic shunts (i.e. extrahepatic shunts in small breeds and intrahepatic shunts in large breeds) than dogs of normally or under-represented breeds. Intrahepatic shunts were diagnosed in a number of Toy and Miniature Poodles. By contrast, the vast majority of congenital PSS in Maltese or Maltese-cross dogs (which make up almost 40% of cases seen at the University Veterinary Centre, Sydney) had extrahepatic shunts arising from the left gastric vein and inserting into the caudal vena cava at the level of the epiploic foramen. This study also showed that dogs of over-represented breeds were more likely to have shunts that could be attenuated.

Congenital PSSs in cats do not follow such obvious guidelines, but extrahepatic shunts are most commonly reported (approximately 80%).

> **WARNING**
>
> Owners of dog breeds that do not commonly present with PSS should be warned that there may be a higher risk of unusual shunt anatomy or a shunt that may not be surgically correctable

Breeds that have been shown to be at risk include a range of terriers (Maltese, Cairn, Yorkshire, Silky, Jack Russell and West Highland White), Bichon Frise, Shih Tzu, Miniature Schnauzer, Irish Wolfhound, Australian Cattle Dog, Border Collie, Old English Sheepdog and Golden Retriever. Anecdotal reports also suggest that Burmese, Siamese, Himalayan and Persian cats are over-represented for PSS. Microvascular dysplasia is most commonly seen in Yorkshire and Cairn Terriers, but can affect other breeds, including the Maltese, Dachshund, Miniature Poodle, Shih Tzu, Lhasa Apso, Cocker Spaniel and West Highland White Terrier.

Pathophysiology

Hepatic encephalopathy

The pathophysiology of abnormalities resulting from PSS is complex. Signs may arise as a direct result of toxins that should normally be processed by the liver reaching the systemic circulation. Perturbations in the balance of endogenous or exogenous substances, such as branched-chain and aromatic amino acids, benzodiazepines and ammonia, have been implicated in the development of neurological and behavioural abnormalities. Hypoglycaemia may exacerbate signs in some animals as a result of their poor hepatic glycogen reserves. Other factors that may precipitate hepatic encephalopathy are listed in Figure 10.5. Inadequate delivery of trophic factors to the liver and reduced deactivation of hormones acting on other body systems may play a role in some of the non-neurological signs.

Aetiological factors
• Increased blood ammonia
• Alterations in monoamine neurotransmitters
• Alterations in amino acid neurotransmitters
• Gamma-aminobutyric acid
• Glutamate
• Increased levels of endogenous benzodiazepines
• Methionine (metabolized to mercaptans)

Precipitating factors
• Various drugs
• High-protein diet
• Hypoglycaemia
• Hypokalaemia (which potentiates renal ammonia production)
• Alkalosis
• Transfusion of stored blood
• Gastrointestinal haemorrhage
• Hypoxia
• Hypovolaemia
• Infection
• Constipation
• Vegetable-based diets in cats (arginine deficiency)
• Sedative and anaesthetic agents

10.5 Factors implicated in hepatic encephalopathy.

Ammonia

Ammonia is produced from the hydrolysis of urea by colonic urease-producing coliforms and anaerobic bacteria and by bacterial deamination of dietary amino acids. Normally ammonia that has been absorbed by the intestines is carried to the liver by the portal vein where it is converted to urea through the Krebs–Henseleit urea cycle. With PSS and hepatic dysfunction, ammonia is no longer adequately metabolized and is diverted to the systemic circulation.

* Ammonia is a key cerebral toxin that exerts direct effects on neurotransmission in the brain.
* The brain lacks an effective urea cycle and thus has limited ability to handle excessive ammonia concentrations.
* Ammonia crosses the blood–brain barrier and is important in astrocyte metabolism; it leads to greater synthesis of glutamine, decreasing osmotic pressure and can result in cell swelling.
* Blood concentrations of ammonia do not directly correlate with the severity of hepatic encephalopathy and many other toxins such as mercaptans and short-chain fatty acids are thought to act synergistically with ammonia.

Mercaptans

Mercaptans are byproducts of dietary methionine degradation by intestinal bacteria. Mercaptans augment the cerebral effects of ammonia and short-chain fatty acids, resulting in depressed cerebral function and coma.

Gamma-aminobutyric acid

Gamma-aminobutyric acid (GABA) is an important inhibitory mediator in the central nervous system (CNS). The intestinal bacteria *Escherichia coli* and *Bacteroides fragilis* produce substances with GABA-like activity. Shunting of portal blood results in increased concentrations of these compounds and gastrointestinal haemorrhage increases their absorption, leading to CNS depression.

> **WARNING**
>
> Precipitating factors of hepatic encephalopathy include various drugs, protein overload, hypokalaemia (which potentiates renal ammonia production), alkalosis, transfusion of stored blood, hypoxia, hypovolaemia, gastrointestinal haemorrhage, infection and constipation

> **WARNING**
>
> Increased sensitivity to sedatives, analgesics, tranquillizers and anaesthetic agents may induce coma in animals with PSS, even when normal doses are given

Clinical signs

Clinical signs seen in animals with PSS (Figure 10.6) include neurological disorders such as disorientation, agitation, ataxia, amaurotic blindness, hepatic coma and seizures. Gastrointestinal signs include chronic vomiting, diarrhoea (uncommonly), pica and capricious appetite. Hypersalivation and lacrimation may occur. Urinary signs include polyuria, polydipsia and cystitis, resulting from ammonium urate urolithiasis or recurrent urinary tract infection. Urethral obstruction is not uncommon in male dogs. In addition, animals may display recurrent episodes of fever, lethargy and inappetence, suggesting systemic infection or toxaemia. Some animals simply present for unduly prolonged effects of administered drugs such as thiobarbiturates. In others, a shunt may be found co-incidentally while evaluating other problems.

Considering the major metabolic perturbations that occur in animals with PSS, the reasons why some animals show marked clinical signs and others seem only mildly affected is unclear. It would seem sensible to assume that the shunt fraction (the proportion of portal blood flow passing through the hepatic sinusoids) is related to clinical signs, but this has not been proven conclusively. Likewise, the relative size of the shunt does not seem to have an obvious correlation with severity of clinical signs or prognosis after surgery.

Cats are not affected with PSS as commonly as dogs, but cases are encountered sporadically. Neurological signs, hypersalivation and copper-coloured irises (Figure 10.7) are traditionally considered to be common features of the clinical presentation. However, the presence or absence of copper-coloured irises is not a definitive indication of congenital PSS.

System affected	Clinical signs
Neurological	Lethargy, depression, behavioural changes, disorientation, pacing, evidence of hepatic encephalopathy (e.g. blindness, head pressing, seizures and coma)
Gastrointestinal	Anorexia, vomiting, polyphagia, ascites, diarrhoea
Urinary	Ammonium biurate stones and crystalluria (which may cause urethral obstruction), polyuria and polydipsia
Miscellaneous	Ptyalism (hypersalivation), lacrimation, copper-coloured irises (cats), poor growth rate, weight loss, hair loss, prolonged sedation effect from anaesthetic or sedative drugs

10.6 Clinical signs associated with portosystemic shunts.

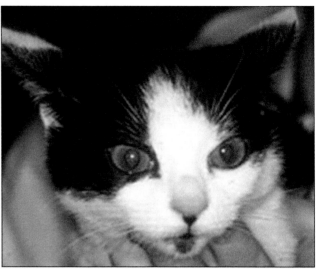

10.7 Copper-coloured irises in a 9-month-old Domestic Shorthaired cat with an extrahepatic portosystemic shunt.

Preoperative considerations

Diagnosis

(The diagnosis of PSS is discussed in greater detail in the *BSAVA Manual of Canine and Feline Gastroenterology*.) Although signalment, presenting signs and non-specific biochemical changes (Figure 10.8) may suggest a congenital PSS, diagnosis is contingent on demonstrating biochemical (pre- and postprandial serum bile acids, ammonia tolerance test), scintigraphic, radiographic (venous portography) or ultrasonographic evidence of portosystemic shunting. Unlike dogs, cats with PSS usually have normal haematology, and hypoalbuminaemia is less common. Abnormalities on urinalysis include decreased urine specific gravity and ammonium biurate crystalluria (reported in 21–74% of dogs and 16–42% of cats).

Haematology	Mild microcytic anaemia Occasional leucocytosis
Biochemistry	Hypoalbuminaemia Hypoglycaemia Hypocholesterolaemia Low urea Slight elevation in serum alkaline phosphatase (ALP) Moderate increase in alanine aminotransferase (ALT)
Urinalysis	May have low specific gravity Ammonium biurate crystals (21–74% of dogs; 16–42% of cats)

10.8 Non-specific but common haematological and biochemical abnormalities seen in cases of portosystemic shunts.

Liver function tests

Liver function tests, such as evaluation of pre- and postprandial bile acids, are more definitive for diagnosing hepatic disease than routine biochemistry profiles, but serum bile acid values cannot differentiate between liver diseases because abnormal values overlap widely. Serum bile acid concentrations are dependent on adequate hepatoportal circulation, functional hepatic mass and normal intestinal absorption. Abnormal serum bile acids in the absence of jaundice and abnormal liver enzyme activity indicate metabolically quiet liver disease associated with hepatoportal perfusion abnormalities or severely reduced hepatic mass. In animals with PSS, serum bile acids are typically elevated before and after feeding, with a steep rise in levels over a sampling period of 2 hours following feeding, but in some cases the preprandial levels may be normal. The same is true for serum ammonia levels. Bile acids are equivalent to blood ammonia concentrations in detecting deficiencies in hepatic mass or circulation but, unlike ammonia, they are not labile in blood and are easily quantified in samples handled routinely.

Coagulation profiles

Patients with PSS may have an increased activated partial thromboplastin time (aPTT) and, if secondary liver damage is severe, they may experience excessive bleeding during surgery. However, the majority of patients do not show clinical signs of a coagulopathy.

Animals with microvascular dysplasia or developmental abnormalities leading to portal hypertension (e.g. portal vein hypoplasia, hepatic arteriovenous fistula) may present in almost identical ways to those animals with single, macroscopic shunts. It may or may not be possible to differentiate these cases using the techniques mentioned above.

Biochemistry and scintigraphy will detect the presence of shunting but do not usually define the anatomical basis. Arteriovenous fistulae can usually be detected ultrasonographically. Preoperative detection of a macroscopic intrahepatic or extrahepatic shunt assists surgical decision-making, but in the author's experience up to 25% of shunts will not be identified by ultrasonography. Dogs with macroscopic shunts, microvascular dysplasia and portal vein hypoplasia all display microhepatica and, thus, can only be differentiated by demonstration of a macroscopic shunt. Contrast-enhanced CT (CT angiography) is one of the most sensitive and specific ways to confirm PSS anatomy.

PRACTICAL TIP

Intrahepatic shunts are often more readily identified on ultrasound examination than extrahepatic shunts. The presence of gas or fluid in the stomach or intestines may obscure an extrahepatic shunt

Regardless of the method chosen to confirm the presence of portosystemic shunting, a broad-based biochemical screen should be performed in all patients to establish a baseline against which postoperative results can be measured. Useful indicators of changes in hepatic mass and function, and resolution of secondary abnormalities, include urea, cholesterol, creatinine and liver enzymes. Abnormalities of serum bile acids and ammonia tolerance may persist postoperatively in animals that have developed multiple acquired shunts, but improvements in the parameters listed above indicate the magnitude of improvement in hepatic function and usually reflect clinical improvement.

Preoperative management

In the author's experience, it is rarely necessary to perform PSS occlusion as an emergency. Diagnosis of a PSS in an overtly encephalopathic animal should be followed by attempts at medical stabilization prior to subjecting the

patient to anaesthesia and surgery. Medical management has a number of components, some or all of which may be required in a given case. These components are dietary protein restriction, glucose supplementation, enteral lactulose and oral antibiotics. Adjunctive treatments, such as parenteral fluid administration, sedation for animals with severe encephalopathy (see Palliation of neurological signs, below) and treatment of urinary tract infections, may also be required.

Reduction in dietary protein intake and/or substitution with highly digestible protein sources, such as cottage cheese and egg, is indicated in animals with clinical signs as a result of their condition. Some severely affected animals, and those animals with anorexia or marked gastrointestinal signs, will benefit from 24 hours of complete starvation. Carbohydrate-rich foods (e.g. apples, bananas) are often well tolerated for short periods of time; indeed many animals show a particular preference for this type of food.

WARNING

It should be remembered that animals with PSS have markedly reduced hepatic glycogen reserves, due to their small liver mass, and should be provided with glucose either orally or parenterally

Administration of oral or rectal lactulose is easily achieved; it has beneficial effects through its purgative action and alterations in intestinal pH, favouring retention of ammonia within the intestinal lumen. Lactulose is sweet and most animals will tolerate it in food, or will lick it from a syringe. The usual dose is 0.5 ml/kg two or three times daily, but this should be introduced gradually to avoid precipitating severe diarrhoea. Lactulose may be given as a retention enema in vomiting or severely neurologically affected animals.

Oral antibiotics (Figure 10.9) reduce intestinal bacterial load and hence reduce the amount of ammonia produced within the gut. These may be used acutely or chronically in the food of animals requiring long-term medical management.

Drug	Dose: dogs	Dose: cats
Neomycin	20 mg/kg 3–4 times daily	10–20 mg/kg twice daily
Ampicillin	20 mg/kg thrice daily	20 mg/kg thrice daily
Amoxicillin	20 mg/kg twice daily	20 mg/kg twice daily
Metronidazole	20 mg/kg 2–3 times daily	10 mg/kg twice daily

10.9 Oral antibiotics most commonly used in patients with portosystemic shunts.

Editors' note:

The editors do not routinely use metronidazole in PSS patients, owing to its potentially adverse effects of CNS toxicity, especially at higher doses (nystagmus, ataxia, knuckling, head tilt and seizures), and hepatotoxicity

Intravenous fluid supplementation may be required in severely affected animals. Fluid losses from salivation, vomiting and polyuria can be substantial. However, there is evidence in human reports to suggest that fluid homeostatic mechanisms may be deranged as a result of portosystemic shunting, with fluid retention occurring in some cases. Therefore, fluid administration should be undertaken cautiously. Animals with PSS will usually have subnormal levels of albumin, increasing the risk of pulmonary or peripheral oedema. The author has seen a small number of cases develop pulmonary oedema pre- or postoperatively despite judicious use of intravenous fluids.

Palliation of neurological signs

While the mainstays of treatment for hepatic encephalopathy are listed above, some patients become extremely disorientated, displaying vocalization, inappropriate motor activity and seizures. Blood glucose levels should always be checked to rule out hypoglycaemia as a cause of neurological signs in these animals. However, in many cases it is also necessary to consider some form of sedation or anticonvulsant medication. Owing to these animals' poor hepatic function, drugs requiring hepatic metabolism will have a prolonged duration of action. This may not affect the initial dose, but adjustments should be made in subsequent doses and frequency. The pathophysiology of hepatic encephalopathy is complex, and reports suggest that a variety of chemical mediators are important. For this reason, it has been suggested that certain anaesthetic and sedative agents are inappropriate and may exacerbate signs of hepatic encephalopathy. These theoretical considerations are valid but have not been demonstrated clinically. Hence, the author prefers to treat the neurological consequences of hepatic encephalopathy or post-ligation neurological disorders using intravenous infusions, such as propofol or midazolam, that can be titrated to effect. However, phenobarbital and diazepam, and acepromazine maleate (ACP), have reportedly been used successfully.

Treatment of an acute encephalopathic crisis

- Place an intravenous cannula and start administration of a balanced electrolyte solution. Avoid fluid overload, which will worsen cerebral oedema.
- Measure serum blood glucose and supplement fluids if required.
- Ensure that the animal is not hypokalaemic.
- *Nil per os* for at least 48 hours.
- Check for presence of abnormalities leading to gastrointestinal blood loss (such as ulceration, coagulopathy, renal failure).
- If the patient is conscious and capable of swallowing safely, administer lactulose (0.5 ml/kg).
- Perform a cleansing enema to decrease colonic toxin production and absorption.
- If the patient is not capable of swallowing, then administer 0.5 ml/kg lactulose as a retention enema.
- Administer a parenteral antibiotic (see Figure 10.9).
- To control seizures use a bolus of propofol at 1–5 mg/kg to abolish seizure activity (repeated if necessary), then maintain the animal on 0.1–1 mg/kg/min infusion. The infusion is continued for 12–24 hours. Intubation may be required in some animals, and some may require 72 hours of anaesthesia to resolve seizure activity.
- Consider starting anticonvulsant therapy (e.g. phenobarbital, potassium bromide, levetiracetam or a combination of these in dogs; phenobarbital in cats).

> **WARNING**
>
> Concerns about the ability of ACP to lower the seizure threshold mean that it should be used with great care and only in an environment of adequate anticonvulsant drug levels

> **WARNING**
>
> Potassium bromide should NOT be used in cats owing to the potential for respiratory complications

Anaesthesia for portosystemic shunt ligation

Concerns about the role of various neurotransmitters in the pathophysiology of hepatic encephalopathy have led to different recommendations regarding appropriate anaesthetic agents for use in animals with PSS. The chosen agents should not cause liver damage and should ideally not be dependent on hepatic metabolism. They should also not cause major haemodynamic changes, because measurement of haemodynamic variables is an important component of surgical decision-making during shunt attenuation.

Premedication

Previous reports indicate that pre-treatment with anticonvulsant medications reduces the likelihood of post-ligation neurological sequelae. Phenobarbital (10 mg/kg i.m.) may be used as a premedicant. Phenobarbital is continued parenterally or orally for at least 3 days postoperatively to reduce the risk or severity of post-ligation neurological disorders, particularly seizures (Tisdall *et al.*, 2000). Surprisingly, despite marked reduction in hepatic function, most animals do not display prolonged recovery from anaesthesia as a result of phenobarbital administration. A recent report showed a significant reduction in neurological sequelae in dogs treated with levetiracetam *versus* those that did not receive any anticonvulsant treatment (Fryer *et al.*, 2011). An opioid is also usually administered preoperatively. Atropine is given routinely, to reduce the chance of major changes in heart rate and cardiac output that would confound the intraoperative assessment of portal pressure and intestinal perfusion.

Induction of anaesthesia

Anaesthesia is induced using intravenous propofol or alfaxalone. It should be noted that the latter is available in Australia as alfaxolone in cyclodextrin. This is not the same preparation as alfaxalone/alfadolone.

Anaesthesia is maintained with isoflurane in oxygen and nitrous oxide. All anaesthetic agents are used at published dose rates.

Infusion or incremental doses of a narcotic, such as morphine or fentanyl, may be used as required during surgery. Intravenous fluids should contain glucose; alternatively, serum glucose should be measured regularly and a separate infusion started if hypoglycaemia occurs. Many animals will require regulation of plasma oncotic pressure using plasma or colloid solutions. (See the *BSAVA Manual of Canine and Feline Anaesthesia and Analgesia* for a more detailed description of anaesthetic techniques for this condition.)

> **Editors' note:**
>
> Both editors routinely use propofol for the induction of anaesthesia in cats undergoing surgery for PSS

Current techniques for extrahepatic shunts

The advantages and disadvantages of current techniques are described in Figure 10.10. Most surgeons agree that slow, complete occlusion of congenital PSS yields superior results to partial occlusion. The potential reasons for this include reduced risk of life-threatening portal hypertension, speculation that slow occlusion may reduce the risk of post-ligation neurological dysfunction, reduced operating time, less extensive intraoperative monitoring and the fact that animals undergoing complete shunt occlusion have a better long-term prognosis than those undergoing partial attenuation only.

Technique	Advantages	Disadvantages
Cellophane banding	Slow complete occlusion Reduced risk of portal hypertension	May develop multiple acquired shunts May require second procedure (rare)
Ameroid constrictor	Slow complete occlusion Reduced risk of portal hypertension	Rate of occlusion not completely predictable Weight/size of ring in small dogs and cats may kink shunt vessel May develop multiple acquired shunts
Ligation with silk ligatures	Possibility of complete and rapid occlusion	Careful monitoring of portal pressures Portal hypertension May require second procedure if only partial attenuation is achieved

10.10 Current techniques for extrahepatic shunts.

Two methods of slow occlusion using extravascular techniques have been trialled: the Ameroid constrictor (Research Instruments & Manufacturing, Corvallis, Oregon, USA) and cellophane bands (see Operative Technique 10.1). Results of both techniques have been encouraging, although a high incidence of multiple acquired shunts has been identified in published studies and anecdotal reports (Hunt *et al.*, 2004; Mehl *et al.*, 2005).

> **WARNING**
>
> Cellophane banding and Ameroid constrictors are not suitable for multiple acquired shunts, or shunts associated with portal vein atresia or aplasia

Cellophane banding

Cellophane banding of a congenital PSS in a dog was first described by Harari *et al.* (1990). Rewarding results in a series of 11 dogs with congenital PSS led to cellophane banding being adopted by the author as the procedure of choice for single extrahepatic shunts in dogs. Cellophane banding is now also employed for congenital PSS in cats.

The effectiveness of cellophane banding is based on production of a foreign body reaction around the implanted cellophane. Deposition of fibrous tissue within the cellophane band causes slow occlusion of the thin-walled vessel. The rate of occlusion seems to depend on the diameter of the cellophane band. Experimentally,

complete occlusion has been confirmed only after placement of bands of 3 mm diameter or less, but some published clinical reports and anecdotal observations suggest that wider bands will also promote eventual occlusion.

Cellophane banding is suitable for all extrahepatic shunts in which the portal vasculature is patent, and those intrahepatic shunts in which it is possible to dissect around the shunt or the portal vein branch leading to the shunt (see Figure 10.4a).

> **WARNING**
>
> Check whether the product you are planning to use is actually cellophane *versus* a synthetic substance such as polypropylene. Synthetic plastic sheeting can also promote slow occlusion, but results may vary from those of published reports if the thin film is something other than cellophane

Ameroid constrictor placement

The technique for placement of an Ameroid constrictor (Figure 10.11) is similar to that described for cellophane banding (see Operative Technique 10.1). Placement of the Ameroid ring requires narrowing of the shunt vessel to allow the ring to be placed. This can be readily achieved either by use of two Rummel tourniquets fashioned from 3 metric (2/0 USP) polypropylene or by gentle pressure using right-angled forceps. The rings may be quite bulky in small patients, although they are available in a range of sizes from 3.5 mm up to 11 mm (the 11 mm constrictor is available by special order only). It is most common to use a constrictor of either 3.5 mm or 5 mm diameter. In the original report by Vogt *et al.* (1996) constrictors were placed to cause an initial reduction of 50% or greater in the diameter of the shunt vessel. Owing to the incidence of portal hypertension, this advice was later modified to recommend placement of a constrictor that caused no more than 25% initial reduction in shunt vessel diameter.

One editor [JW] has extensive experience using the Ameroid constrictor and has only had to remove one postoperatively, when the size of the ring led to kinking of the shunt vessel and subsequent portal hypertension. The published clinical results after attenuation using the Ameroid ring have been similar to those experienced after cellophane banding, with >80% of animals showing resolution of clinical signs and major biochemical evidence of hepatic dysfunction. However, a proportion of animals continue to show evidence of portosystemic shunting, presumably due to the development of multiple acquired shunts (Mehl *et al.*, 2005).

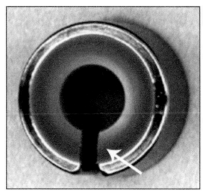

10.11 Ameroid constrictor. The internal diameter of this constrictor is 5 mm, while the overall diameter is more than twice that, making the device bulky in small patients. A small round 'key' or cylinder of Ameroid clay is placed in the hole (arrowed) to secure the device once it has been positioned around a blood vessel.

Ameroid constrictors have been shown experimentally to have variable closure rates. Some may achieve complete occlusion as rapidly as 2 weeks after placement. Others may take 6–8 weeks to occlude the shunt vessel

Attenuation using silk ligatures

Conventional attenuation of extrahepatic shunts using silk or other materials yields a success rate of >70% (Hunt and Hughes, 1999; Kummeling *et al.*, 2004). However, the procedure tends to be more time-consuming than either cellophane banding or Ameroid constrictor placement, owing to the necessity of carefully monitoring portal venous pressure and other haemodynamic parameters to ensure that the degree of attenuation does not exceed safe guidelines.

Outcomes of shunt attenuation in cats

Several papers have now documented short- and long-term outcomes after shunt attenuation in cats (Kyles *et al.*, 2002; Lipscombe *et al.*, 2007; Cabassu *et al.*, 2011). In general, outcomes are somewhat worse for cats than dogs. Up to 40% of cats develop neurological complications following shunt attenuation, ranging from twitching to generalized motor seizures, hence owners should be carefully counselled prior to surgery. Nevertheless, up to 75% of cats that survive surgery may be expected to have a good to excellent outcome.

Current techniques for intrahepatic shunts

Surgical approach

A variety of techniques for surgical attenuation of intrahepatic shunts have been reported. As with extrahepatic shunts, techniques resulting in slow complete occlusion are preferable; however, owing to the anatomical location and nature of the shunts, it is often not possible to place a slow occlusion device. Shunts are often buried within the liver parenchyma, making access and evaluation of shunt anatomy difficult (Figures 10.12 and 10.13). In the author's experience, intrahepatic shunts are rarely amenable to total ligation, hence partial ligation is performed in the majority of cases and published prognoses reflect this (White *et al.*, 1998). Due to the highly variable nature of intrahepatic shunts, the range of published techniques should be considered as a repertoire for experienced surgeons to embrace, with each type of shunt being suited to a particular technique and *vice versa*. The most promising advance in intrahepatic shunt attenuation has been development of the extravascular anastomosis technique, in which the original shunt is located and totally occluded using the most appropriate technique and an extrahepatic anastomosis is created between the portal vein and the splenic vein or caudal vena cava (White *et al.*, 1996; Kyles *et al.*, 2001). This extrahepatic shunt may then be occluded over time using the slow occlusion devices previously mentioned.

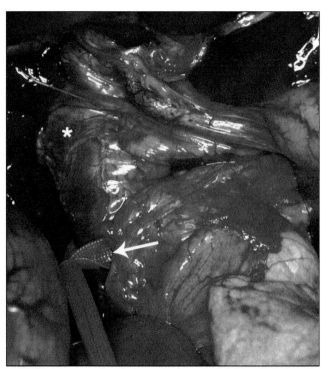

10.12 Intraoperative photograph of a central-divisional intrahepatic shunt. A Rummel tourniquet (white arrow) has been placed around the portal vein in preparation for portal venotomy and transvenous attenuation. Dilatation of the portal vein (*) indicates the point of origin of the intrahepatic shunt, although its course and its insertion into the systemic venous circulation are obscured by the hepatic parenchyma.

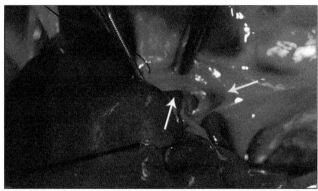

10.13 Intraoperative photograph of transvenous attenuation of a central-divisional intrahepatic shunt. A portal venotomy has been performed in the dilated region of the portal vein from which the shunt is arising (yellow arrow). The window-like shunt (white arrow) can be seen deep inside the dilated segment. The opening of the left branch of the portal vein cannot be seen in this view but must be identified prior to placing the attenuating suture.

Minimally invasive approach

As a less invasive and safer alternative to surgical attenuation, intrahepatic shunts are more commonly being attenuated using thrombogenic coils (Leveille *et al.*, 2003; Weisse *et al.*, 2003). There is growing experience with minimally invasive treatment of extrahepatic shunts in dogs, and a small number of case reports of intravenous attenuation of extrahepatic shunts in small dogs and cats. Owing to the size of the equipment available, and the technical skills and imaging required for successful coil embolization, larger breed dogs with intrahepatic shunts are currently considered to be the best candidates. However, as experience grows, it is likely that this technique will become feasible for all patients with congenital PSS.

In brief, contrast-enhanced CT is performed to confirm the presence of a shunt and to define its anatomy. Measurements of the shunt opening and diameter of the caudal vena cava are obtained. A woven, expandable stent is placed in the caudal vena cava, spanning the shunt opening. A catheter is passed through the meshed wall of the stent and into the shunt, and a series of thrombogenic coils deployed to reduce blood flow through the shunt. Portal pressure is measured after deployment of each coil, and the procedure is continued until portal pressures begin to rise, indicating a clinically significant reduction in blood flow (and hence shunt fraction).

Anecdotal experience suggests that the majority of patients do not experience complete shunt attenuation following a single coil insertion procedure. However, the reduction in shunt fraction and increase in hepatic blood flow result in liver growth, improvement in biochemical parameters, and reduction in the severity of clinical signs. Many owners report a good to excellent result, even if the shunt remains patent.

In general, the anatomy and biological behaviour of intrahepatic shunts can be very variable. Intraoperative localization and attenuation of intrahepatic shunts may be difficult and surgical success depends on the experience of the surgeon and the range of techniques with which they are familiar. For this reason, owners of animals suspected of having intrahepatic shunts should be offered referral to an appropriate specialist to ensure the best possible outcome.

Postoperative management

> **WARNING**
>
> If appropriate postoperative care cannot be provided, surgery for congenital PSS should not be attempted

After shunt attenuation, patients are allowed to recover normally with appropriate pain management. It is preferable to perform 24-hour monitoring for the first 72 hours, paying close attention to haemodynamic variables and neurological status. Phenobarbital administration (2–5 mg/kg i.v., orally q12h) is continued during this time. The majority of major complications will occur within the first 3 days after surgery. Intravenous fluids with dextrose added should be continued until the animal is eating, to ensure that hypoglycaemia does not occur. Many animals are polyuric and polydipsic and the rate of fluid administration should reflect this. The risk of portal hypertension should be very low if slow methods of attenuation are used or safe guidelines adhered to. The necessity for medical management after surgery depends on the severity of the preoperative clinical signs and the expected time required for liver function to return to normal. Owing to the variability in closure rates following shunt attenuation, many surgeons routinely keep animals on antibiotics and lactulose in the postoperative period, in addition to dietary management. If the animal is doing well clinically, and examination and biochemical parameters are improving, the antibiotics are stopped. If the owner notices no apparent change in the animal over the following 2 weeks, the lactulose is stopped. If no changes are noticed in the animal following cessation of lactulose therapy, the diet is gradually changed back to one with a higher protein concentration. Animals presenting initially with gastrointestinal signs are also placed on an H2 blocker for the first 7–10 days postoperatively. Animals with persistent portosystemic shunting may benefit from lifelong treatment with H2 blockers.

Post-ligation neurological dysfunction

> **WARNING**
>
> Post-ligation neurological dysfunction continues to be a major problem despite pre-treatment with anticonvulsant drugs

A form of post-ligation neurological dysfunction may be expected in approximately 5–18% of dogs and up to 22% of cats, regardless of shunt type or method of attenuation (Tisdall et al., 2000). Cats and Maltese dogs appear to be at increased risk. Animals may begin to have seizures without warning, or they may display progressively deteriorating neurological function with ataxia, disorientation and vocalization, progressing to generalized motor seizures in the absence of treatment. The prognosis for recovery after post-ligation neurological dysfunction is variable; in the author's experience up to 75% of patients will survive with vigorous treatment, although the recovery period can be prolonged (weeks) and some animals will require ongoing anticonvulsant medication. Some animals may also display residual neurological deficits such as blindness or personality changes. Dogs surviving post-ligation neurological dysfunction can usually be expected to regain normal liver function after surgery.

References and further reading

Cabassu J, Seim HB, MacPhail CM and Monnet E (2011) Outcomes of cats undergoing surgical attenuation of congenital extrahepatic portosystemic shunts through cellophane banding: 9 cases (2000–2007). *Journal of the American Veterinary Medical Association* **238**, 89–93

Center SA (1996) Hepatic vascular diseases. In: *Strombeck's Small Animal Gastroenterology*, ed. WG Guilford et al., pp.802–846. WB Saunders, Philadelphia

Fryer KJ, Levine JM, Peycke LE, Thompson JA and Cohen ND (2011) Incidence of postoperative seizures with and without levetiracetam pretreatment in dogs undergoing portosystemic shunt attenuation. *Journal of Veterinary Internal Medicine* **25**, 1379–1384

Hall EJ, Simpson JW and Williams DA (2005) *BSAVA Manual of Canine and Feline Gastroenterology, 2nd edn*. BSAVA Publications, Gloucester

Harari J, Lincoln J, Alexander J and Miller J (1990) Lateral thoracotomy and cellophane banding of a congenital portoazygous shunt in a dog. *Journal of Small Animal Practice* **31**, 571–573

Heldmann E, Holt DE, Brockman DJ, Brown DC and Perkowski SZ (1999) Use of propofol to manage seizure activity after surgical treatment of portosystemic shunts. *Journal of Small Animal Practice* **40**, 590–594

Hunt GB and Hughes J (1999) Outcomes after extrahepatic portosystemic shunt ligation in 49 dogs. *Australian Veterinary Journal* **77**, 303–307

Hunt GB, Kummeling A, Tisdall PLC et al. (2004) Outcomes of cellophane banding for congenital portosystemic shunts in 106 dogs and 5 cats. *Veterinary Surgery* **33**, 25–31

Kummeling A, Van Sluijs FJ and Rothuizen J (2004) Prognostic implications of the degree of shunt narrowing and of the portal vein diameter in dogs with congenital portosystemic shunts. *Veterinary Surgery* **33**, 17–34

Kyles AE, Gregory CR, Jackson J et al. (2001) Evaluation of a portocaval venograft and Ameroid ring for the occlusion of intrahepatic portocaval shunts in dogs. *Veterinary Surgery* **30**, 161–169

Kyles AE, Hardie EM, Mehl M and Gregory C (2002) Evaluation of Ameroid ring constrictors for the management of single extrahepatic portosystemic shunts in cats: 23 cases (1996–2001). *Journal of the American Veterinary Medical Association* **220**, 1341–1347

Lamb CR and White RN (1998) Morphology of congenital intrahepatic portacaval shunts in dogs and cats. *Veterinary Record* **142**, 55–60

Leveille R, Johnson SE and Birchard SJ (2003) Transvenous coil embolization of portosystemic shunt in dogs. *Veterinary Radiology and Ultrasound* **44**, 32–36

Lipscombe VJ, Jones HJ and Brockman DJ (2007) Complications and long-term outcomes of the ligation of congenital portosystemic shunts in 49 cats. *Veterinary Record* **160**, 465–470

Mehl ML, Kyles AE, Hardie EM *et al.* (2005) Evaluation of ameroid ring constrictors for single extrahepatic portosystemic shunts in dogs: 168 cases (1995–2001). *Journal of the American Veterinary Medical Association* **226**, 2020–2030

Seymour C and Duke-Novakovski T (2007) *BSAVA Manual of Canine and Feline Anaesthesia and Analgesia, 2nd edn.* BSAVA Publications, Gloucester

Tisdall PLC, Hunt GB, Youmans KR and Malik R (2000) Neurological dysfunction in dogs following attenuation of congenital extrahepatic portosystemic shunts. *Journal of Small Animal Practice* **41**, 539–546

Tobias KM (2003) Portosystemic shunts and other hepatic vascular anomalies. In: *Textbook of Small Animal Surgery, 3rd edition*, ed. DH Slatter, pp.727–751. WB Saunders, Philadelphia

Vogt JC, Krahwinkel DJ, Bright RM *et al.* (1996) Gradual occlusion of extrahepatic portosystemic shunts in dogs and cats using the Ameroid constrictor. *Veterinary Surgery* **25**, 495–502

Weisse C, Solomon JA, Holt D, Nicholson M and Cope C (2003) Percutaneous transvenous coil embolization of canine intrahepatic portosystemic shunts: short term results in 14 dogs. *Veterinary Surgery* **32**, 499 [Abstract]

White RN, Burton CA and McEvoy FJ (1998) Surgical treatment of intrahepatic shunts in 45 dogs. *Veterinary Record* **142**, 358–365

White RN, Trower ND, McEvoy FJ, Garden OA and Boswood A (1996) A method for controlling portal pressure after attenuation of intrahepatic portacaval shunts. *Veterinary Surgery* **25**, 407–413

OPERATIVE TECHNIQUE 10.1

Attenuation of an extrahepatic portosystemic shunt

POSITIONING

Dorsal recumbency.

ASSISTANT

Essential.

EQUIPMENT EXTRAS

Fine thumb forceps (DeBakey); right-angled dissecting forceps (Lahey bile duct forceps); cellophane band and haemostatic clips; Ameroid constrictors (various sizes).

SURGICAL TECHNIQUE

Approach

Ventral midline laparotomy.

Surgical manipulations: locating the portosystemic shunt

1   Perform a ventral midline laparotomy with the incision extending from just cranial to the xiphoid to the pubis.

2   Resect the falciform ligament to provide as much access as possible to the liver and diaphragm.

> **WARNING**
>
> Note that, rarely, extrahepatic shunts have been reported within the falciform ligament, and therefore dissection should proceed carefully in order to avoid accidental division

3   Retract the abdominal viscera to the right using the mesocolon, and inspect the paravertebral gutter and left kidney. Multiple acquired shunts are often most prominent in this location. Inspect the crura of the diaphragm. Portoazygous shunts can usually be identified at this location (see Figure 10.3).

4   Retract the abdominal viscera to the left using the mesoduodenum, and trace the caudal vena cava cranially from the confluence of the common iliac veins to the point where it disappears dorsal to the liver, confirming that the caudal vena cava anatomy is normal and that it does not continue as the azygous vein. The left and right renal veins should be the only visible major vessels entering the caudal vena cava within the abdominal cavity. Note that the smaller phrenicoabdominal veins that cross the adrenal glands enter the vena cava cranial to the renal veins; they may, however, be surrounded by retroperitoneal fat.

→ **OPERATIVE TECHNIQUE 10.1 CONTINUED**

5   Locate the epiploic foramen, created by the fold of tissue containing the hepatic artery and portal vein. Retraction of the hepatic artery and portal vein to the left will permit inspection of the prerenal caudal vena cava between the right renal vein and the liver. This is the most common location for extrahepatic shunts in dogs and cats (see Figure 10.2 and Chapter 9).

6   Confirm the presence of a hepatic portal vein extending to and arborizing at the porta hepatis of the liver. Identify the right branches of the portal vein (leading to the right lateral and right medial liver lobes) and the left branch of the portal vein. Dilatation of any of these branches may indicate the presence of an intrahepatic shunt.

7   Return the viscera to their normal positions and perforate the ventral leaf of omentum to gain access to the omental bursa. Retraction of the stomach cranially will usually reveal a dilated branch of the portal venous system in animals with extrahepatic shunts. Identify the portal vessel from which this dilated branch is arising and trace to its entry into the systemic circulation.

8   If no shunt has been identified, consider the possibility of an intrahepatic shunt or microvascular dysplasia. If this seems unlikely, divide the crura of the diaphragm and inspect the caudal mediastinum for evidence of a portoazygous shunt. If no shunt vessel is identified, perform an intraoperative portogram by catheterizing a jejunal vein and injecting a water-soluble iodine-based contrast medium, and ideally monitoring with fluoroscopy.

9   Once the shunt has been identified, retract the viscera in the most appropriate way to provide access for dissection and attenuation. This will vary according to the shunt anatomy.

WARNING

Dissection should be performed as close as possible to the systemic vascular insertion of the shunt, to avoid the possibility of small portal branches entering distal to the attenuation point.

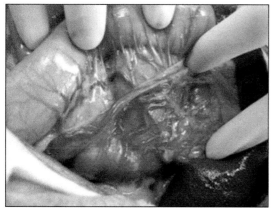

Multiple acquired shunt vessels.

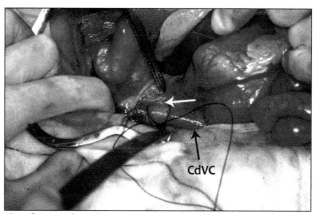

Identification of extrahepatic PSS. Ventral midline laparotomy view with the animal's head towards the left of the photograph. The hepatic artery has been retracted using a Poole suction tip and a silk ligature placed around the shunt (white arrow) as it enters the caudal vena cava (CdVC).

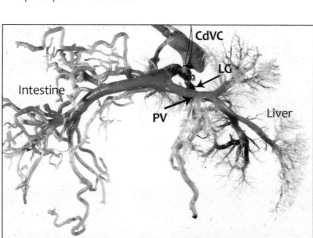

Corrosion cast of the portal vasculature in a dog with an extrahepatic shunt. Right lateral view with the dog's head positioned towards the right. A silk ligature has been placed around the shunt between the left gastric vein (LG) and the caudal vena cava (CdVC). A well developed portal vein (PV) can be seen travelling towards the liver and arborizing into the different liver lobes.

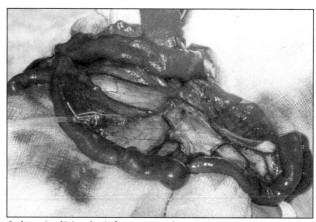

Catheterized jejunal vein for portography or water manometry.
(Courtesy of J Niles)

→ **OPERATIVE TECHNIQUE 10.1 CONTINUED**

Surgical manipulations: placement of a cellophane band

Cellophane is purchased from a stationery or paper company in sheet form. The sheets should not be too flimsy (to maximize handling strength) or too thick (which would distort the fragile vessel when passed around it). Cellophane should be pre-sterilized with ethylene oxide. Steam or chemical sterilization is not recommended. Repeated sterilization using ethylene oxide appears to increase cellophane fragility and should also be avoided.

1　After dissection around the vessel to be attenuated, place a suture of 3 or 3.5 metric (2/0 or 0 USP) polypropylene.

2　The anaesthetist then takes a series of baseline measurements, including heart rate and direct or indirect systolic arterial pressure (and central venous pressure if a catheter has been placed).

3　Inspect the intestines and pancreas for colour, motility and signs of venous congestion. In dogs weighing >10 kg, and for all dogs with intrahepatic shunts, portal pressure is also measured via a catheter placed in a jejunal vein and attached to a water manometer.

4　Tighten the polypropylene suture temporarily using a Rummel tourniquet and repeat the above observations after 5 minutes. The shunt is considered to be refractory to complete occlusion if the heart rate is elevated by >20 beats per minute, the systolic arterial pressure falls by >10 mmHg, the central venous pressure falls by >1 mmHg, and the portal pressure rises by >10 cmH$_2$O or reaches a maximum of 20 cmH$_2$O. Congestion and cyanosis of the pancreas and intestines, and a substantial increase in intestinal motility, are also considered indications of unacceptable portal hypertension.

　　In animals weighing <10 kg, observation of the above-described changes should result in placement of a cellophane band of 3 mm diameter. Absence of change suggests a shunt that could be totally occluded if necessary; in these animals a 2 mm diameter band is placed. All dogs and cats displaying changes between the two extremes receive a cellophane band of 2.5 mm diameter. Placement of cellophane bands between 2 and 3 mm in diameter causes substantial shunt attenuation. However, the author has encountered only one dog that developed life-threatening portal hypertension necessitating cellophane band removal; in this instance a small thrombus was found to have lodged suddenly at the attenuation site 3 days after surgery. Surgeons should also be aware that cellophane bands of greater diameter may cause complete eventual occlusion, obviating the need to produce shunt occlusion intraoperatively, but this has not yet been proven by controlled experimental study.

5　Once the shunt has been dissected and an appropriate cellophane band diameter chosen, fold a strip of cellophane (1.2 cm wide and about 15 cm long) lengthwise to produce a three-layered band 4 mm in width and 15 cm in length. This configuration is chosen because it was the type of band tested experimentally in early studies. The multiple layers impart extra strength to the cellophane band, which is easily torn when it becomes wet. Cut the end of the strip obliquely to facilitate passage through the perivascular tissue.

6　Carefully pass the cellophane band around the shunt vessel, avoiding incorporation of a large amount of perivascular tissue. The band should be placed as close to the shunt's insertion into the systemic vasculature as possible.

7　Hold the two ends of the band by hand and place a stainless steel pin of appropriate diameter inside the band, next to the shunt vessel.

8　Position a pair of haemostatic forceps (clip) across the two sides of the cellophane strip and apply whilst holding the cellophane band tight around both the stainless steel pin and the shunt. This results in fixation of the cellophane band at the predetermined diameter.

9　Withdraw the stainless steel pin from the cellophane band, allowing the shunt to expand to the diameter of the pin.

10　Note haemodynamic parameters and the appearance of the viscera to ensure that safe limits have not been exceeded. These limits include an elevation of heart rate by >20 beats per minute, reduction in mean arterial pressure by >10 mmHg, reduction in central venous pressure by >2 cmH$_2$O and elevation of portal pressure by >10 cmH$_2$O (to a maximum of 20 cmH$_2$O).

11　Cut the cellophane band, leaving an end of approximately 1 mm protruding beyond the surgical clip to reduce the risk of the clip dislodging. The cellophane band may then be gently manipulated so that it sits comfortably without kinking or distorting the shunt vessel or impinging on other vessels in the local area.

12　Leave the polypropylene suture in place and tied loosely. Its ends are left 4 cm long. This is to enable easy identification if subsequent surgery is required owing to persistent signs of hepatic dysfunction or portosystemic shunting.

　　As a result of fibrous tissue formation, it may not be possible to dissect around the shunt a second time, but the polypropylene suture may be grasped and pulled tight to check whether the original shunt is closed or patent. If the shunt has remained patent for some reason, it may then be possible to attenuate the polypropylene suture further without having to disturb the shunt itself. Although recommending this course of action, the author has never been faced with the necessity to attenuate a shunt further in a dog using this method.

→

→ **OPERATIVE TECHNIQUE 10.1 CONTINUED**

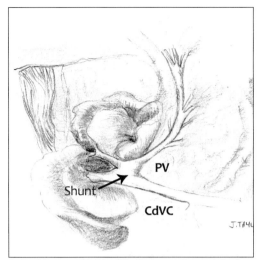

A shunt (arrowed) is identified between the portal vein (PV) and caudal vena cava (CdVC) at the level of the epiploic foramen.

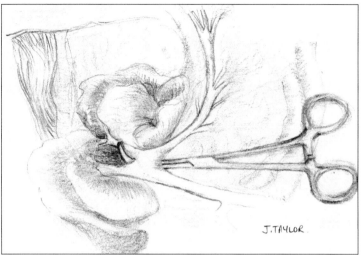

The shunt is carefully dissected with Lahey bile duct forceps, close to its insertion into the caudal vena cava.

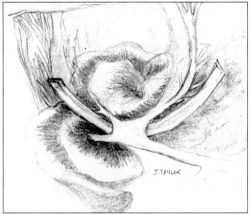

A 4 mm wide strip of cellophane, folded into three layers, is passed around the shunt.

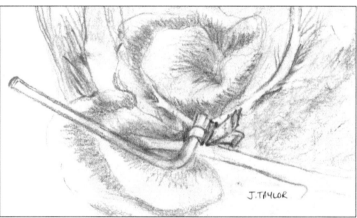

The cellophane is tightened around the shunt and a stainless steel pin of predetermined diameter is secured using a surgical clip.

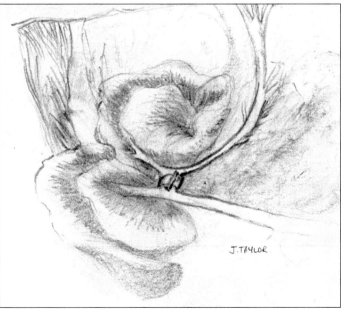

The stainless steel pin is withdrawn, allowing the shunt to expand to the diameter of the cellophane band. This causes partial immediate attenuation of the shunt without increasing portal pressure to dangerous levels. The cellophane band is trimmed close to the clip and manipulated into a position where it sits flat and does not distort or kink the shunt.

→ **OPERATIVE TECHNIQUE 10.1 CONTINUED**

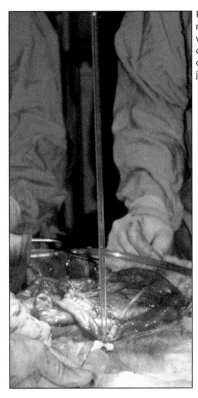

Portal venous pressure measurement using a water manometer connected to a catheter placed in a jejunal vein.

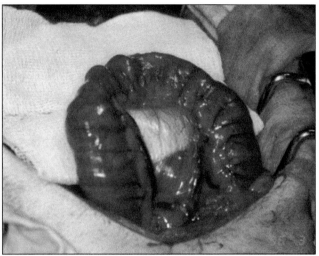

Intestines showing signs of portal hypertension. Note dark cyanotic colour, the dilated veins and hypersegmentation of the intestine.

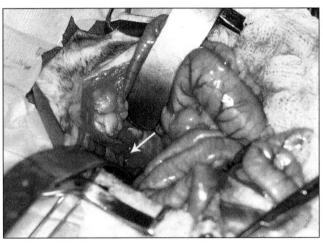

Cellophane banding (arrowed) of a congenital extrahepatic shunt in a Maltese dog.

Surgical manipulations: placement of an Ameroid constrictor

The initial steps are the same as preparation for placement of a cellophane band. An Ameroid constrictor is chosen that ideally should not cause >25–50% reduction in the diameter of the shunt vessel. This is not always possible and, once the constrictor has been placed, the surgeon must assess for evidence of portal hypertension.

1 Place the 'key' from the Ameroid constrictor safely on a sterile swab on the instrument tray.

2 Use a pair of right-angled forceps, such as Lahey's, to dissect around the shunt vessel.

3 Place either two Rummel tourniquets fashioned from 2 metric (3/0 USP) polypropylene and 18 G intravenous catheters to occlude the shunt vessel or, by spreading the jaws of the right-angled forceps, it may be possible to flatten the vessel temporarily. This allows the Ameroid constrictor to be passed over the shunt vessel

4 Rotate the Ameroid constrictor as necessary to allow the key to be placed in the 'keyhole', so as to prevent the constrictor falling off the vessel.

→ **OPERATIVE TECHNIQUE 10.1 CONTINUED**

5   Replace the intestines in the abdominal cavity and assess over 5 minutes for any evidence of portal hypertension. Particular attention should be paid to the pancreas. Prior to closure, take a liver biopsy (see Chapter 9).

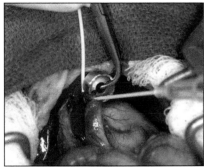
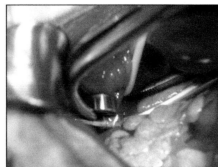
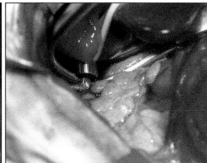

Placement of an Ameroid constrictor around a collapsed extrahepatic shunt vessel using Rummel tourniquets fashioned from 2 metric (3/0 USP) polypropylene and 18 G intravenous catheters.
(Courtesy of J Niles)

Right-angled forceps being using to collapse the shunt vessel gently while the Ameroid constrictor is applied.
(Courtesy of J Niles)

Wound closure

This is routine. Skin sutures should be left in place for at least 12–14 days, owing to the risk of poor wound healing in patients with hepatic dysfunction.

POSTOPERATIVE MANAGEMENT

Administer glucose-containing intravenous fluids, prophylactic anticonvulsant medication and a protein-restricted diet (see text for details).

- Monitor for signs of portal hypertension (distended abdomen, abdominal pain, bloody diarrhoea, poor capillary refill, tachycardia, weak pulse, collapse). Signs are most often seen early in the postoperative period. Mild signs can be managed with intravenous fluids and analgesia. Although rarely seen, severe signs require emergency surgery to remove the cellophane band or Ameroid constrictor from the shunt vessel.
- Monitor for signs of post-ligation neurological dysfunction (see main text).
- Monitor for signs of hypoglycaemia, particularly in animals that are slow to recover from anaesthesia and begin eating.

Chapter 11

The pancreas

Floryne O. Buishand and Jolle Kirpensteijn

The pancreas is a glandular organ in the cranial abdomen that has both endocrine and exocrine functions. The islet cells of the endocrine pancreas produce the hormones insulin and glucagon, which regulate glucose metabolism, and the acinar cells of the exocrine pancreas produce digestive enzymes. The exocrine pancreas also secretes bicarbonate, which is essential to buffer stomach acid.

Pancreatic surgery can be challenging and can be associated with serious complications, if not conducted *lege artis* (i.e. according to all the principles of the art of surgery). Therefore, a comprehensive knowledge of pancreatic anatomy, physiology and its surgical diseases is of utmost importance in order to perform any pancreatic surgery safely. This chapter covers those diseases of the pancreas that benefit from surgical intervention.

Anatomy

The pancreas in dogs and cats consists of a right and a left lobe that are united at the pancreatic body (Figure 11.1). The angle formed with the pancreatic body by the left and right lobes is smaller in cats than in dogs. The right or duodenal lobe is located in the peritoneal fold of the descending duodenum. In contrast to the canine pancreas, the distal third of the feline right lobe curves cranially, giving it a hook-like appearance, and ends close to the vena cava. The right lobe is easily exposed by retraction of the duodenum ventrally and medially into the abdominal incision (duodenal manoeuvre; see Chapter 1). The left lobe is positioned in a dorsal fold of the omentum. It begins at the pylorus and extends along the greater curvature of the stomach to the dorsal extremity of the spleen. Exposure of the left lobe is best achieved by retraction of the stomach and greater omentum cranially, while retracting the transverse colon caudally. Alternatively, a fenestration can be made in the omentum immediately caudal to the greater curvature of the stomach. This fenestration, followed by cranial retraction of the stomach, will reveal the left lobe of the pancreas. The body of the pancreas is adjacent to the proximal duodenum.

Vascular supply

The arterial blood supply to the pancreas is tripartite (see Figure 11.1). The largest inflow vessel is the cranial pancreaticoduodenal artery, a terminal branch of the gastroduodenal artery, which enters the body of the pancreas,

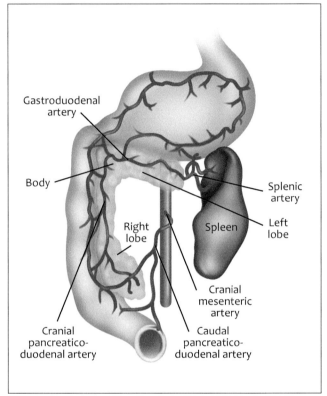

11.1 Anatomy and blood supply to the pancreas and adjacent structures.

courses through the right pancreatic lobe, and also supplies the duodenum after exiting the pancreas. The pancreatic artery, which branches from the splenic artery in 80% of dogs, supplies the left lobe of the pancreas. In the remaining 20% of dogs the pancreatic artery originates from the cranial mesenteric artery.

> **PRACTICAL TIP**
>
> The pancreatic artery should always be identified at surgery, so that the specific surgical procedure is carried out with knowledge of the location of the arterial supply

The third and smallest source of arterial inflow is the caudal pancreaticoduodenal artery, which arises from the cranial mesenteric artery and supplies and courses through the distal portion of the right pancreatic lobe. The cranial and caudal pancreaticoduodenal arteries anastomose within the right lobe of the pancreas. The pancreaticoduodenal vein drains the right lobe of the pancreas, and the body and left lobe are drained via the splenic vein.

Innervation

The pancreas is directly innervated by vagal fibres that, when stimulated, cause an increase in pancreatic juice production and secretion. The coeliac and superior mesenteric plexus innervate the blood vessels of the pancreas.

Pancreatic ducts

Pancreatic duct anatomy varies between dogs and cats. Dogs typically have two pancreatic ducts (Figure 11.2). The accessory pancreatic duct carries secretions from the right pancreatic lobe to the minor papilla in the duodenum. The smaller pancreatic duct transports secretions from the left lobe and enters the major duodenal papilla next to the common bile duct, approximately 5 cm from the pylorus. Some dogs are found to have only an accessory pancreatic duct, and three duodenal openings have also been reported. In 80% of cats, a single pancreatic duct is present that joins the common bile duct before entering the major duodenal papilla. In the remaining 20% of cats, an accessory pancreatic duct is present, which, as in dogs, opens into the minor duodenal papilla.

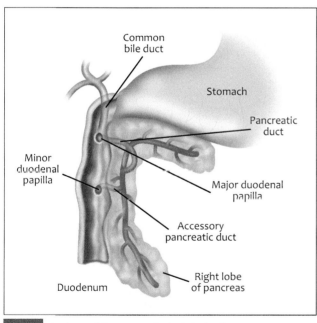

11.2 Anatomy of the pancreatic ducts in the dog.

Physiology

Digestion

The acinar cells of the pancreas secrete:

* Amylase
* Proteases: trypsinogen, chymotrypsinogen, proelastase, procarboxy peptidase A and B
* Lipases: pancreatic lipase, phospholipase A2 and cholesterol esterase.

These enzymes are responsible for the digestion of carbohydrate, protein and fat. In order to prevent auto-digestion of the pancreas, the proteolytic enzymes and phospholipase A2 are secreted in inactive forms. These proenzymes require activation in order to exert their enzymatic function. After delivery of the proenzymes to the duodenum, they become activated through cleavage of activation peptides from the proenzymes by trypsin and enterokinase. Besides enzymes, pancreatic juice contains bicarbonate for neutralization of gastric acid, factors that facilitate absorption of cobalamin, zinc and colipase C and antibacterial factors.

Glucose metabolism

Unlike the exocrine pancreas, where acinar cells secrete all types of enzymes, islet cells specialize in the secretion of one hormone type. Insulin, which is secreted by beta cells, is the best-studied pancreatic hormone. Insulin secretion is tightly regulated by the blood glucose concentration. In contrast to most other cells, the entrance of glucose into beta cells via facilitative glucose transporters (GLUTs) is insulin independent. With increasing blood glucose concentrations, insulin secretion gradually increases, eventually reaching a plateau. When blood glucose concentrations decrease, insulin secretion is inhibited. The function of insulin is to decrease blood glucose levels, through inhibition of gluconeogenesis, glycogenolysis, fatty acid breakdown and ketogenesis and stimulation of glycogenesis and protein synthesis. The actions of insulin are opposed by glucagon, which is secreted by alpha cells. Glucagon increases hepatic glycogenolysis and gluconeogenesis. Finally, ghrelin, which is secreted by epsilon cells, influences glucose metabolism by inhibiting the beta-cell response to glucose, leading to a decrease in insulin release.

Surgical techniques

Pancreatic biopsy

Surgical biopsy (see Operative Technique 11.1) and fine needle aspiration can be performed either via an open surgical procedure or through a laparoscopic procedure (see Chapter 3 for details on laparoscopic pancreatic biopsy). Pancreatic biopsies have not commonly been performed historically, owing to the perceived high risk of potential complications, though this risk is in fact negligible (Barnes et al., 2006; Spillman, 2013). In cats, particularly because there is a broad range in the sensitivity and specificity of feline pancreatic lipase immunoreactivity in the diagnosis of feline pancreatitis, pancreatic biopsy is often indicated (Cosford et al., 2010). The decision whether or not to take pancreatic biopsy samples should be made on a case-by-case basis, and the technique should be carried out with care and precision to minimize any risk of complications (Cosford et al., 2010; Spillman, 2013).

> **PRACTICAL TIP**
>
> It is not uncommon to find multiple small fibrotic nodules (1–2 mm) in the pancreas of older dogs and cats. These are usually incidental findings and probably result from previous bouts of pancreatitis. These usually do not need to be biopsied unless necessary to solve a clinical dilemma in the patient

Partial pancreatectomy

Partial pancreatectomy (see Operative Technique 11.2) is indicated in cases of focal pancreatic trauma, or where there are isolated pancreatic masses, pseudocysts or abscesses. Up to 75–90% of the pancreas can be removed without affecting exocrine or endocrine function, provided that the duct to the remaining portion of the pancreas is left intact and the remainder of the pancreas is healthy (Thomson, 2003).

> **WARNING**
>
> Total pancreatectomy should not be attempted by an inexperienced surgeon, because it is extremely difficult to remove the right pancreatic lobe while sparing the shared blood supply to the duodenum

Pancreatic drainage

Pancreatic drainage can be achieved in several ways, depending on the indication. Ultrasound-guided aspiration of fluid-containing masses is indicated for pancreatic pseudocysts. However, if repeated ultrasound examinations reveal persistence or enlargement of the pancreatic lesion, surgical exploration is indicated (see Operative Technique 11.3). In patients with pancreatic abscesses without diffuse peritonitis, a Jackson–Pratt or sump drain can be used. In cases where pancreatic abscesses occur together with severe diffuse peritonitis, open abdominal drainage or the use of vacuum-assisted closure (VAC) is indicated (Buote and Havig, 2012).

> **WARNING**
>
> To prevent devastating ascending infections in patients with open abdomens or external drains, use of aseptic technique is critical when bandaging these patients (see Chapter 18)

Surgical conditions

Insulinoma
Pathophysiology

Insulinoma originates from endocrine beta cells in the islets of Langerhans, and is the most common pancreatic endocrine tumour in the dog. In 95% of cases, insulinomas are considered to be malignant, because they almost always tend to metastasize to the regional lymph nodes and the liver. Insulinomas hypersecrete insulin, producing an increased insulin concentration in the blood. The clinical signs of hyperinsulinaemia are induced by hypoglycaemia, and include seizures, generalized weakness, posterior paresis, lethargy, ataxia and muscle tremors. The clinical signs of canine insulinoma often occur intermittently and in the initial stages fasting, exercise, excitement or stress often precedes hypoglycaemic episodes.

Diagnosis

The presumptive diagnosis of canine insulinoma is commonly based on signalment and history, combined with the fulfilment of Whipple's triad:

> **Whipple's triad**
> * Presence of clinical signs associated with hypoglycaemia (usually neurological signs)
> * Fasting blood glucose concentration <2.2 mmol/l (<40 mg/dl)
> * Relief of clinical signs after glucose administration or feeding

While Whipple's triad diagnoses hypoglycaemia, it is not definitive for insulinoma. The next step is to exclude differential diagnoses by determining the plasma insulin concentration. In cases with insulinoma, circulating insulin concentrations are typically within the reference range or higher, despite hypoglycaemia. The simultaneous occurrence of blood glucose <3.5 mmol/l and plasma insulin >70 pmol/l is diagnostic for insulinoma.

Diagnostic imaging techniques, including trans-abdominal ultrasonography, computed tomography (CT), single-photon emission CT (SPECT) and somatostatin receptor scintigraphy (SRS), have been shown to help in the identification and preoperative staging of insulinoma. Ultrasonography was found to have a low sensitivity in detecting canine insulinoma (Robben et al., 2005) with only 5 of 14 primary insulinomas correctly identified, and no lymph node metastases were detected. Similar results were obtained using SPECT. CT proved to be the most sensitive method, correctly identifying 10 of 14 primary tumours and 2 of 5 lymph node metastases. However, conventional pre- and post-contrast CT was not found to be a very specific method, because it also identified many false-positive lesions (Figure 11.3). More recently, dual-phase CT angiography (CTA) techniques have been developed, and the accurate use of dynamic CTA for the presurgical localization of insulinoma in four dogs has been reported (Iseri et al., 2007; Mai and Caceres, 2008). With CTA, after an intravenous injection of contrast medium, CT images are acquired during the arterial and venous phases. CT images of canine insulinoma are hyperattenuating during the arterial phase in 55% of cases (Mai and Caceres, 2008), compared with the normal pancreas.

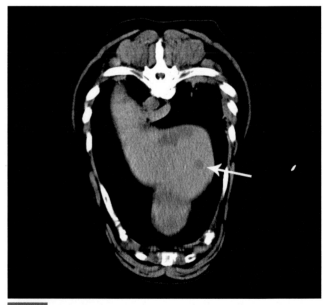

11.3 CT image showing insulinoma liver metastasis (arrowed).

Surgical treatment

Insulinoma therapy can be divided into medical management and surgical treatment. Partial pancreatectomy (see Operative Technique 11.2) is considered the treatment of choice because it has been associated with the longest survival times. However, most dogs are also managed medically at some point in the disease course (i.e. postoperative treatment of residual disease).

If clinical signs of hypoglycaemia occur in the immediate preoperative period, a 50% glucose solution should be administered intravenously (small dogs: 2.5–5 ml; large dogs: 8–15 ml, administered slowly to effect over 10 minutes; Buishand and Kirpensteijn, 2013). During anaesthesia, dogs should receive a continuous intravenous infusion of a balanced electrolyte solution containing 2.5–5.0% dextrose, and continuous blood glucose monitoring is required. Glucose infusion is normally stopped as soon as the insulinoma is removed. Normoglycaemia is typically restored but hyperglycaemia may occur. This is due to atrophy of the normal beta cells by feedback inhibition, and is induced within minutes after insulinoma resection.

> **WARNING**
>
> Excessive manipulation of an insulinoma during surgery should be minimized, because this can trigger increased insulin secretion, leading to a more profound hypoglycaemia

> **WARNING**
>
> Persistent hypoglycaemia indicates the presence of residual tumour tissue or undetected metastases. Reoperation should be considered. Otherwise, continued medical management of hypoglycaemia is necessary to elevate serum glucose levels

Postoperative considerations

In addition to standard postoperative management after surgical manipulation of the pancreas (see Operative Technique 11.1), it is essential to monitor blood glucose concentrations closely (see Operative Technique 11.2). In some dogs, hyperglycaemia may occur as a consequence of atrophy of the normal beta cells caused by feedback inhibition. Hyperglycaemia may be transient and resolve with time. If hyperglycaemia persists, administration of insulin is required. In most cases, normal pancreatic endocrine function should eventually resume; however, some dogs require lifelong insulin therapy. If these dogs no longer require insulin at a certain point, because their glucose concentrations are returning to reference values, this may indicate the growth of insulinoma (micro)metastases.

Prognosis

Prognostic indicators for insulinoma are the tumour, node, metastasis (TNM) stage, tumour size, age, postoperative blood glucose concentrations and the Ki67 index. Ki67 is a proliferation marker that is expressed during the active phases of the cell cycle and is absent from resting cells. Dogs with a negative Ki67 index, with insulinomas confined to the pancreas or with primary tumours smaller than 2 cm, survive significantly longer postoperatively compared with dogs with a positive Ki67 index, with insulinomas that have spread to lymph nodes and distant sites or with larger tumours. Young dogs have been shown to have a worse prognosis than older dogs, and dogs that are hyperglycaemic or normoglycaemic immediately postoperatively survive significantly longer than dogs with hypoglycaemia postoperatively (Buishand et al., 2010).

Gastrinoma
Pathophysiology

Gastrinoma is a very rarely reported and diagnosed malignant tumour of the dog and cat that is characterized by hypersecretion of gastrin, derived from D cells in the islets of Langerhans. The secretion of excessive amounts of gastrin results in gastric acid hypersecretion, and is associated with clinical signs of severe vomiting, melaena, anorexia, depression and weight loss.

Diagnosis

The presence of the above clinical signs, in combination with hypergastrinaemia in fasted patients, is highly suggestive of gastrinoma. Endoscopic examination of the stomach and duodenum often reveals ulceration. Ultrasonography frequently fails to identify the tumour, because gastrinomas are very small. In human medicine, SRS has been reported to be the most sensitive diagnostic imaging modality for diagnosing gastrinomas. The same technique has been successfully used to diagnose metastatic gastrinoma in one dog (Altschul et al., 1997).

Surgical treatment

Surgical resection of the gastrinoma by partial pancreatectomy may provide a cure in cases where metastasis is not present. However, 72% of canine gastrinomas have already metastasized at the time of surgery. Surgery also offers a chance to excise gastrointestinal ulcers that otherwise could perforate and lead to peritonitis.

Prognosis

The long-term prognosis for dogs with gastrinomas is grave, ranging from 1 week to 18 months (mean 4.8 months; Lurye and Behrend, 2001), although one case report documented a survival time of 26 months (Hughes, 2006).

Glucagonoma
Pathophysiology

Glucagonoma in dogs is a very rare glucagon-secreting neuroendocrine carcinoma of pancreatic alpha cells. Serum glucagon levels become elevated and, secondary to this, glucagon mediates a decrease in plasma amino acids. Furthermore, increased glucagon levels reduce the amount of albumin in the blood, leading to a relative deficiency of zinc and essential fatty acids, because these substances are normally carried by albumin. Although the exact pathogenesis is uncertain, the changes in plasma levels of zinc and fatty acids are suggested to directly cause the cutaneous manifestation of glucagonoma syndrome: erosions, ulceration and hyperkeratosis of the footpads; and crusting and alopecia around the mucocutaneous junctions. Additionally, lethargy, anorexia, polyuria and polydipsia have been reported in dogs with glucagonoma.

Diagnosis

Glucagonomas are often missed on abdominal ultrason-ography. Recently, the use of CT has been reported for the diagnosis of lymph node, splenic and hepatic gluca-gonoma metastases that were not identified on ultra-sonography (Oberkirchner *et al.*, 2010). Skin biopsy samples demonstrate histological changes characteristic of metabolic epidermal necrosis in dogs. However, in 90% of canine cases with metabolic epidermal necrosis, the skin condition is associated with severe liver dysfunction, rather than the presence of a glucagonoma. Furthermore, plasma glucagon levels can also be increased in hepato-cutaneous syndrome, without the presence of a gluca-gonoma. Therefore, liver disease, and other dermatological differential diagnoses, need to be ruled out before the diagnosis of glucagonoma can be confirmed.

Surgical treatment

Partial pancreatectomy and surgical debulking of meta-static lesions is the treatment of choice. Furthermore, dogs should be fed a high-protein diet, which can be supple-mented with zinc and fatty acids. In two cases of canine non-resectable glucagonomas, the dogs were treated palliatively with the somatostatin analogue octreotide, which inhibits glucagon secretion. In one of the dogs, the ocretotide treatment resulted in improvements in skin lesions within 10 days. However, after 6 weeks this dog had to be euthanased owing to progressive metastatic disease (Oberkirchner *et al.*, 2010).

Prognosis

Three cases of canine glucagonoma have been described that were treated surgically. Surgical resection of the pan-creatic masses resulted in severe acute postoperative pancreatitis in two cases. These dogs died 3 days after surgery. The third dog survived for 9 months after surgery, whereafter skin lesions recurred and the dog was eutha-nased without post-mortem examination (Gross *et al.*, 1990; Torres *et al.*, 1997).

Exocrine pancreatic neoplasia
Pathophysiology

Pancreatic (adeno)carcinomas are highly malignant tumours that originate from acinar or duct epithelial cells. These tumours most commonly occur in older animals that present with weight loss, anorexia, abdominal pain, ascites, vomiting and icterus. Benign pancreatic adeno-mas are extremely rare and are often incidental findings.

Diagnosis

Abdominal ultrasonography often detects a mass in the pancreatic area, but neither ultrasonography nor gross examination of the pancreas allows an adenocarcinoma to be distinguished from pancreatitis.

PRACTICAL TIP

Histopathology is required to differentiate between pancreatic adenocarcinoma and chronic fibrosing pancreatitis

---

Surgical treatment

In most cases surgical resection of pancreatic adenocarci-noma is not possible, owing to the advanced stage of the disease, because these tumours rapidly spread to the liver, lungs, peritoneum and local lymph nodes.

Prognosis

In cases where surgery is feasible, most animals survive <3 months postoperatively. One-year survival after diagno-sis, regardless of treatment, has not been reported.

Pancreatitis
Pathophysiology

Pancreatitis can be acute, when inflammation of pancre-atic tissue is sudden in onset and reversible, or chronic, when inflammation is often subclinical with irreversible fibrosis and atrophy. Most cases of pancreatitis are idio-pathic in origin but, regardless of the underlying cause, following initiation of pancreatitis, autodigestion of the gland starts to occur. The most common clinical signs of pancreatitis in dogs are anorexia, vomiting, weakness, abdominal pain and diarrhoea. In contrast to dogs, pan-creatitis only causes vomiting in a minority of cats, and diarrhoea is not observed. In cats the most common clini-cal signs associated with pancreatitis are anorexia and lethargy, which are not specifically indicative of gastro-intestinal disease.

Diagnosis

In most cases the diagnosis of pancreatitis is based on the clinical signs, together with increased serum pan-creatic lipase levels. On ultrasound examination, the echodensity of the pancreas can be decreased, or increased with pancreatic fibrosis. A mass lesion might be seen within the pancreas, a cystic mass in the case of a pancreatic pseudocyst, or an abscess. The echodensity of the surrounding mesentery is often hyperechoic in acute pancreatitis, as a result of inflammation. Pancreatic biopsy (see Operative Technique 11.1) can be performed to confirm the diagnosis.

Surgical treatment

Whether surgery is the appropriate treatment for pancrea-titis remains controversial. Frequently patients with severe pancreatitis are poor anaesthetic and surgical risks, and medical treatment is preferred. However, in certain cases surgery is more appropriate. Indications for surgery are:

- Confirmation of diagnosis
- Failure to respond to aggressive medical therapy
- Presence of pancreatic abscess/cyst
- Presence of extrahepatic biliary obstruction
- Presence of septic peritonitis.

Prior to surgery, attention should be paid to factors that could increase the complication rate, including age, sepsis, hypoproteinaemia, disseminated intravascular coagulation (DIC) and diabetes mellitus. Any abnormal-ities in fluid and electrolyte balance, coagulation, oncotic pressure or plasma glucose levels should be corrected preoperatively. Furthermore, although septic complica-tions are rare in cases of pancreatitis, it is often recom-mended to initiate antibiotic therapy in febrile patients.

Surgical objectives are:

* To determine the type and extent of pancreatic disease and associated abdominal problems
* To resect necrotic pancreatic tissue
* To flush and drain cysts or abscesses
* To perform cholecystoduodenostomy in cases of complete permanent bile duct obstruction
* To consider placement of a jejunostomy tube.

PRACTICAL TIPS

* Handle the pancreas gently; it is reasonable to touch and palpate the pancreas but pinching should be avoided
* It is essential to maintain excellent tissue perfusion during surgery to prevent pancreatic ischaemia and postoperative pancreatitis
* Perform thorough abdominal lavage with large volumes of sterile isotonic fluid prior to closure, to dilute and reduce the level of free intraperitoneal proteases

Prognosis

In a case series of 37 dogs with acute pancreatitis that were treated surgically, the overall survival rate was 63% (Thompson *et al.*, 2009). Within this group, dogs with extrahepatic biliary obstruction that had undergone resection of necrotic tissue had a better prognosis than dogs with pancreatic abscesses. The severity of the clinical signs at initial diagnosis was not correlated with clinical outcome.

Pancreatic abscesses and pseudocysts

Pathophysiology

Pancreatic abscesses are mucopurulent necrotic exudates within the pancreatic parenchyma, with or without extension into adjacent tissue. In contrast to human pancreatic abscesses, bacteria are only rarely isolated in canine cases. A pancreatic abscess is usually a sequel to pancreatitis, and therefore the clinical signs of abscesses closely parallel those of pancreatitis. Pancreatic abscesses can also occur if parts of the pancreas are devoid of a pancreatic duct; for example, as a result of leaving a distal part of the pancreas intact during partial resection.

Pancreatic pseudocysts are collections of pancreatic secretions, debris and blood in a non-epithelialized fibrous tissue sac (Figure 11.4). The exact pathogenesis of pseudocysts is unknown; however, it has been suggested that premature activation of digestive enzymes might result in autodigestion of the pancreatic parenchyma, leading to inflammation and necrosis. Pancreatic pseudocysts may be asymptomatic, or animals may be presented with signs attributed to pancreatitis.

Diagnosis

Ultrasonography may reveal a fluid-filled mass in the area of the pancreas, but imaging alone cannot differentiate pseudocysts from abscesses. To make a definitive diagnosis, fluid acquired by percutaneous fine-needle aspiration should be examined. However, fine-needle aspiration of cavitary pancreatic masses is not without risk, and this risk must be weighed against the advantage of a preoperative diagnosis.

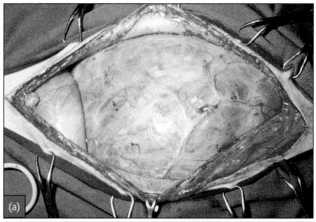

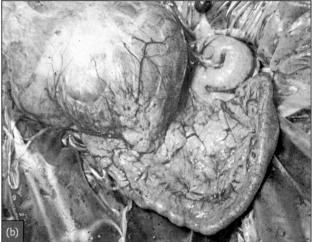

11.4 (a) A large pancreatic pseudocyst in a dog obliterates the view of the internal organs. (b) The pancreatic pseudocyst and small intestines have been externalized from the abdomen.

Surgical treatment

Pancreatic pseudocysts do not always necessitate treatment. Only if they increase in size, or if clinical signs of pancreatitis worsen, is ultrasound-guided aspiration of the lesion recommended. After percutaneous drainage the pseudocyst may resolve completely. If the pseudocyst fails to resolve after repeated drainage, surgical intervention may be necessary (see Operative Technique 11.3). Pancreatic abscesses are treated by complete excision, if possible, or by surgical drainage and omentalization.

Prognosis

The prognosis for dogs with pancreatic abscesses is guarded; survival rates range from 14–55% postoperatively. The prognosis for dogs that undergo surgical treatment (including repeated percutaneous aspiration) of pancreatic pseudocysts is better, with a 75% survival rate reported (Smith and Biller, 1998; VanEnkevort *et al.*, 1999; Anderson *et al.*, 2008; Thompson *et al.*, 2009).

References and further reading

Allenspach K, Arnold P, Glaus B *et al.* (2000) Glucagon-producing neuroendocrine tumour associated with hypoaminoacidaemia and skin lesions. *Journal of Small Animal Practice* **41**, 402–406

Altschul M, Simpson KW, Dykes NL *et al.* (1997) Evaluation of somatostatin analogues for the detection and treatment of gastrinoma in a dog. *Journal of Small Animal Practice* **38**, 286–291

Anderson JR, Cornell KK, Parnell NK *et al.* (2008) Pancreatic abscess in 36 dogs: a retrospective analysis of prognostic indicators. *Journal of the American Animal Hospital Association* **44**, 171–179

Barnes RF, Greenfield CL, Schaeffer DJ *et al.* (2006) Comparison of biopsy samples obtained using standard endoscopic instruments and the harmonic scalpel during laparoscopic and laparoscopic-assisted surgery in normal dogs. *Veterinary Surgery* **35**, 243–251

Buishand FO, Kik M and Kirpensteijn J (2010) Evaluation for clinico-pathological criteria and the Ki67 index as prognostic indicators in canine insulinoma. *The Veterinary Journal* **185**, 62–67

Buishand FO and Kirpensteijn J (2013) Canine and feline insulinoma. In: *Small Animal Soft Tissue Surgery, 1st edn*, ed. E Monnet, pp.32–42. Wiley-Blackwell, Ames

Buote NJ and Havig ME (2012) The use of vacuum-assisted closure in the management of septic peritonitis in six dogs. *Journal of the American Animal Hospital Association* **48**, 164–171

Cosford KL, Myers SSL, Taylor SM *et al.* (2010) Prospective evaluation of laparoscopic pancreatic biopsies in 11 healthy cats. *Journal of Veterinary Internal Medicine* **24**, 104–113

Etue SM, Penninck DG, Labato MA *et al.* (2001) Ultrasonography of the normal feline pancreas and associated anatomic landmarks: a prospective study of 20 cats. *Veterinary Radiology and Ultrasound* **42**, 330–336

Gross TL, O'Brien TD, Davies AP *et al.* (1990) Glucagon-producing pancreatic endocrine tumors in dogs with superficial necrolytic dermatitis. *Journal of the American Veterinary Medical Association* **197**, 1619–1622

Hughes SM (2006) Canine gastrinoma: a case study and literature review of therapeutic options. *New Zealand Veterinary Journal* **54**, 242–247

Iseri T, Yamada K, Chijiwa K *et al.* (2007) Dynamic computed tomography of the pancreas in normal dogs and in a dog with pancreatic insulinoma. *Veterinary Radiology and Ultrasound* **48**, 328–331

Kim JP and Byrne JJ (1971) Segmental venous drainage of the canine pancreas. *Journal of Surgical Research* **11**, 559–562

Knol JA, Strodel WE and Eckhauser FE (1987) Blood flow and distribution in the canine pancreas. *Journal of Surgical Research* **43**, 278–285

Lurye JC and Behrend EN (2001) Endocrine tumours. *Veterinary Clinics of North America: Small Animal Practice* **31**, 1083–1110

Mai W and Caceres AV (2008) Dual-phase computed tomographic angiography in three dogs with pancreatic insulinoma. *Veterinary Radiology and Ultrasound* **49**, 141–148

Oberkirchner U, Linder KE, Zadrozny L *et al.* (2010) Successful treatment of canine necrolytic migratory erythema (superficial necrolytic dermatitis) due to metastatic glucagonoma with octreotide. *Veterinary Dermatology* **21**, 510–516

Probst A and Kneissl S (2001) Computed tomographic anatomy of the canine pancreas. *Veterinary Radiology and Ultrasound* **42**, 226–230

Robben JH, Pollak YW, Kirpensteijn J *et al.* (2005) Comparison of ultrasonography, computed tomography, and single-photon emission computed tomography for detection and localization of canine insulinoma. *Journal of Veterinary Internal Medicine* **19**, 15–22

Smith SA and Biller DS (1998) Resolution of a pancreatic pseudocyst in a dog following percutaneous ultrasonographic-guided drainage. *Journal of the American Animal Hospital Association* **34**, 515–522

Spillman T (2013) Pancreatic biopsies. In: *Canine and Feline Gastroenterology*, ed. RJ Washabau and MJ Day, p.329. Elsevier, St Louis

Thompson LJ, Seshadri R and Raffe MR (2009) Characteristics and outcomes in surgical management of severe acute pancreatitis: 37 dogs (2001-2007). *Journal of Veterinary Emergency and Critical Care* **19**, 165–173

Thomson M (2003) Alimentary tract and pancreas. In: *Textbook of Small Animal Surgery, 3rd edn*, ed. D. Slatter, pp.2368–2376. Saunders, St Louis

Torres SMF, Caywood DD, O'Brien TD *et al.* (1997) Resolution of superficial necrolytic dermatitis following excision of a glucagon-secreting pancreatic neoplasm in a dog. *Journal of the American Animal Hospital Association* **33**, 313–319

Van Enkevort BA, O'Brien RT and Young KM (1999) Pancreatic pseudocysts in 4 dogs and 2 cats: ultrasonographic and clinicopathologic findings. *Journal of Veterinary Internal Medicine* **13**, 309–313

Van Schilfgaarde R, Gooszen HG, Overbosch EH *et al.* (1983) Arterial blood supply of the left lobe of the canine pancreas. I. Anatomic variations relevant to segmental transplantation. *Surgery* **93**, 545–548

Wouters EG, Buishand FO, Kik M *et al.* (2011) Use of a bipolar vessel-sealing device in resection of canine insulinoma. *Journal of Small Animal Practice* **52**, 139–145

OPERATIVE TECHNIQUE 11.1

Pancreatic biopsy

POSITIONING

Dorsal recumbency.

ASSISTANT

Optional.

EQUIPMENT EXTRAS

Suction; electrocautery; haemostatic gelatin sponge; malleable retractors; laparotomy swabs.

SURGICAL TECHNIQUE

Approach

Perform a ventral midline abdominal incision, extending from the xiphoid cartilage to caudal to the umbilicus.

Surgical manipulations

1   Retract the free portion of the greater omentum cranially and cover it with moist sponges. Grasp the descending duodenum and place it in the surgical field to expose the right pancreatic lobe. In order to expose the left pancreatic lobe, the omental leaf overlying the pancreas can be fenestrated. Isolate the intended biopsy site with laparotomy swabs.

→ **OPERATIVE TECHNIQUE 11.1 CONTINUED**

Handle the pancreatic tissue as gently as possible and lavage the tissue frequently with warm sterile isotonic saline

2 If diffuse pancreatic disease is present, the least traumatic and easiest method of obtaining a biopsy specimen is to remove a small portion of the tip of the right pancreatic lobe, using the suture–fracture technique. Incise the mesoduodenum or omentum on each side of the pancreas at the desired area, and pass a suture of a slowly absorbable suture material (e.g. polydioxanone) around the pancreas. Tighten the ligature, allowing it to crush though the pancreatic parenchyma, ligating the vessels and ducts. Then, excise the pancreatic tissue distal to the ligature. If minor bleeding persists at the biopsy site, place an absorbable gelatin sponge on the area.

PRACTICAL TIP

Avoid the use of rapidly absorbable suture materials (e.g. polyglactin 910 or poliglecaprone 25), because they are quickly digested by pancreatic enzymes

3 In the case of focal lesions not located at the caudal aspects of the pancreatic lobes, the biopsy sample can be taken using the dissection–ligation technique. The pancreatic capsule is incised and bluntly dissected down to the pancreatic duct and vessels. The duct and vessels are individually ligated, using double ligatures, and then transected between the two ligatures.

PRACTICAL TIPS

* Given that pancreatitis can be a localized or a multifocal disease, multiple biopsy samples should be taken if there are no obvious pancreatic lesions
* Alternatively, blood vessel-sealing devices (e.g. LigaSure™, or Harmonic® scalpel) and surgical staplers can be used to obtain large pancreatic biopsy specimens

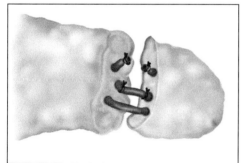

The pancreatic vessels are individually ligated and transected between the double ligatures.

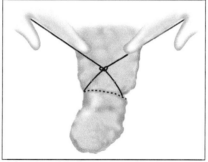

Tightening of the ligatures crushes the pancreatic parenchyma.

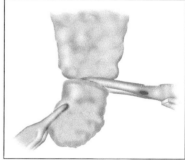

Pancreatic tissue distal to the ligature is transected.

Wound closure

Routine abdominal closure is performed.

POSTOPERATIVE MANAGEMENT

Although, historically, it has been suggested that food should be withheld for 24–48 hours after surgery to reduce pancreatic secretions, there is no evidence that this is the case. In the authors' experience, offering a bland diet immediately after recovery is well sustained by patients. If a patient refuses to eat, balanced electrolyte solutions should be administered intravenously until oral intake of food and water resumes. Furthermore, in cases where patients show clinical signs of pancreatitis (i.e. abdominal pain, lethargy, vomiting and anorexia) for more than 24 hours postoperatively, further diagnostics, including measurement of serum lipase activity, should be performed. In patients with vomiting and inappetence, additional therapy with ranitidine, maropitant and metoclopramide is indicated for several days. Care should be taken when using metoclopramide because it may induce vasoconstriction and potentially exacerbate pancreatitis.

OPERATIVE TECHNIQUE 11.2

Partial pancreatectomy

POSITIONING

Dorsal recumbency.

ASSISTANT

Essential.

EQUIPMENT EXTRAS

Suction; electrocautery; haemostatic gelatin sponge; malleable retractors; laparotomy swabs.

SURGICAL TECHNIQUE

Approach

Perform a ventral midline abdominal incision, extending from the xiphoid cartilage to caudal to the umbilicus.

Surgical manipulations

1 Thoroughly examine and gently palpate the entire pancreas to detect masses. In addition, thoroughly explore the rest of the abdomen with an emphasis on the regional lymph nodes and liver, to check for any possible metastases.

> **WARNING**
>
> If tumours cannot be identified on careful inspection and palpation of the pancreas, an intravenous infusion of methylene blue (3 mg/kg, administered over 30–40 minutes) reveals most neoplastic tissue. However, since intravenous methylene blue has been found to induce fatal haemolytic anaemia or acute renal failure, its use is not routinely recommended. Alternatively, intraoperative ultrasonographic examination of the pancreas can be useful

2 If an electrothermal bipolar device (e.g. LigaSure™ V) or Harmonic® scalpel is not available, remove the mass by the suture–fracture method, as described in Operative Technique 11.1. If the mass is located in the body of the pancreas, or in the most proximal portions (i.e. close to the body) of the right and left lobes, local enucleation using the dissection–ligation technique should be considered.

> **WARNING**
>
> Extreme caution should be taken to prevent damage to the ductal system and the pancreaticoduodenal arteries when a mass has to be resected from the corpus or the most proximal portions of the right and left pancreatic lobes

3 If using an electrothermal bipolar device (e.g. Ligasure™ V), the pancreatic parenchyma is grasped with the jaws of the device. A calibrated force is applied to the tissue by closing the jaws of the device. Coagulation is initiated and haemostasis is obtained at the same time as the tissue is sealed. Cutting is carried out by the device when the audible signal indicates the correct impedance of the pancreatic tissue, indicating that the vessels and ducts are sealed. The procedure is repeated until the entire nodule is freed from pancreatic tissue (nodulectomy) or the pancreatic lobe is severed in a perpendicular fashion.

> **WARNING**
>
> Although it might be tempting to remove a mass located in the middle of either pancreatic lobe *en bloc* with the surrounding pancreatic tissue while leaving the most distal part of the pancreas in place, such segmental pancreatectomy is not indicated. The distal part of the pancreas may still have an adequate blood supply but often has no ductal structure that leads to the duodenum. Therefore there is a high risk of local pancreatitis or sterile pancreatic abscesses after segmental pancreatectomy

→ **OPERATIVE TECHNIQUE 11.2 CONTINUED**

4 After removal of the primary pancreatic mass, remove enlarged local lymph nodes. Potential macrometastatic nodules in the liver, identified as round white to yellowish foci, should also be removed. Hepatic nodules can be removed by partial or complete lobectomy (see Chapter 9); however, ablating the nodules using the non-contact mode of an Nd:YAG (neodymium-doped:yttrium–aluminium–garnet) 1064nm surgical laser is preferred by the authors.

5 Prior to closure, lavage the abdomen with copious volumes of warm, sterile saline.

Wound closure

Abdominal closure is routine.

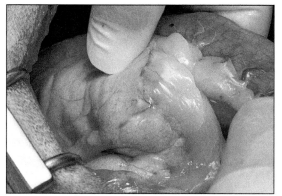

Outprojection of a canine insulinoma in the right pancreatic lobe.

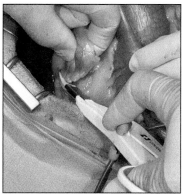

The electrothermal biopolar device allows rapid resection of the insulinoma.

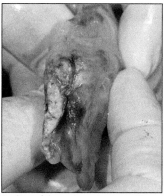

Sealing of the removed pancreatic lobe following application of the bipolar device.

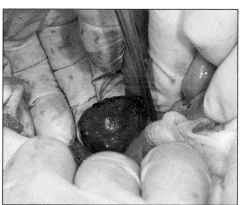

Removal of an enlarged pancreaticoduodenal lymph node in a dog with an insulinoma. Excision and histopathology of the node revealed metastasis of the insulinoma.

POSTOPERATIVE MANAGEMENT

After insulinoma resection, blood glucose levels should be closely monitored. If glucose levels are very low (<2 mmol/l) and the patient refuses to eat or demonstrates clinical signs of hypoglycaemia, the dog should be stabilized by intravenous infusion of a balanced electrolyte solution containing 5% dextrose. Therapy with diazoxide (5–30 mg/kg q12h) should also be initiated. Intravenous glucose can be discontinued if the animal has a stable and normal glucose level, or if the patient becomes hyperglycaemic.

OPERATIVE TECHNIQUE 11.3

Debridement/omentalization of pancreatic abscesses or pseudocysts

POSITIONING

Dorsal recumbency.

ASSISTANT

Essential.

EQUIPMENT EXTRAS

Suction; electrocautery; haemostatic gelatin sponge; malleable retractors; laparotomy swabs; culture swabs.

SURGICAL TECHNIQUE

Approach

Perform a ventral midline abdominal incision, extending from the xiphoid cartilage to caudal to the umbilicus.

Surgical manipulations

1 Expose the right pancreatic lobe by retracting the duodenum ventrally into the abdominal incision.

2 Expose the left pancreatic lobe by retracting the stomach and greater omentum cranially, while retracting the transverse colon caudally.

3 Carefully explore the abdomen and gently examine the pancreas for masses and abscesses. Gently remove omental adhesions to the pancreatic lesion using a combination of blunt and sharp dissection. Take care not to disrupt the pancreatic blood supply, pancreatic ducts or common bile ducts during dissection.

> **PRACTICAL TIP**
>
> It is essential to collect samples of fluid or tissue for bacterial culture and sensitivity testing. All tissues should be submitted for histopathology

4 Carefully debride necrotic tissue and purulent pancreatic areas. Flush with warm sterile saline.

5 After debridement, consider omentalization of pancreatic abscesses or cysts. Omentum should be mobilized, packed into the cystic area and sutured to the cyst wall with simple interrupted sutures (preferably using polydioxanone).

6 Gently express the gallbladder to determine whether the common bile duct is patent. If the common bile duct is obstructed, catheterize the duct (see Chapter 9). Consider performing a cholecystoenterostomy if patency of the bile duct cannot be obtained by catheterization.

7 If generalized peritonitis is present, thoroughly lavage the peritoneal cavity with copious volumes of warm sterile saline.

Wound closure

If severe septic peritonitis is present, consider establishing abdominal drainage by placing a Jackson–Pratt or sump drain, or by leaving the abdomen open. Alternatively, close the abdomen routinely, following lavage.

POSTOPERATIVE MANAGEMENT

Continue medical treatment for pancreatitis (intravenous fluids, analgesics, antibiotics if infection is found, and a diet low in protein and fat to limit stimulation of pancreatic secretions).

Chapter 12

The spleen

Jacqui D. Niles

Surgical conditions of the spleen are commonly encountered in small animal practice. In some instances splenic biopsy or partial splenectomy may be warranted, but in most cases splenectomy is the treatment of choice. The spleen is a part of the reticuloendothelial system and, although it has several important functions, it is not essential for life. Overwhelming septicaemia, occasionally observed in humans after splenectomy, has not been reported following splenectomy in dogs or cats.

Anatomy

The spleen is suspended by the greater omentum and is attached to the greater curvature of the stomach by the gastrosplenic ligament (Figure 12.1). The spleen is usually located in the left cranial quadrant of the abdomen in the dog and cat, although the position can vary owing to the mobile nature of the abdominal organs. It can be located under the rib cage if the stomach is empty but in the presence of gastric distension it may move to a more caudal position within the abdomen.

The spleen is normally firm and red, but it may have white fibrin deposits or yellowish-brown siderotic plaques (iron and calcium deposits) on its surface (Figure 12.2). The blood supply is via the splenic artery, which arises from the coeliac artery and supplies branches to the left lobe of the pancreas as it courses to the splenic hilus (Figure 12.3). As the splenic artery terminates at the spleen, it divides into a dorsal and ventral branch. The dorsal branch

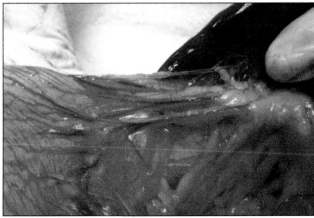

12.1 Gastrosplenic ligament containing the short gastric arteries and veins.

continues to the dorsal portion of the spleen and gives off the short gastric arteries. The ventral branch gives off the left gastroepiploic artery before it contacts the spleen. Venous drainage from the spleen is via the gastrosplenic vein, which empties into the portal vein.

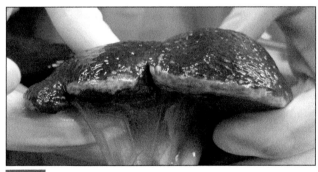

12.2 Siderotic plaques on the tail of the spleen.

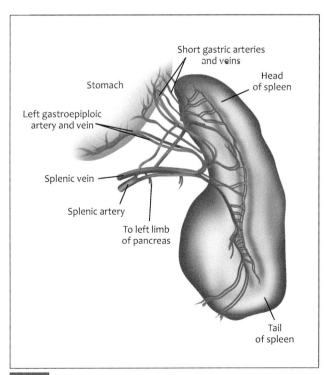

12.3 The blood supply to the spleen.

Short gastric arteries and veins

Head of spleen

Stomach

Left gastroepiploic artery and vein

Splenic vein

Splenic artery

To left limb of pancreas

Tail of spleen

The spleen is composed of a capsule (elastic and smooth muscle fibres), internal trabeculae (collagen, elastin and smooth muscle fibres) and parenchyma (white and red pulp). Unlike in the human spleen, the abundance of smooth muscle cells in the spleen of cats and dogs enables it to contract and relax under the control of alpha-adrenergic receptors.

Function

The two components of the splenic parenchyma have separate functions. The white pulp is lymphoid tissue, and is a major site of trapping and immunological recognition of blood-borne antigens and antibody production. The red pulp is composed of venous sinuses and cellular tissue (consisting of red and white blood cells, megakaryocytes and macrophages) filling the intravascular spaces. It serves as a reservoir of erythrocytes and platelets and is also a highly efficient filter that clears circulating blood of particulate matter, such as bacteria and aged or damaged blood cells. The functions of the spleen include the following:

- Blood filtration
- Phagocytosis of aged or damaged red blood cells, parasites, bacteria and other particles
- Extramedullary haemopoiesis. This function normally ceases after birth and the bone marrow takes over the role; however, if bone marrow haemopoiesis is disrupted (e.g. myeloproliferative diseases, immune-mediated haemolysis, immune-mediated thrombocytopenia, chronic inflammatory or infectious diseases) the spleen can resume a limited degree of haemopoietic activity
- Erythrocyte and platelet storage. Dog and cat spleens have large sinusoidal spaces that can store between 10% and 20% of the circulating red blood cell mass and 30% of the total platelet mass. Splenic contraction mobilizes the stored blood under conditions of stress, hypoxaemia or blood loss to maintain appropriate circulating volume and oxygen-carrying capacity
- Immune functions. The spleen produces the majority of B and T lymphocytes in adult animals and the germinal centres of the spleen are the major sites of immunoglobulin M production
- Miscellaneous functions, including iron metabolism, regulation of angiotensin-converting enzyme levels, storage and activation of factor VIII.

Surgical techniques

Surgical biopsy

See Operative Technique 12.1. Indications for splenic biopsy include:

- Evaluation of nodular or focal masses
- Evaluation of clinically significant diffuse splenomegaly or abnormal ultrasonographic echogenicity
- Confirmation of any suspected metastatic lesions of the spleen.

Via a ventral midline laparotomy, biopsy samples from focal lesions may be taken with a core biopsy needle or using a skin biopsy punch (see Chapter 9).

Partial splenectomy

Partial splenectomy is indicated in animals with traumatic or focal lesions of the spleen, such as an isolated abscess. Although performed rarely, a partial splenectomy (see Operative Technique 12.1) allows preservation of splenic function. It is not recommended for splenic neoplasia even though the tumour mass may grossly involve only one portion of the spleen. Several techniques have been reported, differing in the method by which the parenchyma is transected and handled.

Splenectomy

Complete splenectomy is the most commonly performed splenic surgery (see Operative Technique 12.2). The two most commonly performed techniques involve either individual ligation of the hilar vessels or ligation of the major splenic arteries and veins as well as the short gastric arteries. Individual ligation of the hilar vessels is time-consuming and studies have shown that gastric blood flow is not compromised by ligation of the short gastric arteries and veins, or the left gastroepiploic artery and vein.

Absorbable monofilament suture material is most widely used for vessel ligation when performing splenectomy but there are a variety of other techniques available, including the use of metal haemostatic clips, mono- and bipolar electrocautery and ultrasonic-activated scalpels (see Chapter 9). Haemostatic clips can be placed rapidly but can be un-stable and may be removed or dislodged easily. They should only be used on vessels less than 3–4 mm in diameter. Ultrasonic scalpels can seal vessels up to 5 mm in diameter; thus, ligatures are required for adequate haemostasis of the splenic artery and vein in large dogs. Recently, the use of a bipolar vessel sealant device was described for splenectomy in dogs (Rivier and Monnet, 2011). These devices involve an electrothermal bipolar sealing system, which achieves haemostasis by compression of vessels in the jaws of the instrument and heat-induced fusion of collagen and elastin in the vessel walls. In human patients, vessels up to 7 mm in diameter can be safely coagulated. In the report by Rivier and Monnet (2011), the splenic artery was sealed three times with an overlap of the seals, and the vein was sealed twice. None of the dogs required any vessel ligation with suture material but one dog developed a haemoabdomen postoperatively. Until more studies are performed, the routine use of bipolar vessel-sealing devices cannot currently be recommended for ligation of the main splenic artery and vein.

Indications for total splenectomy include:

- Splenic neoplasia
- Splenic rupture secondary to trauma
- Splenic torsion.

In the USA, elective splenectomy may be performed in dogs used as blood donors to prevent the spread of infections involving *Haemobartonella canis* or *Babesia canis*.

The major disadvantages of splenectomy are the loss of the reservoir, immuno defence, haemopoiesis and filtration functions. Splenectomy is contraindicated in patients with immune-mediated haemolytic anaemia or thrombocytopenia unless other forms of treatment (e.g. immunosuppressive drugs) have failed. It is also contraindicated for patients with bone marrow hypoplasia; in these patients the spleen is the main site of haemopoiesis.

Laparoscopy

Splenic biopsy and partial and complete splenectomy using laparascopic equipment has been described in both the dog and the cat (Khalaj *et al.*, 2012; Radhakrishnan and Mayhew, 2013). These techniques are not applicable in cases where emergency treatment of a haemoabdomen associated with a ruptured splenic mass is required.

Splenic conditions

In the majority of cases, splenic disease results in either diffuse or focal splenic enlargement (Figure 12.4). It is worth noting that dogs more frequently have focal splenic enlargement while cats more frequently have diffuse splenic enlargement. A wide range of conditions can cause diffuse splenomegaly (Figure 12.5). Causes of focal splenic enlargement are listed in Figure 12.6. In one study, the pathological findings in 87 dogs with splenic abnormalities revealed that the most common diagnosis was splenic neoplasia (*n* = 38) and the most frequently recognized canine splenic neoplasm was haemangiosarcoma (HSA; 17 of 38 cases). Benign splenic enlargement secondary to nodular hyperplasia, haematoma or non-specific changes, including congestion, haemorrhage, extramedullary haemopoiesis and haemosiderin deposition, was also recognized (Day *et al.*, 1995).

Clinical signs and diagnosis

Clinical signs are variable and often non-specific in animals with splenic disease. Subtle signs, such as abdominal distension, anorexia, lethargy, polydipsia, vomiting or

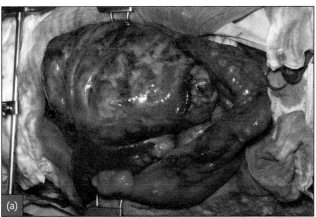

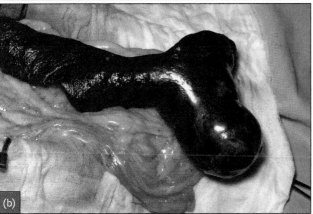

12.4 (a) Diffuse splenomegaly due to an undifferentiated sarcoma. (b) Focal splenomegaly due to a splenic haemangiosarcoma.

Infiltrative [a]	• Neoplastic – leukaemia, lymphoma, systemic mastocytosis, multiple myeloma, malignant histiocytosis (dogs) • Non-neoplastic – extramedullary haemopoiesis, hypereosinophilic syndrome (cats)
Infectious	• Bacterial – septicaemia • Viral – feline infectious peritonitis (caused by feline coronavirus; cats), infectious canine hepatitis (dogs) • Parasitic – *Haemobartonella* • Fungal – histoplasmosis and blastomycosis (USA)
Hyperplastic	• Immune-mediated – haemolytic anaemia or thrombocytopenia • Hypersplenism – can be primary but splenomegaly is usually secondary to an underlying disease process that causes any combination of anaemia, leucopenia and thrombocytopenia, with secondary bone marrow hyperplasia and resolution of cytopenia following splenectomy
Congestive	• Splenic torsion – alone or in conjunction with gastric dilatation and volvulus (GDV) • Portal hypertension – secondary to right-sided heart failure or caudal vena cava obstruction • Drug-induced – barbiturates or tranquilizers

12.5 Causes of diffuse splenic enlargement. [a] Most common causes of splenomegaly.

Neoplastic (primary or metastatic)
• Haemangiosarcoma • Haemangioma • Sarcoma
Non-neoplastic
• Nodular hyperplasia (can be single or multiple benign accumulations of lymphoid cells and is the most commonly encountered splenic mass in dogs) • Haematoma (may be the result of trauma) • Abscess (rare) • Fibrohistiocytic nodules (hyperplastic lymphoid proliferation containing distinct population of spindle cells)

12.6 Causes of focal splenic enlargement.

depression, may be noted, or the patient may present with acute signs of weakness or collapse associated with haemorrhage from a ruptured HSA. In these cases the history may also reveal intermittent episodes of weakness or collapse, often with spontaneous recovery within 12–24 hours. These episodes are associated with haemorrhage and subsequent blood reabsorption.

Physical examination findings in animals with splenic disease include:

* Abdominal distension (due to either splenic enlargement or haemorrhage)
* Pain on abdominal palpation
* Pale mucous membranes
* Petechiae or ecchymoses
* Enlarged peripheral lymph nodes
* Fever.

The normal spleen can be palpated in many animals and splenomegaly may often be detected on abdominal palpation. Additional diagnostic imaging modalities are frequently required for definitive diagnosis of splenic enlargement. Care should be taken when assessing splenic size in the anaesthetized patient because the use of barbiturates and propofol may lead to significant splenomegaly.

Radiography and ultrasonography

Abdominal radiographs often reveal an abdominal mass; however, ultrasonography is regarded as more useful in all cases and particularly when there is a significant haemo-abdomen. Ultrasonography is especially useful for localizing a mass to the spleen, performing needle aspiration and evaluating the rest of the abdomen for the presence of metastasis (Figure 12.7). Additionally, the parenchyma of the spleen and vasculature can be assessed, which may aid in the diagnosis of splenic torsion. Advanced imaging techniques, such as computed tomography (CT) (Figure 12.8) or magnetic resonance imaging (MRI), readily demonstrate splenic enlargement but their use is rarely necessary or practical.

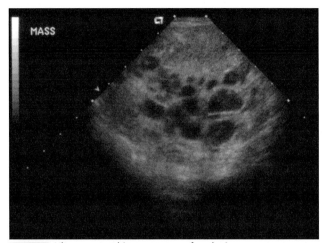

12.7 Ultrasonographic appearance of a splenic haemangiosarcoma.

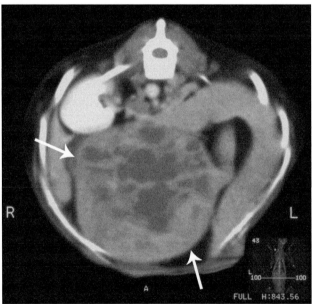

12.8 CT scan showing a large splenic mass localized to one end of the spleen (arrowed).

Biopsy

Splenic biopsy is indicated to ascertain the cause of clinically significant splenomegaly or to evaluate suspected metastatic lesions. Biopsy may be performed percutaneously by fine-needle aspiration, or at surgery. Use of ultrasound guidance improves the likelihood of obtaining diagnostic samples percutaneously because it allows focal lesions to be targeted; it is also of diagnostic value for diffuse lesions, but it should be noted that some focal lesions may be missed. The technique for fine-needle aspiration is as follows:

1. Place the animal in right lateral or dorsal recumbency, using manual restraint or mild sedation. Avoid using phenothiazine tranquillizers or barbiturates, because the resultant splenic congestion may cause a non-diagnostic sample due to blood dilution.
2. Surgically prepare a small area on the side of the abdomen and isolate the spleen.
3. Using a syringe attached to a 23–25 G needle (2.5–3.5 cm; 1–1.5 inches), penetrate the abdominal wall and advance the needle into the spleen. Apply suction several times.
4. Before removing the needle from the abdomen, relieve suction on the syringe to prevent aspiration of the contents of the needle into the syringe.

WARNING

Splenic aspiration is contraindicated in animals with cavitary lesions. The lesions may rupture during the procedure and this may be fatal, especially in animals with coagulopathies

Splenic torsion

Splenic torsion, or rotation of the spleen about its vascular pedicle, is an uncommon condition most frequently reported in large- or giant-breed dogs. German Shepherd Dogs and Great Danes appear to be predisposed (Neath *et al.*, 1997). It is frequently associated with gastric dilatation and volvulus (GDV; see Chapter 6) but can also occur in the absence of GDV. Primary splenic torsion occurs in both acute and chronic forms and can be difficult to diagnose, owing to the non-specific and sometimes chronic or intermittent clinical signs.

Acute splenic torsion usually causes severe abdominal pain and cardiovascular collapse over a few hours.

- Signs include weakness, salivation, retching and collapse.
- Dogs may present with pale mucous membranes, poor capillary refill, tachycardia and abdominal splinting.
- An enlarged spleen may be palpable.
- Bloodwork is often unremarkable.

In *chronic splenic torsion* the signs are vague:

- Dogs present with lethargy, depression and anorexia. They may also vomit intermittently or have diarrhoea
- Acute deterioration can occur
- Reported bloodwork abnormalities include anaemia, leucocytosis, haemoglobinaemia, and elevated serum alkaline phosphatase (ALP) and alanine aminotransferase (ALT) levels. Pancreatic enzyme concentrations (amylase and lipase) may also be elevated.

Radiographs often show a cranial to mid-abdominal mass, absence of the normal splenic silhouette, or a C-shaped spleen (Figure 12.9a). In cases of chronic splenic torsion, infarction and ischaemia can lead to gas densities in the region of the spleen. Abdominal detail may be poor as a result of peritoneal effusion. Ultrasonography may reveal diffuse splenomegaly and a hypoechoic pattern in the splenic parenchyma. Colour-flow Doppler ultrasonography is most reliable for diagnosis. In a study by Neath *et al.* (1997), decreased blood flow in the splenic veins was demonstrated in 92% of cases, and intravascular thrombi in 50% of cases. In cases where abdominal radiography and ultrasonography are not conclusive, contrast-enhanced CT has been used to demonstrate torsion of the splenic pedicle (Patsikas *et al.*, 2001). A corkscrew-like soft tissue mass representing the splenic pedicle, in conjunction with lack of contrast enhancement of the splenic parenchyma, is considered pathognomonic for the condition.

Treatment of acute or chronic splenic torsion is by splenectomy (Figure 12.9b). Animals that present with acute collapse and hypotension should be stabilized prior to surgery, and careful monitoring for cardiac arrhythmias should be carried out in the pre-, peri- and immediate postoperative period.

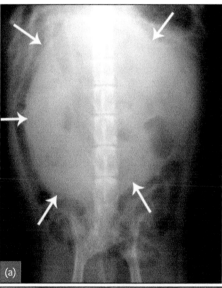

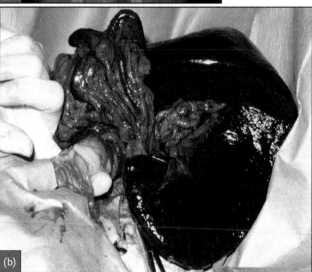

12.9 Splenic torsion. (a) Ventrodorsal abdominal radiograph of a dog with splenic torsion. Note the C-shaped spleen (arrowed). (b) Splenic pedicle; note the 'corkscrew' appearance.
(b, Courtesy of S Birchard)

> **WARNING**
>
> The splenic pedicle should not be untwisted prior to splenectomy. This can cause the release of thrombi, free radicals, toxins and vasoactive compounds such as tumour necrosis factor from the ischaemic spleen into the portal circulation

The splenic pedicle should be gradually divided and ligated to achieve adequate haemostasis. Mass ligation should be avoided.

> **PRACTICAL TIP**
>
> Although the relationship between splenic torsion and GDV is not clear, it has been suggested that repeated episodes of gastric dilatation may stretch the gastrosplenic ligament sufficiently to allow splenic hypermotility. Since deep-chested breeds of dog present with splenic torsion, prophylactic gastropexy should be considered at the time of splenectomy

The prognosis for acute splenic torsion is variable and dogs may develop splenic necrosis, sepsis, pancreatitis, peritonitis and/or disseminated intravascular coagulation (DIC). Chronic splenic torsion usually carries a good prognosis because these cases tend to have a lower incidence of cardiovascular shock and toxaemia than cases of acute splenic torsion.

Splenic infarction

Splenic infarction can occur in association with splenic torsion, but infarction without torsion is a rarely described condition. In one retrospective study (Hardie *et al.*, 1995), 16 dogs with splenic infarction were identified. These dogs often had multiple concurrent diseases, including cardiac, renal or liver disease, neoplasia, or evidence of sepsis, coagulopathy or vasculitis. Clinical findings included anorexia, intermittent vomiting, lethargy, diarrhoea, pale mucous membranes, abdominal mass, effusion or pain, cardiac arrhythmias, polyuria, polydipsia and fever. However, it was difficult to determine which findings were due to splenic infarction and which were due to the concurrent disease.

Ultrasound examination findings include thrombosis within a splenic vein, loss of blood flow to a section of spleen, a diffuse 'lacy' appearance throughout the spleen, or an enlarged hypoechoic ventral extremity.

At surgery infarctions can be nodular or wedge-shaped with the base at the periphery (Figure 12.10) and can involve an extremity or the entire organ. Given that

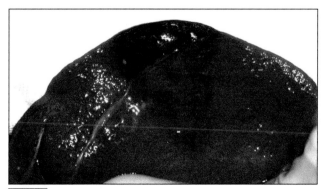

12.10 Wedge-shaped splenic infarct.

splenic infarction is regarded as an indicator of altered blood flow and coagulation abnormalities, rather than as a primary disease, surgery carries a high mortality rate in these patients. Medical management is often preferable to splenectomy. Surgery should be reserved for animals with life-threatening complications such as haemoperitoneum or sepsis.

Splenic trauma

Traumatic injury to the spleen is uncommonly reported. Mild trauma can result in the formation of a subcapsular haematoma. Major trauma may result in deep parenchymal lacerations or crush injury associated with life-threatening haemorrhage. If the animal fails to respond to conservative therapy, partial or complete splenectomy may be indicated. In humans, preservation of splenic function is of primary importance. Splenic lacerations can be repaired with absorbable sutures or by 'splenic wrapping', which involves wrapping the spleen in a mesh bag made from absorbable suture material.

Splenic trauma can lead to dissemination of splenic tissue throughout the abdominal cavity and the subsequent development of 'splenosis', in which pieces of splenic tissue remain viable, suspended within the omentum. This is often found incidentally during abdominal exploratory surgery.

Splenic neoplasia

Splenic neoplasia is the most common reason for performing a total splenectomy in general practice. Tumours of the spleen may arise from a variety of tissues, including blood vessels, lymphoid tissue, smooth muscle and connective tissue. Non-neoplastic lesions include hyperplastic lymphoid nodules (which can be single or multiple, and are an uncommon problem in cats), haemangiomas, hamartomas and haematomas. The most common malignant splenic tumour in dogs is HSA, accounting for up to 80% of splenic malignancies identified (Weinstein *et al.*, 1989). Other malignant neoplasms include lymphosarcoma, mast cell tumour, leiomyosarcoma, fibrosarcoma, liposarcoma, osteosarcoma, chondrosarcoma, myxosarcoma, rhabdomyosarcoma and fibrous histiocytoma. In a recent study of 249 dogs with splenic masses, 117 dogs (47%) had non-malignant masses (nodular hyperplasia, haematoma, splenitis) and 132 dogs (53%) had malignant tumours, among which HSA was the most common (Eberle *et al.*, 2012). Splenic tumours reported in cats include lymphosarcoma and mast cell tumours, but HSAs are rare.

Haemangiosarcoma

HSA is a highly malignant tumour derived from vascular endothelial cells and is characterized by early and aggressive metastasis. It is usually seen in older large-breed dogs, but there are sporadic reports of HSAs occurring in younger animals. German Shepherd Dogs are predisposed. Other commonly reported breeds include Golden Retriever, Pointer, Boxer, Labrador Retriever, English Setter, Great Dane, Poodle and Siberian Husky (Brown *et al.*, 1985).

HSAs can arise in any tissue with blood vessels, but the most common sites in dogs are the spleen (50–60%), right atrium (3–25%), subcutaneous tissues (13–17%) and liver (5–6%) (Brown, 1985).

> **WARNING**
>
> HSAs tend to metastasize rapidly via haematogenous routes to the liver, omentum (Figure 12.11), mesentery and lungs; overt metastasis is present in >80% of canine patients at clinical presentation (MacEwen, 2001)

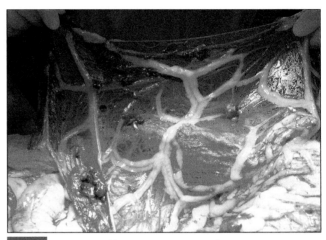

12.11 Metastasis of haemangiosarcoma to the omentum.

In dogs, HSA is considered the sarcoma most likely to metastasize to the brain. Splenic and atrial masses coexist in up to 25% of dogs with HSA (Walters *et al.*, 1988), although whether one site is primary or whether multicentric HSA has developed is usually undetermined.

HSAs can be single or multiple in any organ and vary in size. They may contain areas of haemorrhage or necrosis, are poorly circumscribed and non-encapsulated and often adhere to adjacent organs.

> **WARNING**
>
> Splenic haematoma and haemangioma must be differentiated from HSA. Haematomas are also seen in older large-breed dogs and have a clinical appearance that resembles HSA. It is not possible to differentiate between these lesions by direct visualization

Histopathological examination of tissues is required to diagnose HSA or any other tumour type definitively. An excisional biopsy is preferred because it is both a diagnostic and a therapeutic procedure.

Clinical signs: Clinical signs most commonly reported in association with HSA include:

- Weakness
- Distension of the abdomen
- Increased pulse and respiratory rate
- Pale mucous membranes
- Tachypnoea
- Weight loss
- Sudden death.

Dogs with concurrent right atrial HSA may develop pericardial effusion and present with muffled heart sounds, arrhythmias and signs of right-sided heart failure.

The majority of all naturally occurring deaths from HSA are associated with haemorrhage due to tumour rupture, or DIC. Haematological abnormalities in dogs with splenic HSA are listed in Figure 12.12.

Abnormality	Percentage
Anaemia	68%
Thrombocytopenia	51%
Increased reticulocyte count	22%
Neutrophilia	67%
Increase in band neutrophils	70%

12.12 Haematological abnormalities in dogs with splenic haemangiosarcoma.

Treatment: Splenectomy is the treatment of choice for an animal with a suspected splenic HSA (see Operative Technique 12.2). The surgery should be as radical as possible to remove all locally affected tissue. Additionally, a biopsy should be performed on any suspicious lesions in the liver or omentum. Animals that present in acute hypovolaemic shock should be stabilized initially. Management of patients with haemoperitoneum is discussed below.

Prognosis: The prognosis for dogs with splenic HSA following surgery alone is very poor, with median survival times of 19–86 days (MacEwen, 2001). Death is usually due to metastatic disease. With the addition of chemotherapy following splenectomy, survival times of 141–179 days have been reported (MacEwen, 2001). Despite aggressive surgery and/or chemotherapy, survival times are short for almost all forms of primary HSA, with <10% of dogs surviving a year or longer.

Haemoperitoneum

Numerous diseases can result in a haemoperitoneum (Figure 12.13). The most common differential diagnoses include a bleeding neoplasm (HSA, hepatoma), coagulopathy (rodenticides) and trauma. Specific treatments are indicated for each final diagnosis. In general, neoplasia, GDV, splenic torsion and liver lobe torsion are treated surgically. Coagulopathy disorders are considered nonsurgical. Trauma is usually managed conservatively. If the patient fails to stabilize, abdominal exploratory surgery may be warranted.

Traumatic
- Damage to the liver, spleen or kidneys can occur from blunt or penetrating trauma
- Breakdown in surgical haemostasis
- Haemorrhage from a biopsy site

Non-traumatic
- Neoplasia – splenic (HSA/haematoma), hepatic, renal, adrenal gland
- Other diseases – GDV, splenic torsion, liver lobe torsion
- Coagulopathies – congenital, acquired

12.13 Causes of haemoperitoneum.

Initially, the patient presenting with haemoperitoneum may be difficult to differentiate from other causes of acute abdomen (see Chapter 18). However, these patients usually present with pale mucous membranes, prolonged capillary refill time, severe lethargy or collapse, distended abdomen, fluid wave on ballottement, weak peripheral pulses, tachycardia and tachypnoea. A thorough history should be obtained immediately upon patient presentation. It may reveal recent trauma or surgery, documented splenic masses, episodes of collapse, coagulopathy or rodenticide consumption (Spangler and Kass, 1997). Patient signalment is inconsistent, but breed and age predilections exist for some neoplastic and congenital coagulopathy disorders.

Diagnosis

Confirming a suspected haemoperitoneum when a large amount of free abdominal fluid is evident on physical examination simply requires abdominocentesis.

Diagnosis of the underlying cause is often more complicated. Cytological evaluation of the fluid will reveal numerous red blood cells, though occasionally neoplastic cells may be identified. It is important to remember that false negatives can occur with this technique. The abdomen has a tremendous capacity for absorbing and storing fluid. Failure to obtain blood on aspiration does not rule out haemoperitoneum. Diagnostic peritoneal lavage (DPL) is typically performed if abdominocentesis results are negative (see Chapter 18).

Haematology

A complete blood count may reveal changes in PCV. It is important to note that such changes can be variable, depending on the hydration status of the patient, underlying disease processes and time since onset of haemorrhage. For instance, dehydration may cause both PCV and total protein to increase owing to haemoconcentration. Patients with dehydration and haemorrhage may have a normal PCV. Persistent underlying diseases may contribute to an anaemia of chronic inflammatory disease, making a single PCV result difficult to interpret. Additionally, splenic contraction (a normal canine response to increased circulating catecholamines) may release enough red blood cells systemically to maintain a normal PCV for a short time in the face of acute haemorrhage. Perhaps more beneficial in the diagnosis of ongoing bleeding related to haemoperitoneum is serial monitoring of PCV and total protein. A recent study showed that dogs with splenic HSAs had significantly lower total protein and platelet counts than dogs with other splenic masses (Hammond and Pesillo-Crosby, 2008).

Less precipitous reductions of PCV can also suggest active bleeding. Moreover, serial PCVs, taken 10–30 minutes apart, may allow the clinician to decide whether medical or surgical intervention is most appropriate. Lastly, a serum chemistry panel and urinalysis need to be performed to evaluate the patient for any underlying disease processes.

> **PRACTICAL TIP**
>
> A coagulation panel should be performed for all patients with haemoperitoneum

Cardiac abnormalities

Cardiac auscultation may reveal a heart murmur. Left-sided physiological heart murmurs are commonly heard in patients with anaemia. An electrocardiogram (ECG) monitor may reveal cardiac arrhythmias. Ventricular premature contractions are commonly observed in patients with several disease processes, including haemoperitoneum, HSA, GDV, pancreatitis, trauma and mesenteric volvulus.

Diagnostic imaging

Frequently, abdominal masses can be diagnosed on plain abdominal radiographs, although fluid in the abdomen can reduce abdominal detail and give a 'ground glass' appearance. Patients that have suffered trauma, have abdominal masses or have a suspected coagulopathy should undergo thoracic radiography to rule out additional problems in the chest. Ultrasonography may be a more useful modality for imaging of a haemoperitoneum. Importantly, free abdominal fluid does not distort the image. Additionally, ultrasonography can be used to guide a needle for abdominocentesis. Serial abdominal ultrasound examinations have been used to determine whether there is ongoing abdominal haemorrhage.

Management

Patients with haemoperitoneum may have numerous presentations, depending on the disease process and rate of haemorrhage. Some patients are critical at presentation, while others are very stable. However, all haemoperitoneum cases should be treated very seriously. Typically, rapid therapeutic measures, including administration of intravenous crystalloids, colloids and blood products, should be initiated (see Chapter 4 and the *BSAVA Manual of Canine and Feline Emergency and Critical Care* for further information).

Oxygen support should always accompany resuscitation of a haemorrhaging patient. Severely anaemic patients lack adequate oxygen-carrying capacity, and 100% oxygen can be supplemented via a face cone, nasal catheter or oxygen cage to improve the partial pressure of oxygen. Surgery is indicated in patients with haemoperitoneum due to a bleeding splenic neoplasm. Suction should be used to clear the abdominal cavity, and the spleen, liver, kidneys and omentum should be checked thoroughly. Following identification of a bleeding splenic neoplasm, the spleen should be removed as efficiently as possible. Splenectomy is often complicated by the presence of omental adhesions (Figure 12.14). If possible, the omentum should not be peeled off the spleen; rather, it should be divided, ligated and removed concurrently.

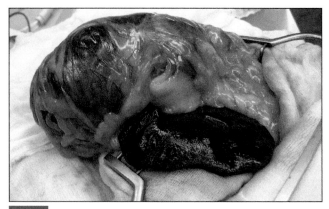

12.14 Omental adhesions to a splenic haemangiosarcoma.

Postoperative considerations

After splenectomy, fluid therapy should be continued until the animal is haemodynamically stable and can maintain its own hydration. The PCV should be monitored and blood transfusions administered if indicated. Septic complications after splenectomy in dogs and cats are rare and antibiotic therapy can be discontinued postoperatively or within 24 hours in most animals.

Complications

Serious complications following splenectomy are rare. Haemorrhage secondary to ligature displacement is the most common complication. In a study by Brown *et al.* (1985), haemorrhage was the most common reason for immediate postsurgical death of dogs undergoing splenectomy for non-neoplastic conditions. Surgical intervention may be required with decreasing PCV, worsening clinical condition and evidence of blood in the abdominal cavity. Anaemia after splenectomy is often self-limiting in the presence of normally functioning bone marrow. Other infrequent complications include damage to the vasculature of the stomach or pancreas, which can cause ischaemic necrosis of those organs. In addition, pancreatitis may result from traumatic handling of the pancreas during surgery.

Cardiac arrhythmias

Cardiac arrhythmias have been reported in dogs following splenectomy, and a study by Marino *et al.* (1994) indicated that there is a high incidence of rapid ventricular tachycardia following splenectomy. Monitoring for ventricular arrhythmias is helpful; however, intermittent ECG monitoring is not reliable for detecting ventricular arrhythmias and continuous monitoring is recommended if possible. Ventricular arrhythmias can result in haemodynamic instability and potentially progress to fatal arrhythmias. Institution of anti-arrhythmic therapy should be performed if indicated (see Chapter 6 and the *BSAVA Manual of Canine and Feline Emergency and Critical Care*).

References and further reading

Brockman DJ, Mongil CM, Aronson LR and Brown DC (2000) A practical approach to haemoperitoneum in the dog and cat. *Veterinary Clinics of North America: Small Animal Practice* **30**, 657–668

Brown NO (1985) Hemangiosarcoma. *Veterinary Clinics of North America: Small Animal Practice* **15**, 569–575

Brown NO, Patnaik AR and MacEwen EG (1985) Canine hemangiosarcoma: retrospective analysis of 104 cases. *Journal of the American Veterinary Medical Association* **186**, 56–58

Day MJ, Lucke VM and Pearson H (1995) A review of pathological diagnoses made from 87 canine splenic biopsies. *Journal of Small Animal Practice* **36**, 426–433

Dye T (2003) The acute abdomen: a surgeon's approach to diagnosis and treatment. *Clinical Techniques in Small Animal Practice* **18**, 53–65

Eberle N, von Babo V, Nolte I, Baumgartner W and Betz D (2012) *Tierärztliche Praxis. Ausgabe K, Kleintiere/Heimtiere* **40**, 250–260

Hammond TN and Pesillo-Crosby SA (2008) *Journal of the Veterinary Medical Association* **232**, 553–558

Hardie EM, Vaden SL, Spauling K and Malarkey DE (1995) Splenic infarction in 16 dogs: a retrospective study. *Journal of Veterinary Internal Medicine* **9**, 141–148

Khalaj A, Bakhtiari J and Niasari-Naslaji A (2012) Comparison between single and three portal laparoscopic splenectomy in dogs. *BMC Veterinary Research* **8(1)**, 161

King L and Boag A (2007) *BSAVA Manual of Canine and Feline Emergency and Critical Care, 2nd edn.* BSAVA Publications, Gloucester

Ledgerwood AM and Lucas CE (2003) A review of studies on the effects of hemorrhagic shock and resuscitation on the coagulation profile. *Journal of Trauma: Injury, Infection, and Critical Care* **54**, S68–S74

MacEwen EG (2001) Miscellaneous tumours: hemangiosarcoma. In: *Small Animal Clinical Oncology, 3rd edn*, ed. SJ Withrow and EG MacEwen, pp.295–297. Lea and Febiger, Philadelphia

Marino DJ, Matthiesen, Fox PR, Lesser MB and Stamoulis ME (1994) Ventricular arrhythmias in dogs undergoing splenectomy: a prospective study. *Veterinary Surgery* **23**, 101–106

Mazzaferro EM (2003) Triage and approach to the acute abdomen. *Clinical Techniques in Small Animal Practice* **18**, 1–6

Neath PJ, Brockman DJ and Sanders HM (1997) Retrospective analysis of 19 cases of isolated torsion on the splenic pedicle in dogs. *Journal of Small Animal Practice* **38**, 387–392

Patsikas MN, Rallis T, Kladakis SE and Dessitis AK (2001) Computed tomography diagnosis of isolated splenic torsion in a dog. *Veterinary Radiology and Ultrasound* **42**, 235–237

Radhakrishnan A and Mayhew PD (2013) Laparoscopic splenic biopsy in dogs and cats: 15 cases (2006–2008). *Journal of the American Animal Hospital Association* **49(1)**, 41–45

Rivier P and Monnet E (2011) Use of a vessel sealant device for splenectomy in dogs. *Veterinary Surgery* **40(1)**, 102–105

Spangler WL and Kass PH (1997) Pathologic factors affecting post splenectomy survival in dogs. *Journal of Veterinary Internal Medicine* **11**, 166–171

Waldron DR and Robertson J (1995) Partial splenectomy in the dog: a comparison of stapling and ligation techniques. *Journal of the American Animal Hospital Association* **31**, 343–348

Walters DJ, Caywood DD, Hayden DW and Klausner JS (1988) Metastatic pattern in dogs with splenic haemangiosarcomas: clinical implications. *Journal of Small Animal Practice* **29**, 805–814

Weinstein MJ, Carpenter JL and Schunk CJ (1989) Nonangiogenic and nonlymphomatous sarcomas of the canine spleen: 57 cases (1975–1987). *Journal of the American Veterinary Medical Association* **195**, 784–788

OPERATIVE TECHNIQUE 12.1

Splenic biopsy and partial splenectomy

POSITIONING

Dorsal recumbency.

ASSISTANT

Useful but not essential.

EQUIPMENT EXTRAS

Topical haemostatic agent; large abdominal swabs; two large non-crushing forceps (i.e. Doyens); suction; electrocoagulation unit (optional); stapling equipment (optional).

SURGICAL TECHNIQUE

Approach

Perform a routine ventral midline abdominal incision from the xiphoid process to cranial to the pubis. Place a self-retaining retractor (e.g. Balfour retractor) to retract the abdominal wall and expose the abdominal viscera.

Surgical manipulations: splenic biopsy

During coeliotomy, biopsy of splenic lesions may be performed using a variety of techniques, including Tru-Cut needles or a Keyes punch biopsy. A topical haemostatic agent (see Chapter 2) may be beneficial in maintaining haemostasis.

Surgical manipulations: removal of focal lesions

1   For focal lesions near the centre of the spleen, make an oval incision through the capsule and into the parenchyma to an adequate depth to remove the lesion.

2   Close the splenic capsule by placing simple interrupted or mattress sutures of an absorbable 1.5 or 2 metric (4/0 or 3/0 USP) suture material.

3   For focal lesions near the splenic margins, use the overlapping mattress suture technique (see Operative Technique 9.1).

➜ **OPERATIVE TECHNIQUE 12.1 CONTINUED**

Surgical manipulations: partial splenectomy

1 Exteriorize the spleen and pack off with laparotomy swabs.

2 Define the area of the spleen to be removed.

3 Double ligate and incise the hilar vessels supplying the area. Note the extent of ischaemia that develops; this can be used as a guideline for the resection.

4 Squeeze the splenic tissue at the line of demarcation and milk the splenic pulp towards the ischaemic area using the thumb and forefingers.

5 Place forceps on the flattened portion and divide the spleen between the forceps.

6 Close the cut surface of the spleen adjacent to the forceps using an absorbable 1.5 or 2 metric (4/0 or 3/0 USP) suture material in a simple continuous pattern. Alternatively, two rows of mattress sutures in a continuous overlapping fashion can be placed across the line of demarcation. Any ongoing haemorrhage can be controlled by oversewing the end of the spleen with a continuous suture pattern or by using electrocautery.

Automatic stapling devices, such as a thoracoabdominal stapler, may also be used for partial splenectomy. The stapling device is placed across the spleen near the line of colour demarcation. It is important to place the double row of staples in the perfused, non-ischaemic portion of the spleen. Stainless steel staples 3.5 mm or 4.8 mm in size are recommended. Use of staples that are too long or too short may result in failure of the staples to hold and subsequent haemorrhage. In a study comparing stapling and ligation techniques for partial splenectomy, blood loss was equally low, as determined by clinical observation and comparison of PCV and total protein. Stapling techniques significantly decrease the surgery time. Other techniques that can be used to divide the splenic parenchyma include CO_2 lasers and ultrasonic cutting devices such as the Harmonic® scalpel (see Chapter 9).

Wound closure

Routine abdominal closure is performed.

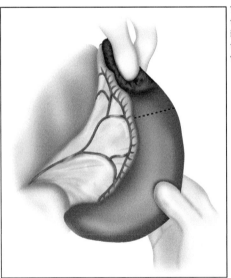

The portion of spleen to be removed is identified and the transection line is visualized.

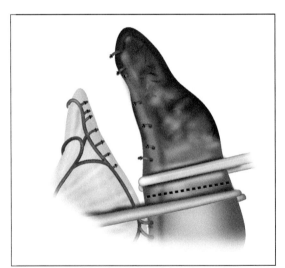

The vessels supplying the portion of the spleen to be removed are ligated and divided. Crushing forceps are placed across the tissue to be removed and atraumatic forceps (such as Doyen forceps) are placed across the remaining portion of the spleen. The spleen is then divided between the two pairs of forceps.

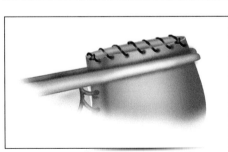

The cut surface of the spleen is oversewn with a continuous suture pattern. Alternatively, a double row of overlapping horizontal mattress sutures can be placed just proximal to the cut edge to ensure haemostasis.

POSTOPERATIVE MANAGEMENT AND COMPLICATIONS

See main text.

OPERATIVE TECHNIQUE 12.2

Splenectomy

POSITIONING

Dorsal recumbency.

ASSISTANT

Useful but not essential.

EQUIPMENT EXTRAS

Surgical suction to aspirate abdominal fluid or haemorrhage. Metal haemostatic clips or automated stapling devices may be useful for total splenectomy. The author routinely uses the a ligate-and-divide stapler (e.g. LDS™) for rapid ligation of smaller vessels.

SURGICAL TECHNIQUE

Approach

Ventral midline coeliotomy extending from the xiphoid process to the pubis.

Surgical manipulations

1   Thoroughly explore the abdomen for the presence of metastasis. In some cases a complete exploration may not be possible until the spleen has been removed.

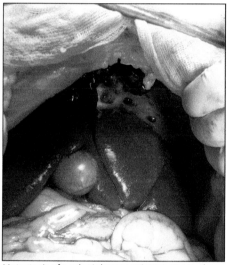

Metastasis of a splenic haemangiosarcoma to the diaphragm.

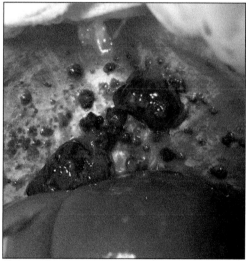

Close-up view.

PRACTICAL TIP

A routine biopsy sample should be taken from the liver in any patient undergoing splenectomy because of the presence of a splenic mass. Although the presence of hepatic nodules may indicate metastasis in dogs with splenic masses, the hepatic nodules may also represent nodular hyperplasia

2   Exteriorize the spleen and pack off with laparotomy swabs.

3   Begin hilar vessel ligation with dissection and isolation of splenic vessels as they branch to enter the splenic parenchyma. This is usually started from the tail of the spleen, working carefully towards the head of the spleen.

→ **OPERATIVE TECHNIQUE 12.2 CONTINUED**

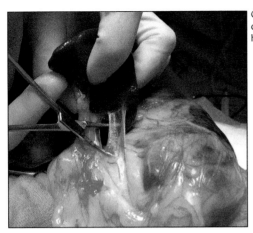

Curved forceps are used to dissect the vessels along the hilus of the spleen.

4 Double ligate the main branches of the splenic artery and vein with one circumferential and one transfixation ligature before transection to decrease the risk of postoperative haemorrhage.

5 Vascular occlusion can be achieved with absorbable or non-absorbable sutures or a variety of haemostatic clips:

- Metal haemostatic clips can supplement ligatures or be used as the primary method of vessel occlusion. A ligate-and-divide automatic stapling device places metallic clips on both sides of a pedicle and then cuts between them. This works especially well in dividing mesenteric or omental adhesions, but it is necessary to use well tied ligatures on vessels of substantial size. Haemostatic clips are appropriate for use on vessels up to 3 mm in size. A bipolar vessel-sealing device (e.g. LigaSure™) or Harmonic® scalpel, can be used to rapidly seal vessels, decreasing surgical time. Haemostatic clips or electrosurgical devices should not be used on the main splenic arteries and veins.

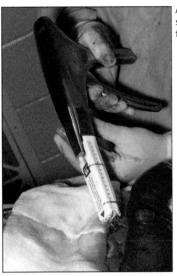

A ligate-and-divide stapler being used for a splenectomy.

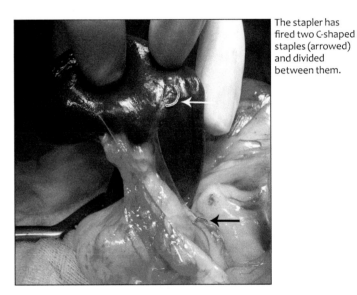

The stapler has fired two C-shaped staples (arrowed) and divided between them.

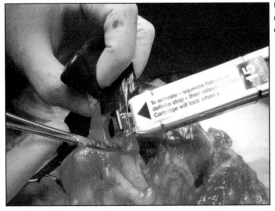

Use of a ligate-and-divide stapler for complete splenectomy.

→ **OPERATIVE TECHNIQUE 12.2 CONTINUED**

PRACTICAL TIP

Attention to ligature placement and careful application of vascular clips can reduce the likelihood of intra- or postoperative haemorrhage

- A faster technique for total splenectomy involves opening up the omental bursa and identifying the splenic artery and vein. These vessels or major branches can be double ligated and transected. It is important to identify and preserve the branches supplying the left limb of the pancreas when using this technique.

WARNING

This technique is often not possible in cases where splenic anatomy is grossly distorted owing to neoplasia or omental adhesion and it is safer to identify and transect vessels at the splenic hilus, rather than risk development of ischaemic pancreatitis

WARNING

In cases of chronic splenic torsion there can be significant fibrosis of the splenic pedicle, which can make identification of the vessels very difficult; however, mass ligation of the pedicle often fails to achieve adequate haemostasis and should be avoided

Wound closure

Routine abdominal closure is performed.

POSTOPERATIVE MANAGEMENT AND COMPLICATIONS

See main text.

Chapter 13

The adrenal glands

Catherine Sturgeon

The increasing availability of advanced imaging techniques coupled with more veterinary surgeons (veterinarians) developing and refining the skills of ultrasonography has meant that adrenal masses are more frequently diagnosed and their removal contemplated. Adrenalectomy, however, can be a daunting prospect owing to the complex physiology of functional adrenal masses, their deep location within the abdomen and their close proximity to the vena cava and abdominal aorta. Careful planning prior to surgery can alleviate some of the anticipated hurdles, ensure the selection of a suitable candidate for surgery and allow preparation for any intra- or postoperative complications that may arise.

Anatomy

The adrenal glands are located at the cranial aspect of each kidney (Figure 13.1). Both adrenal glands are normally beige in colour and are located within the retroperitoneal space. The size of the adrenal glands can be determined by ultrasound examination, and varies in dogs and cats (Figure 13.2). The phrenicoabdominal vein courses over the ventral surface of each gland and the phrenicoabdominal artery lies on the dorsal aspect of each gland. There is often a section of retroperitoneal fat lying over the glands. The right adrenal gland is usually more cranially located than the left adrenal gland, situated beneath the 13th thoracic vertebra and with the

Species	Range	Source
Dog	0.19–1.2 cm wide; 1–5 cm long	Douglass et al., 1997
Cat	0.29–0.53 cm wide; 0.45–1.37 cm long	Zimmer et al., 2000

13.2 Normal range of adrenal gland size as determined by ultrasonography.

vena cava adherent to it medially. The right adrenal gland is further obscured from view by the right lateral liver lobe. The left adrenal gland is located in the region of the 2nd lumbar vertebra with the abdominal aorta medially and its caudal pole in close proximity to the left renal artery.

The adrenal glands are divided into two very distinct sections: the outer cortex and the inner medulla. The arterial supply to each adrenal gland is made up of small tributaries from the renal, lumbar and phrenicoabdominal arteries, and also has a direct contribution from the aorta. A plexus is formed, sending branches into the cortex and medulla. There is a single adrenal vein, with the left adrenal vein emptying into the left renal vein and the right adrenal vein into the vena cava.

Physiology

The cortex and the medulla are functionally separate endocrine glands. The adrenal cortex produces 30 different hormones, but these can be grouped according to their predominant actions into: mineralocorticoids, such as aldosterone, which are important in electrolyte and blood pressure homeostasis; and glucocorticoids, which regulate metabolism by promoting gluconeogenesis. Glucocorticoids also enhance protein catabolism and suppress the immune and inflammatory responses. There are also small quantities of sex hormones that have weak androgenic activity. The adrenal medulla produces the catecholamines noradrenaline (norepinephrine) and adrenaline (epinephrine), which act primarily to promote a response to acute stress and to regulate metabolism. Functional adrenal masses, whether from the cortex or medulla in origin, can trigger varied clinical signs and have different implications for adrenalectomy (see the *BSAVA Manual of Canine and Feline Endocrinology*). Very rarely, patients can have concurrent functional cortical and medullary masses (Hylands, 2005; Calsyn et al., 2010).

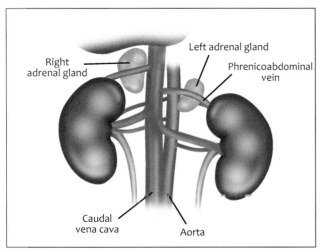

13.1 Anatomy of the adrenal glands and surrounding structures.

Right adrenal gland

Left adrenal gland

Phrenicoabdominal vein

Caudal vena cava

Aorta

Adrenalectomy

Adrenalectomy may be considered in the following situations:

* Functional adrenocortical tumours
* Functional adrenomedullary tumours
* Large masses that may be prone to rupture
* Masses that are increasing in size on serial ultrasonographic examinations.

Hyperadrenocorticism

Hyperadrenocorticism (HAC), also known as Cushing's disease, can be either pituitary- or adrenal-dependent. Adrenocortical tumours can be unilateral or bilateral, benign or malignant, and account for approximately 20% of spontaneous cases of HAC. Adrenal adenomas tend to be well circumscribed, not locally invasive and approximately 50% are calcified. Adrenocortical carcinomas are usually large, haemorrhagic, necrotic and 50% may be calcified. Adrenal carcinomas have a locally invasive rate of 11% (Kyles *et al.*, 2003) and a distant metastatic rate of 14% (Anderson *et al.*, 2001). Although patients with HAC may often have obvious clinical signs (Figures 13.3 and 13.4), it can be a very difficult condition to diagnose.

Routine biochemistry, haematology and urinalysis can often flag up the suspicion of HAC. Adrenocorticotropic hormone (ACTH) stimulation tests, low-dose dexamethasone suppression tests (LDDST) and endogenous ACTH assays all have a place in trying to diagnose and differentiate between pituitary- and adrenal-dependent HAC (see the *BSAVA Manual of Canine and Feline Endocrinology*). Functional adrenal adenomas and carcinomas secrete excessive amounts of cortisol independent of the pituitary gland. The negative feedback mechanism to the hypothalamus ultimately reduces the circulating ACTH concentration, but it will not suppress further cortisol secretion from functional tumours. The contralateral adrenal gland in this situation would be expected to atrophy. Dogs with adrenal-dependent HAC do not have suppressed cortisol levels during an LDDST. It is worthy of note, however, that 40% of dogs with pituitary-dependent HAC also do not suppress cortisol during an LDDST (Feldman *et al.*, 1996). An endogenous ACTH assay can also be very useful for detecting dogs with a functional adrenal mass; these cases would commonly have low (10 pg/ml; normal 20–80 pg/ml) or undetectable levels of ACTH.

A novel method for detecting the presence of HAC in humans involves the serum inhibin concentration. Inhibin is a glycoprotein synthesized predominantly by the gonads, but the adrenal glands are an extragonadal source of inhibin. Secretion of inhibin has been identified from adrenocortical tumours in humans, with the highest secretion rates in cortical adenomas associated with HAC. In dogs, adrenocortical tumours and pituitary-dependent HAC have been associated with increased serum inhibin concentrations. This diagnostic test may also prove very useful when trying to detect the presence of a phaeochromocytoma. Undetectable levels of inhibin are highly supportive of a phaeochromocytoma in neutered dogs with adrenal tumours (Bromel *et al.*, 2013).

Phaeochromocytoma

Phaeochromocytoma is a tumour of the adrenal medulla. It can be responsible for a variety of non-specific, sometimes vague, clinical signs which are often attributable to the release of catecholamines, mainly adrenaline (Figure 13.5). The secretion of catecholamines, however, can be sporadic and intermittent, making many phaeochromocytomas clinically silent for periods of time, which adds to the challenge of reaching a diagnosis.

Clinical signs (Figure 13.6) can also be attributed to the mass itself, local invasion of the surrounding structures such as the vena cava and/or distant metastatic disease. Rarely, but worthy of note, a haemoabdominal crisis can arise from a ruptured phaeochromocytoma in dogs. Haemorrhage has been reported from tumours of both adrenocortical and adrenomedullary origin (Whittemore *et al.*, 2001).

---

* Polyuria and polydipsia
* Polyphagia
* Potbellied appearance
* Alopecia/comedones
* Liver enlargement
* Muscle wasting
* Exercise intolerance

13.3 Common clinical signs of canine hyperadrenocorticism.

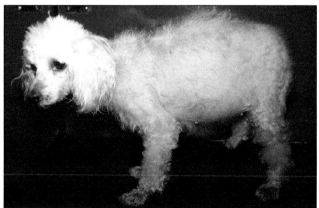

13.4 A 6-year-old Poodle bitch with pituitary-dependent hyperadrenocorticism. Note the abdominal distension, muscle wasting, alopecia and thin skin.
(Reproduced from the *BSAVA Manual of Canine and Feline Endocrinology, 4th edn*)

---

* Increased blood glucose concentrations
* Inhibition of insulin secretion
* Increased force of cardiac contraction
* Vasodilatation of skeletal muscle arterioles, coronary arteries and all veins
* Gastrointestinal smooth muscle relaxation
* Urine retention
* Pupil dilatation
* Central nervous system excitation

13.5 Actions of adrenaline.

---

* Weakness
* Lethargy
* Polydipsia and polyuria
* Collapse
* Panting
* Anorexia
* Weight loss
* Seizures
* Tachyarrhythmia
* Tachypnoea
* Abdominal pain
* Pyrexia
* Hypertension

13.6 Historical and clinical signs that can be associated with a phaeochromocytoma.

Often, frustratingly, there are no specific or consistent abnormalities on routine blood or urine profiles in association with a phaeochromocytoma. In human patients, measurement of plasma-free metanephrines is the test of choice to identify phaeochromocytomas. Work to validate this test in dogs has been carried out, with promising results for an effective and minimally invasive means of identifying dogs with phaeochromocytomas in the future (Gostelow *et al.*, 2013).

Phaeochromocytomas are reported to be locally invasive in between 39% and 71% of patients (Gilson *et al.*, 1994; Barthez *et al.*, 1997; Herrera *et al.*, 2008). They can also produce metastases in 13% of patients (Barthez *et al.*, 1997). Common sites for metastases include the regional lymph nodes, kidney, liver, lung, spleen and bone. Dogs with phaeochromocytomas can also have a high frequency (54%) of concurrent neoplasia (Barthez *et al.*, 1997).

The presumptive diagnosis of a phaeochromocytoma has to rely upon suspicion raised by the history, detection of one or more of the appropriate abnormalities, possible demonstration of hypertension and ultimately identification of an adrenal mass.

> **PRACTICAL TIP**
>
> Ultrasonography or advanced imaging that documents an adrenal mass with a normally sized contralateral adrenal gland, coupled with normal adrenal function tests, is strongly indicative of a phaeochromocytoma

Imaging of the adrenal glands

Radiography

Radiography often raises the suspicion of adrenal pathology if there is adrenal calcification. Calcification of the adrenal glands is uncommon in clinically healthy dogs and dogs with pituitary-dependent HAC. If calcification is seen, however, it does not distinguish between functional and non-functional disease or between carcinomas and adenomas (Penninck *et al.*, 1988). Survey thoracic radiographs to check for pulmonary metastases should always be taken immediately prior to surgery if recent computed tomography (CT) images of the thorax are not available.

Ultrasonography

Ultrasonography is the most popular and readily available modality for identifying an adrenal mass. 'Incidentalomas' are adrenal masses found during an abdominal ultrasound examination performed for other reasons when adrenal pathology has not been suspected. If the enlargement is marginal, it is prudent to consider whether an enlarged adrenal gland is of true significance to the patient. Successive ultrasonographic examinations are important to document any further size increase in those patients that have no corresponding clinical signs. A slightly bulbous appearance at one of the adrenal poles does not necessarily mean that there is a neoplastic mass. This can be normal in some dogs, or may represent cystic change, hyperplasia of normal tissue or a small haematoma. If a newly found and clinically unsuspected adrenal mass is deemed to be of a significant size then testing to determine its functional status is extremely important prior to any surgical intervention.

> **PRACTICAL TIP**
>
> An adrenal gland of a dog is considered abnormal if the **width** of the adrenal gland is more than 1.5 cm and the gland is asymmetrical in shape and size when compared with the contralateral adrenal gland

The diagnosis of an adrenal mass in a dog is made when the maximum width of the adrenal gland exceeds 1.5 cm, the gland loses its typical 'kidney-bean' shape and the gland is asymmetrical in shape or size compared with the other adrenal gland (Figure 13.7). An adrenal mass is more likely to be malignant if it is large, with a thickness >2 cm (Besso *et al.*, 1997), invading into surrounding tissue and vasculature, and if there are other masses present. Regional vascular invasion may be as high as 71% for phaeochromocytomas (Herrara *et al.*, 2008) and 11% for adrenocortical tumours (Kyles *et al.*, 2003). In the hands of specialist diagnostic imagers, ultrasonography can identify 86% of vascular invasion correctly (Davis *et al.*, 2012). Most dogs that have vena cava invasion have an extension of the thrombus from the phrenicoabdominal vein overlying the adrenal gland, rather than direct invasion via erosion of the vascular wall (Kyles *et al.*, 2003). Subtleties of invasion into vessel walls or small adjacent vessels such as the phrenicoabdominal vein or renal vein, however, can be challenging with ultrasonography alone. Tumours abutting adjacent vessels, surrounding the vessel or narrowing the vessel as it courses by should raise suspicion of vascular invasion (Davis *et al.*, 2012).

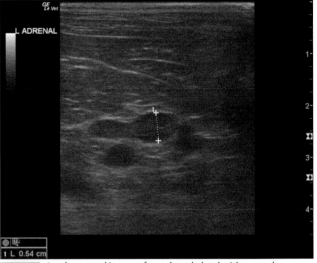

13.7 An ultrasound image of an adrenal gland with normal dimensions.
(Courtesy of J Shimali)

CT and MRI

The use of CT (Figure 13.8) and magnetic resonance imaging (MRI) can complement the initial ultrasonographic examination or can be used as the primary imaging modality. Using contrast-enhanced CT imaging, vascular invasion can be correctly identified in 91% of patients with adrenal masses. Thinly collimated (1–2 mm) images from at least 1 cm cranial and caudal to the adrenal mass, including the phrenicoabdominal and renal vasculature, as well as the adjacent caudal vena cava and kidneys, are recommended (Schultz *et al.*, 2009). Incorporating

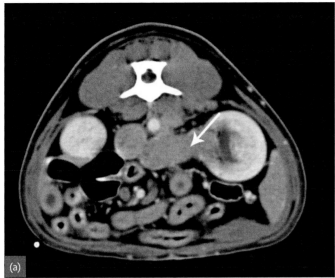
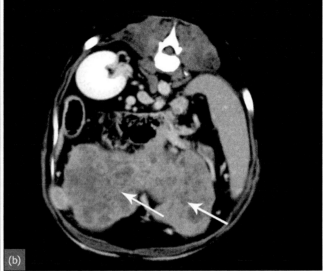

13.8 (a) CT image showing an adrenal mass invading the renal vein (arrowed). (b) CT image showing extensive abdominal metastases (arrowed) from a phaeochromocytoma.
(a, courtesy of F McConnell)

10-minute delayed post-contrast images will document the presence of a contrast-enhancing intraluminal tumour. Contrast enhancement suggests the presence of a neoplastic mass rather than a thrombus. CT will also reveal any extension into the hypaxial and epaxial musculature, which may render the mass inoperable. In humans, CT is the preferred imaging modality to evaluate adrenal masses, with the primary objective being to differentiate benign from malignant disease.

Preoperative and postoperative considerations for adrenalectomy

Considerations applicable to patients with either HAC or phaeochromocytoma

- **Surgical equipment:** Adrenalectomy is challenging as a consequence of the deep and cranial location of the glands, particularly in the case of a right-sided adrenal mass. Ensure that there are sufficient laparotomy swabs to 'pack off' surrounding viscera that constantly encroach upon the surgical field. Balfour self-retaining retractors and hand-held malleable retractors can prove useful. The best form of retraction uses the hands of an assistant. Mixter forceps and right-angled Lahey cholecystectomy clamps are used for dissection through connective tissue and around vessels. Satinsky clamps, Potts vessel scissors and nylon tape for potential venotomy should also be available. Haemostatic clips are essential, and vessel-sealing devices if available; see section on Haemostasis (below).
- **Muscle relaxants** can enhance the exposure for the often deep surgical dissection required for adrenalectomy. Atracurium is the author's preferred choice, at a dose rate of 0.25–0.5 mg/kg i.v., providing 30–40 minutes of relaxation. Neuromuscular blocking agents paralyse all skeletal muscles including respiratory muscles, so it is essential that the patient is intubated and under a stable plane of anaesthesia, facilities for controlled ventilation are used and that a peripheral nerve stimulator is on hand to monitor the blockade (see the *BSAVA Manual of Canine and Feline Anaesthesia and Analgesia*).

> **Editors' note:**
> Neither of the editors routinely use muscle relaxants for patients undergoing adrenalectomy

- **Blood products and coagulation:** Considerable blood loss is possible, so it is ideal to have the patient blood typed, a coagulation profile run and blood products available for transfusion. (See the *BSAVA Manual of Canine and Feline Haematology and Transfusion Medicine*.)
- **Central venous catheters:** These can be a very useful accessory if the patient is likely to require a prolonged period of intravenous fluid therapy and blood sampling postoperatively.
- **Analgesia and enteral feeding:** Gentle retraction of the pancreas will be necessary in some patients and this may cause mild pancreatitis, perhaps requiring a more prolonged period of analgesia. If opiate analgesia seems insufficient then a lidocaine continuous rate infusion (CRI) at 0.025–0.05 mg/kg/min could be considered in more severely affected individuals. Non-steroidal anti-inflammatory drugs must not be used in patients with HAC because they will be receiving supplementary exogenous steroids intra- and postoperatively. If the pancreas has undergone extensive manipulation or the patient is debilitated, enteral feeding support should be considered with the placement of an oesophagostomy tube prior to recovery from anaesthesia.

Specific considerations for HAC

- **Trilostane:** Most patients with adrenal-dependent HAC will be already receiving this medication prior to adrenalectomy. Trilostane is a synthetic steroid with no innate hormonal activity. It blocks adrenal synthesis of glucocorticoids, mineralocorticoids and sex hormones and thereby aids correction of some of the endocrine-triggered metabolic abnormalities. In patients with functional adrenocortical neoplasia where adrenalectomy is considered too high a risk, or is declined by the owners, continued medical management with trilostane can be considered (Eastwood *et al.*, 2003).

- **Diabetes mellitus:** 5–15% of dogs with HAC have steroid-induced diabetes mellitus; it is important to be aware of the presence of this concurrent condition when planning anaesthesia and postoperative care.
- **Hypertension:** Patients with HAC can have hypertension due to the increased activation of angiotensin I. An angiotensin-converting enzyme inhibitor can be used to reduce peripheral vasoconstriction and aldosterone secretion.
- **Pulmonary thromboembolism (PTE):** A complication that can be seen in patients with HAC after the removal of the adrenal tumour. PTE is typically noted within 72 hours after surgery and is associated with a high mortality rate. Treatment involves the use of oxygen supplementation and anticoagulants such as heparin. Common signs are dyspnoea, tachypnoea and lethargy, with coughing, haemoptysis and collapse with sudden death seen less frequently. Auscultation of the thorax may reveal crackles, and alveolar infiltration is often seen on radiography. Routine coagulation profiles can be normal. Hypoxaemia and hypocapnia are seen on blood gas analysis. To try to minimize the incidence of thromboembolism, heparinized plasma (35 IU/kg of heparin added to 10 ml/kg of canine plasma) is given intravenously during surgery as a source of antithrombin III. After surgery, subcutaneous heparin (35 IU/kg) is given twice more q8h on day 1, then 25 IU/kg q8h on day 2, then 15 IU/kg q8h (Adin and Nelson, 2012). Alternatively, unfractionated heparin at 50–100 IU/kg s.c. q8–12h or low molecular weight heparin at 100–150 IU/kg s.c. q24h can be used. However, it has not yet been proven that preoperative anticoagulation decreases the incidence of postoperative thromboembolism. The decision to heparinize is a matter for the clinician's judgement, based on experience and available clinical evidence. Allowing the patient to walk around in a reasonable time frame following surgery will also improve the circulation and minimize clot formation. Careful choice of analgesia protocols is warranted to allow patients to be comfortable but alert and ambulatory 4–6 hours following surgery.

> **Editors' note:**
> Neither of the editors routinely use heparinization for patients undergoing adrenalectomy

- **Hypoadrenocorticism – glucocorticoids:** The contralateral adrenal gland will normally be atrophied in the presence of a cortisol-secreting adrenal mass. Once this mass is removed, it can take a few months before the atrophied adrenal gland secretes a normal level of glucocorticoids. All patients have low circulating levels of cortisol once the cortisol-secreting mass is removed. At anaesthetic induction and immediately postoperatively give dexamethasone at 0.1 mg/kg intravenously to compensate for the anticipated drop in glucocorticoid secretion. Injectable dexamethasone should be given at a lower tapering dose of 0.05 mg/kg q24h until the patient is eating. Use prednisolone at 0.5 mg/kg q12h for 7–14 days, then 0.2 mg/kg q24h for 14 days, tapering accordingly during the weeks and months that follow.

> **Editors' note:**
> Dogs that have had unilateral adrenal gland tumours removed should eventually be able to produce endogenous cortisol from the remaining adrenal gland, allowing discontinuation of glucocorticoid therapy. The decision to stop therapy is based on the results of postoperative ACTH stimulation tests, which are performed every 2–4 weeks as needed until normal results are obtained

- **Mineralocorticoids:** Electrolyte measurements are important before and after adrenalectomy for patients with HAC. Hyponatraemia and hyperkalaemia are common during the first 3 days but usually normalize as the exogenous supplementary glucocorticoids are reduced and the patient starts to eat.

Specific considerations for phaeochromocytoma

- **Hypertension:** Phaeochromocytomas secrete catecholamines, which can cause generalized vasoconstriction. Further manipulation of the adrenal tumour during surgery can cause surges of catecholamines, producing acute episodes of hypertension, ventricular tachycardia, arrhythmias and even cardiac arrest (Adin and Nelson, 2012). The use of phenoxybenzamine, an alpha-adrenergic receptor blocker, preoperatively can reduce perioperative mortality from 48% to 13% in dogs with a phaeochromocytoma (Herrera *et al.*, 2008). If there is a strong suspicion of a phaeochromocytoma, phenoxybenzamine should be initiated 2 weeks before surgery at a dose rate of 0.5 mg/kg q12h. It is difficult to make dose adjustments during this period on the basis of any improvements in clinical signs or blood pressure because the catecholamine surges can be intermittent, causing fluctuating clinical signs and blood pressure measurements. Intraoperatively, arterial hypertension may require administration of a short-acting alpha antagonist such as phentolamine at 0.02–0.1 mg/kg as an intravenous bolus followed by a CRI, or the direct vasodilator nitroprusside at 0.1–3 µg/kg/min, starting at the lowest rate.
- **Tachycardia:** Persistent tachycardia can be seen in patients with phaeochromocytoma. Preoperatively they may require a beta-adrenergic antagonist such as propranolol at 0.2–1 mg/kg orally q8h or atenolol at 0.2–1 mg/kg q12–24h. Note that phenoxybenzamine must be in use prior to starting beta-blockers. For severe and ongoing intraoperative tachycardia use propranolol at 0.3–1 mg/kg i.v. or esmolol at 0.05–0.5 mg/kg slowly i.v. every 5 minutes until a total cumulative dose of 0.5 mg/kg is reached, or 25–200 µg/kg/min CRI.
- **Arrhythmias:** Ventricular premature complexes with runs of 15 abnormal complexes or more require intravenous boluses of lidocaine at 2 mg/kg to a total dose of 8 mg/kg to test whether the patient is responsive to this medication. Note that 1 mg/kg is 0.05 ml/kg of a 2% solution. If the patient is responsive, continue lidocaine as a CRI of 0.025–0.1 mg/kg/min (see the *BSAVA Small Animal Formulary*).

Intraoperative management

Surgical approaches

Ventral midline

This is the most common surgical approach used and gives the greatest exposure for adrenalectomy. Although very rarely needed, an additional paracostal incision can be made, branching off the coeliotomy incision, if further exposure of the dorsal retroperitoneal space is required. Many patients with an adrenal mass associated with concurrent HAC have swollen liver lobes, with hepatomegaly making removal of the adrenal gland even more challenging; a coeliotomy gives more exposure than a flank approach. Occasionally, if there is invasion into the renal vein, a nephrectomy should be performed and a venotomy into the vena cava may be necessary to remove a thrombus, therefore adequate surgical exposure is of paramount importance (see Operative Technique 13.1).

Flank

A flank, sometimes termed paralumbar, approach can only be advised for small, unilateral tumours with no evidence of any invasion into surrounding structures. A patient undergoing a flank approach must have advanced imaging prior to surgery to be certain that this approach is appropriate. If in doubt, a coeliotomy should be performed.

Laparoscopy

Laparoscopic removal of an adrenal gland can be performed by those familiar and confident with laparoscopy. Right- or left-sided adrenal masses without vena caval thrombi can be removed with success from both dogs and cats (Pelaez *et al.*, 2008; Smith *et al.*, 2012). Adrenal carcinomas are very friable and ruptures can occur even with open surgery. Removal of an adrenal mass in multiple fragments via laparoscopy does raise concern regarding tumour seeding, and retrieval bags should be used to limit this risk during laparoscopy.

Caval invasion

Caval invasion can occur in 25% of dogs with adrenal gland tumours.

> **WARNING**
>
> Adrenal tumours can be very aggressive and may invade the lumen of the cranial vena cava, making resection difficult or even impossible in some cases

Caval tumour thrombi can develop from left- or right-sided adrenal masses. With careful surgical planning, caval thrombi associated with adrenal gland tumours may be amenable to adrenalectomy and thrombectomy without significantly increased morbidity or mortality (Kyles *et al.*, 2003; Rose *et al.*, 2007; see Operative Technique 13.1).

Haemostasis

Haemorrhage is the most common complication during adrenalectomy. Neoplastic masses will have a plethora of additional small arteries and veins coursing in and around the adrenal capsule. These vessels are not very amenable to ligature placement for haemostasis (Figure 13.9). Bipolar diathermy can also fail, in the author's experience, because these vessels are very fragile and, although small, bleed profusely on contact with the diathermy forceps. Surgical clips (Figure 13.10) and vessel-sealing devices are ideal accessories for adrenalectomy. The surgical clips are titanium staples, available in small, medium and large sizes, and are applied with reusable applicators that allow straight or right-angled delivery. The single-use devices containing multiple clips are more expensive but are less likely to be dropped while advancing towards the vessel, and some have rotating handles that facilitate application. The Harmonic® scalpel (Figure 13.11) can seal vessels <5 mm and the LigaSure™ device can seal vessels <7 mm. While these devices are expensive, surgical clips can be purchased for a very reasonable cost. Both haemostatic clips and vessel-sealing devices are very useful for a variety of abdominal and thoracic surgical procedures.

- Soft loading system clips (Mediplus)
- Ligaclip® (Ethicon Inc.)
- Surgiclip® (Covidien Inc.)
- Harmonic® scalpel (Ethicon Inc.)
- LigaSure® (Covidien Inc.)

13.9 Alternative options to ligatures for haemostasis.

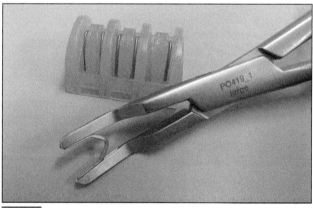

13.10 Haemostatic surgical clips.

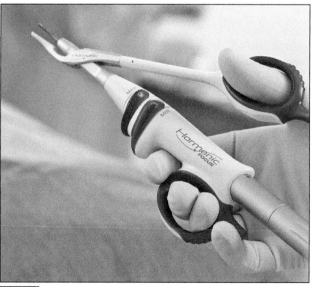

13.11 Harmonic® scalpel. (© Ethicon Inc.)

Prognosis

Historically, adrenalectomy has been associated with high mortality rates, with 60% reported in a cohort of 25 dogs in one study (Scavelli *et al.*, 1986). The most common complications are haemoabdomen, PTE, acute pancreatitis, renal failure and hypoadrenocorticism. However, with the advancement in surgical techniques, haemostasis accessories and preoperative medical support, more recently reported mortality rates have reduced to 13.5% in 52 dogs (Massari *et al.*, 2011), and 22% in 40 and 41 dogs (Kyles *et al.*, 2003; Schwartz *et al.*, 2008), respectively. Median survival times of 935 days (range 0–1941 days), with 65% surviving 1 year or more following adrenalectomy, have been reported (Massari *et al.*, 2011). Survival time is not associated with the side of the adrenalectomy or duration of surgery (Massari *et al.*, 2011).

A study published in 2003 found there to be no significant difference in morbidity or mortality between dogs with or without tumour thrombi (Kyles *et al.*, 2003). However, a more recent study found a generally poorer prognosis associated with venous thrombi (median survival time 2.5 days; range 1–981 days), adrenal masses >5 cm in length (median survival time 156 days; range 1–1279 days) and the presence of metastases (median survival time 120 days; range 1–941 days) (Massari *et al.*, 2011). Shorter survival times have been reported in dogs with preoperative weakness, lethargy, thrombocytopenia, increased blood urea nitrogen (BUN), prolonged prothrombin time (PTT), elevated aspartate aminotransferase (AST) and hypokalaemia (Schwartz *et al.*, 2008).

Successful management of adrenalectomy patients requires a strong emphasis on adopting a thorough approach to all aspects of the patient's treatment. From the initial diagnostic investigation, surgical planning, ensuring that a surgeon is available with expertise and familiarity with the anatomy, provision of the appropriate preoperative medical support, to the immediate postoperative period, this is a surgical procedure that needs careful consideration.

Adrenalectomy in cats

Adrenal conditions are rare in cats; however, pituitary- and adrenal-dependent HAC, primary hyperaldosteronism and signs attributed to a phaeochromocytoma have been described in cats (Watson and Herrtage, 1998; Rose *et al.*, 2007; Calsyn *et al.*, 2010). Adrenalectomy, although associated with a risk of postoperative mortality, is still the treatment of choice for cats with a functional adrenal mass. No consistent medical treatment has been found effective for cats with HAC. Cats with pituitary-dependent HAC receiving trilostane showed a reduction in their clinical signs and an improvement in endocrine test results, but all continued to have signs of hypercortisolaemia and, for those with concurrent diabetes mellitus, the insulin requirement did not change (Neiger *et al.*, 2004). Bilateral adrenalectomy is the advised surgical procedure for cats with pituitary-dependent HAC. The surgery can be performed via a ventral coeliotomy or laparoscopy.

> **WARNING**
>
> Left untreated, cats with HAC experience a very poor prognosis and often die within months of the diagnosis

Worthy of note is that, unlike dogs, a high proportion of cats with HAC (50–80%) have concurrent diabetes mellitus (Feldman and Nelson, 1994; Watson and Herrtage, 1998). This fact undoubtedly has an impact on the complexity of managing these patients. Unlike dogs, cats do not possess a glucocorticoid-induced alkaline phosphatase (ALP) isoenzyme, and thus cats with HAC do not show a marked elevation in ALP. Cats with HAC do not always display hepatomegaly and interestingly 30% of normal cats have calcified adrenal glands (Myers and Bruyette, 1994).

Pre- and postoperative consideration should be given to stabilizing any electrolyte and glucose imbalance. The provisional need for enteral feeding should be taken seriously, even for those cats with the classically increased appetite encountered with HAC. Large or obese cats that become acutely inappetent following surgery are in danger of developing hepatic lipidosis. An oesophagostomy tube not only provides a method of feeding but affords excellent access for administering medications to cats in the recovery period. Fludrocortisone (0.2 mg q24h) should be commenced on the morning of surgery and used for the life of the cat when a bilateral adrenalectomy has been performed. Prednisolone can also be used long term for those patients with lethargy and poor appetite following bilateral adrenalectomy.

The prognosis for cats undergoing bilateral adrenalectomy for treatment of pituitary HAC has been reported, with variable survival times. One report describes one cat surviving 15 months and another surviving more than 5 years (Watson and Herrtage, 1998). Neither of these cats had concurrent diabetes mellitus. Early recognition and diagnosis of HAC in cats should theoretically increase the success of surgery because this limits the debility caused by chronically high circulating levels of corticosteroids and other concurrent conditions.

References and further reading

Adin CA and Nelson RW (2012) Adrenal glands. In: *Veterinary Surgery: Small Animal*, ed. KM Tobias and SA Johnston, pp.2033–2042. Elsevier Saunders, Missouri

Anderson CR, Birchard SJ, Powers BE *et al.* (2001) Surgical treatment of adrenocortical tumours: 21 cases. *Journal of the American Animal Hospital Association* **37**, 93–97

Barthez PY, Marks SL, Woo J *et al.* (1997) Pheochromocytoma in dogs: 61 cases. *Journal of Veterinary Internal Medicine* **11**, 272–278

Besso JG, Penninck DG and Gliatto JM (1997) Retrospective ultrasonographic evaluation of adrenal lesions in 26 dogs. *Veterinary Radiology and Ultrasound* **38**, 448–455

Bromel C, Nelson RW, Feldman EC *et al.* (2013) Serum inhibin concentration in dogs with adrenal gland disease and in healthy dogs. *Journal of Veterinary Internal Medicine* **27**, 76–82

Calsyn JDR, Green RA, Davis GJ *et al.* (2010) Adrenal pheochromocytoma with contralateral adrenocortical adenoma in a cat. *Journal of the American Animal Hospital Association* **46**, 36–42

Davis MK, Schochet RA and Wrigley R (2012) Ultrasonographic identification of vascular invasion by adrenal tumours in dogs. *Veterinary Radiology and Ultrasound* **53**, 442–445

Day M and Kohn B (2012) *BSAVA Manual of Canine and Feline Haematology and Transfusion Medicine, 2nd edn.* BSAVA Publications, Gloucester

Douglass JP, Berry CR and James S (1997) Ultrasonographic adrenal gland measurements in dogs without evidence of adrenal disease. *Veterinary Radiology and Ultrasound* **38**, 124–130

Eastwood JM, Elwood CM and Hurley KJ (2003) Trilostane treatment of a dog with functional adrenocortical neoplasia. *Journal of Small Animal Practice* **44**, 126–131

Feldman EC and Nelson RW (1994) Comparative aspects of Cushing's syndrome in dogs and cats: endocrinology and metabolism. *Veterinary Clinics of North America: Small Animal Practice* **23**, 671–691

Feldman EC, Nelson RW and Feldman MW (1996) Use of low and high dose dexamethasone tests for distinguishing pituitary dependent and adrenal dependent hyperadrenocorticism in dogs. *Journal of the American Veterinary Medical Association* **209**, 772–775

Gilson SD, Withrow SJ and Orton EC (1994) Surgical treatment of pheochromocytoma: technique, complications and results in six dogs. *Veterinary Surgery* **23**, 195–200

Gostelow R, Bridger N and Syme HM (2013) Plasma free metanephrine and free normetanephrine measurement for the diagnosis of pheochromocytoma in dogs. *Journal of Veterinary Internal Medicine* **27**, 83–90

Herrera MA, Mehl ML, Kass PH *et al.* (2008) Predictive factors and the effect of phenoxybenzamine on outcome in dogs undergoing adrenalectomy for pheochromocytoma. *Journal of Veterinary Internal Medicine* **22**, 1333–1339

Hylands R (2005) Malignant phaeochromocytoma of the left adrenal gland invading the caudal vena cava, accompanied by a cortisol secreting adrenocortical carcinoma of the right adrenal gland. *Canadian Veterinary Journal* **46**, 1156–1158

Kyles AE, Feldman EC, De Cock HEV *et al.* (2003) Surgical management of adrenal gland tumours with and without associated tumour thrombi in dogs: 40 cases. *Journal of the American Veterinary Medical Association* **5**, 654–662

Massari F, Nicoli S, Romanelli G *et al.* (2011) Adrenalectomy in dogs with adrenal gland tumours: 52 cases. *Journal of the American Veterinary Medical Association* **239**, 216–221

Mooney C and Peterson M (2012) *BSAVA Manual of Canine and Feline Endocrinology, 4th edn.* BSAVA Publications, Gloucester

Myers NC and Bruyette DS (1994) Feline adrenocortical diseases: part 1 – hyperadrenocorticism. *Seminars in Veterinary Medicine and Surgery (Small Animal)* **9**, 137–143

Neiger R, Witt AL, Noble A *et al.* (2004) Trilostane therapy for treatment of pituitary dependent hyperadrenocorticism in 5 cats. *Journal of Veterinary Internal Medicine* **18**, 160–164

Pelaez MJ, Bouvy BM and Dupre GP (2008) Laparoscopic adrenalectomy for treatment of unilateral adrenocortical carcinomas: technique, complications and results in seven dogs. *Veterinary Surgery* **37**, 444–453

Penninck DG, Feldman EC and Nyland TG (1988) Radiographic features of canine

hyperadrenocorticism caused by autonomously functioning adrenocortical tumours: 23 cases. *Journal of the American Veterinary Medical Association* **192**, 1604–1608

Ramsey I (2014) *BSAVA Small Animal Formulary, 8th edn.* BSAVA Publications, Gloucester

Rose SA, Kyles AE, Labelle P *et al.* (2007) Adrenalectomy and caval thrombectomy in a cat with primary hyperaldosteronism. *Journal of the American Animal Hospital Association* **43**, 209–214

Scavelli TD, Peterson ME and Matthieson DT (1986) Results of surgical treatment for hyperadrenocorticism caused by adrenocortical neoplasia in the dog: 25 cases. *Journal of the American Veterinary Medical Association* **189**, 1360–1364

Seymour C and Duke-Novakovski T (2007) *BSAVA Manual of Canine and Feline Anaesthesia and Analgesia, 2nd edn.* BSAVA Publications, Gloucester

Schultz RM, Wisner ER, Johnson EG *et al.* (2009) Contrast enhanced computed tomography as a preoperative indicator of vascular invasion from adrenal masses in dogs. *Veterinary Radiology and Ultrasound* **50**, 625–629

Schwartz P, Kovak JR, Koprowski A *et al.* (2008) Evaluation of prognostic factors in the surgical treatment of adrenal gland tumours in dogs: 41 cases. *Journal of the American Veterinary Medical Association* **1**, 77–84

Smith RR, Mayhew PD and Berent AC (2012) Laparoscopic adrenalectomy for management of a functional adrenal tumour in a cat. *Journal of the American Veterinary Medical Association* **3**, 368–372

Watson PJ and Herrtage ME (1998) Hyperadrenocorticism in six cats. *Journal of Small Animal Practice* **39**, 175–184

Whittemore JC, Preston CA and Kyles AE *et al.* (2001) Nontraumatic rupture of an adrenal gland tumour causing intra-abdominal or retroperitoneal haemorrhage in four dogs. *Journal of the American Veterinary Medical Association* **3**, 329–333

Zimmer C, Horauf A and Reusch C (2000) Ultrasonographic examination of the adrenal gland and evaluation of the hypophyseal-adrenal axis in 20 cats. *Journal of Small Animal Practice* **41**, 156–160

OPERATIVE TECHNIQUE 13.1

Adrenalectomy including venotomy of the caudal vena cava

POSITIONING

Dorsal recumbency.

ASSISTANT

Essential in large, deep-chested dogs or dogs with highly vascular adrenal masses/masses with caval invasion; two assistants are ideal.

EQUIPMENT EXTRAS

Adrenalectomy

Laparotomy swabs; Balfour retractors; malleable retractors; surgical haemostatic clips; bipolar diathermy; Harmonic® scalpel or LigaSure™ vessel-sealing devices can be used if available; Mixter forceps; long-handled DeBakey forceps and Metzenbaum scissors; surgical suction.

Venotomy of the caudal vena cava

Satinsky clamp; right-angled Lahey cholecystectomy clamps; Potts or DeBakey vessel scissors; 6 mm nylon tape; blood giving set for Rummel tourniquet; blood and blood giving sets in preparation for intraoperative blood transfusion.

→ **OPERATIVE TECHNIQUE 13.1 CONTINUED**

SURGICAL TECHNIQUE

Approach

Count all swabs and then make a ventral midline abdominal incision from the xiphoid to an appropriate point caudal to the umbilicus, which will subsequently allow maximal lateral retraction of the abdominal wall. Place moistened swabs around the borders of the incision and use the Balfour retractors to achieve the first step in the abdominal exposure.

Use moistened laparotomy and more conventionally sized swabs to carefully 'pack off' the surrounding viscera. In combination with these swabs, use malleable retractors and the assistant's hands to hold the swabs in place. It can take several minutes to establish optimal retraction to provide the best surgical access.

Surgical manipulations: adrenalectomy

1. If recently acquired CT images have been interpreted in detail by a diagnostic imager, there should be no need to examine both adrenal glands for a concurrent lesion. If advanced imaging has not been used then a thorough exploratory examination should be performed to check for local invasion and distant metastases.

2. Identify the adrenal gland to be removed; retract the liver lobes cranially, kidney caudally and the vena cava medially.

3. Isolate the phrenicoabdominal vein using curved mosquito or Mixter forceps. Carefully tease away the connective tissue surrounding the vein to enable smooth passage of the forceps. The small tunnel created will then allow haemostatic clip devices to encircle the vein. Apply a clip towards the vena cava and one towards the adrenal gland. The vein can then be transected. Many large adrenal masses have extensive neovascularization and require the application of multiple haemostatic clips. The phrenicoabdominal vein can be removed *en bloc* with the adrenal gland.

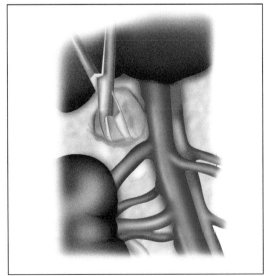

The adrenal gland is exposed by carefully dissecting the peritoneum and fatty tissue away from the gland.

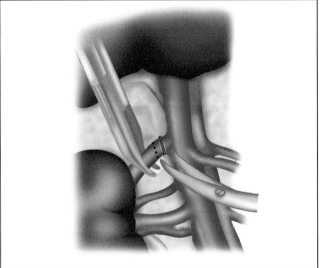

The phrenicoabdominal vein is dissected from surrounding structures and attachments. Vessels are ligated with haemoclips prior to being divided.

➜ **OPERATIVE TECHNIQUE 13.1 CONTINUED**

WARNING

Extreme care should be taken to ensure that the renal vein is not inadvertently ligated

4   The adrenal gland is carefully teased from the surrounding connective tissues and retracted medially to expose the multiple penetrating vessels on the dorsal aspect of the gland. A stay suture can be placed into the gland or non-traumatic forceps used on the adrenal capsule to aid manipulation of the gland. Try to not fragment the gland because this could seed neoplastic cells into the abdomen. Once haemostasis is achieved, gently free the adrenal gland from its caudal attachments to the renal vessels and the remaining attachments to the vena cava and aorta.

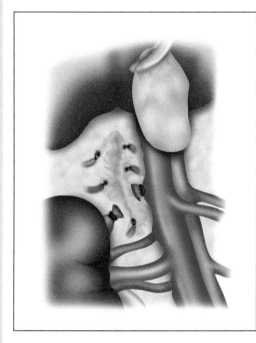

The adrenal gland is then removed and the surgical site examined for haemorrhage.

5   Local invasion into the renal vasculature or structure of the neighbouring kidney will warrant a concurrent ureteronephrectomy at this stage.

6   Double-check the surgical site to ensure that haemostasis has been achieved. If there is just a generalized slow oozing from the capillaries in the connective tissues, then collagen or gelatin sponges can be laid into and left in this tissue to aid haemostasis and degrade naturally. Count all swabs back out of the abdomen.

Surgical manipulations: venotomy of the caudal vena cava

1   The adrenal gland is exposed and the vena cava is dissected around carefully using curved haemostatic forceps and right-angled Lahey cholecystectomy clamps to create two tunnels, cranial and caudal to the tumour thrombus. Rummel tourniquets are then passed around the vena cava and left loose. The adrenal gland is dissected as described above, but any attachments to the area where the thrombus enters the vena cava are left intact.

2   The Rummel tourniquets are tightened and a venotomy is performed with a longitudinal incision in the vena cava adjacent to where the thrombus enters the vein. Continue the venotomy using Potts scissors, taking care not to incise the opposing wall of the vena cava. Use surgical suction to clear the surgical field. The thrombus is then removed, ideally still attached to the phenicoabdominal vein and adrenal gland, *en bloc*.

3   To minimize air emboli in the vena cava after the closure of the venotomy site, allow a small amount of blood to trickle into the venotomy site by slightly releasing one of the Rummel tourniquets. A Satinsky clamp is then placed across the venotomy site to partially occlude the vena cava. The Rummel tourniquets are released and the venotomy site is repaired using 1 metric (5/0 USP) polypropylene in a simple continuous suture pattern. The Satinsky clamp is then released.

→ **OPERATIVE TECHNIQUE 13.1 CONTINUED**

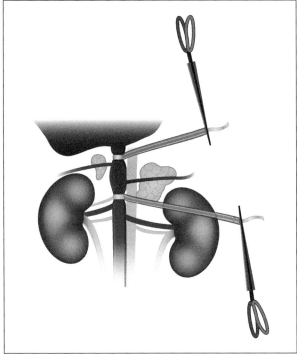

Removal of a left-sided adrenal mass with a thrombus extending into the vena cava. Rummel tourniquets are placed and a venotomy is made into the vena cava.

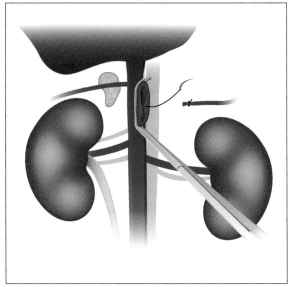

The thrombus and adrenal mass are removed *en bloc*. The Satinsky clamp is placed over the venotomy site, allowing restoration of blood flow once the Rummel tourniquets have been removed.

PRACTICAL TIP

There is no cited time limit for temporarily occluding a vena cava that is already experiencing a chronic change in blood flow dynamics due to the presence of a thrombus. However, it would be prudent to complete the thrombectomy and application of the Satinsky clamp in a timely manner, ensuring that the venotomy is closed with precision

Wound closure

The linea alba is closed with polypropylene in patients with HAC and polydioxanone in patients with a phaeochromocytoma.

POSTOPERATIVE MANAGEMENT

All patients must be monitored very carefully during the first 3 days following adrenalectomy. The patient should be clinically assessed for any signs of haemorrhage, dyspnoea, pancreatitis or discomfort. Blood samples should be taken daily to detect any electrolyte or metabolic imbalances. Electrocardiography and blood pressure monitoring should be performed intermittently during the initial postoperative period. See text on pre- and postoperative considerations for more specific comments and medications for patients with HAC and phaeochromocytoma. An ACTH stimulation test is performed the first day postoperatively in patients with HAC and then every 2–4 weeks until normal.

Chapter 14

The upper urinary tract

Mary McLoughlin and Brian A. Scansen

Surgical procedures involving the upper urinary tract of small animal patients are indicated for a variety of diagnostic, prognostic or therapeutic reasons. Patients with diseases of the upper urinary tract frequently present with clinical signs of renal disease or renal failure. Successful surgery relies on appropriate evaluation, diagnosis and medical stabilization of patients that are azotaemic or uraemic. Knowledge of the regional anatomy, including vascular supply and nervous innervation, is extremely important, as are specific evaluation of renal function and choice of appropriate anaesthetic agents. In addition, application of appropriate surgical techniques to minimize soft tissue trauma is essential. Important considerations for successful urinary tract surgery include:

- Minimize haemorrhage
- Maintain luminal diameters
- Establish a watertight seal
- Eliminate tension
- Use appropriate size and type of suture materials.

Evaluation of the patient

Diseases involving the upper urinary tract may be acute or chronic in nature. A complete and thorough history and physical examination of patients with suspected upper urinary tract disorders is an essential part of the minimum database (Figure 14.1). Specific examination and external evaluation of the upper urinary system is somewhat limited. The abdominal cavity should be palpated to evaluate kidney and bladder location and relative size, and to identify mass lesions or the presence of abdominal fluid. Small or moderate amounts of abdominal fluid may be difficult to detect by abdominal palpation alone. The presence of fluid within the abdominal cavity, although supportive, is not diagnostic for urinary tract injury or disease. Further diagnostic evaluation is indicated to determine the aetiology of the abdominal fluid. Palpation of the urethra rectally or externally in addition to examination of the external genitalia should be included as part of the complete physical examination.

Although physical examination may provide information to support the diagnosis of upper urinary tract disease, injury or obstruction, it is not generally considered to be a completely reliable evaluation when used alone. Specific evaluation of the presence and extent of upper urinary tract disorders is indicated prior to considering the administration

- History
  - Past history
    - Medical illness
    - Injuries
    - Surgeries
    - Medications
  - Vaccination, neutering and preventive medicine history
  - Current history
    - Medical illness
    - Injury
    - Surgery
    - Medications
  - Dietary history
    - Type of diet or supplements
    - Appetite
    - Vomiting, regurgitation, diarrhoea
    - Body condition score
  - Water consumption history
    - Polyuria/polydipsia
    - Quantitative (daily intake)
  - Urinary history
    - Haematuria
    - Pollakiuria
    - Stranguria
    - Anuria
    - Inappropriate urination
- Complete physical examination
- Haematology (complete blood count)
- Serum chemistry profile
- Collection of urine samples – cystocentesis
- Urinalysis
- Aerobic bacteriological culture
- Urine protein:creatinine ratio

14.1 Minimum database for patients with upper urinary tract disease.

of general anaesthesia and possible surgical intervention. A number of non-invasive and minimally invasive diagnostic techniques are available to evaluate and image the structure and function of the upper urinary system (Figure 14.2).

Technique	Details
Plain abdominal radiography	
Contrast radiography	Intravenous urogram (see Figure 14.3) Positive contrast cystogram Double contrast cystogram Retrograde urethrocystogram Retrograde vaginourethrogram
Contrast-enhanced computed tomography	

14.2 Specific diagnostic techniques for upper urinary tract evaluation. (continues) ▶

Technique	Details
Ultrasonography	Kidneys Renal pelvis Ureters Bladder
Uroendoscopy (luminal evaluation)	Vestibule Cranial vaginal vault Urethra Bladder Ureters – distal aspect (if dilated)
Nuclear scintigraphy	Global and differential glomerular filtration rate – ^{99m}Tc-DPTA

14.2 (continued) Specific diagnostic techniques for upper urinary tract evaluation.

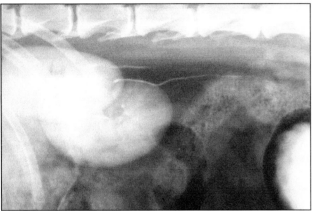

14.3 A normal intravenous urogram showing both kidneys and contrast medium filling the proximal ureters.

The kidneys

Renal biopsy procedures

Biopsy of the kidney is indicated for diagnosis or prognosis in small animal patients with documented renal disease or renal failure.

Ultrasound-guided percutaneous biopsy

Renal biopsy samples are frequently obtained in small animal patients using an ultrasound-guided percutaneous biopsy needle, ranging in size from 14 to 18 G. Ultrasonographic evaluation of the kidneys provides valuable information with regard to renal size, shape, parenchymal architecture, echogenicity and blood flow. Ultrasonographic orientation and visualization of the biopsy site provides a relatively safe and accurate means of obtaining a sample of renal tissue in small animal patients under light sedation.

> **WARNING**
>
> Patients must be carefully monitored for clinical signs of continued renal haemorrhage following percutaneous renal biopsy

Surgical biopsy

Indications for surgical or 'open' biopsy of a kidney (see Operative Technique 14.1) include:

- Patients undergoing exploratory coeliotomy for other reasons

- When a suitable percutaneous biopsy sample cannot be obtained
- Patients with potential bleeding disorders or coagulopathies
- When a larger tissue specimen is desired for evaluation.

Small animal patients undergoing renal biopsy procedures are typically azotaemic and/or proteinuric. Evaluation of renal parameters, including the serum concentration of urea nitrogen and creatinine as well as serum electrolytes and albumin, is an essential part of the presurgical evaluation. Administration of appropriate intravenous fluid therapy to maintain hydration, correct electrolyte disturbances and establish diuresis prior to the administration of general anaesthesia is indicated.

Nephrotomy

Nephroliths (Figure 14.4), fungal granulomas (USA), tissue debris and renal parasites can accumulate within the renal pelvis, resulting in obstruction to urine outflow, increased renal intrapelvic pressures, hydronephrosis and subsequent parenchymal damage. Removal of obstructive lesions from the renal pelvis can be surgically accomplished by either nephrotomy or pyelotomy.

Nephrotomy involves surgical incision through the renal parenchyma, exposing the renal pelvis, to remove calculi or other obstructive lesions directly from the renal pelvis.

> **WARNING**
>
> Incision through the renal parenchyma is associated with significant haemorrhage; therefore temporary vascular occlusion is required to perform this procedure

The renal fraction of the cardiac output is typically between 21 and 30% in normal individuals. In addition, the potential for nephron loss due to local parenchymal tissue injury and hypoxia, severing of the intersegmental vessels and scar tissue formation has been reported to diminish renal function, temporarily or permanently, by as much as 20–50% (Gahring et al., 1977). A comparison of renal function and parenchymal injury following two types of nephrotomy procedure described for clinical use in small animal patients (bisectional and intersegmental nephrotomy) was performed in normal dogs (Stone et al., 2002). This study concluded that neither bisectional nor intersegmental nephrotomy resulted in alteration of renal

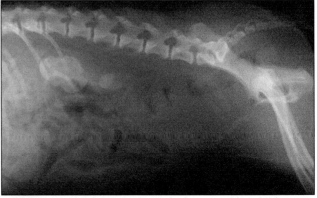

14.4 Lateral abdominal radiograph of a 4-year-old Pug bitch diagnosed with bilateral nephroliths.

function in normal dogs and the extent of healing was similar for both procedures by 4 weeks after surgery. Bisectional nephrotomy is simpler to perform (see Operative Technique 14.2), requiring less time and less meticulous parenchymal dissection than the intersegmental procedure.

Bilateral renal obstruction

Azotaemic patients with bilateral renal obstruction present an extremely challenging dilemma. Evaluation of individual renal function is essential. If bilateral nephrotomy is indicated, staging the surgical procedures approximately 4 weeks apart may reduce the risk of inducing acute renal failure by further insulting the compromised kidneys with general anaesthesia, vascular occlusion and surgical trauma.

Pyelotomy

When significant dilatation of the renal pelvis and proximal ureter occurs, it may be possible to remove a moderate-sized nephrolith by incising directly into the renal pelvis (Figure 14.5). Pyelotomy procedures avoid the complications associated with temporary vascular occlusion and surgical trauma to the renal parenchyma, but there are disadvantages: significant dilation of the pelvis is required; surgical exposure is limited; and meticulous closure of the pelvis, creating a watertight seal while avoiding luminal obstruction, is critical.

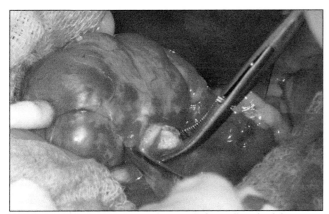

14.5 Pyelolithotomy: surgical removal of a small nephrolith through a pyelotomy incision.

Lithotripsy

Minimally invasive alternatives to traditional surgical techniques for the removal of upper urinary tract calculi are gaining popularity in small animal patients. Lithotripsy refers to the crushing or fragmentation of uroliths using shock waves or laser energy (Adams *et al.*, 2008). The two most common types of lithotripsy reported for clinical management of urinary calculi in human and small animal patients are extracorporeal shock wave lithotripsy (ESWL) and intracorporeal endoscopic laser lithotripsy utilizing a Ho:YAG (holmium:yttrium–aluminium–garnet) laser.

Factors that impact the choice of lithotripter and specific procedure to be performed include:

- Availability and cost of equipment
- Operator expertise
- Location of urolith(s)
- Number and size of urolith(s)

- Species (canine *versus* feline)
- Size of patient
- Sex of patient
- Medical status of the patient
- Procedural cost.

The clinical application of endoscopic laser lithotripsy in small animal patients is increasing with the availability of equipment and trained operators at both academic institutions and specialty practices (see Operative Technique 14.3). Urolithiasis is commonly recognized in both dogs and cats. Resolution of urolithiasis through medical management and dietary dissolution cannot always be achieved or may require an extended period of time. Owners may be reluctant to endure the clinical signs, including haematuria, stranguria and pollakiuria, commonly associated with cystoliths (Figure 14.6) and urethroliths. In addition, infection and partial or complete urinary outflow obstruction can be sequelae of chronic urolithiasis.

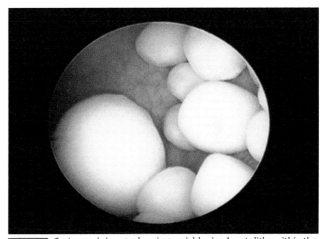

14.6 Cystoscopic image showing variably sized cystoliths within the bladder lumen.

Extracorporeal shock wave lithotripsy

ESWL involves the fragmentation or implosion of uroliths using high-energy shock waves generated outside the body and directed across tissue planes with the assistance of a focusing device. Imaging modalities, either fluoroscopy or ultrasonography, are used to localize the urolith within the treatment site. Nephroliths should be treated if obstruction is associated with chronic or recurrent urinary tract infection or chronic haematuria, without other identifiable aetiologies within the urogenital system. The number of shock waves, delivered to implode and powder nephroliths, is based on the type of lithotripter used as well as the size and composition of the nephroliths. The therapeutic goal of ESWL is to fragment uroliths, permitting spontaneous passage of smaller particles (generally ≤1 mm in diameter) with urine outflow. Ureteral stenting may be warranted to promote passive dilation of the ureters, facilitating passage of these smaller particles. ESWL has revolutionized the treatment of urolithiasis in humans and is considered to be the standard of care for treatment of upper urinary tract calculi. ESWL is ideally suited for uroliths that are confined to a small tissue space, such as the renal pelvis or ureters, preventing movement away from the focal field as shock waves are applied. Two types of shock wave lithotripters, based on coupling medium, are available for clinical use in humans and small animal patients: water-bath and dry lithotripters. Both types of ESWL have been successfully used to fragment nephroliths and ureteroliths in dogs and uretero-liths in cats. Technological advances in the development of dry lithotripters have improved the size and power of the focal zone, thus improving the efficiency of stone fragmentation. Water-bath lithotripters are currently very limited in availability for clinical use.

Current recommendations for the use of ESWL in small animal patients are focused on the treatment of nephro-liths in dogs, with consideration for obstructing ureteroliths in cats. Although both nephroliths and ureteroliths are recognized with increasing frequency in cats, the diameter of a non-dilated feline ureter ranges between 0.3 and 0.4 mm, potentially prohibiting passage of small stone fragments, and resulting in obstruction at a distal site. It has been reported that ESWL can be performed safely for ureteroliths less than 5–10 mm in dogs and less than 3–5 mm in cats (Berent, 2011). ESWL is performed with the patient under general anaesthesia to eliminate movement once the urolith is positioned within the focal zone. ESWL is well tolerated; however, transient haematuria can be observed after treatment. Renal injury is dose-dependent and a transient reduction in glomerular filtration rate (GFR) can occur, which typically resolves within 7 days of therapy. Concerns have been expressed that the feline kidney may be more sensitive to the effects of ESWL than that of the dog. Further investigation of the effects of ESWL on obstructed or diseased kidneys is warranted. Additional complications may include pancreatitis, diarrhoea and abdominal discomfort.

Intracorporeal laser lithotripsy

Intracorporeal endoscopic laser lithotripsy using a Ho:YAG laser was first reported for clinical use in humans in 1995. This modality is now recognized as the standard of care for management of human ureteroliths, cystoliths and urethroliths, with reported success rates exceeding 90% (Bevan et al., 2009). Intracorporeal lithotripsy using a Ho:YAG laser has been more recently reported for successful treatment of cystoliths and urethroliths in both male and female dogs and female cats. The Ho:YAG laser is a solid-state pulsed laser emitting light at a wavelength of 2100 nm that can be applied in a fluid medium. Infrared energy is emitted from an active medium of holmium, a rare earth element, and a yttrium, aluminium and garnet (YAG) crystal. Laser energy is transmitted via small diameter optical quartz fibres (200, 365 and 550 μm) that can be accommodated through the biopsy channel of varying sizes of rigid and flexible endoscopes, making this ideal for uroendoscopic surgery and lithotripsy (Lulich et al., 2009b; Figure 14.7). Stone fragmentation using the Ho:YAG laser is mainly photothermal and involves thermal drilling, versus the shock wave effect applied by the extracorporeal lithotripters. The effect of the pulsed laser on uroliths results when vapour, created by the pulse of laser energy travelling through the fluid medium from the tip of the quartz fibre, is trapped within a bubble (Adams et al., 2008). Rapid expansion and collapse of vaporization bubbles at the surface of the stone shear the stone into fragments as a result of thermal decomposition (Lulich et al., 2009a). If the laser tip is greater than 0.5 mm away from the urolith, the vapour bubble collapses and the fluid medium will absorb the laser energy. Fragmentation of uroliths can only occur when the laser tip is in direct contact or within 0.5 mm of the surface of the stone (Figure 14.8). As a result of poor absorption of pulsed laser energy by the surrounding uroendothelial structures, endoscopic laser lithotripsy has been shown to be a safe

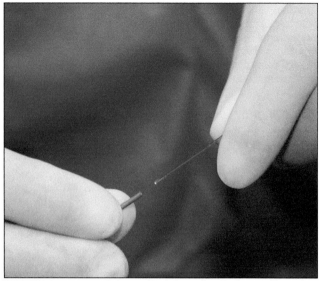

14.7 Laser energy is transmitted via small optical quartz fibres that pass through the biopsy channel of rigid and flexible endoscopes. Insertion of a 365 μm laser fibre into the open end of a catheter sheath, which protects the laser fibre as it passes through the endoscope.

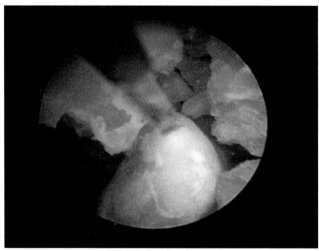

14.8 The open-ended catheter sheath is passed through the biopsy channel located on the bridge of the rigid endoscope.

and efficient method of treatment for cystoliths, urethroliths and ureteroliths (Davidson et al., 2004).

Ureteronephrectomy

Ureteronephrectomy is excision of the kidney and ureter (see Operative Technique 14.4). It is indicated when the kidney is non-functional, severely traumatized, infected, haemorrhagic, hydronephrotic or neoplastic.

It is important to establish normal renal function in the contralateral kidney prior to performing ureteronephrectomy (Figure 14.9). Determination of acceptable renal function in the contralateral kidney can be challenging in azotaemic patients. Serum parameters of renal function, including urea nitrogen and creatinine, remain within the normal range until approximately 75% of total renal function is compromised. Therefore evaluation of these parameters alone is not an accurate method for evaluating function of the contralateral kidney when considering ureteronephrectomy. Evaluation using plain radiography or ultrasonography may provide insight into the relative size and shape of the contralateral kidney but does not determine renal function.

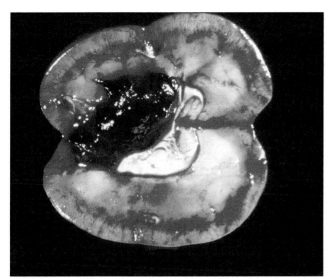

14.9 Excised kidney from a 6-year-old mixed-breed dog diagnosed with idiopathic renal haematuria. Note the large blood clot filling the renal pelvis.

global renal function as well as individual function of the affected and contralateral kidney (Figure 14.10). As nuclear scintigraphy is not widely available in the practice setting, intravenous urography (see Figure 14.3) is frequently used as a crude method of establishing qualitative renal function in the contralateral kidney. Assessment of the functional capacity of the kidneys is based on the ability of each kidney to filter and excrete contrast medium (Figure 14.11). Compromised renal function, any form of outflow obstruction or systemic hypotension will result in decreased clearance and excretion of the contrast medium.

> **WARNING**
>
> Prolonged renal excretion of contrast medium has been reported to cause renal damage

Specific evaluation of the GFR can be determined in a non-invasive manner with nuclear scintigraphy. This is the most accurate method for clinically assessing

Ureteronephrectomy can be performed from a flank or ventral midline coeliotomy. Most surgeons choose the midline approach because it facilitates exposure of the distal aspect of the ureter for ligation, transection and removal, and facilitates exposure of the retroperitoneal space for removal of neoplastic masses involving the kidney and ureter (see Operative Technique 14.4).

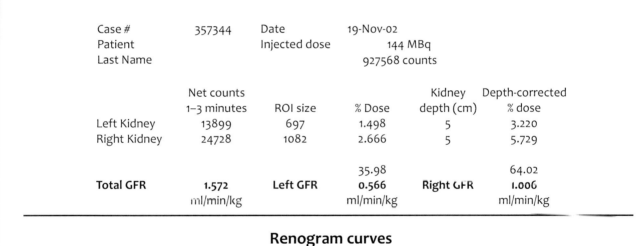

	Case #	357344	Date	19-Nov-02		
	Patient		Injected dose	144 MBq		
	Last Name			927568 counts		

	Net counts 1–3 minutes	ROI size	% Dose	Kidney depth (cm)	Depth-corrected % dose
Left Kidney	13899	697	1.498	5	3.220
Right Kidney	24728	1082	2.666	5	5.729

				35.98		64.02
Total GFR	**1.572** ml/min/kg	**Left GFR**	0.566 ml/min/kg		**Right GFR**	1.006 ml/min/kg

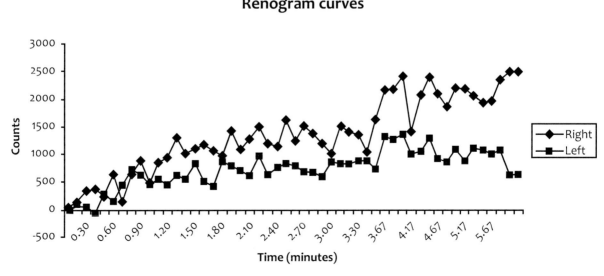

Renogram curves

Legend: Right, Left

Y-axis: Counts (−500 to 3000)
X-axis: Time (minutes) (0.30, 0.60, 0.90, 1.20, 1.50, 1.80, 2.10, 2.40, 2.70, 3.00, 3.30, 3.67, 4.17, 4.67, 5.17, 5.67)

14.10 Calculation of total and individual glomerular filtration rate (GFR) with nuclear scintigraphy. ROI = region of interest.

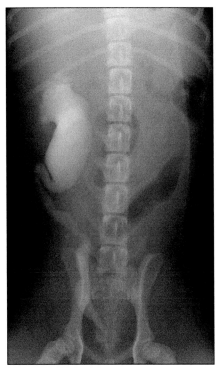

14.11

Ventrodorsal abdominal radiograph of a 7-month-old mixed-breed bitch presented for urinary incontinence. Intravenous urogram demonstrates severe right hydronephrosis, pyelectasia and dilatation of the ureter associated with an ectopically displaced ureter. The left kidney is non-functional and cannot be visualized.

Nephrolithiasis

Optimal management of upper urinary calculi in dogs and cats remains controversial. Removal of nephroliths and ureteroliths is recommended if stones are increasing in size or positioned to create a partial or complete urinary outflow obstruction, resulting in dilatation of the renal pelvis, hydronephrosis, parenchymal loss, reduced renal function, haematuria, infection, fever or abdominal discomfort (DeFarges et al., 2013). Determination of urinary outflow obstruction in the persistently azotaemic patient is confirmed by imaging modalities, including ultrasonography, fluoroscopy, contrast pyelography and contrast-enhanced computed tomography (CT).

Initial stabilization and medical management of patients with upper urinary tract obstruction is focused on careful fluid diuresis and critical monitoring of hydration status using central venous pressure, serial bodyweight measurements, urine output and changes in the concentration of serum electrolytes. Crystalloid fluid therapy is administered at maintenance rates using 0.45% saline and 2.5% dextrose with additional replacement fluids using an isotonic, balanced crystalloid solution, avoiding excessive sodium, to correct patient hydration status and establish diuresis. Additional medical therapies may be warranted, including a continuous rate infusion (CRI) of mannitol promoting further osmotic diuresis, and administration of either amitriptyline or an alpha-adrenergic receptor antagonist (prazosin or tamsulosin) to induce smooth muscle relaxation of upper urinary tract structures, thus facilitating dislodgement of obstructive urolith(s) (Berent, 2011).

Failure of medical therapies to dislodge obstructing uroliths, with worsening azotaemia and decreased urine output, within 24 hours is an indication to consider alternative options for urolith removal or fragmentation. Decompression of the obstructed urinary outflow tract is essential and delay is related to loss of renal function. Historically, surgery has been the mainstay for management of obstructive nephrolithiasis in both dogs and cats. Surgical procedures for the removal of nephroliths include nephrotomy, pyelotomy and ureteronephrectomy. Depending on the degree of obstruction, surgical intervention may be indicated for one or both kidneys. Challenges and risks of invasive renal surgery include providing general anaesthesia to unstable patients with renal dysfunction, control of haemorrhage, preservation of functional nephrons and prevention of urine leakage. Minimally invasive techniques (e.g. lithotripsy) can also be used (see above).

Renal neoplasia

Renal neoplasia is relatively uncommon in small animal patients, accounting for 0.06–1.7% of all reported neoplasia (Klein et al., 1988). Malignant renal neoplasia is recognized more frequently than benign tumours in both dogs and cats (Figure 14.12). Primary or metastatic lymphoma has been shown to be the most common malignant renal tumour in cats, but renal carcinomas are frequently recognized. Tubular cell carcinomas are the most common primary malignant renal tumours recognized in dogs. The incidence of renal carcinoma increases with age and it has been shown to occur more often in males.

Renal neoplasia is frequently not identified until an advanced stage, resulting in enlargement of the kidney, haematuria or obstruction. Bilateral renal involvement is recognized in approximately 30% of dogs with primary renal neoplasia. The metastatic potential of malignant renal tumours to sites including the local lymph nodes, liver, lung, adrenal glands and bone is high. Capsular disruption and local spread to the surrounding retroperitoneal space, adrenal gland and renal vasculature has been reported.

Thoracic radiographs and ultrasonographic evaluation of the abdomen will assist in staging the patient for evidence of bilateral renal involvement or metastatic disease. Surgical treatment of primary renal neoplasia typically involves complete or partial nephrectomy, based on the extent of the disease and renal function. Adjunct chemotherapy may be indicated after surgery, depending on the tumour type and staging.

	Malignant	Benign
Dogs	Carcinoma • Tubular cell carcinoma • Transitional cell carcinoma Haemangiosarcoma Fibrosarcoma Chondrosarcoma Liposarcoma Rhabdomyosarcoma Leiomyosarcoma Nephroblastoma Undifferentiated tumours • Sarcoma • Carcinoma	Adenoma Haemangioma Osteoma Lipoma Teratoma
Cats	Lymphoma • Primary • Metastatic – alimentary Carcinoma • Transitional cell carcinoma • Squamous cell carcinoma Fibrosarcoma Leiomyosarcoma Haemangiosarcoma Nephroblastoma Undifferentiated sarcoma	Adenoma Lipoma

14.12 Primary renal tumours in dogs and cats.

Renal trauma

Traumatic injuries to the kidney requiring surgical intervention are infrequently recognized in small animal patients. The relative rarity of serious renal injuries is explained by regional anatomy. The kidneys lie in a retroperitoneal position, covered with a fibrous capsule and embedded in perirenal adipose tissue. The location of the kidneys renders them well protected by the ribs, epaxial musculature and spine. Classifications of renal injuries have been developed in both human and veterinary medicine to describe the detailed range of renal pathology that results from trauma and to develop guidelines for patient care (Figure 14.13). Early recognition and characterization of renal injuries has become more detailed with improved diagnostic imaging modalities, including intravenous urography (Figure 14.14), angiography and contrast-enhanced CT.

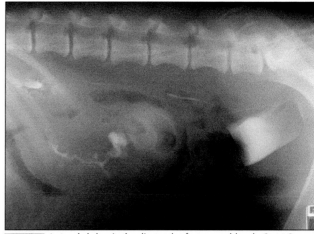

14.14 Lateral abdominal radiograph of a 1-year-old male Great Dane presented for abdominal pain and lethargy. Intravenous urogram demonstrates a rupture of the caudal pole of the left kidney and extravasation of contrast medium into the retroperitoneal space.

> **PRACTICAL TIP**
>
> Gross or microscopic haematuria following blunt or penetrating abdominal trauma indicates injury to the urinary tract but is not specific to either the upper or lower urinary structures

Uncontrolled renal haemorrhage or extravasation of urine into the retroperitoneal space or peritoneal cavity can occur as a result of any form of blunt or penetrating abdominal trauma. Severe renal trauma can result in an acute haemorrhagic diathesis and death prior to emergency presentation. In patients with suspected abdominal trauma that are haemodynamically unstable at the time of presentation, the first medical priority involves stabilization of the cardiovascular system and treatment of hypovolaemic shock. A cursory physical examination and assessment of the vital parameters is performed while a central venous catheter is placed for the administration of crystalloid fluids at a shock dosage. In addition, a peripheral venous catheter can be placed for the administration of additional fluids, colloids, blood products or other medications needed for patient stabilization. If possible, the urinary bladder is catheterized to characterize urine output. Lack of appropriate urine output may be indicative of:

- Severe bilateral upper urinary tract injury
- Accumulation of urine within the retroperitoneal space or peritoneal cavity due to rupture of the urinary tract
- Urethral disruption
- Hypovolaemic shock
- Primary renal failure.

Serial monitoring of vital parameters and haematocrit is performed at regular intervals over the first 2–6 hours to evaluate the patient's status and response to fluid therapy. Fluid therapy is adjusted based on the results of central venous pressure monitoring, indirect blood pressure monitoring and urine output. When the haematocrit and total solids do not stabilize but continue to decrease and vital parameters are not improving with the appropriate fluid support, continuing haemorrhage is likely. Transfusion with whole blood or packed red blood cells and colloids should be performed. The site of haemorrhage must be identified and controlled.

Diagnosis

Diagnosis of intra-abdominal haemorrhage is confirmed by abdominocentesis (see Chapter 18). When the haematocrit of an abdominal fluid sample is similar to the peripheral haematocrit, intra-abdominal haemorrhage has occurred. The diagnosis of intra-abdominal haemorrhage does not determine the severity or the aetiology of bleeding.

The specific diagnosis of renal injury is made by contrast radiography (intravenous urography or angiography), contrast-enhanced CT (Figure 14.15) or exploratory laparotomy. Minor renal injuries, including contusions, superficial lacerations and perinephric or subcapsular haematomas, comprise the majority of renal trauma cases. They are typically self-limiting and do not require invasive medical or

Trauma	Description
Bruising and ecchymosis	Simple bruising followed by subcapsular ecchymosis is the most common lesion resulting from a blow to the kidney. The haemorrhage generally arrests spontaneously and the subcapsular blood is absorbed. Microscopic haematuria may occur
Haematoma	Break in the fibrous capsule allowing blood to accumulate in the perinephric region between the capsule and renal fascia. Bleeding may arrest spontaneously. Following the injury, the haematoma will liquefy to a clear amber liquid and absorb (perirenal cyst) or become infected (perirenal abscess). In the latter case, perinephric infection may require surgical drainage. Microscopic haematuria may be present with haematomas
Fissure	Complete tear of the parenchyma extending through the capsule, creating a perinephric haematoma. Microscopic haematuria is noted. If the fissure involves the renal pelvis, gross haematuria will be present. Active bleeding stops with onset of clot formation and the tear scars over
Laceration	Occurs when a contusion is of such force that a tear develops in the renal fascia and capsule and extends into the renal parenchymal tissue, allowing blood to empty directly into the retroperitoneal space or peritoneal cavity. If the tear involves the renal hilum and pelvis, extravasation of blood and urine ensues. Either form of tear is associated with marked haematuria
Rupture of vascular pedicle	Rarely, there is disruption of the renal vascular pedicle, which allows massive haemorrhage to occur. Due to blood loss and hypovolaemic shock, this condition can be rapidly fatal

14.13 Classification of renal trauma.
(Modified from Thornhill and Cechner, 1981)

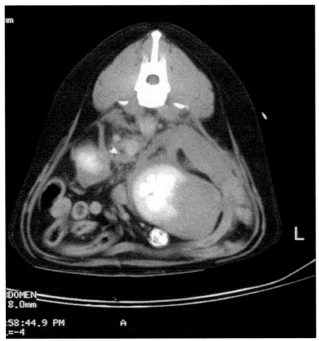

14.15 Spiral contrast-enhanced CT scan of a 4-year-old neutered Gordon Setter bitch presenting with acute abdominal pain. Note loss of integrity of the convex surface of the left kidney and contrast medium leakage into the area of soft tissue.

surgical intervention. A major renal injury generally results in the leakage of blood and/or urine into the retroperitoneal space or peritoneal cavity. Major renal injuries include deep lacerations of the parenchyma, extravasation of urine from the collecting system or pelvis, moderate to large haematomas, renal pedicle injuries, renal parenchymal fragmentation and generalized crushing of parenchymal tissue. Identification of widening or streaking within the retroperitoneal space on plain abdominal radiographs may be indicative of fluid accumulation in this region (Figure 14.16).

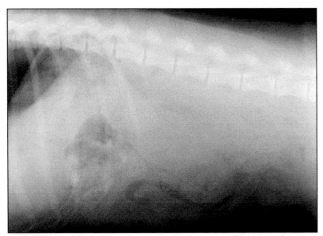

14.16 Lateral abdominal radiograph of a 4-year-old neutered Gordon Setter bitch with acute abdominal pain. Widening and streaking of the retroperitoneal space is suggestive of fluid accumulation in this region.

WARNING

Accumulation of urine or blood in the retroperitoneal space is not typically diagnosed by abdominal palpation or abdominocentesis, often resulting in a delay in the diagnosis of major renal injury

Surgery

Exploratory coeliotomy is indicated on an emergency basis in veterinary patients with uncontrolled intra-abdominal haemorrhage. Accurate assessment of renal function and stabilization of the patient are critical prior to surgical intervention and general anaesthesia.

1. Perform a ventral midline coeliotomy.
2. Use suction to clear the abdominal cavity of accumulated blood.
3. Explore the entire abdominal cavity to identify sites of active haemorrhage. Persistent intra-abdominal haemorrhage frequently results from parenchymal injury of organs or vascular disruption.
4. Once a site of active bleeding is identified, use digital pressure initially to control the haemorrhage until haemostatic forceps can be applied.
5. In the event of renal haemorrhage, atraumatic vascular occlusion of the renal pedicle is indicated to control bleeding and allow complete assessment of the injuries to the kidneys and urinary tract.
6. If the retroperitoneal space is intact, use blunt dissection to expose the kidney. Rotate the convex surface of the kidney medially to expose the dorsal aspect of the hilus and evaluate the renal vascular pedicle.

WARNING

Maceration, oedema and haemorrhage of retroperitoneal tissues make gross evaluation of the renal pedicle and ureter extremely difficult

7. Leave undisturbed any lacerations of the renal capsule and parenchyma that are clotted with no evidence of active bleeding at surgery.
8. If active parenchymal bleeding is apparent, sutures can be placed through the ruptured edges of the renal capsule. Continued haemorrhage from the parenchyma will accumulate under the renal capsule, forming a subcapsular haematoma. In addition, sutures can be placed directly into the renal parenchyma in a mattress pattern to compress the intersegmental vessels at the site to control haemorrhage.

Severe fractures of the renal parenchyma may necessitate complete ureteronephrectomy (see Operative Technique 14.4) or partial nephrectomy. Although infrequently performed in veterinary patients, partial nephrectomy is indicated to preserve functional renal tissue when parenchymal injury is localized to a pole of the kidney.

Technique for partial nephrectomy:

1. Following vascular occlusion of the renal pedicle with atraumatic vascular forceps or a tourniquet, excise the damaged parenchymal tissue.
2. To accomplish haemostasis, individually ligate the interlobar vessels supplying the local parenchymal tissues. Blood flow through the renal pedicle is re-established and the exposed renal parenchyma is evaluated for bleeding.
3. If a portion of the renal capsule is available, it can be sutured over the excision site. Otherwise, use omentum to cover the exposed renal parenchyma. Mattress sutures through the renal parenchyma or capsule can be used to secure the omentum to the kidney.

An alternative technique for performing a partial nephrectomy is shown in Figure 14.17.

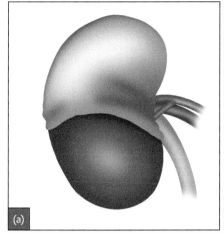

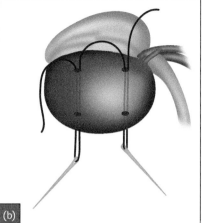

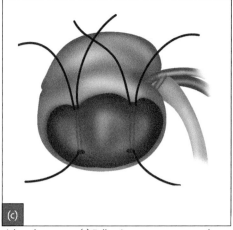

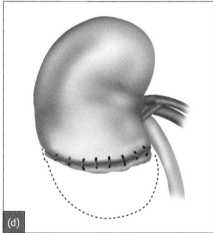

14.17 Alternative surgical procedure for partial nephrectomy. (a) Following temporary vascular occlusion of the renal pedicle, the renal capsule is peeled away from the parenchyma to be resected. (b) Long, straight needles are used to pass an absorbable suture through the parenchyma at the proposed resection site. (c) The suture is cut and then tied in three separate ligatures, taking care not to damage the ureters or renal vessels. (d) The parenchyma distal to the ligatures is excised and the capsule is sewn back over the end of the kidney.

Complete or partial disruption of the renal pedicle results in significant haemorrhage, often necessitating ureteronephrectomy in veterinary patients as a life-saving effort.

Postoperative considerations

Patients should be carefully monitored after surgery. Administration of intravenous fluids and colloids is continued and serial evaluation of vital parameters is indicated every 2–4 hours until the patient is haemodynamically stable. Continued assessment for additional injuries resulting from trauma is warranted during this period of postoperative stabilization and monitoring.

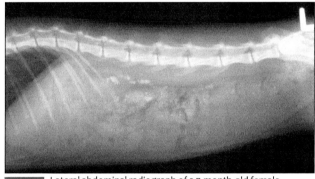

14.18 Lateral abdominal radiograph of a 7-month-old female neutered Domestic Shorthaired cat presented for polyuria and polydipsia. Multiple bilateral calcium oxalate ureteroliths are present.

The ureters

Ureteral obstruction

Common causes of ureteral obstruction in small animal patients include urolithiasis, strictures, neoplasia, trauma, inflammatory disease, fibrosis, polyps, foreign bodies, blood clots and inadvertent surgical ligation. Ureterolithiasis is currently recognized with increasing frequency in both dogs and cats. Radiodense ureteroliths may be identified as an incidental finding on plain abdominal radiographs. Non-obstructive ureteroliths with no associated clinical signs are left untreated. Struvite and calcium oxalate are currently the most common ureteroliths identified in small animal patients (Figure 14.18). Neoplasia of the ureter is rare in small animal patients, but transitional cell carcinoma, leiomyoma, leiomyosarcoma and benign polyps of the ureter have been reported.

Diagnosis and management of ureteral obstruction can be extremely challenging. The degree of upper urinary tract injury is based on a number of factors, including chronicity and extent of obstruction as well as the presence of urinary tract infection. Acute complete or severe partial obstruction of both ureters produces post-renal azotaemia and uraemia that, if not corrected, can be fatal within 3–6 days (Hosgood and Hedlund, 1993). Obstruction in the face of urinary tract infection is devastating, resulting in hydronephrosis, pyelonephritis, septicaemia and potential death. Complete obstruction of one ureter and the associated kidney in the absence of infection is often not identified until an advanced stage. Clinical signs of uraemia do not occur if the contralateral kidney is functional and remains unobstructed. Progressive dilatation of the upper urinary tract proximal to the site of obstruction occurs, resulting in dilatation of the renal pelvis, hydronephrosis, damage to or loss of renal parenchyma and reduced renal function, in the absence of medical, surgical or minimally invasive intervention.

Resolution of the ureteral obstruction can result in return of renal function, depending on the severity and duration of the obstruction. Experimental and clinical studies evaluating the effects of complete unilateral ureteral obstruction for periods of 1, 2, 4 and 6 weeks have shown that varying degrees of recovery of renal function occur. Following the release of a complete unilateral ureteral obstruction for 1 week, the GFR returned to 68% of the normal value. However, following the release of complete unilateral ureteral obstructions that had lasted for 2, 4 and 6 weeks, the return to renal function was shown to be 38.7%, 9.8% and 2%, respectively. Recovery of renal function is inversely related to the duration of the obstructive event (Osborne and Polzin, 1986).

> **WARNING**
>
> Early recognition, with medical, surgical or minimally invasive intervention to relieve ureteral obstruction or provide temporary urinary diversion, such as nephrostomy drainage, is critical to preserving renal function

Ureterolithiasis

The diagnosis of upper urinary calculi is often delayed until ureterolith(s) become obstructive. Most ureteroliths in dogs (>30–60%) and cats (>98%) are composed of calcium oxalate and identifiable on plain abdominal radiographs (DeFarges et al., 2013). Improved imaging modalities, including ultrasonography, contrast radiography (intravenous urography and positive contrast pyelography) and contrast-enhanced CT, help confirm and characterize the degree of secondary pathology including pyelectasia, hydronephrosis and ureteral dilatation proximal to the site of obstruction. The rate of migration of ureteroliths is variable. Ureteroliths are frequently irregular, adhering to the ureteral mucosa. Prolonged presence of calculi within the ureter may result in necrosis and rupture of the ureteral wall.

Treatment options

The use of medical management alone is discussed under Nephrolithiasis (see above).

Options for surgical management include:

- Retrograde flushing of calculi into the renal pelvis for removal via pyelotomy or nephrotomy
- Ureterotomy
- Resection of the obstructed distal ureteral segment and neoureterostomy
- Ureteral resection and anastomosis
- Ureteronephrectomy
- Placement of a subcutaneous ureteral bypass.

Minimally invasive surgery includes:

- ESWL (see above)
- Antegrade or retrograde ureteral stenting.

Therapeutic decision-making should be individualized and based on the clinical presentation, degree of azotaemia and renal pathology, determination of partial or complete obstruction, involvement of one or both ureters, and the specific location of the obstruction. Medical management is initiated to stabilize the azotaemic patient and attempt to dislodge obstructing ureterolith(s). Medical management alone has been shown to be effective in only a limited number of feline patients (13% of cats; Kyles et al., 2005). If clinical improvement has not occurred within 24 hours, alternative approaches to treatment should be implemented to remove the obstruction to urine outflow, thus decompressing the renal pelvis. Historically, surgery has been the mainstay of treatment for patients with obstructing ureterolithiasis. Ureteral surgery requires a very high level of surgical skill and training; it is optimally performed with surgical magnification.

> **PRACTICAL TIP**
>
> Magnification of the operative field, using surgical magnifying telescopes (x3.5) or an operating microscope, is essential for ureteral surgery

The location of an obstructing ureterolith generally dictates the surgical procedure chosen. Ureterotomy is most commonly performed to remove ureteroliths located in the proximal one-third to one-half of the ureter. Ureteroliths positioned more distally are generally removed by resection of the ureter proximal to the obstruction and neoureterocystotomy. Avoiding tension on the shortened ureter to promote primary healing without leakage or stricture formation is essential for surgical success. Tension-relieving procedures such as renal descensus (caudal displacement of the kidney) and psoas muscle cystopexy can also be performed. These procedures are adapted from human surgery and focus on reducing the physical distance between a shortened ureter and the site of bladder reimplantation, and are performed as follows:

1. Gently free the kidney from the retroperitoneal space without disrupting the renal vascular pedicle, permitting increased mobility.
2. The kidney can be displaced (descended) several centimetres in a caudal direction without kinking or excessive tension of the renal pedicle.
3. 'Pexy' the kidney at this caudal location with several mattress sutures placed through the renal capsule and adjacent epaxial musculature. Avoid placement of suture material into the renal parenchyma, which could potentially injure functional nephrons.
4. Ureteral reimplantation and neoureterocystotomy can be performed at any site on the bladder wall between the trigone and the apex.
5. Movement and positional changes of the bladder related to micturition must be considered when choosing the site for reimplantation.
6. With the bladder under moderate cranial traction, the dorsal bladder wall is fixed, or pexied, to the adjacent psoas musculature, minimizing extreme movements during bladder filling and contraction. It is not uncommon to relocate a shortened ureter into the bladder apex to eliminate tension.

The postsurgical complication rate and perioperative mortality rate have been reported to be as high as 31% and 18%, respectively, in a study of 153 cats with ureteral obstruction (Kyles et al., 2005). Complications of ureteral surgery are reported more commonly in cats than in dogs. Leakage of urine, uroabdomen, persistent or recurrent ureteral obstruction and renal insufficiency are the most frequently recognized short- and long-term complications after surgery. Despite the challenges and potential complications associated with ureteral surgery, survival rates for cats 12–24 months after surgery are significantly greater than for cats receiving medical management alone.

Ureterotomy

Retrograde flushing of ureteral calculi into the renal pelvis for removal is generally considered preferable to direct removal of calculi from the ureter, avoiding complications associated with ureteral surgery. However, obstructive ureteral calculi are frequently adherent to the ureteral mucosa and are not movable. In these situations, ureterotomy is performed using a longitudinal or transverse incision over the calculus. Following removal of ureteral calculi, the proximal and distal ureteral segments should be gently flushed to remove blood clots and debris. Ureterotomy closure can be performed longitudinally or transversely, or the longitudinal incision may be closed in a transverse manner to prevent luminal narrowing (Figure 14.19).

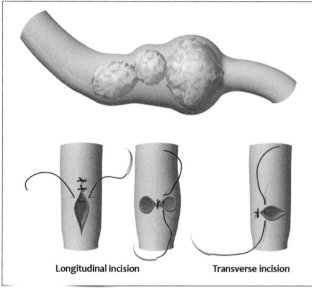

14.19 Ureterotomy. The surgical incision can be made directly over the ureterolith. The incision can be closed longitudinally or transversely.

> **WARNING**
>
> Precise closure of the ureterotomy incision is critical

Ureterotomy incisions are closed using a 0.5–0.7 metric (7/0–6/0 USP) monofilament suture material in an interrupted or continuous pattern; appositional closure creates a watertight seal. The submucosa is the surgical holding layer of the ureter. In spite of successful closure and healing without urine leakage, chronic inflammatory mucosal changes or intraluminal scar tissue may limit urine flow through the site.

Nephrostomy tubes

Percutaneous or surgically placed nephrostomy tubes have been advocated as a method of maintaining continuous decompression of the renal pelvis and establishing urinary diversion prior to surgical intervention or minimally invasive stenting. Urinary diversion using nephrostomy tube drainage may also be indicated after invasive surgery, to direct urine flow away from the surgical incision in the

ureter for a period of 3–7 days, allowing local inflammation to resolve and restoring luminal diameter.

1. Position the nephrostomy tube through the body wall and convex surface of the kidney into the renal pelvis.
2. Position the tip of the tube in the proximal ureter.
3. 'Pexy' the kidney to the body wall to prevent premature displacement of the nephrostomy catheter.
4. Collect urine into a closed urinary collection system.
5. Prior to removal of the nephrostomy tube, evaluate the patency of the ureter by administering a radiographic contrast medium through the tube; this permits evaluation of the ureterotomy site for patency and leakage of urine (Figure 14.20).
6. Continue administration of intravenous fluid therapy after surgery.
7. Evaluate renal function parameters on a daily basis until renal function is stable and the patient can maintain its hydration status with only oral intake of water, or subcutaneous fluid supplementation.

Appropriate antibiotic therapy is indicated, based on the results of aerobic bacteriological culture of the urine. Mineral analysis of the calculi should be performed.

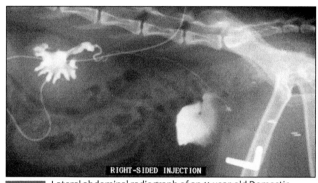

RIGHT-SIDED INJECTION

14.20 Lateral abdominal radiograph of an 11-year-old Domestic Shorthaired cat after bilateral ureterotomies to remove multiple ureteroliths. A nephrostomy drainage catheter was placed for urinary diversion. Contrast medium injection through the nephrostomy catheter demonstrates that the ureter is patent. The proximal ureter and renal pelvis are significantly dilated.

Ureteral stenting

Minimally invasive placement of ureteral stents for the treatment of obstruction is rapidly gaining interest for clinical use in small animal speciality practice and has been the focus of numerous recent clinical investigations in both dogs and cats. Minimally invasive or surgically assisted ureteral stent placement provides the benefits of immediate decompression of the renal pelvis and re-establishing urine outflow while avoiding the risks and complications associated with more invasive surgical interventions such as ureterotomy, ureteral resection, reimplantation, neoureterocystotomy, ureteronephrectomy or renal transplantation. Minimally invasive ureteral stenting is ideally performed in a dedicated interventional surgical suite (Figure 14.21). This area is maintained for aseptic surgery and can accommodate a C-arm for fluoroscopic and radiographic imaging, ultrasonography, endoscopy and a Ho:YAG laser. Highly skilled technical staff are also necessary because multiple modalities may be necessary in the treatment protocol of a given patient.

Double-pigtail ureteral stents are completely intracorporeal and can be placed by minimally invasive techniques (uroendoscopy and fluoroscopy) alone in most

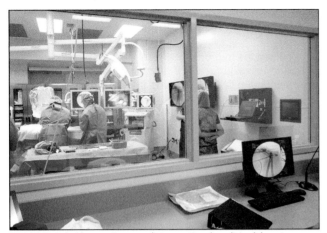

14.21 Hybrid operating room/interventional medicine laboratory where both percutaneous and hybrid interventional procedures are performed. The room functions as a sterile theatre, with fluoroscopic imaging, an array of catheters, wires, devices and stents immediately accessible, and multiple monitors to display real-time imaging and patient monitoring data to the veterinary surgeons, nursing staff and observers.

dogs, but generally require surgical assistance (cystotomy to access the ureteral orifice within the bladder, open pyelocentesis or nephrostomy) for placement in cats and small dogs (<7 kg). Double-pigtail ureteral stents are manufactured in a variety of sizes from 2 to 6 Fr for specific use in small animal patients (Figure 14.22). These polymer stents are multi-fenestrated with variable length pigtail loops located on each end to secure placement within the renal pelvis and the bladder lumen (Figure 14.23). A hydrophilic coating on the surface of the stent facilitates passage in either an anterograde or a retrograde manner. Ureteral stent placement provides both intraluminal and extraluminal flow of urine and promotes passive dilation of the ureters, thus facilitating the passage of obstructive ureteroliths or fragmented nephroliths. Placement of ureteral stents has

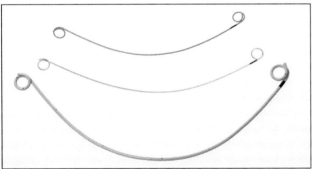

14.22 Varying sizes (2–6 Fr) of double-pigtail ureteral stents are commercially available for minimally invasive or surgically assisted placement in dogs and cats.

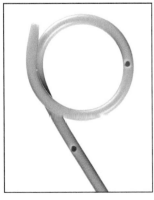

14.23 Close-up view of one of the looped ends of a double-pigtail ureteral stent catheter with multiple fenestrations.

been advocated in patients diagnosed with nephrolithiasis in preparation for ESWL. Passive dilation of the ureter is warranted to prevent more distal obstruction with smaller stone fragments following lithotripsy. This pre-emptive procedure should be considered for dogs with large or multiple nephroliths, and for small dogs and cats if ESWL is attempted to fragment ureteroliths. Surgical placement of ureteral stents may also be considered following invasive surgical procedures involving the ureters, to divert urine flow away from the surgical incision, thus enhancing primary healing without leakage or stricture.

Minimally invasive retrograde placement of ureteral stents can be performed in most dogs and some female cats (Figure 14.24).

1. The procedure is performed in the anaesthetized patient using both uroendoscopy and fluoroscopy.
2. An appropriately sized cystoscope is used to evaluate the lower urinary tract, identifying the C-shaped ureteral orifices. Identification of the ureteral orifices is facilitated by using only moderate fluid distension of the bladder, permitting the orifices to protrude slightly within the bladder lumen (Figure 14.25).
3. A flexible hydrophilic guidewire is passed through the biopsy channel and advanced through the ureteral orifice into the distal ureter.
4. The cystoscope is removed from the lower urinary tract, carefully maintaining the guidewire in position within the ureters and allowing the excess length of the guidewire to pass through the biopsy channel as the endoscope is retracted.

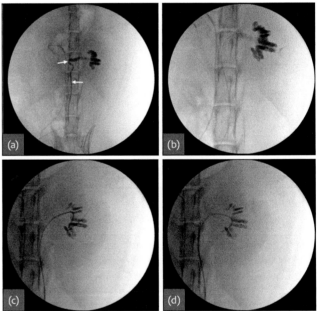

14.24 Images obtained during retrograde ureteral stent placement in a 6-year-old female cat with bilateral obstructing ureteroliths. This procedure is performed as a hybrid approach with surgical exposure and fluoroscopic imaging. (a) The right ureteral stent has already been placed. A dilator is advanced into the left ureteral orifice following ventral cystotomy. Iodinated contrast medium is infused to highlight the left ureter and renal pelvis. The left renal pelvis is dilated and multiple filling defects (arrowed) represent the ureteroliths. (b) A hydrophilic guidewire is advanced up the ureter and directed into the left renal pelvis. Optimally, the wire is curled into the renal pelvis with one or two loops, to afford a stable position prior to stent advancement. (c) The stent is advanced over the wire and into the renal pelvis. (d) As the wire is withdrawn, the proximal portion of the stent forms a loop (pigtail) constraining the stent within the renal pelvis and ureter. The guidewire is then fully withdrawn, the distal loop of the stent placed within the bladder, and the cystotomy site and abdomen closed routinely.

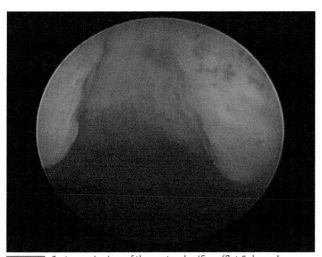

14.25 Cystoscopic view of the ureteral orifices (flat C-shaped openings) normally positioned within the trigone region of the bladder.

5. An open-ended ureteral catheter is introduced over the guidewire and advanced into the distal ureter under fluoroscopic guidance.
6. The guidewire is removed. Positive contrast retrograde pyelography is performed to identify and evaluate the obstructive pathology using fluoroscopy.
7. Replace the guidewire, passing it through the lumen of the open-ended ureteral catheter.
8. Using fluoroscopy, the guidewire is manipulated past the site of the obstruction and into the renal pelvis.
9. Once the guidewire is in position, the open-ended ureteral catheter is removed.
10. An appropriately sized double-pigtail ureteral stent is inserted over the guidewire and gently advanced, positioning the proximal end with at least one complete pigtail loop within the renal pelvis. The guidewire is partially withdrawn to visualize the formation of the loop and verify appropriate positioning within the renal pelvis.
11. The stent fills the ureteral lumen and the distal pigtail loop forms within the bladder lumen upon complete removal of the guidewire (Figure 14.26)

Small bitches (<7 kg) and cats may require surgical access to expose the ureteral orifices (hybrid approach) using a ventral midline cystotomy. Retrograde placement of the double-pigtail ureteral stent is performed as described above, with direct visualization of the ureteral orifice when manually passing the guidewire, opened ureteral catheter and double-pigtail stent. Fluoroscopy facilitates manipulation and placement of the stent during an open procedure.

Anterograde placement of ureteral stents is more frequently performed in male dogs and cats, small bitches (<6 kg) and queens when endoscopic access to the distal ureteral orifice is unavailable owing to patient size, equipment availability and anatomical or pathological limitations. Anterograde ureteral stenting is indicated to establish urine outflow in patients with obstructive transitional cell carcinoma (TCC) within the bladder trigone. This procedure is preferred to the hybrid approach because it avoids direct contact with the tumour, thus reducing the risk of tumour seeding. Anterograde stent placement is performed using minimally invasive techniques or surgical approaches to access the renal pelvis.

Minimally invasive or surgically assisted (hybrid) anterograde placement of ureteral stents (Figure 14.27) involves the following steps.

1. Anterograde ureteral stent placement is performed with the patient under general anaesthesia, using fluoroscopy and ultrasonography.
2. For a minimally invasive technique, ultrasound-guided pyelocentesis is performed using an over-the-needle intravenous catheter or renal access needle.
3. Surgical access affording exposure to the renal pelvis for pyelocentesis is accomplished by a ventral midline coeliotomy (exposure of one or both kidneys) or a paracostal approach (exposure of one kidney).
4. Positive contrast pyelography is performed by injection of aqueous contrast medium through the access needle in the renal pelvis, allowing evaluation of the site of obstruction and related pathology.
5. A flexible hydrophilic guidewire is passed through the access needle into the proximal ureter and manipulated past the obstruction, assisted by fluoroscopy.
6. The guidewire is advanced into the urinary bladder and guided out of the urethra.
7. An open-ended sheath and dilator are passed over the guidewire in a *retrograde* manner to dilate the ureteral orifice and distal ureter.
8. The dilator is removed and an appropriately sized double-pigtail ureteral stent is passed through the sheath over the guidewire in a *retrograde* manner to avoid trauma and leakage at the access site within the renal pelvis.

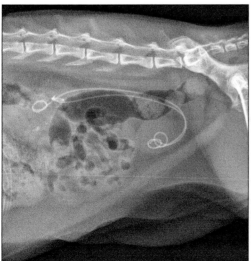
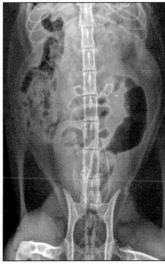

14.26 Lateral and ventrodorsal radiographs taken of the cat in Figure 14.24 after the procedure. The double-pigtail appearance of the ureteral stents can be seen, spanning from the renal pelvis to the bladder lumen. Multiple nephroliths remain in the left kidney; however, passive ureteral dilation around the stent may help to facilitate their passage if they enter the ureter.

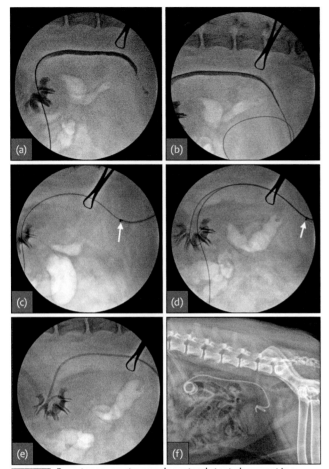

14.27 Percutaneous anterograde ureteral stent placement in a 10-year-old male dog with TCC of the bladder and proximal urethra. (a) Percutaneous renal access has been obtained and iodinated contrast medium highlights the left renal pelvis and ureter. An end-hole catheter is advanced down the ureter over a hydrophilic guidewire, and contrast medium highlights the complete obstruction to ureteral flow at the ureterovesicular junction. (b) The guidewire is manipulated across the ureterovesicular junction and curled in the bladder. (c) After the guidewire has been manipulated out of the urethra, a long vascular sheath (arrowed) is advanced from the urethra and retrograde up the ureter over the guidewire. (d) A second guidewire is advanced up the sheath and curled in the renal pelvis (arrowed). The first guidewire serves as a safety wire in case ureteral access is lost during stent deployment. (e) The ureteral stent is then advanced within the sheath, over the guidewire, and as the guidewire is withdrawn the proximal loop of the stent forms in the renal pelvis. The sheath and wire are then carefully withdrawn to deploy the distal loop in the bladder. (f) Lateral postoperative radiograph of the final stent position spanning the tumour and decompressing the ureteral obstruction.

9. The ureteral stent is manipulated into the renal pelvis, forming a pigtail loop as the guidewire is withdrawn.
10. The second pigtail loop within the bladder is formed as the guidewire and sheath are removed from the urethra.

Complications and risks associated with ureteral stent placement include failure to complete placement as a minimally invasive procedure, requiring conversion to a surgically assisted approach, perforation or disruption of the ureter or renal pelvis with a guidewire or stent, and inability to pass a guidewire or stent beyond the site of obstruction. Once ureteral stents are in position in dogs and cats, they are left in place for long term management. Ureteral stents are completely intracorporeal, requiring uroendoscopy for removal from the bladder lumen. Minor complications including dysuria, stranguria and haematuria have been reported but are often medically controlled with anti-inflammatory therapy. The

long-term impact of ureteral stents in small animal patients is currently under investigation.

Subcutaneous ureteral bypass

Initially proposed as a salvage procedure for failed ureteral interventions, subcutaneous ureteral bypass (SUB) techniques are now used by some practitioners as a first-line therapy in cats with ureteral obstruction, owing to the relative ease of placement of the device compared with ureteral stents. The SUB device consists of a locking-loop pigtail nephrostomy tube placed in the renal pelvis and a cystostomy tube placed in the urinary bladder, both connected to a double-sided shunting port that is implanted subcutaneously.

Surgical placement of a SUB device (Figure 14.28) involves the following steps.

1. SUB device placement is performed through a ventral midline coeliotomy with the animal under general anaesthesia.
2. The caudal pole of the affected kidney is exposed and perinephric fat removed to allow a smooth surface for adherence of the nephrostomy tube cuff.
3. An 18 G over-the-needle catheter is used to gain access to the renal pelvis and a guidewire is advanced through this catheter into the renal pelvis under fluoroscopic guidance.
4. The nephrostomy tube is advanced over this wire and the pigtail formed upon withdrawal of the guidewire and stylet, making certain that the radiopaque band on the nephrostomy tube is within the renal pelvis.
5. The pigtail loop of the nephrostomy tube is locked by tightening the string, which is kept taut until placement on the port.
6. The Dacron cuff of the nephrostomy tube is advanced until it is flush with the renal capsule and sterile cyanoacrylate tissue glue is placed on this cuff to facilitate adherence to the renal capsule.
7. A purse-string suture is placed in the apex of the bladder and a stab incision made in the centre of this suture line for advancement of the cystostomy tube.
8. The purse-string is tightened around the cystostomy tube and the cuff of the cystostomy tube is both sutured and glued to the bladder apex.
9. Both tubes are brought through the body wall with blunt haemostats, taking care to maintain tension on the string of the nephrostomy tube.
10. A site is chosen for placement of the shunting port by dissection of the subcutaneous tissue adjacent to the coeliotomy incision. Optimally, a site should be selected that is cranial enough for ease of access in the conscious animal and that allows for both tubes to enter the body wall at a gentle angle to avoid kinking.
11. The tubes are advanced on to the shunting port, with the string of the nephrostomy tube kept taut during advancement on to the first rung and then cut prior to complete advancement on to the port. Exposure of string will result in leakage and should be avoided.
12. The port is sutured to the body wall with non-absorbable suture material and the system checked for leaks prior to abdominal closure

The animal is kept with a soft wrap on the abdomen for the first 24–28 hours to minimize seroma formation. The owner should be advised to prevent any jumping and not to pick up the animal by the abdomen to avoid risking dislodgement of the SUB device connections. Once in place, the SUB device is flushed every 3–6 months with aqueous contrast medium or normal saline under fluoroscopic or ultrasonographic visualization to maintain patency, using a standard 22 G Huber needle. Complications of SUB device placement can be catastrophic and include uroabdomen or subcutaneous urine leakage secondary to avulsion, or seepage around the connections, and familiarity with the technique is paramount to a successful outcome. In addition, obstruction of the SUB device may occur as a result of kinking/obstruction of the system, most commonly at the body wall entry site, which can be detected by serial radiography and avoided by using care during placement to minimize acute angulation of the tubes.

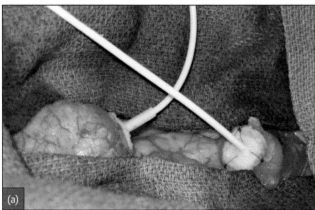

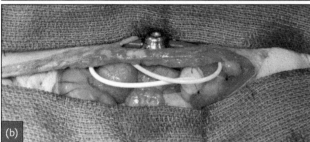

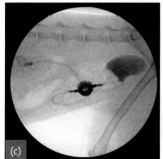
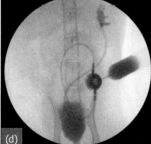

14.28 SUB device placement in a cat with obstructive ureterolithiasis. (a) The locking loop nephrostomy tube and cystostomy tube both have Dacron cuffs that are advanced to the renal capsule and bladder, respectively. The bladder cuff is both sutured and glued, while the renal cuff is glued and held in place by a plastic retainer around the tube. (b) Both tubes are bluntly directed through the abdominal wall and attached to the shunting port, leaving sufficient space on either side for a gentle angulation of the tube into the abdomen to avoid kinking. (c) Radiographic image of the SUB device in place. Note that the nephrostomy tube is fully advanced until the radiographic marker is within the renal pelvis and the pigtail is locked via a string that is held taut by the shunting port. Typically, the nephrostomy tube is connected to the caudal end and the cystostomy tube to the cranial end of the shunting port to maintain gentle curvature of the tubing. (d) The SUB device is flushed and assessed for any evidence of leakage by inserting a 22 G Huber needle into the shunting port and injecting saline or aqueous contrast medium. The port may also be used for urine sampling as needed.

The bladder

Cystotomy

Cystotomy is one of the most frequently performed surgical procedures in small animal practice (see Operative Technique 14.5). It is indicated for a variety of non-neoplastic and neoplastic disorders (Figure 14.29). Access to the luminal surface of the bladder permits direct visualization of questionable lesions, biopsy, culture, removal of calculi (Figure 14.30), closure of traumatic injuries, resection of mass lesions including neoplasia, polyps, chronic inflammation or infection, and evaluation of the proximal urethra and upper urinary tract.

Historically, cystotomy has been the treatment of choice for cystoliths in small animal patients. A ventral midline cystotomy provides direct visualization of the bladder lumen for complete removal of cystoliths. Additional uroliths lodged along the length of the urethra can be displaced into the bladder lumen for removal using retrograde urohydropulsion. Cystotomy is considered to be a basic surgical procedure and is routinely performed at all levels of veterinary surgical skill. Complications associated with cystotomy in small animal patients are infrequently reported but include postsurgical pain or discomfort, haematuria, dysuria, urinary outflow obstruction, dehiscence, leakage of urine, calculogenesis secondary to exposed or extruded suture material and incomplete removal of uroliths at the time of surgery.

Non-neoplastic indications
• Urolithiasis
• Cystic
• Ureteral
• Urethral
• Trauma
• Ruptured bladder/urethra
• Ureteral injury/rupture
• Congenital abnormalities
• Diverticulum
• Patent urachus
• Ureterocele
• Ectopic ureter
• Trigonal defect
• Biopsy/culture
• Inflammation/infection
• Foreign body removal
• Evaluation of upper urinary tract
• Idiopathic renal haematuria
• Ureteral obstruction
• Ureteral stent
• Obstruction
• Neoplasia
• Haematoma
• Urolithiasis
• Ureteral transposition
• Congenital disorder
• Distal obstruction

Neoplastic indications
• Bladder neoplasia: benign
• Polypoid cystitis
• Ureteral polyp
• Bladder neoplasia: malignant
• Epithelial neoplasia (transitional cell carcinoma, squamous cell carcinoma)
• Mesenchymal neoplasia
• Leiomyosarcoma
• Rhabdomyosarcoma
• Botyrorhabdomyosarcoma
• Haemangiosarcoma

14.29 Surgical indications for cystotomy.

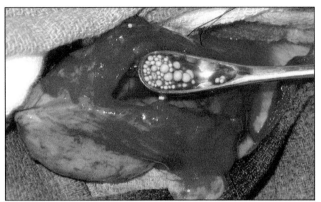

14.30 Surgical removal of cystic calculi through a ventral midline cystotomy. A bladder spoon is used for retrieval of calculi.

Bladder healing

The urinary bladder is considered a 'compound' organ because of its distinct tissue layers, including mucosa, submucosa, muscularis and serosa. The submucosa is the surgical holding layer of the bladder. The urinary bladder is unique with respect to other tissues of the body, because it has the capacity to regain 100% of its presurgical strength within 21–28 days after a wound or incision is made.

Appositional or inverting suture patterns, such as Cushing and Lembert suture patterns, are considered appropriate for bladder wall closure. Regardless of the choice of suture pattern, care should be taken to avoid placement of any suture material through the mucosa, exposing the suture within the bladder lumen. Suture materials, especially braided ones, may act as a nidus for chronic infection and may become calculogenic. Synthetic absorbable monofilament suture materials of appropriate size (1.5 or 2 metric; 4/0 or 3/0 USP) are considered ideal for bladder wall closure.

The urinary bladder is lined by a highly regenerative epithelial surface. Complete re-epithelialization of the luminal surface of the bladder occurs within 10–30 days by migration of transitional epithelium from the ureteral orifices. In situations of bladder trauma, devitalized tissue is resected and the bladder is closed routinely.

Percutaneous cystolithotomy

Minimally invasive and minimally assisted approaches to transabdominal removal of cystoliths and urethroliths have been described. The focus of these procedures is to eliminate cystoliths with reduced surgical trauma and exposure in an effort to enhance recovery with reduced pain and discomfort. Minimally invasive transabdominal approaches are advantageous if intracorporeal lithotripsy cannot be considered because of patient size, sex, lack of availability of laser equipment, technical expertise or cost. Transabdominal laparoscopic removal of cystoliths should be performed aseptically in a dedicated surgical or interventional room. It requires creation of a pneumoperitoneum and multiple portals for instrumentation and endoscopic viewing. Expertise in laparoscopic procedures and tissue manipulation is essential. Percutaneous cystolithotomy (PCCL) is a similar minimally assisted procedure that avoids the creation of a pneumoperitoneum for direct visualization and manipulation of the bladder. Pneumoperitoneum has been associated with pain and discomfort following minimally invasive procedures.

1. PCCL is performed with the patient under general anaesthesia and positioned in dorsal recumbency.
2. A transurethral catheter is aseptically placed with the tip in the bladder lumen.
3. The ventral abdomen is clipped, aseptically prepared and draped for sterile surgery.
4. The bladder is insufflated to distension with sterile fluid injected through the urethral catheter.
5. A 2 cm incision is made through the ventral body wall directly over the apex of the bladder, guided by transabdominal palpation.
6. Digital palpation within the peritoneal cavity confirms the position of the distended bladder.
7. The bladder apex is gently grasped with atraumatic forceps (Babcock forceps) and manipulated to the body wall incision.
8. The bladder is drained of fluid and refilled several times through the urethral catheter to flush small cystoliths (<3–4 mm) from the bladder lumen. All fluid drained from the lower urinary tract should be filtered to retrieve uroliths.
9. The apex of the bladder is held in gentle traction at the surgical incision. Three or four stay sutures (using a 3.0 metric (2/0 USP) suture material) are placed in a circular fashion just below the apex to assist with traction.
10. The bladder apex is retracted through the incision and packed off with gauze sponges to absorb any urine leakage.
11. A stab incision is made into the bladder lumen at the apex and a 6 mm threaded laparoscopic cannula with a diaphragm is inserted and positioned to engage the bladder wall.
12. A rigid cystoscope with a biopsy channel is inserted through the diaphragm of the cannula into the bladder lumen. The rigid cystoscope provides direct visualization of the luminal surface of the entire bladder and proximal urethra (Figure 14.31).

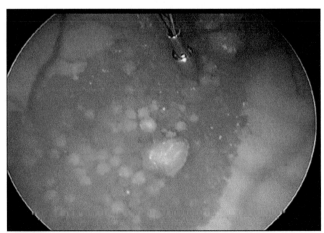

14.31 Percutaneous cystolithotomy: transabdominal view of multiple cystoliths within the bladder lumen. Small cystoliths (<3 mm) can be removed by transurethral flushing or urohydropulsion. Larger cystoliths (>5 mm) require laser fragmentation or basket retrieval using the endoscope.

13. Sterile fluid ingress through the cystoscope maintains intraluminal distension and an optically clear environment.
14. The urethral catheter is maintained in place to provide drainage and prevent over-distension of the bladder.
15. Cystoliths >5 mm can be removed using a basket retrieval device passed through the biopsy channel of the cystoscope (Figure 14.32).
16. Smaller particles and debris can be removed by careful flushing using the urethral catheter and suctioning with the tip of a suction instrument carefully positioned against the wall of the bladder cannula, avoiding damage to the bladder wall.
17. Upon complete removal of all uroliths and debris, the bladder is emptied and the trocar removed.
18. The bladder is closed in an appositional or inverting pattern using 2.0 metric (3/0 USP) absorbable monofilament suture material.
19. The abdominal incision is closed in a routine manner.
20. Plain abdominal radiographs are obtained to check that all radiodense uroliths have been removed.

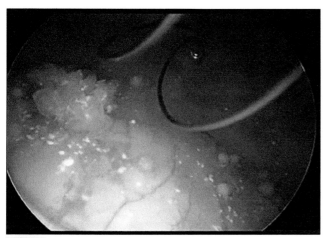

14.32 Percutaneous cystolithotomy stone basket.

Bladder neoplasia

The most common form of canine bladder tumour is the TCC. Other types of tumour (see Figure 14.29) are much less common. Bladder cancer is extremely rare in cats. TCCs are infiltrative tumours that are most often located in the trigone. Due to the location of the tumour, dogs frequently present with partial or complete urinary outflow obstruction. Other signs, including haematuria, dysuria and pollakiuria, may have been present for weeks to months prior to presentation.

Diagnosis of TCC

- *Rectal examination:* may reveal thickening of the urethra and/or enlargement of the iliac lymph nodes.
- *Urinalysis:* neoplastic cells may be present in the urine of 30% of dogs (Norris *et al.*, 1992) but these cells are often indistinguishable from reactive epithelial cells associated with inflammation.
- *Contrast cystography:* reveals a filling defect, usually in the area of the trigone.
- *Ultrasonography:* reveals a mass within the bladder lumen and is also useful for evaluating local lymph nodes.

- *Uroendoscopy:* allows direct visualization and biopsy.
- *Histopathology:* tissue for histopathological examination may be obtained by traumatic catheterization, uroendoscopy or cystotomy.

Treatment of TCC

Complete surgical excision of TCC is not possible, owing to the most common location within the trigone and bladder neck. There are currently no acceptable urinary diversion procedures developed for small animal patients that permit bladder exenteration without life-threatening clinical complications. The infiltrative and expansile nature of TCC can result in obstruction of ureteral outflow into the bladder lumen. Malignant obstruction can be palliated by minimally invasive anterograde placement of ureteral stents, as previously described. Neoplasia located in the apical region of the bladder can be surgically debulked by partial cystectomy, but this is rarely curative. Numerous chemotherapy protocols have been tried but the response of TCCs to agents such as cisplatin and carboplatin is poor. The best clinical response is to non-steroidal anti-inflammatory drugs (NSAIDs) such as piroxicam, which has anti-neoplastic activity against TCC in dogs. Further discussion is beyond the scope of this book and the reader is referred to the *BSAVA Manual of Canine and Feline Oncology*.

Clinical signs of progressive stranguria and urethral outflow obstruction are commonly reported in dogs with TCC, ultimately affecting quality of life and limiting survival periods. Limited options are available for the palliative management of urethral obstruction resulting from TCC. The use of chronic indwelling transurethral catheters or tube cystotomy is associated with tedious maintenance by owners and numerous complications including chronic urinary tract infections, haematuria, discomfort, kinking, obstruction and dislodgement. Intracorporeal self-expanding metallic urethral stents (SEMS) have been developed in a variety of sizes for small animal patients. SEMS are composed of nitinol, a metal alloy containing nickel and titanium that demonstrates unique properties of shape memory and super-elasticity (Figure 14.33). Urethral stents are placed using minimally invasive techniques.

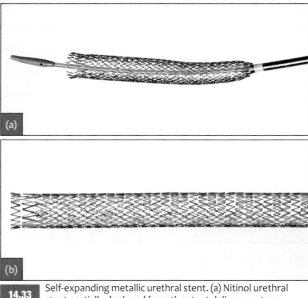

14.33 Self-expanding metallic urethral stent. (a) Nitinol urethral stent partially deployed from the stent delivery system. (b) Close-up view of the stent.

Urethral stenting: SEMS (nitinol) are positioned and deployed to alleviate obstruction within the urethral lumen with the assistance of fluoroscopy (Figure 14.34).

1. Stent placement is performed with the patient under general anaesthesia in lateral recumbency.
2. The perivulvar or preputial region is clipped and aseptically prepared.
3. A measuring catheter is placed within the lumen of a 12 or 14 Fr urethral catheter and gently inserted into the rectum and advanced into the distal colon to assist with stent sizing and adjustment for radiographic magnification.
4. A hydrophilic guidewire is inserted through the external urethral orifice and gently passed into the bladder lumen under fluoroscopic visualization.

5. An introducer sheath sized for the stent delivery system is passed into the urethra using the guidewire. The guidewire is removed and the catheter positioned in the distal urethra.
6. A positive contrast urethrocystogram is performed, maximally distending both the bladder and urethra.
7. External pressure is placed on the bladder to assist with maximal distension and facilitate evaluation of the vesicourethral junction for narrowing. The maximal urethral diameter and length of obstruction are measured to determine stent size and length.
8. A SEMS is chosen by adding an additional 10–15% to the maximal urethral diameter at the site of obstruction; the length should not allow it to protrude more than 1 cm proximal or distal to the obstruction site (Weisse *et al.*, 2006).
9. The appropriately sized stent is introduced over the guidewire, positioned at the site of obstruction and deployed with fluoroscopic guidance.
10. It is essential to determine that the urethra remains patent and the patient can void urine following stent placement.

Recent investigations have reported successful placement of nitinol SEMS for palliative treatment of urethral obstruction secondary to malignancy. Although urinary outflow obstruction was relieved in more than 90% of the affected dogs (Figure 14.35), complications including urinary incontinence, re-obstruction, stranguria, urinary tract infection, stent displacement and tumour ingrowth were reported.

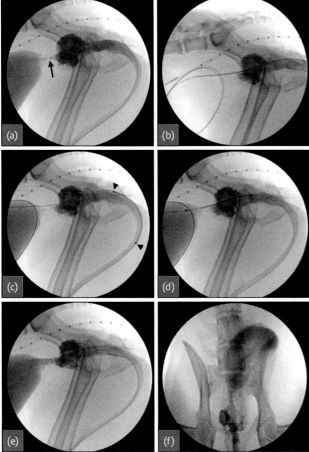

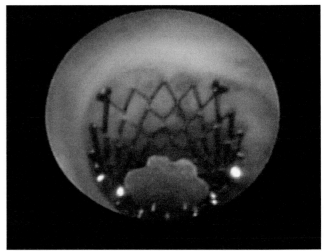

14.35 Endoscopic view of a self-expanding metallic urethral stent placed within the urethra.

14.34 Images from a dog with obstructive TCC of the bladder trigone. (a) A contrast urethrogram is performed to localize the site of obstruction (arrowed) and to obtain measurements of urethral diameter and the length of the obstruction. The calibrated marker catheter in the colon serves as a reference measure of the degree of radiographic magnification in the image to normalize measurements. Maximal distension of the non-affected portion of the urethra is achieved and a stent chosen that is the same diameter as the urethra, or slightly larger, and of a length sufficient to span the obstruction fully. (b) A hydrophilic guidewire is advanced across the obstruction and curled within the urinary bladder. (c) The stent delivery system is then advanced over the guidewire. The stent can be seen between the platinum marker bands (arrowheads). (d) The stent is gradually expanded under fluoroscopic visualization and opened to span from the bladder trigone to beyond the filling defect of the tumour/obstruction. (e) Once the stent has been deployed, a repeat urethrogram shows improved patency through the site of obstruction. (f) Ventrodorsal fluoroscopic image of the final stent position shows external compression by the tumour. The stent will continue to exert a radial force on the tumour and will probably open further with time.

References and further reading

Adams LG, Berent AC, Moore GE and Bagley DH (2008) Use of laser lithotripsy for fragmentation of uroliths in dogs: 73 cases (2005–2006). *Journal of the American Veterinary Medical Association* **232(11)**, 1680–1687

Barthez PY, Begon D and Delisle F (1998) Effect of contrast medium dose and image acquisition timing on ureteral opacification in the normal dog as assessed by computed tomography. *Veterinary Radiology and Ultrasound* **39**, 524–527

Berent AC (2011) Ureteral obstructions in dogs and cats: a review of traditional and new interventional diagnostic and therapeutic options. *Journal of Veterinary Emergency and Critical Care* **21(2)**, 86–103

Bevan JM, Lulich JP, Albasan H and Osborne CA (2009) Comparison of laser lithotripsy and cystotomy for the management of dogs with urolithiasis. *Journal of the American Veterinary Medical Association* **234(10)**, 1286–1294

Bjorling DE (1984) Traumatic injuries of the urogenital tract. *Veterinary Clinics of North America: Small Animal Practice* **14**, 61–76

Blackburn AL, Berent AC, Weisse CW and Brown DC (2013) Evaluation of outcome following urethral stent placement for the treatment of obstructive carcinoma of the urethra in dogs: 42 cases (2004–2008). *Journal of the American Veterinary Medical Association* **242(1)**, 59–68

Brandes SB and McAninch JW (1999) Reconstructive surgery for trauma of the upper urinary tract. *Urology Clinics of North America* **26**, 183–199

Davidson E, Ritchey J, Higbee R *et al.* (2004) Laser lithotripsy for the treatment of canine uroliths. *Veterinary Surgery* **33(1)**, 56–61

DeFarges A, Dunn M and Berent A (2013) New alternatives for minimally invasive management of uroliths: lower urinary tract uroliths. *Compendium on Continuing Education for Practicing Veterinarian* **35(1)**, E1

Dobson J and Lascelles D (2011) BSAVA *Manual of Canine and Feline Oncology, 3rd edn.* BSAVA Publications, Gloucester

Evans HE and Christensen GC (1993) The urogenital system. In: *Miller's Anatomy of the Dog, 3rd edn*, p.494. WB Saunders, Philadelphia

Gahring DR, Crowe DT and Powers TE (1977) Comparative renal function studies of nephrotomy closure with and without sutures in dogs. *Journal of the American Veterinary Medical Association* **171**, 537–541

Hosgood G and Hedlund CS (1993) Urethral disease and obstructive uropathy. In: *Disease Mechanisms in Small Animal Surgery, 2nd edn*, ed. MJ Bjorab, p.528. Lea and Febiger, Malvern

Klein MK, Cockerell GL, Harris CK *et al.* (1988) Canine primary renal neoplasms: a retrospective review of 54 cases. *Journal of the American Animal Hospital Association* **24**, 443–452

Kyles AE, Hardie EM, Wooden BG *et al.* (2005) Management and outcome of cats with ureteral calculi: 153 cases (1984–2002). *Journal of the American Veterinary Medical Association* **226(6)**, 937–944

Kyles AE, Stone EA, Gookin J *et al.* (1998) Diagnosis and surgical management of obstructive ureteral calculi in cats: 11 cases (1993–1996). *Journal of the American Veterinary Medical Association* **213**, 1150–1156

Lanz OI and Waldron DR (2000) Renal and ureteral surgery in dogs. *Clinical Techniques in Small Animal Practice* **15**, 1–10

Lulich JP, Adams LG, Grant D, Albasan H and Osborne CA (2009a) Changing paradigms in the treatment of uroliths by lithotripsy. *Veterinary Clinics of North America: Small Animal Practice* **39(1)**, 143–160

Lulich JP, Osborne CA, Albasan H and Bevan JM (2009b) Efficacy and safety of laser lithotripsy in fragmentation of urocystoliths and urethroliths for removal in dogs. *Journal of the American Veterinary Medical Association* **234(10)**, 1279–1285

McLoughlin MA (2000) Surgical emergencies of the urinary tract. *Veterinary Clinics of North America: Small Animal Practice* **30**, 581–602

McLoughlin MA and Bjorling DE (2002) Surgery of the ureter. In: *Textbook of Small Animal Surgery, 3rd edn*, ed. DH Slatter, pp.1619–1627. WB Saunders, Philadelphia

McMillan S, Knapp D, Ramos-Vara J *et al.* (2012) Outcome of urethral stent placement for the management of urethral obstruction secondary to transitional cell carcinoma in dogs: 19 cases (2007–2010). *Journal of the American Veterinary Medical Association* **241**, 1627–1632

Norris AM, Laing EJ, Valli VEO *et al.* (1992) Canine bladder and urethral tumours: a retrospective study of 115 cases (1980–1985). *Journal of Veterinary Internal Medicine* **6**, 145–153

Osborne CA and Finco DR (1979) Urinary tract emergencies and renal care following trauma. *Veterinary Clinics of North America: Small Animal Practice* **9**, 259

Osborne CA and Polzin DJ (1986) Nonsurgical management of canine obstructive urolithopathy. *Veterinary Clinics of North America: Small Animal Practice* **16**, 333–347

Stone EA and Mason LK (1990) Surgery of ectopic ureters: types, method of correction, and postoperative results. *Journal of the American Animal Hospital Association* **26**, 81–88

Stone EA, Robertson JL and Metcalf MR (2002) The effect of nephrotomy on renal function and morphology in dogs. *Veterinary Surgery* **31**, 391–397

Thornhill JA and Cechner PE (1981) Traumatic injuries to the kidneys, ureters, bladder and urethra. *Veterinary Clinics of North America: Small Animal Practice* **11**, 157–169

Vaughan ED, Sorenson EJ and Gillenwater JY (1970) The renal hemodynamic response to chronic unilateral complete ureteral occlusion. *Investigative Urology* **8**, 78–90

Wiesse C, Berent A, Todd K *et al.* (2006) Evaluation of palliative stenting for management of malignant urethral obstructions in dogs. *Journal of the American Veterinary Medical Association* **229(2)**, 226–234

OPERATIVE TECHNIQUE 14.1

Renal biopsy

POSITIONING

Dorsal recumbency.

ASSISTANT

Useful.

EQUIPMENT EXTRAS

Fine DeBakey thumb forceps and Metzenbaum scissors; suction; cautery unit; needle biopsy device.

SURGICAL TECHNIQUE

The kidneys and ureters are located separately within the peritoneal cavity within the retroperitoneal space. Visual and digital inspection of both kidneys should be routinely performed as part of the complete abdominal surgical exploration. Biopsy samples are obtained using a needle biopsy or tissue wedge technique. Presence of an obvious lesion or abnormality involving only one kidney will dictate the specific kidney for biopsy.

> ### PRACTICAL TIP
>
> When both kidneys have a similar gross appearance the left kidney should be chosen for biopsy, because it is more easily accessible owing to its more caudal position within the abdominal cavity

The goal of surgery is to obtain an adequate tissue specimen with minimal injury to the surrounding renal parenchyma. Position and depth are critical for obtaining a tissue sample that will provide diagnostic information. To be considered appropriate for evaluation of renal pathology, specimens *must* contain multiple glomeruli. The largest concentration of glomeruli is located within the renal cortex and the corticomedullary junction.

→ **OPERATIVE TECHNIQUE 14.1 CONTINUED**

Approach

A routine ventral midline coeliotomy from the xiphoid process to the pubis should be performed to examine all the structures of the urinary tract.

Surgical manipulations: needle biopsy

A 14 or 18 G needle biopsy device can be used during surgery to obtain small core tissue specimens. The biopsy instrument is oriented at the site of a gross lesion or from the caudal renal pole longitudinally along the convex surface, avoiding the renal pelvis and major blood vessels entering at the hilus. Spring-loaded or manual biopsy needle instruments are commercially available.

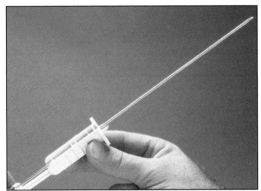

Core (needle) biopsy instrument.

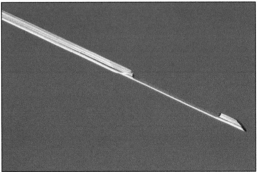

Biopsy rod extended, demonstrating site for core biopsy specimen.

1 With the biopsy rod fully retracted and covered by the outer cutting cannula, insert the trocar point of the biopsy instrument through the renal capsule into the renal parenchyma in a controlled manner.

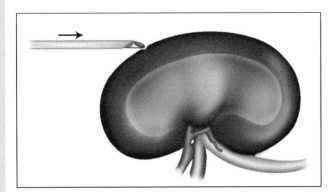

2 Advance the inner biopsy rod through the renal parenchyma.

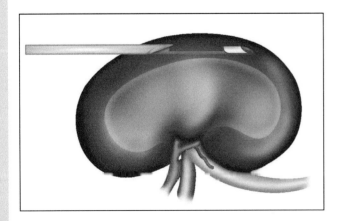

➜ **OPERATIVE TECHNIQUE 14.1 CONTINUED**

3   Fire or advance the outer cutting cannula to cut a core-shaped specimen of renal tissue from its attachments.

4   Remove the biopsy needle from the kidney, with the outer cutting cannula covering and protecting the biopsy specimen.

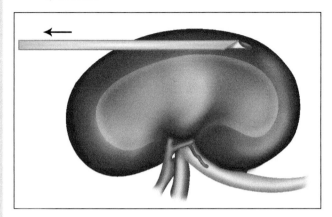

5   As the instrument is removed from the kidney, brisk haemorrhage will occur. Apply digital pressure for 5 minutes or place a single 1.5 metric (4/0 USP) monofilament absorbable suture in the renal capsule at the biopsy site to control renal haemorrhage. Accumulation of blood under the renal capsule will result in a haematoma at the biopsy site.

6   Advance the biopsy rod from the outer cannula to retrieve the core biopsy specimen.

7   Gently transfer the small tissue core sample to a biopsy container, using a 25 G needle.

WARNING

Grasping or manipulating the small tissue specimen with surgical instruments will result in crushing artefacts

---

Surgical manipulations: wedge biopsy

A No. 10, 11 or 15 scalpel blade is used to obtain a wedge-shaped sample of renal parenchyma for biopsy, culture or other analysis. Depth and location are critical for obtaining valuable diagnostic information. A larger tissue sample provides additional opportunity for the pathologist to make a specific diagnosis. Wedge biopsy samples can be obtained from either kidney.

1   Rotate the kidney ventrally and medially to expose the convex surface.

2   Make two small (1.5–2 cm) incisions along the greater curvature to remove a wedge-shaped piece of renal tissue approximately 0.5–1 cm in depth.

3   Use monofilament absorbable suture material of appropriate size (1.5 metric; 4/0 USP) for closure of the renal capsule in a continuous or interrupted pattern to control parenchymal haemorrhage.

4   Inspect biopsy sites for continued haemorrhage prior to abdominal closure.

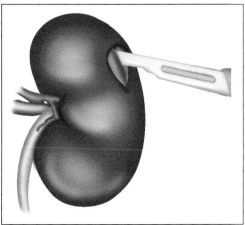

Excision of a 1.5 cm wedge of tissue from the convex surface of the kidney.

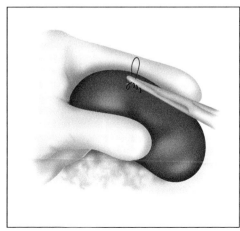

Closure of the biopsy site in the renal capsule using 1.5 metric (4/0 USP) absorbable suture material in an interrupted or continuous pattern.

→ **OPERATIVE TECHNIQUE 14.1 CONTINUED**

Wound closure

Routine midline abdominal closure.

- Intravenous fluid therapy should be administered for 12–24 hours following general anaesthesia and surgical biopsy.
- Evaluation of heart rate, mucous membrane colour and haematocrit is recommended 4–6 hours after the biopsy procedure to verify that renal haemorrhage is controlled. Gross or microscopic haematuria is frequently noted for 24 hours after renal biopsy procedures.
- Appropriate pain management is indicated for 24–72 hours after abdominal surgery and renal biopsy.

OPERATIVE TECHNIQUE 14.2

Bisectional nephrotomy

POSITIONING

Dorsal recumbency.

ASSISTANT

Ideal.

EQUIPMENT EXTRAS

Standard surgical pack with a Balfour retractor; Rummel tourniquet or vascular occluding forceps (essential); suction and cautery (helpful).

SURGICAL TECHNIQUE

Approach

Ventral midline coeliotomy from the xiphoid process to the pubis. Place a self-retaining retractor (e.g. Balfour retractor) to retract the abdominal wall and expose the abdominal viscera.

Surgical manipulations

1 Carefully examine both kidneys. The left kidney is exposed by lifting the descending colon and using the mesentery to retract the intestinal loops towards the right. The right kidney is exposed by retracting the descending duodenum.

2 Examine the liver and remaining abdominal viscera and palpate for metastatic lesions or other abnormalities.

3 Expose the affected kidney from the retroperitoneal space by blunt dissection.

4 Gently strip the perirenal adipose tissue from the kidney with a surgical swab.

PRACTICAL TIP

Rotate the kidney medially to expose the dorsal aspect and renal hilus. Identify and isolate the renal artery and vein. The renal artery is located dorsal to the renal vein. Apply atraumatic vascular forceps or a Rummel tourniquet on the renal artery and vein to occlude blood flow during the nephrotomy procedure. Renal vascular occlusion should be <10 minutes

5 Make an incision through the renal capsule and parenchyma along the convex surface of the kidney with a No. 10 scalpel blade. The incision is continued into the renal pelvis and should be of adequate length to gain exposure of the renal pelvis.

→ **OPERATIVE TECHNIQUE 14.2 CONTINUED**

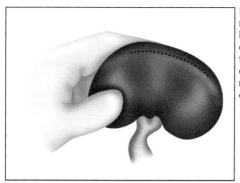

Following mobilization of the kidney, an incision of about two-thirds of the length of the kidney is made along its convex surface.

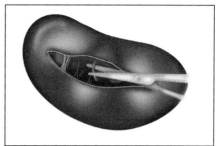

The renal parenchyma can be bluntly separated with a scalpel handle and arcuate or interlobar vessels can be ligated and severed.

6 Use suction to clear the surgical site of blood. Gently explore the renal pelvis and remove all obstructive material or calculi.

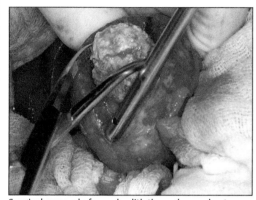

Surgical removal of a nephrolith through a nephrotomy incision. Temporary vascular occlusion is performed with a Rummel tourniquet.

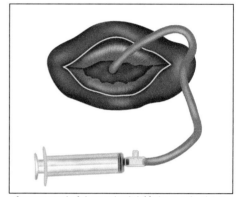

After removal of the nephrolith(s) the renal pelvis is flushed with warm saline to remove any debris.

7 Obtain aerobic bacterial culture samples from the renal pelvis, which should be thoroughly irrigated and suctioned.

8 Place a small catheter through the vesicoureteral orifice of the associated ureter to flush any debris from the proximal ureter into the renal pelvis for removal. Submit any calculi for mineral analysis.

9 Obtain a renal biopsy specimen by removing a 2–4 mm slice of the renal parenchyma along the incised edge of the nephrotomy incision.

10 Apply digital pressure to close the two sides of the nephrotomy incision.

11 Use monofilament absorbable suture material of suitable size (1.5 metric; 4/0 USP) to close the renal capsule in a continuous pattern. Once closed, release the tourniquet to restore blood supply to the kidney.

Wound closure

Standard abdominal wound closure.

POSTOPERATIVE MANAGEMENT

- Patients should be monitored closely after nephrotomy.
- Continue administration of intravenous fluid therapy at maintenance rates or greater to establish diuresis. Administer intravenous fluids for 24–48 hours after surgery.
- Carry out serial monitoring of vital parameters, haematocrit and urine output for the first 24 hours or as patient status dictates. Gross haematuria may be evident for several days after surgery.
- Monitor renal function parameters in patients with renal disease.
- Exercise restriction for 10–14 days after surgery.
- Appropriate pain management is indicated for 24–72 hours after abdominal surgery.

OPERATIVE TECHNIQUE 14.3

Intracorporeal endoscopic laser lithotripsy

POSITIONING

Bitches and queens: lateral or dorsal recumbency (operator preference).
Male dogs: lateral recumbency.

ASSISTANT

Essential.

EQUIPMENT EXTRAS

Uroendoscopy equipment

Rigid cystoscope – various sizes are helpful:

- Adult cystoscope (for bitches ≥6 kg):
    - 4.0 mm telescope with a 6.7 mm outer sheath
    - 4 Fr biopsy channel
    - 0- or 30-degree view
    - 30 cm length
    - Ingress and egress ports.
- Paediatric cystoscope (for bitches <6 kg and queens):
    - 2.0 mm telescope with a 4.0 mm outer sheath
    - 4 Fr biopsy channel
    - 0- or 30-degree view
    - 19 cm length
    - Ingress and egress ports.

Flexible endoscope:

- Flexible ureteroscope (for male dogs ≥6 kg; must be able to pass an 8 Fr urethral catheter):
    - 3.0 mm tip
    - 100 cm length
    - 4 Fr biopsy channel
    - Fluid ingress only
    - Tip moves in one direction.

- Xenon light source.
- Light cable.
- Three-chip camera.
- Videoendoscopy capture unit for a permanent record of all endoscopic procedures.

Lithotripsy equipment

- Ho:YAG laser.
- Quartz laser fibres (200, 365, 550 μm).
- Protective sheath: 4 Fr open-ended ureteral catheter.
- Laser protection goggles.

PATIENT PREPARATION

- Uroendoscopy is performed with the patient under general anaesthesia.
- All endoscopes, cameras, light cables and laser fibres should be gas-sterilized prior to the procedure.
- The perineal and perivulvar region of bitches and queens or the preputial region of male dogs is clipped and aseptically prepared. The prepared region is surgically draped to maintain asepsis during the procedure.
- Operators are gowned and gloved, wearing laser protection goggles when indicated.

→ **OPERATIVE TECHNIQUE 14.3 CONTINUED**

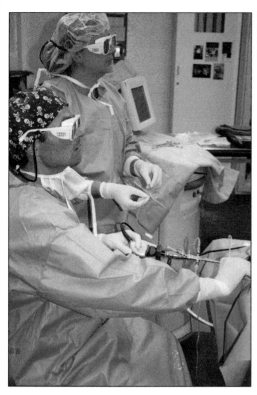

Surgeons performing laser lithotripsy. The patient is aseptically prepared and surgically draped. The surgeons are gowned and gloved and wear laser eye protection during the procedure.

Surgical manipulations: rigid endoscopy in bitches and queens

Knowledge of lower urogenital anatomy and basic uroendoscopy skills are essential. (For information on endoscopy in the male dog, the reader is referred to the *BSAVA Manual of Canine and Feline Endoscopy and Endosurgery*.)

1. Assemble the endoscopic unit (telescope, outer sheath and bridge) in a sterile manner. Attach the light cable and camera to the endoscope and carefully hand the adaptors to a non-sterile assistant. Turn on the light source, white balance the camera and focus the image.

2. Apply sterile lubricant to the outer edges of the endoscope sheath.

3. Gently introduce the tip of the endoscope into the vestibule and initiate fluid insufflation. Fluid insufflation during uroendoscopy is provided by gravity flow of sterile 0.9% saline or lactated Ringer's solution through the ingress port on the bridge. Litre bags of sterile irrigation fluid can be stored in a small refrigerator and made available for use in situations of mucosal haemorrhage that might occur during the procedure. Cold irrigation promotes vasoconstriction and flushes small clots to maintain an optically clear visual field.

4. Using the non-dominant hand, manually occlude the vulvar lips around the endoscope to prevent fluid drainage and permit distension of the urogenital tract for visualization.

5. Perform a complete examination of the lower urinary tract to identify the presence of uroliths and any anatomical or pathological abnormalities.

6. If a urolith is partially or completely occluding the urethral lumen, prohibiting a complete examination of the lower urinary tract, use the endoscope to gently displace the urethrolith into the bladder lumen or use lithotripsy to fragment the uroliths within the urethra, providing immediate relief from the obstruction.

Surgical manipulations: laser lithotripsy procedure

The authors very infrequently perform laser lithotripsy on queens due to size limitations of the equipment and the retrieval size of the stone fragments, which must be extremely small (<1–2 mm) to prevent urethral obstruction. Surgical removal of uroliths is recommended in both male and female cats.

1. Pass a 4 Fr open-ended ureteral catheter through the biopsy channel of the endoscope. The ureteral catheter acts as a sheath and guides the passage of the laser fibre through the biopsy channel and protects the endoscope.

➜ **OPERATIVE TECHNIQUE 14.3 CONTINUED**

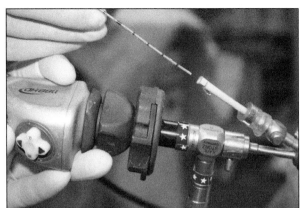

The open-ended ureteral catheter sheath is passed through the biopsy channel of the cystoscope to facilitate and protect the laser fibre as it is passed.

2   Select an appropriate laser fibre based on the type of endoscope being used, the procedure being performed, the size of the patient and the number of uroliths that require fragmentation. Open and handle the pack of laser fibres in an aseptic manner. Gently hand the laser connector to the circulating assistant for attachment to the laser console.

3   Inspect and prepare the laser fibre prior to each use. Ensure that the fibre is not bent or kinked; there should be no fractures in the covering of the fibre. Approximately 3 mm at the end of the fibre is exposed to form a tip with no external covering.

4   Hold the laser fibre tip next to a non-reflective surface to ensure that a circular red spot appears. If the red spot is not completely circular, re-cleave the fibre tip using ceramic scissors by making a perpendicular cut across the laser fibre approximately 5–6 mm from the end. Using a stripping device, remove the outer covering from the most distal aspect of the laser fibre to form an operative tip. Recheck to ensure that the newly cleaved tip forms a circular red spot.

5   Carefully insert the laser fibre into the biopsy channel of the endoscope through the ureteral catheter and gently advance until the tip is visible in the optical field. Only a very small collar of the insulated covering of the laser fibre should be visible. The laser fibre should be retracted into the biopsy channel when the endoscope is being moved and manipulated within the lower urinary tract to protect the laser tip.

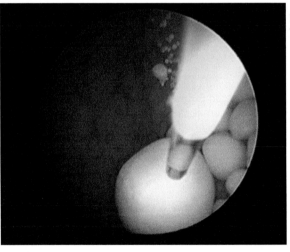

Endoscopic image of the tip of the laser fibre. Only a small collar of the insulated covering is visible.

6   Pass the endoscope within 5 mm of the urolith and extend the laser fibre from the biopsy channel.

7   Place the laser tip in direct contact with the surface of the urolith. Use the red aiming beam to orientate the laser fibre perpendicular to the urolith to achieve fragmentation.

8   Perform urolith fragmentation with the Ho:YAG laser set at 0.6–0.8 J and 6–8 Hz. The energy setting may be increased if necessary to achieve fragmentation. Settings >1 J and 12 Hz are rarely needed to fragment the type of uroliths most frequently found in small animal patients (Lulich *et al.*, 2009ab).

9   Repeatedly fragment the uroliths to achieve particle sizes that can be safely evacuated through a distended urethra using fluid lavage, urohydropulsion or endoscopic basket retrieval.

→ **OPERATIVE TECHNIQUE 14.3 CONTINUED**

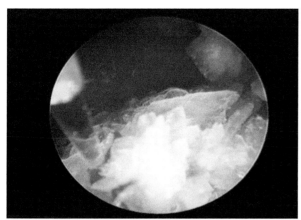

Endoscopic image of the laser fibre orientated perpendicular to and touching the cystolith to be fragmented.

Care should be taken to avoid damage to the urothelial surfaces resulting from manipulation of the endoscope or direct laser injury. Most patients with partial or full-thickness injuries to the urethra can be managed with placement of a transurethral catheter, providing continuous closed urinary drainage for 2–7 days, depending on the severity of the injury. Complete perforation of the bladder wall may necessitate conversion of a minimally invasive procedure to an open cystotomy for surgical repair of the injury.

Surgical manipulations: removal of urolith fragments

- Small urolith fragments (1–2 mm) – these fragments can be flushed from the lower urinary tract of bitches and queens with the egress fluid used during the procedure. The receptacle used to collect the egress fluid should be emptied through a paper coffee filter to separate the fluid from the small stone particles.
- Medium urolith fragments (<5 mm in male dogs and queens; ≤7 mm in bitches) – these fragments are generally removed by voiding urohydropulsion.
- Large urolith fragments (≥5 mm in male dogs; >7 mm in bitches) – these fragments may need to be removed from the bladder or urethra using endoscopic basket retrieval.

Endoscopic basket removal

1 Pass the endoscopic basket through the biopsy channel of the endoscope after lithotripsy is complete and the laser fibre and sheath have been removed.

2 Position the endoscope to visualize the largest urolith fragment. Extend a three- or four-wire basket retrieval instrument from the biopsy channel into the visual field adjacent to the fragment.

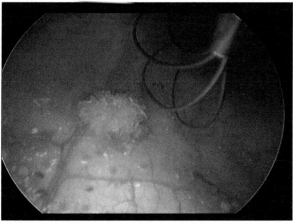

Endoscopic view of the four-wire stone retrieval basket device being positioned for cystolith retrieval.

3 Manually open the basket and extend the wires to form a cage-like orientation. Gently manipulate the instrument to surround and cradle the urolith fragment.

4 Gently close the basket and retract to position the urolith fragment at the end of the endoscope sheath.

5 Withdraw the endoscope from the lower urinary tract, removing the fragment. If any resistance is encountered upon removal of the endoscope with the urolith fragment, immediately release the stone, preventing urethral trauma. In these cases, additional fragmentation may be required.

→

→ **OPERATIVE TECHNIQUE 14.3 CONTINUED**

6   Repeat this procedure until all large fragments have been removed.

7   Obtain abdominal radiographs to check that all radiodense uroliths have been removed.

Voiding urohydropulsion

1   Position the endoscope within the bladder lumen or proximal urethra.

2   Infiltrate the bladder with sterile fluid via the ingress port until the bladder is distended and externally palpable.

3   Remove the endoscope and, with the help of an assistant, lift the patient to a vertical position relative to the table. Manually palpate and gently agitate the bladder to help dislodge small stone fragments and crystalline material.

4   Manually express the bladder by applying steady digital pressure transabdominally. Maintain abdominal compression to facilitate the flow of urine and urethral distension. The voided fluid should be collected and filtered to collect urolith fragments.

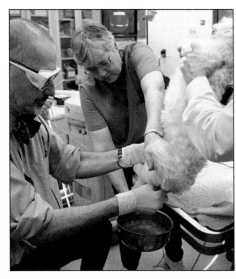

Urohydropulsion is performed after laser lithotripsy to removed stone fragments that are ≤5–7 mm. The bladder is distended with sterile fluid through the cystoscope. The cystoscope is removed and the patient is raised to a vertical position. Manual palpation and gentle agitation of the bladder is performed to dislodge small fragments. Manual expression of the bladder is performed by applying constant pressure to the abdominal wall in the region of the bladder. All urine should be collected and filtered to remove the stone material.

5   Repeat the procedure until the lower urinary tract is cleared of all urolith fragments and crystalline material.

6   Obtain abdominal radiographs to check that all radiodense uroliths have been removed.

OPERATIVE TECHNIQUE 14.4

Ureteronephrectomy

POSITIONING

Dorsal recumbency.

ASSISTANT

Optional.

EQUIPMENT EXTRAS

Balfour retractor; malleable retractors; haemoclips; topical haemostatic swab; abdominal swabs; long-handled DeBakey thumb forceps; Metzenbaum scissors; right-angled forceps; suction; cautery unit.

→

→ **OPERATIVE TECHNIQUE 14.4 CONTINUED**

SURGICAL TECHNIQUE

Approach

Routine ventral midline abdominal incision from the xiphoid process to just cranial to the pubis. Place a self-retaining retractor (e.g. Balfour retractor) to retract the abdominal wall and expose the abdominal viscera.

PRACTICAL TIP

In many pathological states requiring nephrectomy, the kidney is enlarged and supplied by extensive neovascularization. Make a large enough abdominal incision to facilitate manipulation of the kidney and achieve accurate haemostasis

Surgical manipulations

1   Carefully examine both kidneys.

2   Examine the liver and remaining abdominal viscera and palpate for metastatic lesions or other abnormalities. Examine both adrenal glands. Large hand-held retractors (e.g. malleable retractors) can be used to retract the liver cranially if necessary.

3   Expose the affected kidney from the retroperitoneal space by blunt dissection.

4   Gently strip the perirenal adipose tissue from the kidney capsule with a surgical swab. Alternatively, digital dissection can be used to peel the peritoneum from the kidney. In areas where the peritoneum is tightly adherent to the kidney, sharp dissection should be used to free it. Small vessels can be cauterized; larger vessels should be ligated or haemoclips applied.

5   Rotate the kidney medially to expose the dorsal aspect and renal hilus, exposing the renal artery and vein. The perirenal fat may need to be reflected from the ventromedial surface of the kidney to expose the vessels and the ureter.

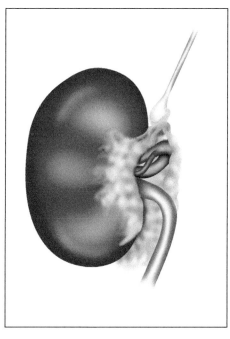

Kidney being rotated medially to locate the renal artery and vein.

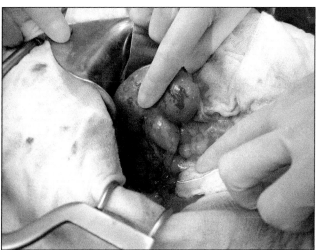

A 6-year-old male Bulldog undergoing ureteronephrectomy. The dog presented with gross haematuria due to a proximal ureteral tumour.

6   Multiple renal arteries, supplying blood to a single kidney, may be present. Double ligate or transfix the renal artery close to its attachment to the aorta with silk or a non-absorbable monofilament suture material of an appropriate size.

7   Place haemostatic forceps on the renal artery close to the kidney. Transect the renal artery between the ligatures and the haemostatic forceps.

8   Repeat the same procedure for the renal vein.

9   Inspect the vascular pedicles for bleeding.

→ **OPERATIVE TECHNIQUE 14.4 CONTINUED**

10 Check that the bladder is not rotated and that the correct ureter is identified as it empties into the bladder. It should be transected between two ligatures of an absorbable monofilament suture material, as close to the bladder as possible.

11 Then the ureter may be dissected from the retroperitoneum or simply stripped out, pulling gently on the freed kidney.

12 After removal of the kidney, the surgical field should be carefully examined for haemorrhage. All tissues should be submitted for histopathology (with or without culture). Biopsy of potential metastatic masses in the liver should also be performed.

Wound closure

Standard abdominal closure.

POSTOPERATIVE MANAGEMENT AND COMPLICATIONS

- Administer intravenous fluid therapy for 24 hours and monitor vital parameters, including urine output.
- Appropriate pain management is indicated for 24–72 hours after abdominal surgery.
- Exercise restriction for 10–14 days until suture removal.

OPERATIVE TECHNIQUE 14.5

Cystotomy/cystectomy

POSITIONING

Dorsal recumbency.

ASSISTANT

Optional.

EQUIPMENT EXTRAS

Suction and electrocoagulation (helpful).

SURGICAL TECHNIQUE

Approach

Ventral midline coeliotomy from the umbilicus to the pubis to expose the urinary bladder.

Surgical manipulations: cystotomy

1 Place a 3 metric (2/0 USP) silk or polypropylene stay suture through the apex of the bladder for manipulation.

2 Isolate the bladder by packing moistened laparotomy swabs beneath it. If the bladder is distended with urine, use a syringe and needle or suction to remove the majority of the urine.

3 Obtain a sterile urine sample for aerobic bacteriological culture.

→ **OPERATIVE TECHNIQUE 14.5 CONTINUED**

PRACTICAL TIP

Cystotomy is performed along the ventral midline to avoid disruption or injury to the ureters and vesicular blood and nerve supply located within the lateral ligaments

4 Use a No. 10 scalpel blade to make a stab incision into the bladder lumen on the ventral midline. Extend the cystotomy incision towards the bladder neck with Metzenbaum scissors.

5 Silk stay sutures can be placed along the incised edges of the bladder for retraction.

6 Visualize and palpate the entire luminal surface of the bladder. Exposure of the bladder neck is critical, to ensure that all cystic and urethral calculi are removed. Assess the ureteral orifices and examine the trigone and vesicourethral junction.

WARNING

If performing a cystotomy to remove cystic calculi, it is important to catheterize the urethra and flush it thoroughly to ensure that all calculi are removed

7 Excise a small full-thickness specimen of tissue along the cystotomy incision for biopsy and culture of the bladder wall.

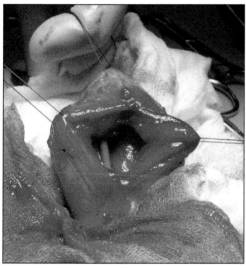

Stay sutures are placed in the apex of the bladder and sides of the cystotomy incision to facilitate examination of the lumen.

Wound closure

Cystotomy incisions are closed in one or two layers. This decision is based on the relative thickness of the bladder wall. The goal of surgical closure is to appose the divided tissues, restoring the integrity of the bladder wall for an adequate period of time to allow healing and to create a watertight seal preventing urine leakage. The submucosa is the surgical holding layer of the bladder. Synthetic absorbable monofilament suture material of appropriate size (1.5 or 2 metric; 4/0 or 3/0 USP) is used to place appositional or inverting suture patterns, such as Cushing and Lembert patterns. Avoid placement of suture material through the mucosa exposing the suture within the bladder lumen. Exposed suture materials may act as a nidus for chronic infection.

PRACTICAL TIP

A single-layer appositional suture pattern is sufficient to close markedly thickened bladder walls

Routine abdominal closure is performed.

Surgical manipulations: cystectomy

Removal of a portion of the bladder wall is not significantly more complicated than performing a cystotomy if the trigone is not affected. Trigonal excision is possible but is a considerably more complicated surgery, involving reimplantation of the ureters into the residual bladder tissue.

→ **OPERATIVE TECHNIQUE 14.5 CONTINUED**

TCCs are typically located in the trigone and complete surgical excision is not possible, since they extend into the proximal urethra

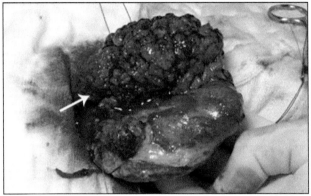

TCC involving approximately 50% of the mucosal surface of the bladder. Note extension of the tumour into the trigone (arrowed).

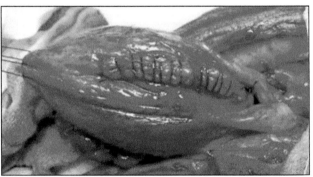

Closure of a cystotomy incision using a one-layer, continuous appositional suture pattern.

Up to 60–75% of the urinary bladder can be resected with minimal clinical signs. The urinary bladder will regain its original size within a few months.

1 Place a 3 metric (2/0 USP) silk or polypropylene stay suture through the apex of the bladder for manipulation.

2 Isolate the bladder by packing moistened laparotomy swabs beneath it. If the bladder is distended with urine, use a syringe and needle or suction to remove the majority of the urine.

3 Gently palpate the bladder wall to identify the mass lesion and incise 1–2 cm away from the mass.

4 Place stay sutures in the unaffected bladder wall to facilitate excision of the mass and reconstruction of the bladder.

WARNING

Ensure that the openings of the ureters are not damaged by the excision or obstructed by closure of the bladder following cystectomy

Wound closure

Closure of the cystectomy bladder incision is similar to cystotomy closure. If a significant portion of the bladder has been resected (>50%), the remaining tissue should be closed around a Foley catheter. This should be left in place for 2–3 days, connected to a closed urine collection system.

PRACTICAL TIP

After excision of a bladder tumour, surgical gloves should be changed and new instruments used to close the bladder and abdominal cavity to prevent seeding of tumour cells

Routine abdominal closure is performed.

POSTOPERATIVE MANAGEMENT AND COMPLICATIONS

- Urination should be monitored closely. Haematuria and pollakiuria are common for 24–48 hours after surgery. Urine leakage and dehiscence are uncommon complications.
- Administration of intravenous fluid therapy is not necessary, provided renal function is normal.
- Appropriate antibiotic therapy is indicated based on results of bacteriological culture and should be administered for 14–21 days if indicated.
- Restrict activity for 10–14 days until sutures are removed.
- Management of pain and discomfort is indicated. The use of NSAIDs may be prudent in patients after cystotomy to provide analgesia and reduce stranguria.

Chapter 15

Urinary incontinence

Alasdair Hotston Moore

The focus of this chapter is on animals in which urinary incontinence is the primary sign, although other urinary abnormalities may be present in some cases. Urinary incontinence is a common problem in dogs (around 5% of adult bitches; Forsee et al., 2013), with many affected animals managed medically in first-opinion practice, often after only minimal diagnostic investigations. There are a number of useful diagnostic procedures that can be undertaken to identify the underlying cause and allow the selection of appropriate surgical management in many cases.

> **PRACTICAL TIP**
>
> The definition of urinary incontinence is the unconscious passage of urine

Anatomy and physiology

The bladder can be considered as a distensible balloon of smooth muscle (the detrusor muscle), covered by serosa and lined by epithelium (urothelium). A remarkable feature of the bladder is the extent to which it can change in size as it fills and empties. The ureters enter the bladder at the caudodorsal aspect in a region known as the trigone. Each ureter passes into the bladder at a slight angle so that the ureter has a short section that is tunnelled within the thickness of the bladder wall (intramural portion). On the urothelial aspect, each ureter enters the lumen around 2 cm from the urethra (Rozear and Tidwell, 2003).

At the caudal aspect of the bladder, the lumen narrows rather abruptly to form the bladder neck, which is continuous with the urethra. In normal cats and most dogs the bladder neck is within the abdomen, but in a minority of animals (bitches in particular) the bladder neck may be intrapelvic in position. The urethra is a tube lined with urothelium and contains abundant smooth muscle in its wall. Distally, the urethra terminates at the vaginovulval junction (urethral papilla, females) or the tip of the penis (males). In the terminal part of the urethra there is a small amount of skeletal muscle. The smooth muscle of the urethra functions as the internal urethral sphincter and the skeletal muscle forms the external urethral sphincter.

The blood supply to the bladder derives largely from branches of the internal iliac (cranial vesical arteries to the body of the bladder and caudal vesical arteries to the neck) and partly from the vaginal arteries (in females).

The motor innervation of the detrusor muscle is parasympathetic, from the pelvic nerves, and branches of the hypogastric nerve provide sensory input, giving the sensation of fullness (Figure 15.1). During normal micturition, contraction of the abdominal wall and diaphragm provokes reflex contraction of the detrusor muscle as parasympathetic tone increases.

The principal innervation of the urethral smooth muscle is from branches of the hypogastric nerve and this is sympathetic, with alpha-1 receptors on the smooth muscle. There is also somatic innervation to the external urethral sphincter from the pudendal nerves, although this makes only a minor contribution to urethral outflow resistance in normal animals.

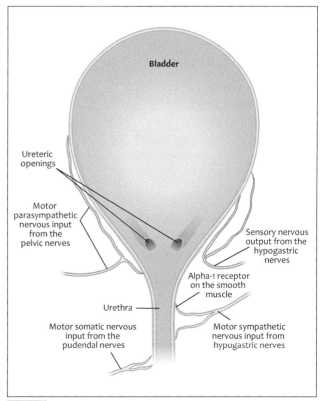

15.1 Innervation of the bladder and urethra.

Investigation of urinary incontinence

History

Sufficient time must be allowed during the consultation to allow a complete history to be gained. In asking about the animal's urination the clinician must attempt to determine whether the animal urinates normally at all (an appropriate volume with a good stream) and to distinguish:

- Incontinence (unconscious passage of urine)
- Polyuria (increased volume of urine produced each day, above the typical volume of 50 ml/kg/day)
- Urinary urgency (urge to urinate with inability to suppress micturition)
- Urinary frequency (increased number of micturition events)
- Inappropriate urination (micturition at a time or place which is not considered normal)
- Dysuria (difficulty in passing urine)
- Polydipsia (increased volume of water intake each day, above a typical maximum of 100 ml/kg/day in dogs and 50 ml/kg/day in cats).

- Urinary urgency is indicated by micturition (usually with behavioural features of normal micturition such as squatting or leg lifting, even if abbreviated). For example, the animal will usually move away from where it is lying, and often urinate close to the exit from the room.
- Inappropriate urination has similar features but often the animal will posture entirely normally although urinate in a place considered unacceptable to the owner (inside the house for example); in such cases, the diagnosis often requires the elimination of pathology as a cause of the behaviour.
- Dysuria is characterized by prolonged attempts at urination, with a poor or absent flow of urine. Signs of urgency and frequency are often also present. If the situation persists, overflow incontinence will develop and by this time detrusor muscle overstretch may have occurred, reducing the reflexes responsible for urgency and frequency.

There is some overlap in these behaviours but every attempt should be made to identify the key signs in each case. For example, animals with both dysuria and incontinence may have a urethral obstruction and the incontinence is actually urinary overflow (overflow incontinence). Treatment aimed at increasing urethral resistance, used for other forms of incontinence, is therefore contraindicated. In addition, in such a case the focus of investigation will be on the urethra (lower urinary tract) rather than the ureters (upper urinary tract; see Chapter 14). Historical indicators associated with true incontinence include urine soiling of the bedding (or where the animal lies) or a steady dripping of urine from the vulva or prepuce.

> **PRACTICAL TIP**
>
> When taking the history, prior medication, and the response to it, should be noted, together with current or recent antibacterial therapy which may interfere with any laboratory testing

Physical examination

As well as examination of the external genitalia for signs of incontinence or morphological abnormalities, the clinician must complete a general examination, abdominal palpation, rectal examination (in both sexes) and a neurological examination focused on the spinal reflexes. Rectal examination (in cats this will usually only be undertaken under anaesthesia at a later time) includes evaluation of the prostate gland (in dogs), the urethra (palpable ventral to and through the vagina) and the completeness of the pelvic diaphragm. Evaluation of spinal reflexes is important because the majority of animals with urinary incontinence due to neurological disease will have abnormalities that can be detected on a neurological examination, prompting a more detailed evaluation of the nervous system (see the *BSAVA Manual of Canine and Feline Neurology*).

Initial tests of spinal reflexes in animals with suspected neurological causes of incontinence

- Postural reactions: hopping, paw placement, visual and tactile placement (tests of proprioception and indicators of upper motor neuron function).
- Anal tone: a test of lower motor neuron function.
- Patellar, withdrawal and perianal reflexes: test the hindlimb spinal reflexes. Reduced activity suggests lower motor neuron or sensory dysfunction; exaggerated responses suggest upper motor neuron dysfunction.

Abnormal findings on these tests should prompt a full evaluation of the neurological system. Details of interpretation and further testing can be found elsewhere (e.g. Platt and Olby, 2013).

Examples of neurological diseases associated with incontinence

- Spinal disease affecting segments T3–L3 (e.g. intervertebral disc disease, vertebral fracture, spinal malformations). Associated with exaggerated spinal reflexes, initial urinary retention and later overflow.
- Spinal disease affecting segments L7–S3 (e.g. lumbosacral stenosis, discospondylitis, neoplasia affecting the cauda equina, spinal bifida). Associated with lower motor neuron dysfunction and urinary incontinence without retention.
- Inflammatory and degenerative neurological diseases (e.g. degenerative myelopathy, radiculoneuropathy). Associated with urinary incontinence with or without retention depending on the balance of lower and upper motor neuron dysfunction.

Systemic diseases (except those causing polydipsia/polyuria) are rare causes of urinary incontinence. For this reason, blood testing is not generally helpful in diagnosis except to rule these out. However, laboratory examination of urine is important. All incontinent animals should have urine submitted for bacteriological culture and sensitivity testing. If the animal is receiving antibacterial medication, this should be withdrawn for 2–5 days before sampling.

Ideally urine samples should be obtained by cystocentesis. Although this occasionally causes microscopic haematuria as a sampling artefact, the microbiology is much more reliable. In severely incontinent animals the bladder may be small, requiring ultrasound-guided cystocentesis or occasionally catheter collection of a sample.

Further investigations (including radiography, ultrasonography, advanced imaging and endoscopy) are discussed later during consideration of the disease conditions.

Differential diagnosis

In considering the causes of incontinence, it is useful to separate affected animals into juvenile and adult groups. Although there is significant overlap in diseases between these groups, age is a guide to the likelihood of certain conditions. Most of the available information relates to dogs (Holt, 1999). Urinary incontinence is rarer in cats of either sex but will be mentioned where information is available.

Important causes of urinary incontinence in juvenile animals

* Ectopic ureters.
* Juvenile urethral sphincter mechanism incompetence.
* Urethral hypoplasia (feline).
* Morphological abnormalities associated with intersex development.
* Urethral diverticulum.
* Congenital spinal disorders (e.g. spina bifida).

Important causes of urinary incontinence in adult animals

* Urethral sphincter mechanism incompetence.
* Ectopic ureters.
* Acquired spinal disease.
* Urethral neoplasia/urethritis.
* Perineal hernia (males > females).
* Trauma/iatrogenic injury (notably ureterovaginal fistula).

Urethral sphincter mechanism incompetence

Urethral sphincter mechanism incompetence (USMI) is a broad diagnostic category and includes all animals where it is considered that there is insufficient urethral sphincter function to maintain continence. It occurs much more frequently in dogs of either sex than cats, and is much commoner in females than males. USMI can present as a congenital or acquired disorder. The underlying pathophysiology is complex because many factors contribute to urethral sphincter function (Noel et al., 2010).

Factors contributing to urethral sphincter function

* Tone of the internal urethral sphincter.
* Tone of the external urethral sphincter.
* Length of the functional sphincter.
* Position of the bladder neck compared with the anatomical limits of peritoneal cavity.
* Presence of folds in the urethral mucosa.
* Oedema within the urethral wall.
* Body size and breed.

The muscular urethral sphincter includes both smooth and skeletal muscle components. Of these, the smooth muscle is considered to make the most important contribution. However, the smooth muscle is not anatomically discrete, in other words it is spread along the urethral length rather than forming a discrete anatomical structure. The smooth muscle is supplied with adrenergic receptors which are themselves induced by the presence of oestrogens. In animals with juvenile USMI (those presenting before sexual maturity), sphincter tone may therefore spontaneously improve at the time of the first oestrus. However, muscle tone tends to reduce with age, and therefore adult USMI becomes increasingly common in older animals. This effect is exacerbated by neutering, with an associated increased incidence of the condition in spayed females (and castrated males). Urinary tract infection may also reduce urethral tone.

The length of the functional sphincter is also important, reflecting the fact that the internal sphincter extends along the urethra. There is a demonstrable link between the incidence of USMI and urethral length (measured radiographically) compared with body size (Holt, 1985).

The position of the bladder neck compared with the pelvic inlet (probably actually the caudal reflection of the peritoneal cavity) is also important. The model explaining this compares the pressure around the bladder neck with that around the urethra. If the bladder neck is intra-abdominal, increases in abdominal pressure act on the bladder and the abdominal urethra, favouring continence. However, if the bladder neck is intrapelvic, raised abdominal pressure (e.g. during recumbency or exercise) will tend to overcome urethral closing pressure, resulting in incontinence (Figure 15.2). In dogs and cats (compared with women, for example), bladder neck position appears to be largely unaffected by age. There is also no evidence that it changes as a result of neutering surgeries (ovariectomy or ovariohysterectomy). However, changes in body fat deposition may change the position of the peritoneal reflection: this may account for improved continence in affected bitches when obesity is controlled. Additionally, rupture of the pelvic diaphragm (perineal hernia formation, typically in male dogs; see Chapter 8), may allow the bladder neck to move caudally and contribute to the incontinence occasionally seen in affected animals.

Longitudinal folds are present in the urethral mucosa of intact, sexually mature bitches. These folds also contribute to normal urethral resistance. These folds are absent in neutered bitches and may play a role in the development of incontinence in neutered animals, and the improvement seen with oestrogen medication. Oestrogens also cause oedema in the urethral submucosa, which is believed to contribute to continence.

There is a recognized breed predisposition to canine USMI. This probably reflects both body size and specific

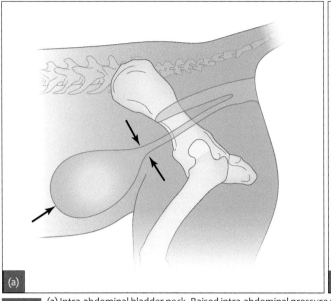
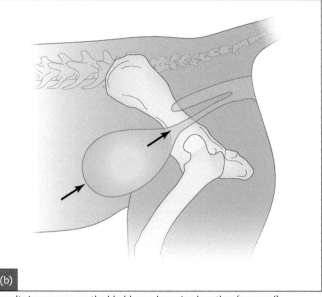

15.2 (a) Intra-abdominal bladder neck. Raised intra-abdominal pressure results in pressure on the bladder and proximal urethra (arrowed), favouring continence. (b) Intrapelvic bladder neck. Raised intra-abdominal pressure favours urine leakage (arrowed).

genetic traits. In general, USMI is more common in large and giant breeds. Particular breeds affected in the UK include the Old English Sheepdog, Rottweiler, Dobermann, Weimaraner and Irish Setter (Holt and Thrusfield, 1993). A similar predisposition is expected in other countries.

Experience of first-opinion practice suggests that most bitches with USMI are managed medically and appear to respond satisfactorily.

> **PRACTICAL TIP**
>
> Many cases in juvenile animals improve after their first oestrus and bitches known to be affected should not be neutered before that time. It is also often recommended that bitches of at-risk breeds should not be neutered prepubertally as a precaution (Holt and Thrushfield, 1993), although this has not been confirmed by clinical trials

Diagnosis

There is no single diagnostic test for USMI. However, several tests can be used to support the diagnosis and it is important to rule out other differential diagnoses. The history and signalment are important guides. Urine bacteriology should always be performed before initiating therapy, or if signs worsen during treatment. To assess the bladder neck position and relative length of the urethra, the most useful test is a retrograde vaginourethrogram (Hotston Moore, 2009; Figure 15.3). Neither ultrasonography nor cystography is useful for this purpose. Pneumocystography in particular causes the bladder to 'float' into a more cranial position. A key differential diagnosis in these cases is ectopic ureter; the most helpful method to confirm that the ureteral orifices are normal in position is urethroscopy (see below). Technology is available to measure intraurethral pressure (urethral pressure prolifometry, UPP). However, this is not widely available and there are significant barriers to its use as a diagnostic (as opposed to research) tool, such as a lack of reliable data, including exclusion of artefacts, and the overlap in measurements between normal (continent) animals and those with USMI.

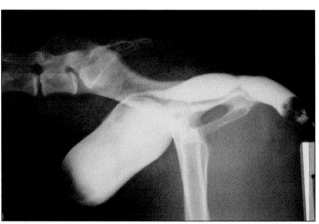

15.3 Retrograde vaginourethrogram of a bitch with a markedly intrapelvic bladder neck.

Medical management

The mainstays of medical management of USMI are alpha-adrenergic agonists and oestrogens (in neutered bitches and perhaps neutered males). Two authorized adrenergic agonists are available: phenylpropanolamine and ephedrine. The manufacturers' dose regimes should be followed. Clinical experience suggests that both are effective in many bitches. It is reasonable to try one agent if the other produces an unsatisfactory result (either lack of efficacy or side effects, such as agitation). The only authorized oestrogen is oestriol. Oestrogenic therapy may produce a number of useful effects in bitches affected by USMI (increase in adrenergic receptor activity, urethral mucosal development, urethral wall oedema) and most affected bitches show a good response. Oestriol may be safer than other (unauthorized) oestrogens because of its short biological half-life, which reduces concerns about oestrogen toxicity (notably bone marrow suppression). The author does not prefer either adrenergic or oestrogen therapy; both, in his experience, seem to have similar overall response rates and incidence of adverse effects.

Surgical management

Several surgical procedures are available as alternatives to medical management. Bitches selected for surgical management are typically those who are relatively young (and often those whose owners are concerned about the adverse effects or cost of prolonged medical management), have not responded adequately to medical management or who develop adverse effects. The most widely used surgical procedures are: colposuspension (see Operative Technique 15.1) and cystourethropexy (see Operative Technique 15.2). Also described, but with limited clinical evidence to date, are urethral sling (Claeys *et al.*, 2010) and artificial sphincter implantation (AUS; Reeves *et al.*, 2013). AUS implantation uses a proprietary silicone device which is wrapped around the urethra during laparotomy, 3 cm caudal to the bladder neck. The AUS has a chamber connected to a subcutaneous port, allowing a degree of inflation postoperatively to increase urethral resistance as required to achieve continence (Figure 15.4). Both colposuspension and cystourethropexy are procedures primarily intended to alter bladder neck position, although they may have some effect on increasing urethral resistance. Despite this, they can improve continence even in bitches with an apparently intra-abdominal bladder neck on radiography. Urethral sling placement and AUS implantation are intended to increase urethral resistance.

USMI is rare in male dogs compared with females. In general, the response to treatment appears to be less than in bitches. No medical therapies are authorized in males, although anecdotally some respond to treatment with adrenergic agents and hormonal therapy (oestrogens or testosterone). Surgical treatment is less well evaluated in males than in females but procedures to alter bladder neck position have been described (see Operative Techniques 15.3 and 15.4; prostatopexy and vas deferensopexy).

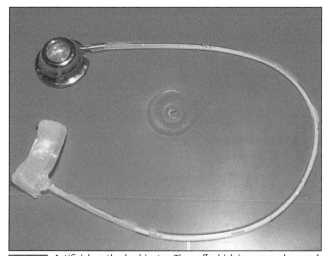

15.4 Artificial urethral sphincter. The cuff which is wrapped around the urethra is to the lower left and the port, which is placed subcutaneously, is to the upper left of the image.

An endoscopic approach to the management of USMI has also described, involving the transurethral submucosal injection of bulking agents such as collagen suspension (Lhermette, 2012; see Operative Technique 15.5). This increases urethral resistance. It can be used as an alternative to surgical techniques or as a second procedure when there is an inadequate response to surgical management (Arnold *et al.*, 1996; Barth *et al.*, 2005). The success rate of submucosal bulking agents is difficult to quantify because many treated bitches are also subjected to medical management. In general, restoration of continence is seen in around half of bitches (Arnold *et al.*, 1996), with improvement in most of the rest. The effect is not permanent (at least when collagen is used), and continence usually deteriorates over the following 9–12 months. Although dysuria is a possible complication of the procedure, it is uncommon. The greatest barrier to wider use of the technique is the cost of the collagen products and the need for repeated treatment.

Ectopic ureter

Ectopic ureter is a congenital abnormality in which one or both ureters do not open into the bladder at the trigone, but elsewhere. The abnormal opening is almost always either into the urethra or, occasionally, close to the urethral papilla in the vagina. There are occasional reports of ectopic ureters entering the vagina elsewhere, or even the uterus. The condition is much commoner in the dog than the cat, and in dogs the ureter typically enters the serosal surface of the bladder in the normal position and then runs within the thickness of the bladder and urethra to open distally (described as intramural ectopic ureter; Figure 15.5a). Less commonly in dogs, but the more common anatomy in affected cats, is that the ureter does not connect to the bladder at all and joins directly to the abnormal location (extramural ectopic ureter; Figure 15.5b). Occasional instances of dual ureteral openings (bladder and urethra) and incompletely closed ectopic ureters (ureteral troughs) are reported, but these are not common.

Pathophysiology

Simplistically, the clinician may assume that affected animals would be constantly incontinent and that incontinence would be apparent early in life. The development of incontinence in affected animals is, however, a balance between the position of the ureteral termination and the urethral pressure distal to it. In many affected animals, there is at times sufficient urethral resistance distal to the ureteric termination to cause urine to flow in a retrograde direction into the bladder, causing bladder filling and preserving continence. Incontinence develops when urethral resistance is overcome, perhaps during recumbency, or reduces, perhaps after neutering or with age.

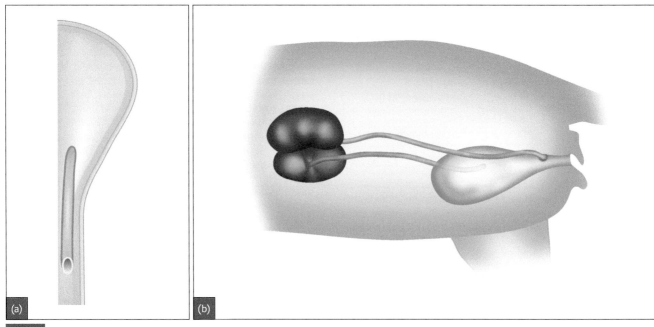

15.5 (a) Intramural ectopic ureter with a submuscosal tunnel opening in the urethra. (b) Extramural ectopic ureter.

Secondary urinary tract infection is also common in affected animals; this may exacerbate incontinence but can also lead to intractable postsurgical infections unless it is eliminated prior to surgery.

A consequence of an ectopic ureteral orifice in many instances is ureteral dilatation, renal pelvic dilatation or hydronephrosis. This does not happen in all cases, but is probably due to a combination of urinary tract infection, resistance to flow and/or intrinsic loss of ureteral motility. In mild cases ureteral and pelvic dilatation may stabilize or even improve after successful treatment, but in marked cases it is considered irreversible and an indication for ureteronephrectomy. Exact guidelines for this decision are not available and are usually based on the clinical experience and judgement of the veterinary surgeon (veterinarian).

Presentation and signalment

Ectopic ureters are most commonly diagnosed in juvenile animals; the diagnosis is commoner in females than males, but it is also the second most frequent diagnosis in adult bitches. Although the clinician might expect affected animals to show continuous incontinence, this is not typical, with many showing intermittent and variable degrees of incontinence. Additionally, many cases have received empirical treatment for USMI before diagnosis and may have responded to this, although often incompletely.

> **PRACTICAL TIP**
>
> The severity of urinary incontinence is variable and cannot be used to determine the location of the ureteral orifice(s) or distinguish between unilateral and bilateral ectopia

Breed predispositions are also well recognized. Breeds suggested to be at increased risk in the UK population are the Border Terrier, Briard, Bulldog, Golden Retriever, Griffon, Labrador Retriever and Skye Terrier (Holt *et al.*, 2000). In other regions the predisposition may be different, and in addition the Siberian Husky is considered predisposed in the USA (Hayes, 1984).

Diagnosis

The physical examination of patients with ureteral ectopia is typically normal, with the exception of moist or urine-stained hair in the perivulvar or preputial region. Perivulvar dermatitis secondary to urine irritation of the surrounding skin may also be observed. Haematological and serum biochemical evaluations are generally within normal limits, unless associated abnormalities of the upper urinary tract that diminish renal function, or pyelonephritis secondary to ascending urinary tract infection, are present.

Given that most ectopic ureters open into the urethra, urethrocystoscopy (Figure 15.6) is a very useful diagnostic tool. This is technically possible in all cats and dogs, although practically limited in male dogs and cats for whom the required equipment is of limited availability. The technique is well described in the *BSAVA Manual of Canine and Feline Endoscopy and Endosurgery*. Cystourethroscopy is used to identify ectopic ureteral orifices and to examine the trigone for normally positioned ureteric openings. Direct catheterization of the ureters allows collection of urine for bacteriology, and occasionally retrograde ureterography is performed. However, cystoscopy alone does not allow

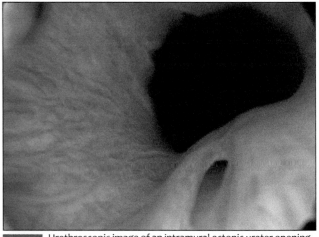

15.6 Urethroscopic image of an intramural ectopic ureter opening into the urethra.

evaluation of ureteral and pelvic dilatation nor of renal changes (hydronephrosis or pyelonephritis), thus a second imaging technique is required, usually ultrasonography.

Conventional radiography (intravenous urography) or computed tomography (CT) can also be used to diagnose ectopia (Hotston Moore, 2009; Schwarz, 2011). These are very useful for examining the kidneys and most of the ureteric length but, with either technique, identifying the position of the ureteric orifice itself can be difficult, even with fluoroscopic evaluation and repeated exposures. The sensitivity can be increased by combining intravenous urography with retrograde (vagino)urethrography (Figure 15.7), and this is strongly recommended when cystourethroscopy is not available. Details of these techniques are available in the *BSAVA Manual of Canine and Feline Abdominal Imaging*.

Ultrasonography has also been used to examine the trigone area for ureteral jets to confirm normal positioning of the ureteral orifices. Although this can be useful when ureteral jets are confidently identified, it is operator dependent and additionally difficult when the bladder neck is intrapelvic, a common condition concurrent with ectopic ureters. Ultrasonography is, however, a very valuable part of the investigation, used to examine the kidneys for secondary changes (with guided aspiration if required).

Urethroscopic repositioning of an ectopic ureteral orifice is a relatively recently described minimally invasive alternative for intramural ectopic ureters (Berent *et al.*, 2012). Transendoscopic laser surgery is used to open the septum between the urethra and ureteric lumen from distally to proximally until the ureter opens at the trigone (Figures 15.8 and 15.9). This technique is often combined with fluoroscopy because the transition of the ureter from intramural to extramural can be hard to assess with cystoscopy alone, and if laser ablation is carried out too far cranially perforation and uroabdomen could occur. Advantages of this technique may include decreased postoperative pain and length of hospitalization; however, the specialized equipment needed limits its application in general practice.

The treatment outcome for patients with ectopic ureters depends partly on the incidence of specific surgical complications (see Operative Techniques 15.4 and 15.5), but largely on the presence of concurrent USMI. This is believed to explain the reported outcome rates of 50% continent, 25% with improved continence and 25% unchanged after surgery (Holt and Hotston Moore, 1995). In persistently incontinent animals, if technical failure and urinary tract infection have been investigated, additional treatment for USMI should be instigated (medical or surgical).

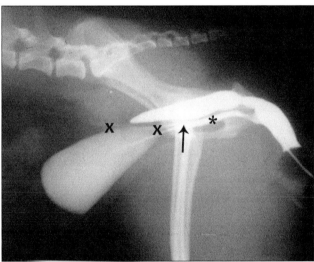

15.7 Retrograde vaginourethrogram demonstrating an intramural ectopic ureter (course indicated by **X** and **X**) entering the urethra (indicated by *****). The approximate point of entry is indicated by the black arrow.

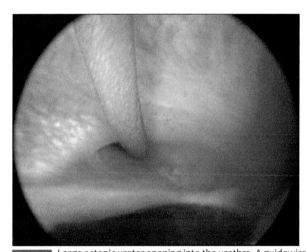

15.8 Large ectopic ureter opening into the urethra. A guidewire has been placed into the ureteral opening.
(Reproduced from Hotson Moore and Ragni (2012) with permission from the publisher)

Treatment

Treatment options consist essentially of repositioning abnormally positioned ureteric openings or removal of the affected kidney/ureter. Ureteronephrectomy is a practical option in certain circumstances, notably when the contralateral kidney is present and demonstrably normal, and the contralateral ureter is normally positioned. If there is uncertainty about any of these factors, ureternephrectomy should be avoided. The technique is described in Chapter 14.

Repositioning of a ureteral orifice can be achieved via surgery (ureteral transplantation) or urethroscopically. Ureteral transplantation can be achieved without transection, if the ureter is intramural in position (the common situation in bitches), described as ureteroneocystotomy (see Operative Technique 15.6). If the ureter is extramural in position (or in male dogs if the prostate gland obscures the bladder neck), ureteral reimplantation is used (see Operative Technique 15.7).

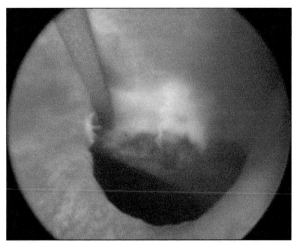

15.9 Laser resection of the ureteral opening back to the trigone.
(Reproduced from Hotson Moore and Ragni (2012) with permission from the publisher)

Urethral hypoplasia

This condition is seen almost invariably in queens. Although it can be considered an extreme form of USMI, it is distinct in that it results from a failure of normal urethral development, resulting in a wide urethra that is continuous with the bladder neck. The diagnosis is best illustrated by retrograde vaginourethrography (Figure 15.10). Surgical treatment consists of excision of a longitudinal strip of urethral wall (which can be reflected cranially to increase the bladder dimensions or discarded), followed by closure of the urethra around a stent, such as a 6 Fr urethral catheter. The technique is described in detail by Holt (2008) and illustrated in Figure 15.11.

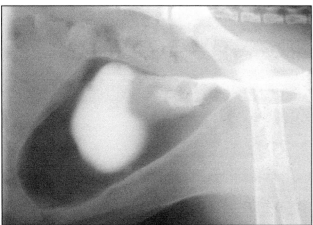

15.10 Retrograde vaginourethrogram showing urethral hypoplasia in a queen.

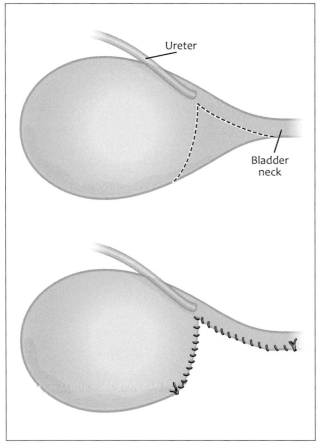

15.11 Bladder neck reconstruction for urethral hypoplasia.

Other congenital urethral abnormalities

A number of other anatomical causes for urinary incontinence have been described. Urethrography is a suitable technique to identify and evaluate these. Of these conditions, urovagina is perhaps the most frequently encountered (Figure 15.12). This is a congenital maldevelopment of the vagina and urethra in which the urethral tube fails to form properly, with a resulting continuation between the bladder neck and vestibule. The vagina appears to be dorsally positioned, with a narrow opening into the vestibule.

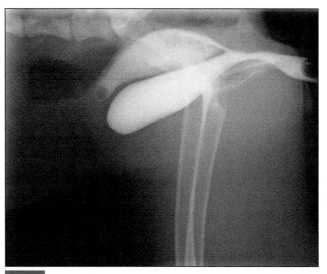

15.12 Retrograde vaginourethrogram illustrating urovagina.

Ureteral vaginal fistulation

Ureteral vaginal fistulation is the most common iatrogenic cause of urinary incontinence and occurs occasionally in both bitches and queens, as a complication of ovariohysterectomy. It happens as a consequence of inadvertent entrapment of the terminal ureter in the vaginal ligature. A typical history in affected animals is an unexpectedly painful postoperative recovery followed by the development of constant urinary incontinence a few days later, when the tissue between the ureter and vaginal lumen has necrosed. Other possible consequences of the same misadventure are hydronephrosis or death, if both ureters are involved.

Diagnosis can be slightly difficult, although the history is extremely helpful (incontinence due to USMI usually does not become apparent for several months after neutering). Cystoscopy will show two normally positioned ureteral orifices, although it may be possible to appreciate the absence of urine jets from the affected ureter. An intravenous urogram may show variable degrees of ureteral dilatation and tortuosity, especially terminally. When a retrograde vaginourethrogram is performed concurrently, continuity of the affected ureter and vaginal stump is apparent (Figure 15.13). Surgical treatment is either by ureteronephrectomy (if the contralateral kidney is normal and if there is marked ureteral dilatation or hydronephrosis) or ureteral reimplantation (as described for the treatment of ectopic ureters in Operative Technique 15.7).

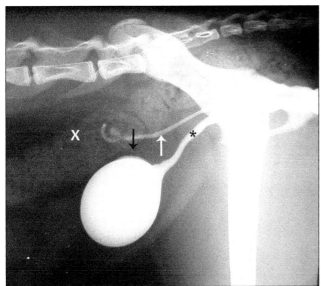

15.13 Ureteral vaginal fistulation in a cat. Combined intravenous urogram and retrograde vaginourethrogram showing the normal ureter entering the trigone (black arrow) and the other ureter (**X**) becoming tortuous and joining the vaginal stump (white arrow). The urethra is shown by the asterisk (*****).

References and further reading

Arnold S, Hubler M, Lott-Stolz G and Rüsch P (1996) Treatment of urinary incontinence in bitches by endoscopic injection of glutaraldehyde cross-linked collagen. *Journal of Small Animal Practice* **37**, 163–168

Barth A, Reichler IM, Hubler M, Hässig M and Arnold S (2005) Evaluation of long-term effects of endoscopic injection of collagen into the urethral submucosa for treatment of urethral sphincter incompetence in female dogs: 40 cases (1993–2000). *Journal of the American Veterinary Medical Association* **226**, 73–76

Berent AC, Weisse C, Mayhew PD *et al.* (2012) Evaluation of cystoscopic-guided laser ablation of intramural ectopic ureters in female dogs. *Journal of the American Veterinary Medical Association* **240**, 716–725

Brissot HN, Dupré GP and Bouvy BM (2004) Use of laparotomy in a staged approach for resolution of bilateral or complicated perineal hernia in 41 dogs. *Veterinary Surgery* **33**, 412–421

Claeys S, de Laval J and Hamaide A (2010) Transobturator vaginal tape inside out for treatment of urethral sphincter mechanism incompetence: preliminary results in 7 female dogs. *Veterinary Surgery* **39**, 969–979

Forsee KM, Davis GJ, Mouat EE, Salmeri KR and Bastian RP (2013) Evaluation of the prevalence of urinary incontinence in spayed female dogs: 566 cases (2003–2008). *Journal of the American Veterinary Medical Association* **242**, 959–962

Hayes HM (1984) Breed associations of canine ectopic ureter: a study of 217 female cases. *Journal of Small Animal Practice* **25**, 501–504

Holt PE (1985) Importance of urethral length, bladder neck position and vestibule–vaginal stenosis in sphincter mechanism incompetence in the incontinent bitch. *Research in Veterinary Science* **39**, 364–372

Holt PE (1999) Diagnosis and management of canine urethral sphincter mechanism incompetence. *Waltham Focus* **9**, 19–23

Holt PE (2008) *Urological Disorders of the Dog and Cat.* Manson, London

Holt PE, Coe RJ and Hotston Moore A (2005) Prostatopexy as a treatment for urethral sphincter mechanism incompetence in male dogs. *Journal of Small Animal Practice* **46**, 567–570

Holt PE and Hotston Moore A (1995) Canine ureteral ectopia: an analysis of 175 cases and comparison of surgical treatments. *Veterinary Record* **136**, 345–349

Holt PE and Thrusfield MV (1993) Association between breed, size, neutering and docking and acquired urinary incontinence due to incompetence of the urethral sphincter mechanism. *Veterinary Record* **133**, 177–180

Holt PE, Thrusfield MV and Hotston Moore A (2000) Breed predisposition to ureteral ectopia in bitches in the UK. *Veterinary Record* **146**, 561

Hotston Moore A (2009) The bladder and urethra. In: *BSAVA Manual of Canine and Feline Abdominal Imaging*, ed. R O'Brien and FJ Barr, pp.205–221. BSAVA Publications, Gloucester

Hotson Moore A and Ragni RA (2012) *Clinical Manual of Small Animal Endosurgery.* Wiley-Blackwell, Chichester

Larson MM (2009) The kidneys and ureters. In: *BSAVA Manual of Canine and Feline Abdominal Imaging*, ed. R O'Brien and FJ Barr, pp.185–204. BSAVA Publications, Gloucester

Lhermette PJ (2012) Urethrocystoscopy and the female reproductive tract. In: *Clinical Manual of Small Animal Endoscopy*, ed. A Hotston Moore and RA Ragni, pp.209–230. Wiley Blackwell, Oxford

Lhermette P and Sobel D (2008) *BSAVA Manual of Canine and Feline Endoscopy and Endosurgery.* BSAVA Publications, Gloucester

McLoughlin MA and Chew DJ (2000) Diagnosis and surgical management of ectopic ureters. *Clinical Techniques in Small Animal Practice* **15**, 17–24

Noel S, Claeys C and Hamaide A (2010) Acquired urinary incontinence in the bitch parts 1 and 2. *The Veterinary Journal* **186**, 10–24

Platt S and Olby N (2013) *BSAVA Manual of Canine and Feline Neurology, 4th edn.* BSAVA Publications, Gloucester

Reeves L, Adin C, McLoughlin M, Ham K and Chew D (2013) Outcome after placement of an artificial urethral sphincter in 27 dogs. *Veterinary Surgery* **42**, 12–18

Rozear L and Tidwell AS (2003) Evaluation of the ureter and ureterovesicular junction using helical CT excretory urography in healthy dogs. *Veterinary Radiology and Ultrasound* **44**, 155–164

Schwarz T (2011) The urinary tract. In: *Veterinary Computed Tomography*, ed. T Schwarz and J Saunders. Wiley, Chichester

White RN (2001) Urethropexy for the management of urethral sphincter mechanism incompetence in the bitch. *Journal of Small Animal Practice* **42**, 481–486

OPERATIVE TECHNIQUE 15.1

Colposuspension

PREPARATION AND POSITIONING

No pre-anaesthetic preparation is required. Clipping: the patient is clipped to include the perineum and abdomen. Place a purse-string suture in the anus. Place a Foley catheter (6–12 Fr) in the urethra and connect to a closed collection system. Douche the vagina with dilute povidone–iodine antiseptic solution. The patient is placed in dorsal recumbency with hindlimbs relaxed (frog-leg position).

ASSISTANT

Yes.

EQUIPMENT EXTRAS

Abdominal retractor (e.g. Balfour or Gosset).

SURGICAL TECHNIQUE

Use a four-quadrant draping to include the vulva in the surgical field. An extra drape is required to cover this area once colposuspension sutures are placed.

1 Make a caudal midline laparotomy incision, extending from the pubic brim cranially to the umbilicus.

2 Place a stay suture of 3 metric (2/0 USP) monofilament material in the cranial pole of the bladder.

3 Bluntly dissect to the left and right of the midline along the ventral aspect of the rectus sheath to identify the prepubic tendon.

4 Identify the internal pudendal vessels as they emerge from caudal to the tendons.

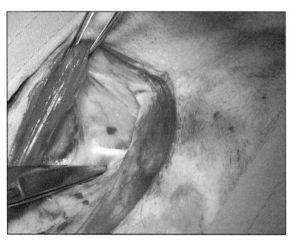

The external pudendal vessels and prepubic tendon should be identified prior to colposuspension (left side shown, caudal is top right and ventral top left of the image, prior to incising the linea alba).

5 Use blunt digital dissection caudal and ventral to the bladder neck between the urethra and vagina. This dissection continues into the retroperitoneal space.

6 Right-handed surgeons should stand to the left of the patient. Lubricate the index finger of the non-dominant hand and place into the vagina. If the bitch is too small to allow this, or a vestibulovaginal stenosis is present, a blunt probe can be used instead.

7 Push the finger cranially and ventrally, displacing the urethra towards the midline. Further blunt dissection is used within the retroperitoneal space to push the fat away until the vaginal wall is visible. Grasp the tissue with Allis tissue forceps, ensuring the urethra is not included (this should be visible and identified by the presence of the urethral catheter). Avoid any large blood vessels in the vaginal wall. Grasp the vagina at its lateral aspect. ➡️

→ **OPERATIVE TECHNIQUE 15.1 CONTINUED**

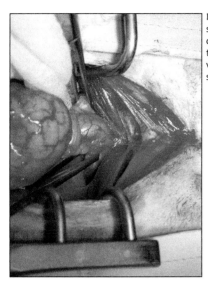

Intraoperative photograph showing the vagina being grasped during colposuspension. Caudal is to the right of the image and the vagina has been grasped on either side of the urethra.

8 Repeat the process on the other side. The vagina should be secured on each side of the urethra.

9 Remove the finger from the vagina. Put on fresh gloves and drape the vulva out of the surgical field.

10 Place the first suture using 3.5 metric (0 USP) monofilament nylon or polypropylene swaged on a taper-cut needle. The needle is passed behind the prepubic tendon, medial to the internal pudendal blood vessels, and into the retroperitoneal space. The needle is re-grasped and then a substantial bite of the vaginal wall taken alongside the Allis forceps, passing craniocaudally. The needle is then passed out from the abdomen immediately cranial to the prepubic tendon, forming a loop around the tendon and through the vaginal wall. Clip the suture with haemostats. Except in small bitches, when only one suture can be placed without compromising the urethra, place two similar sutures on each side.

11 Before tying, pull up firmly on all four sutures. Ensure the urethra is not squeezed by the sutures or vaginal wall: the tip of a pair of needle holders should be able to lie alongside the urethra in the arch formed by the vagina as the sutures are pulled tight. If this is not possible, the sutures must be replaced.

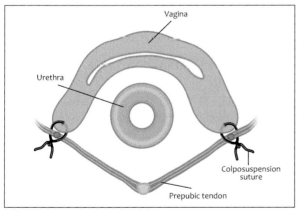

End result of colposuspension (transverse section; dorsal is at the top of image).

12 Tie each suture firmly, taking care to avoid fat becoming entrapped between the vaginal wall and body wall. Check the space around the urethra once more.

13 Close the abdomen routinely. Note: the rectus sheath may not be readily apposed caudally and the caudal part of the laparotomy should be closed with simple interrupted sutures if this is the case.

14 The catheter is removed at the end of surgery.

POSTOPERATIVE MANAGEMENT AND COMPLICATIONS

Routine postoperative analgesia is required (typically opiates for 24 hours and non-steroidal anti-inflammatory drugs (NSAIDs) for 7 days). Perioperative antibiotics are given and continued postoperatively for 10 days (e.g. clavulanate-potentiated amoxicillin (co-amoxiclav).

> ➔ **OPERATIVE TECHNIQUE 15.1 CONTINUED**
>
> Around 10% of bitches have postoperative dysuria. Most commonly this is believed to be due to dyssynergia; if it does not respond to appropriate analgesia, diazepam may be useful (5–15 mg per animal by mouth, three times daily, given 10 minutes before exercise). In a small minority, dysuria persists and a retrograde vaginourethrogram is recommended to ensure that urethral obstruction is not present. If it is not, an indwelling urethral catheter is placed and maintained for 5 days. Postoperative dysuria may be commoner in bitches treated in the previous month with oestrogen therapy, which should therefore be avoided in the preoperative period.
>
> Strict exercise restriction is required for 4 weeks after surgery to allow firm adhesions to develop around the colposuspension sutures: short lead walks only should be taken, with avoidance of stair climbing and jumping. Although some animals show an immediate improvement, the owners should be advised that the effects of this surgery on continence are uncertain for the first 4–6 weeks: some bitches remain incontinent initially and improve after the first few weeks; others are improved initially but begin to leak urine as postoperative swelling reduces. In the long term, 50% of bitches are cured, 40% improved and 10% show no response to colposuspension.
>
> Deterioration of continence after the first few weeks may be due to urinary tract infection, progressive loss of urethral tone with age or (rarely) failure of the surgical technique: if this is suspected, a retrograde vaginourethrogram should be performed.

OPERATIVE TECHNIQUE 15.2

Cystourethropexy

PREPARATION AND POSITIONING

No pre-anaesthetic preparation is required. Clipping: the patient is clipped to include the perineum and abdomen. Place a purse-string suture in the anus. Place a catheter (6–12 Fr) in the urethra and connect to a closed collection system (optional). For this technique, the author prefers a stiff plastic catheter. The patient is placed in dorsal recumbency with hindlimbs relaxed (frog-leg position).

ASSISTANT

Yes.

EQUIPMENT EXTRAS

Abdominal retractor (e.g. Balfour or Gosset).

SURGICAL TECHNIQUE

Use a four-quadrant draping to exclude the vulva from the surgical field.

1 Make a caudal midline laparotomy, extending from the pubic brim cranially to the umbilicus.

2 Place a stay suture in the cranial pole of the bladder.

3 Perform blunt dissection to the left and right of the midline along the ventral aspect of the rectus sheath to identify the prepubic tendon.

4 Identify the internal pudendal vessels as they emerge from caudal to the tendons.

5 Use blunt digital dissection caudal and ventral to the bladder neck between the urethra and pubis. This dissection is into the retroperitioneal space.

6 Identify the bladder neck and urethra.

7 Preplace a suture of 3 or 3.5 metric (2/0 or 0 USP) monofilament nylon or polypropylene caudal to the prepubic tendon on one side, entering the abdomen. Pass the needle transversely, including a partial thickness bite of the ventral urethral wall. The suture is then brought out of the abdomen caudal to the opposite prepubic tendon. Clip the suture and place a second suture 5 mm cranial to the first. ➔

→ **OPERATIVE TECHNIQUE 15.2 CONTINUED**

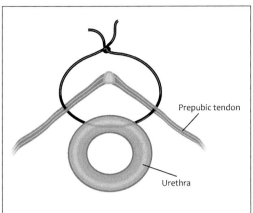

Cross-section showing a urethropexy suture (ventral is to the top and dorsal to the bottom of the image).

Prepubic tendon

Urethra

8   Pull up on the sutures before tying whilst an unscrubbed assistant slides the urethral catheter (if placed) to ensure it is not included in the sutures and that the urethral lumen is not compromised.

9   Tie the urethropexy sutures and close the remainder of the laparotomy routinely.

10   The catheter (if placed) is removed at the end of surgery.

POSTOPERATIVE MANAGEMENT AND COMPLICATIONS

Routine postoperative analgesia is required (typically opiates for 24 hours and NSAIDs for 7 days). Perioperative antibiotics are given and continued postoperatively for 10 days (e.g. clavulanate-potentiated amoxicillin).

A minority of bitches have postoperative dysuria. Most commonly this is believed to be due to dyssynergia; if it does not respond to appropriate analgesia, diazepam may be useful (5–15 mg per animal by mouth, three times daily, given 10 minutes before exercise). In a small minority, dysuria persists and a retrograde vaginourethrogram is recommended to ensure that urethral obstruction is not present. If it is not, an indwelling urethral catheter is placed and maintained for 5 days.

Strict exercise restriction is required for 4 weeks after surgery to allow firm adhesions to develop around the urethropexy sutures: short lead walks only are given, with avoidance of stair climbing and jumping.

Although some animals show an immediate improvement, the owners should be advised that the effects of this surgery on continence are uncertain for the first 4–6 weeks: some bitches remain incontinent initially and improve after the first few weeks; others are improved initially but begin to leak urine as postoperative swelling reduces. In the long term, 50% of bitches are cured, 40% improved and 10% show no response to urethropexy.

Deterioration of continence after the first few weeks may be due to urinary tract infection, progressive loss of urethral tone with age or (rarely) failure of the surgical technique: if this is suspected, a retrograde vaginourethrogram should be performed.

OPERATIVE TECHNIQUE 15.3

Prostatopexy

PREPARATION AND POSITIONING

No pre-anaesthetic preparation is required. Clipping: the patient is clipped to include the perineum and abdomen. Place a catheter (6–12 Fr) in the urethra and connect to a closed collection system. For this surgery, the author prefers a stiff plastic catheter. The prepuce can be retracted and fixed with a towel clip to one side so that is excluded from the surgical field. The patient is placed in dorsal recumbency with hindlimbs relaxed (frog-leg position).

ASSISTANT

Ideally.

→ **OPERATIVE TECHNIQUE 15.3 CONTINUED**

EQUIPMENT EXTRAS

Abdominal retractor (e.g. Balfour or Gosset).

SURGICAL TECHNIQUE

Use a four-quadrant draping to exclude the prepuce from the surgical field.

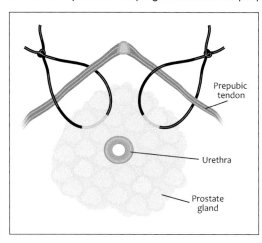

Suture placement in prostatopexy (for clarity, only one suture is shown on each side) (ventral is to the top and dorsal to the bottom of the image).

1   Make a parapreputial approach through the skin and subcutaneous tissues, ligating the preputial blood vessels as required.

2   Use a midline approach into the caudal abdomen.

3   Perform blunt subcutaneous dissection ventral to the rectus sheath on either side of the midline to identify the prepubic tendon and the external pudendal vessels.

4   Bluntly dissect into the retroperitoneal space ventral to the body wall and pubis.

5   Place a stay suture into the cranial pole of the bladder.

6   Identify the prostate gland by palpation from the bladder whilst applying cranial traction on the stay suture.

7   Place the first suture using 3.5 metric (0 USP) monofilament nylon or polypropylene on a taper-cut needle. The needle is passed behind the prepubic tendon, medial to the internal pudendal blood vessels, and into the retroperitoneal space. The needle is re-grasped and then a substantial bite of the prostatic parenchyma is taken, passing craniocaudally. The needle is then passed out from the abdomen immediately cranial to the prepubic tendon, forming a loop around the tendon and through the prostate gland. Clip the suture with haemostats. Two such sutures are placed on each side.

8   Pull up on the sutures and check that the urethra is not compressed against the pubis.

9   Close the abdomen routinely.

10   The catheter is removed at the end of surgery.

POSTOPERATIVE MANAGEMENT AND COMPLICATIONS

Routine postoperative analgesia is required (typically opiates for 24 hours and NSAIDs for 7 days). Perioperative antibiotics are given and continued postoperatively for 10 days (e.g. clavulanate-potentiated amoxicillin).

A minority of dogs have postoperative dysuria. Most commonly this is believed to be due to dysynergia; if it does not respond to appropriate analgesia, diazepam may be useful (5–15 mg per animal by mouth, three times daily, given 10 minutes before exercise). In a small minority, dysuria persists and a retrograde urethrogram is recommended to ensure that urethral obstruction is not present. If it is not, an indwelling urethral catheter is placed and maintained for 5 days.

Strict exercise restriction is required for 4 weeks after surgery to allow firm adhesions to develop around the prostatopexy sutures: short lead walks only are given, with avoidance of stair climbing and jumping.

Although some animals show an immediate improvement, the owners should be advised that the effects of this surgery on continence are uncertain for the first 4–6 weeks.

Deterioration of continence after the first few weeks may be due to urinary tract infection, progressive loss of urethral tone with age or (rarely) failure of the surgical technique: if this is suspected, a retrograde urethrogram should be performed.

OPERATIVE TECHNIQUE 15.4

Vas deferensopexy

PREPARATION AND POSITIONING

No pre-anaesthetic preparation is required. Clipping: the patient is clipped to include the perineum and abdomen. The prepuce can be retracted and fixed with a towel clip to one side so that is excluded from the surgical field. The patient is placed in dorsal recumbency with hindlimbs relaxed (frog-leg position).

EQUIPMENT EXTRAS

Abdominal retractor (e.g. Gosset).

ASSISTANT

Not necessary.

SURGICAL TECHNIQUE

Use a four-quadrant draping to exclude the prepuce from the surgical field.

1   Make a parapreputial approach through the skin and subcutaneous tissues, ligating the preputial blood vessels as required.

2   Use a midline approach into the caudal abdomen.

3   Place a stay suture into the cranial pole of the bladder.

4   Apply cranial traction to expose the prostate gland and identify the paired vasa deferentia emerging from the cranial aspect of the prostate gland.

5   Transect each vas as it leaves the abdomen at the inguinal ring. Place a haemostat on the cut end to identify it.

6   Use blunt dissection with a curved haemostat to create a short tunnel beneath the peritoneum and internal abdominal oblique muscle cranial to the pubic brim on each side, midway between the laparotomy incision and the sublumbar fossa.

7   Draw each vas deferens through the tunnel and suture it to itself, creating a loop through the tunnel and creating tension in the vas to bring the prostate gland into the abdomen.

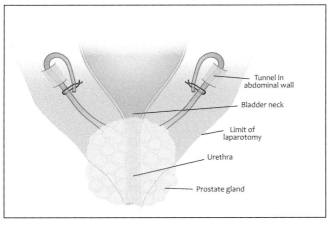

Ventral view of vas deferensopexy (cranial is to the top and caudal to the bottom of the image).

Tunnel in abdominal wall

Bladder neck

Limit of laparotomy

Urethra

Prostate gland

8   Close the abdomen routinely.

POSTOPERATIVE MANAGEMENT AND COMPLICATIONS

Compared with prostatopexy, this technique appears less likely to create a permanent change in the position of the prostate gland, although neither technique has been subject to long-term follow-up studies. Postoperative care and complications are the same as for prostatopexy (see Operative Technique 15.3).

OPERATIVE TECHNIQUE 15.5

Urethral submucosal collagen injection

PREPARATION AND POSITIONING

No pre-anaesthetic preparation is required. Clip the perineum. The animal can be positioned in lateral or dorsal recumbency.

EQUIPMENT EXTRAS

Cystoscope with bespoke injection apparatus and needle.

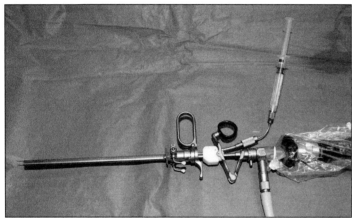

Injection apparatus for urethral collagen injection.

Bulking agent for injection: most commonly collagen suspension, a volume of 3–10 ml should be available.
Note: The technique is possible without the bespoke apparatus, which is only suitable for medium and large bitches because of its diameter, but this is significantly more cumbersome. It is not described here.

SURGICAL TECHNIQUE

1   Complete urethrocystoscopy as normal to rule out other abnormalities. Empty the bladder of urine and flush if necessary to allow excellent visualization.

2   Pass the scope inside its sheath. With the injection apparatus attached, pass it into the urethra and identify the position of the bladder neck. Withdraw 1 cm into the urethra.

3   Extend the needle from the sheath and through the urethral mucosa until the bevel is covered.

4   Inject bulking agent at this depth (submucosal): some leakage may occur alongside the needle. A discrete bulge will form (unless the needle is too deeply inserted). Inject to give a bulge that extends one-third of the diameter of the urethra. A volume of 0.5–1 ml is typically used.

5   At the same level, make two further injections around the circumference of the urethra. The aim is to place three bulges of similar size evenly distributed around the urethra at the same point, which make contact in the centre of the lumen. If this is not achieved, withdraw and repeat 1 cm caudally.

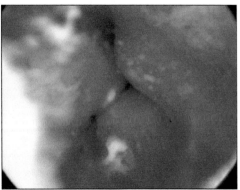

Result of submucosal injection in the urethra. This urethroscopic image shows the urethra closed by three submucosal mounds of collagen.

➜ **OPERATIVE TECHNIQUE 15.5 CONTINUED**

POSTOPERATIVE MANAGEMENT AND COMPLICATIONS

Urinary tract infection is a complication after any urethroscopic manipulation, and postoperative antibiotics (such as clavulanate-potentiated amoxicillin) are provided for 10 days postoperatively. The requirement for analgesia appears to be minimal.

Postoperative dysuria is a possible complication, due to dyssynergia, excessive occlusion by the bulking agent or post-injection swelling, but appears to be rare. After this type of manipulation, it may be several weeks before the benefits of the technique on management of incontinence are clear. The prognosis after this technique is that around half of treated bitches are continent and most of the remainder are improved. If no response is seen, the technique can be repeated.

In most bitches, deterioration in continence is observed after 9–12 months and the technique can then be repeated.

OPERATIVE TECHNIQUE 15.6

Ureteroneocystotomy

PREPARATION AND POSITIONING

No pre-anaesthetic preparation is required. Clipping: the patient is clipped to include the perineum and abdomen. Place a purse-string suture in the rectum. The patient is placed in dorsal recumbency with hindlimbs relaxed (frog-leg position).

ASSISTANT

Yes.

EQUIPMENT EXTRAS

Abdominal retractor (e.g. Gosset) in addition to general pack and fine instruments; magnification is strongly recommended; urinary catheters in sizes 4–10 Fr should be available; fine atraumatic suction tip; sterile cotton buds (Q-tips®).

SURGICAL TECHNIQUE

Use a four-quadrant draping to exclude the vulva from the surgical field.

1 Make a caudal midline laparotomy, extending from the pubic brim cranially to the umbilicus.

2 Place a stay suture in the cranial pole of the bladder.

3 Place an abdominal retractor.

4 Isolate the bladder with laparotomy swabs.

5 Perform a ventral midline cystotomy extending from the bladder neck cranially for 2–4 cm.

6 Place a small self-retaining retractor (eyelid speculum) or stay sutures in the edges of the cystotomy to expose the trigone.

7 Identify the normal ureteral orifice (if present). It may be helpful to place a catheter in it to define its position.

8 Identify the intramural passage of the ectopic ureter at the level of the trigone. In many instances, this is visible as a submucosal bulge. If it cannot be seen, the surgical options are a mucosal incision in the predicted position to look for the ureter, or extension of the cystotomy into the urethra to allow passage of a catheter from the urethral opening of the ureter (or the same by urethroscopy).

9 Make a 5 mm longitudinal incision through the bladder urothelium and identify the intramural portion of the ureter. Careful blunt dissection may be used to isolate the ureter from the muscle until curved forceps can be placed beneath it. Alternatively, lift the wall of the ureter with forceps and pass a swaged-on suture of 3 metric (2/0 USP) monofilament absorbable suture material beneath it.

10 If the ureter has been isolated, place two strands of 3 metric (2/0 USP) monofilament absorbable suture material beneath it. Tie the distal strand to occlude the ureter. Retain the second as a stay suture to elevate the ureter.

➡

→ **OPERATIVE TECHNIQUE 15.6 CONTINUED**

11 Incise the ureter longitudinally to enter the lumen. The incision should be around 3 mm long, and at this stage pass a catheter up the ureter to identify the lumen. Attempt to pass a catheter distally from the ureterotomy to ensure the ureter has been occluded.

12 Place a series of simple interrupted sutures of fine absorbable material (0.7 metric; 6/0 USP) to appose the ureteric mucosa to the bladder urothelium. Start at the cranial aspect and work along either edge.

13 Before completing the anastomosis, tie the second suture around the ureter 2 mm cranially to the first and divide the ureter between the ligatures, ensuring the ends separate.

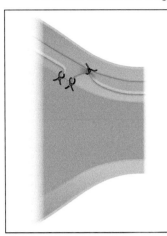

The ureter is stomatized into the bladder at the level of the trigone and ligated just distal to the stoma.

14 Complete the creation of the stoma, closing the bladder urothelium over the knots of the ligatures if possible.

15 If the condition is bilateral, the second ureter can be corrected on the same occasion, unless bladder wall oedema has developed during surgery.

16 Remove the ureteral catheters and close the cystotomy routinely: a continuous appositional pattern is recommended to avoid narrowing at the bladder neck during closure.

Note: A number of variations on the above technique have been described. Some authors recommend that the terminal portion of the ectopic ureter should be dissected from the urethral wall but this has not been shown to improve the outcome. Some authors do not describe double ligation and transection of the ureter, but the present author does this to reduce the possible risk of recanalization. This is more likely to occur if a single ligature is placed and possibly if the ligature is placed using a needle rather than after isolation of the ureter as described above. Another variation is to ligate the distal ureter from outside the dorsal aspect of the bladder with several ligatures. This avoids the suture material being exposed to the bladder lumen and may make ligation more reliable.

POSTOPERATIVE MANAGEMENT AND COMPLICATIONS

Routine postoperative analgesia is required (typically opiates for 24 hours and NSAIDs for 7 days). Perioperative antibiotics are given and continued postoperatively for 10 days (e.g. clavulanate-potentiated amoxicillin). Animals which are operated on in the presence of an active urinary tract infection have a high risk of developing significant postoperative complications due to pyelonephritis and persistent infection; it is important that urinary tract infections are investigated and eliminated before surgery.

A minority of patients have postoperative dysuria. Most commonly this is believed to be due to dyssynergia; if it does not respond to appropriate analgesia, diazepam may be useful (5–15 mg per animal by mouth, three times daily, given 10 minutes before exercise). If dysuria persists an indwelling urethral catheter is placed and maintained for 5 days. This must be placed with great care to avoid disruption of the surgical site (urethroscopy, ultrasonography and/or radiography may be useful). A cystotomy tube is an alternative choice to bypass the surgical site.

Ureteral obstruction is a possible complication but appears to be uncommon after this technique. If bilateral surgery has been performed and obstruction occurs bilaterally, the patient will develop signs of acute renal failure within a few days. Unilateral occlusion, if the contralateral nephroureteric unit is functioning normally, may produce no clinical signs unless massive hydronephrosis becomes apparent in due course.

Although some animals show an immediate improvement, owners should be advised that the effects of this surgery on continence are uncertain for the first 4–6 weeks: some animals remain incontinent initially and improve after the first few weeks; others are improved initially but begin to leak urine as postoperative swelling reduces. In the long term, 50% of patients are cured, 25% improve and 25% show no response to ureteral transplantation.

Persistent incontinence may be due to urinary tract infection, technical failure (recanalization) or concurrent USMI. Recanalization is uncommon but repeated radiography and/or urethroscopy should be used to investigate it. Concurrent USMI is a more common cause of persistent or recurrent incontinence. In intact prepubertal animals, it may improve with sexual maturity. In other instances, medical or surgical management of USMI may be required.

OPERATIVE TECHNIQUE 15.7

Ureteral reimplantation

PREPARATION AND POSITIONING

As for ureteroneocystotomy (see Operative Technique 15.6).

ASSISTANT

Yes.

EQUIPMENT EXTRAS

As for ureteroneocystotomy (see Operative Technique 15.6).

SURGICAL TECHNIQUE

1   Perform steps 1–4 as for ureteroneocystotomy (see Operative Technique 15.6).

2   Identify the extramural ectopic ureter.

3   Ligate the ureter distally. Place a stay suture proximal to the ligature and then transect. Take care not to twist the ureter and avoid traumatic handling of the ureters.

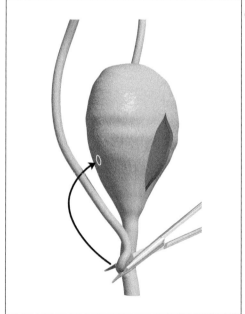

Transection of the distal ureter.
(Redrawn after McLoughlin and Chew, 2000)

4   The ureterocystic anastomosis can be performed through a cystotomy (described here) or through a stab incision in the dorsal wall of the bladder.

5   Perform a cystotomy in the ventral midline. Place small retractors or stay sutures to maintain exposure.

6   Via the cystotomy, make a stab incision in the dorsal bladder wall close to the trigone and pass the tips of mosquito forceps through it.

7   Grasp the stay suture of the transected ureter and bring the ureter into the bladder lumen through the stab incision.

8   Spatulate the ureter by making a short longitudinal incision along its ventral aspect and place a catheter into the lumen to identify it.

→ **OPERATIVE TECHNIQUE 15.7 CONTINUED**

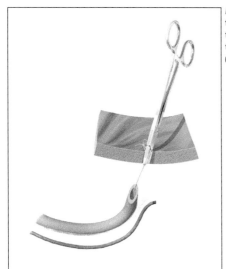

Mosquito forceps are used to create a tunnel through the bladder. The stay suture in the end of the ureter is grasped and the ureter is drawn through the bladder wall into the lumen.
(Redrawn after McLoughlin and Chew, 2000)

9 Use simple interrupted sutures of 0.7 metric (6/0 USP) absorbable suture material to appose the ureteric lining to the bladder urothelium around the stab incision. Use the same material on the dorsal aspect of the bladder to place a partial-thickness tension-relieving suture from the bladder serosa to the outer wall of the ureter.

10 Remove the ureteral catheters and close the cystotomy routinely: a continuous appositional pattern is recommended to avoid narrowing at the bladder neck during closure.

POSTOPERATIVE MANAGEMENT AND COMPLICATIONS

Routine postoperative analgesia is required (typically opiates for 24 hours and NSAIDs for 7 days). Perioperative antibiotics are given and continued postoperatively for 10 days (e.g. clavulanate-potentiated amoxicillin). Animals which are operated on in the presence of an active urinary tract infection have a high risk of developing significant postoperative complications due to pyelonephritis and persistent infection; it is important that urinary tract infection is investigated and eliminated before surgery. Postoperative dysuria is not expected after this surgery.

Ureteral obstruction is a possible complication and appears to be commoner after this technique than after ureteroneocystotomy. If bilateral surgery has been performed and obstruction occurs bilaterally, the patient will develop signs of acute renal failure within a few days. Unilateral occlusion, if the contralateral nephroureteric unit is functioning normally, may produce no clinical signs unless massive hydronephrosis becomes apparent in due course.

Although some animals show an immediate improvement, the owners should be advised that the effects of this surgery on continence are uncertain for the first 4–6 weeks: some animals remain incontinent initially and improve after the first few weeks, others are improved initially but begin to leak urine as postoperative swelling reduces. In the long term, 50% of patients are cured, 25% improve and 25% show no response to ureteral transplantation.

Persistent incontinence may be due to urinary tract infection or concurrent USMI. Concurrent USMI is more common cause of persistent or recurrent incontinence. In intact prepubertal animals, it may improve with sexual maturity. In other instances, medical or surgical management of USMI may be required.

Chapter 16

The male urogenital system

Richard A.S. White

The testicle

Anatomy and physiology

The testes are paired ovoid organs normally located in the scrotum and are responsible for producing both the male hormone (testosterone) and the male gametes (sperm). They contain interstitial (Leydig) cells that secrete and store testosterone and Sertoli cells lining the seminiferous tubules; these produce spermatogenic cells that mature into spermatozoa. The vascular supply to the testicle is via the testicular artery, which is derived from the internal spermatic artery. There is additional supply from the artery of the vas deferens which branches from the urogenital artery. The venous drainage satellites this arrangement, with the addition of the pampiniform plexus surrounding the artery as a cooling mechanism. Lymphatic drainage is via the sublumbar nodes.

Castration

Indications

Surgical castration (orchidectomy, gonadectomy) is one of the most common procedures in small animal practice. The major indications for the procedure include:

- Control of breeding
- Management of perceived behavioural problems (e.g. hypersexuality, aggression, vagrancy)
- Treatment of benign prostatic disease (e.g. hyperplasia (BPH), prostatitis, abscesses and cysts)
- Treatment of testicular disease (e.g. trauma, orchitis, torsion)
- In conjunction with primary herniorrhaphy for the treatment of perineal hernias.

Age

The age at which dogs and cats are castrated tends to attract less controversy than that surrounding ovariectomy and ovariohysterectomy in the bitch. Nevertheless, early (prepubertal) castration may influence development and delays bone maturity, especially in the cat.

Canine castration

See Operative Technique 16.1.

Vasectomy: Elimination of reproductive capacity with retention of male characteristics is sometimes required in 'teasers' or for owners who prefer to avoid orchidectomy for their dog. In such cases, vasectomy can be performed.

1. The patient is prepared as for castration but incisions are made over the scrotal neck to allow localization of the spermatic cords.
2. The common tunics are incised and the ductus deferens retrieved.
3. A section of the ductus is resected and the ends ligated before the tunics and skin are closed.

> **WARNING**
>
> The ejaculate may contain sperm for up to a month after vasectomy and should be assessed microscopically before the dog is used in a stud environment

Testicular prostheses: Silastic prostheses intended to mimic the scrotal testicle following castration are available. The indications and ethics for such a cosmetic procedure are open to considerable debate.

Feline castration

Castration in the cat has fewer surgical options than in the dog.

1. A vertical incision is made through the skin as the testicle is tensed against the surface.
2. The incision is carried through the parietal vaginal tunic, which is then separated from the testicle.
3. The spermatic cord is occluded by ligation or by creating a reef knot between the ductus deferens and the cord.
4. The testicle is resected and the scrotal wound left unsutured.
5. The procedure is repeated for the contralateral testicle through a separate incision.

Cryptorchidism

Aetiology

The failure of normal testicular descent may result from absent or aberrant gubernacular growth. Gubernacular growth and testicular descent are not normally complete until 1–2 months after birth, and failure may be a primary defect or the result of hormonal anomaly. The condition is inherited via an autosomal recessive trait.

A variety of possible anomalies exist:

- Complete failure of testicular differentiation or agenesis of the testicle (rare)
- Reversed outgrowth of the gubernaculum into the abdominal cavity instead of the inguinal canal results in no testicular migration (i.e. the testicle remains in a high abdominal position)
- Mixed intra-abdominal and inguinal outgrowth results in some abdominal migration with the testicle closer to the inguinal canal.

Increasing extra-abdominal growth results in an inguinal or parapenile testicle. The incidence of non-scrotal testicles in the dog ranges from 1 to 10% with smaller breeds (e.g. Poodles, terriers, Pomeranians, Schnauzers, Chihuahuas and Shetland Sheepdogs) at considerably greater risk. The condition may be unilateral or bilateral, although the former is more common; the right to left ratio has been reported as 1.8:1. Abnormal testicular position results in a significantly increased risk of testicular neoplasia (usually Sertoli cell tumours but also seminomas). Intra-abdominal testicles risk the possible development of torsion. Cryptorchidism is less commonly encountered in the cat (2%).

Diagnosis

The absence of the testicle from its normal scrotal position is normally considered to be diagnostic in patients that have reached 10 weeks of age. A testosterone assay may be performed if there is any doubt as to the presence of an intra-abdominal testicle. In the unusual event that remnants are suspected to be present, a chorionic gonadotrophin stimulation test (200–500 IU) should be performed before the testosterone assay.

Management

Cryptorchid relocation: Surgical techniques to mimic the function of the gubernaculum and reposition the testicle in the scrotum are highly questionable for ethical reasons. Similarly, the ethics of administering exogenous hormones are open to debate and, more importantly, the technique is unlikely to be effective.

Cryptorchidectomy: Retained testicles can be difficult to locate and a consistent systematic technique should be employed. Unless diagnostic imaging has definitively identified a high abdominal testicle, the inguinoscrotal region should be explored prior to an abdominal exploration (Figure 16.1). Simple palpation of the inguinal area is often misleadingly negative, and an incision should be made over the inguinal region and the superficial inguinal ring explored for evidence of the spermatic cord, which indicates that the testicle will be found between this point and the scrotum. In the case of abdominal testicles, exploration should begin at the prostate gland to permit the vas deferens to be traced to the testicle. The testicle is usually smaller and softer than a scrotal testicle as a consequence of germinal and interstitial cell hypoplasia. The spermatic vessels are routinely ligated and the testicle resected. Larger testicles are often neoplastic and histopathological examination should always be performed. Laparoscopy can be used to good effect to identify and remove an abdominally retained testicle (see Chapter 3).

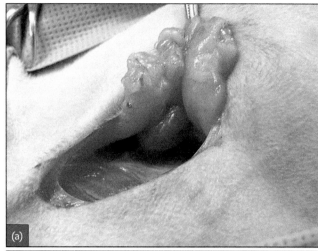
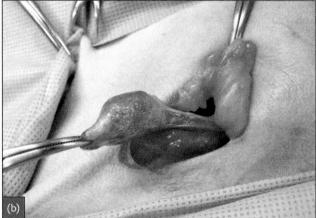

16.1 Incision in the left inguinal region of a cat. (a) The retained left testicle is located under the inguinal fat. (b) Traction on the testicle reveals the spermatic cord and castration is performed routinely. (Courtesy of J. Niles)

> **PRACTICAL TIP**
>
> To locate the retained testicle, identify the vas deferens and follow it caudally towards the inguinal ring

> **WARNING**
>
> Retrieval of abdominal testicles through overly small 'keyhole' laparotomies may be associated with a considerable risk of damage to the prostate gland through inadvertent, non-visualized traction

Testicular tumours

Incidence

Canine testicular tumours occur relatively frequently and represent 5–15% of all male tumours. However, such tumours are rare in cats. Three tumour types predominate in the dog:

- Sertoli cell tumour (SCT)
- Seminoma (SEM)
- Interstitial cell tumour (ICT).

Cryptorchid dogs are at least 10 times more at risk of developing SCT or SEM; this risk factor does not apply to

ICT. About 10% of SCT metastasize to the regional lymph nodes, lung and liver. Metastatic spread is infrequently seen for SEM and very rare for ICT.

Clinical signs and diagnosis

Testicular tumours develop in old dogs (mean age 10 years) although cryptorchid individuals may be affected at an earlier age. The tentative diagnosis of a testicular tumour is based upon the identification of an enlarged testis, with orchitis or trauma as possible differential diagnoses. This enlargement is normally obvious in the fully descended and inguinal testicle but it may be impossible to palpate in cryptorchid individuals with an abdominal testis. Confirmation of the diagnosis by biopsy is rarely performed because it is unlikely to influence the subsequent management of the mass. Where differentiation from orchitis may lead to an attempt to salvage the testicle for breeding purposes, fine-needle aspirates may be helpful in identifying the inflammatory process.

In cases of SCT and some cases of SEM, signs of feminization due to paraneoplastic secretion of oestrogen-like substances may be evident. In some dogs, this paraneoplastic syndrome may be the sole presenting complaint. The 'hyperoestrogenic' or feminizing syndrome includes a range of clinical signs that may occur together or individually.

- Skin changes include a bilaterally symmetrical alopecia affecting particularly the trunk and rear aspects of the thighs, with generalized pruritis in some dogs.
- Gynaecomastia (enlarged mammary glands) and a pendulous prepuce are common. Occasionally, the enlarged mammae may lactate and ectopic nipples may be differentiated from normal sweat glands in the skin.
- The contralateral testicle becomes atrophied and flabby; the prostate gland may be enlarged as a result of squamous metaplasia.
- Characteristically, affected dogs are attractive to other male dogs, have a decreased libido and are lethargic.
- Normochromic, normocytic anaemia develops owing to bone marrow suppression in 15% of cases, and thrombocytopenia may also be present.
- Few clinical signs have been ascribed to ICT and the majority are diagnosed as incidental clinical findings or at post-mortem. However, it is clear that many dogs experience chronic discomfort as the testicle slowly enlarges within its capsule and surgical intervention relieves this.

Sertoli cell tumour: The average age of dogs with SCT is 8–10 years; those with lesions in scrotal testicles are usually older than those with tumours in retained testicles. The incidence of this tumour is greatly increased by cryptorchidism, and 60% of cryptorchid testicular tumours are SCT. The right testicle is at greater risk, reflecting the influence of cryptorchidism. Although SCT develops slowly, the tumour is often quite large and extends beyond the tunic. The surface of the testicle may be irregular and bulging because of cystic changes. Some are oestrogenic, especially if retained. The incidence of malignancy is about 10%, with metastases involving the iliac, sublumbar and inguinal nodes. Distant metastasis to liver, lung, kidney, spleen or pancreas (i.e. predominantly abdominal sites) is less common. There is a possibility of transabdominal or local spread of lesions affecting retained testicles, while the outlook is generally better for scrotal testicles. Oestrogenic signs usually resolve in 1–2

months following castration but the persistence of oestrogenic signs following castration is indicative of functional metastatic deposits. Bone marrow suppression may be prolonged or chronic.

Seminoma: SEM is the least common histological type of testicular tumour and is found in dogs with a mean age of 10 years. Cryptorchidism increases the risk of SEM. These tumours normally cause obvious testicular enlargement and occasionally are oestrogenic. Approximately 5–10% will metastasize, usually regionally to the sublumbar nodes.

Interstitial cell tumour: This is the most common tumour of the descended testicle and tends to affect dogs in an older age group, with a mean age of 11 years. The tumours are usually small: most are less than 1 cm in diameter and rarely disrupt the capsule. Lesions are often light yellow/brown. Up to half are bilateral, and there are often multiple tumours within the same testicle. ICT only rarely results in hormone production *but* one-third to one-half of dogs with perianal tumours have ICT. The prognosis is universally good, with carcinomatous change a rarity.

Management

Cryptorchid dogs should be managed early in life by removal of the retained testicle in order to avoid subsequent tumour development in old age. Surgical removal (castration) is the primary management technique for most testicular tumours. An attempt should be made to examine and, where appropriate, resect the spermatic cord to minimize the risk of residual or metastatic disease. For those dogs presenting with cryptorchid tumours, an inguinal exploration or laparotomy will be necessary to locate and remove the affected testis. Localization of a neoplastic testicle in a non-scrotal site is rarely as complex as that for normal cryptorchid testicles. Exploration of the sublumbar chain of lymph nodes, particularly in the region immediately caudal to the kidney, may be necessary if regional metastasis is suspected.

Prognosis

Surgery is normally highly successful in the management of all tumour types. In the case of secondary abdominal nodal deposits, long-term palliation can often be achieved by nodectomy, and repeat surgery is warranted for recurrent nodal disease. Signs of 'hyperoestrogenism' usually resolve rapidly after surgery; however, if they fail to do so the possibility of a further functional secondary tumour should be considered. Rarely, anaemia may persist after removal of the tumour and can be fatal in those cases where marrow aplasia has been induced.

Orchitis and epididymitis
Aetiology

Testicular infections arise most commonly as a sequel to a retrograde (ascending) infectious process (e.g. prostatitis, urinary tract infection). Infectious agents include the distemper virus, *Escherichia coli*, *Proteus* spp., *Streptococcus* spp., *Staphylococcus* spp., *Mycoplasma* spp., *Nocardia* spp. and, in certain areas of the world, *Brucella canis*. The mode of infection may be through traumatic inoculation (e.g. bite wounds), bacteraemia, venereal, congenital or extension from the peritoneal cavity via the vaginal tunics.

Clinical signs

Swelling of the testicle and epididymis is usually accompanied by scrotal oedema. There is often localized heat with scrotal and/or abdominal pain. Affected patients may lick the scrotum and show reluctance to walk, hindleg stiffness or a straddling gait. In chronic or prolonged disease there is fibrosis and atrophy of the testicle.

Diagnosis

- Confirmation of the diagnosis can be made on cytology and microbiological isolation of fine-needle aspirate samples.
- Semen samples can also be collected by ejaculation for assessment of morphology and function, although this is likely to be uncomfortable for the patient.
- Urine samples should be recovered by cystocentesis for analysis and culture.
- Ultrasound examination of the testicle will confirm the cellulitis and may be useful in identifying discrete collections of pus from which aspirates can be taken. Concurrent prostatic infection is common and should also be assessed by ultrasonography.

Incisional biopsy: Incisional biopsy is occasionally indicated in chronic cases of orchitis that require a histological assessment of infertility.

1. Expose the testicle via a prescrotal incision and incise the tunics to allow access to the parenchyma.
2. Pre-place several fine (0.7 or 1 metric; 6/0 or 5/0 USP) absorbable sutures through the tunic into the parenchyma of the testicle.
3. Remove a thin incisional sample with a scalpel and tie the sutures to pre-empt haematoma formation in the wound that might interfere with any residual sperm production.
4. Repair the tunic and close the skin incision.
5. Patients should be carefully monitored for subsequent testicular swelling.

> **WARNING**
>
> The procedure should only be considered in dogs with an abnormal sperm count because the development of post-biopsy haematoma within the tunic may itself lead to significant damage to the testicle's spermatogenic potential

Treatment

The treatment of choice is normally castration, unless the dog is to be salvaged with intact breeding function. Medical management should be directed towards establishing the identity of the causal organism and its antibiotic sensitivity. Antibiotic selection is based on culture and a bactericidal agent should be used.

Opioids and non-steroidal anti-inflammatory drugs (NSAIDs) can be combined with local ice packing to alleviate pain and discomfort. In cases of obvious abscessation that can be detected on ultrasonography, aspiration or surgical drainage should be performed at an early stage if any fertility is to be salvaged.

Prognosis

In cases that are medically managed, the sperm count should be regularly monitored and may eventually recover. However, the breeding potential is poor in bilaterally affected cases.

Brucellosis
Aetiology and epidemiology

Canine brucellosis is caused by the Gram-negative coccobacillus *Brucella canis* and was first reported in 1966 in the USA, where it is now widespread. Cases have also been reported in Central and South America, Japan and central Europe. The disease affects both female and male dogs, and natural infection can also occur in humans, although the cat is relatively resistant. Serological evidence of exposure to the organism has been found in 1–6% of the canine population in the USA. It is the most frequent cause of abortion in dogs in the USA and represents a significant problem in some breeding kennels. The mode of transmission is via mucous membranes, through:

- Ingestion or oral contact with aborted fetal or placental tissue, vaginal discharge, female genitalia, mammary gland secretions or urine
- Venereal transmission (semen, prostatic fluid)
- Congenital transmission.

Clinical signs

Affected dogs may show epididymitis, orchitis or prostatitis – these sites are normally abundant sources of the bacterium. There may be scrotal and testicular swelling with moist scrotal dermatitis due to excessive licking in response to pain. Cases may also be subclinical without any obvious signs or pyrexia, although a generalized lymph node enlargement is common. Testicular atrophy may develop as a sequel to the acute disease and infertility is an important result in the male. Bacteria may be recovered up to 60 weeks post-infection. In the bitch the most consistent signs of infection are abortion, failure of conception and early embryonic death.

Other forms of the disease: The disease can involve several important non-genital sites, causing discospondylitis, uveitis, generalized lymphadenopathy and prolonged bacteraemia for up to 1–2 years.

Diagnosis

In endemic locations, brucellosis should be considered as part of the differential diagnosis for male infertility, testicular abnormalities and semen anomalies. Culture is the best method of confirmation because chronically infected dogs may be serologically negative but the organism will persist in the prostate gland, epididymis, macrophages and leucocytes. Samples may be recovered from semen, urine, blood, lymph nodes or bone marrow. *Brucella canis* is difficult to grow and successful isolation is dependent on the concentration of the organism submitted in the sample. Serological testing is more rapid but some patients may be negative in the early stages of infection (8–12 weeks). Tests may be non-specific, giving rise to false-positive results.

Treatment

No consistently successful medical treatment regime is known; however, possible options include:

- Quinolone
- Minocycline or doxycycline cycled with quinolone.

Blood should be cultured and serological testing performed 6–8 weeks after treatment is complete. Relapses are common because of the existence of a 'carrier state'. Naturally recovered dogs are immune to reinfection but treated dogs are not solidly immune.

Public health implications

Sporadic cases of human infection have been reported but infections are relatively mild and signs include headaches, fatigue, lymphadenopathy and mild pyrexia. Owners should always be informed of the public health risk and advised to consult their physician.

Control

All positive dogs should be castrated or removed from breeding kennels. Kennels should be disinfected daily and monthly testing of all animals should be performed until three consecutive negative tests are reported.

Testicular trauma

Testicular trauma is remarkably uncommon in small animal species but occasionally penetrating injuries resulting from bite wounds, or crush injuries in road traffic trauma, are encountered. All injuries potentially carry a guarded prognosis: penetrating wounds are likely to permit entry of bacteria leading to the development of orchitis; crush injuries allow leakage of sperm and the development of immune-mediated granulomas that may permanently impair sperm production. There may be haematoma development within the testicle itself or this may extend into a scrotal haematoma. The traumatized testicle is usually enlarged and painful; there is often associated bruising and discoloration of the scrotal tissue and local hypothermia of the tissues. Diagnosis rarely presents a challenge but ultrasonographic examination may be helpful to assess the feasibility of salvage.

In instances of moderate to severe injury, castration represents the most humane and effective management. In breeding dogs, attempts may be made to explore the wound, separately repair minor lacerations in the parietal tunic and tunica albuginea, and provide appropriate analgesia and antibiotic therapy. The prognosis, however, remains uncertain for future breeding potential even after salvage from minor trauma.

Testicular torsion

Torsion of the spermatic cord in the scrotal testicle is a rare event. Affected dogs have rapid and very painful unilateral enlargement of the scrotum. Torsion is more commonly associated with abdominal testicles, particularly those affected by neoplastic change. Patients present with acute abdominal discomfort and may have free fluid in the peritoneal cavity. Diagnosis should be made on surgical exploration for scrotal lesions and on diagnostic imaging followed by exploration in the case of abdominal testicles. Treatment is always resection of the testicle and associated cord.

Inguinoscrotal herniation

Indirect herniation of abdominal contents through the inguinal ring into the scrotal sac (see Chapter 4) is extremely rare in the dog. It has been associated with chondrodystrophism.

Clinical signs

Affected dogs have a unilateral scrotal swelling; reduction of the content may be difficult. Strangulation of the hernia content is common and palpation will cause discomfort in these patients. Differential diagnoses include trauma, neoplastic disease and orchitis.

Management

The hernial sac should be explored via an incision over the inguinal region that permits exploration of the contents' superficial ring. Where the hernia can be reduced, the inguinal ring may be repaired by partial closure of the opening in the aponeurosis of the external abdominal oblique muscle. The vaginal tunic is then closed if breeding potential is to be saved; if not, castration can be performed.

The prostate gland

Anatomy and physiology

The canine prostate gland is a bilobed structure that completely encircles the urethra. It is the sole accessory sex organ of the dog. Prostatic tissue is also found in the cat, partly encircling the urethra. The primary function of the gland is to provide a secretion in the third fraction of the ejaculate that promotes sperm motility and viability. The normal pH of the secretion is 6–6.5; it is rich in zinc, which is antibacterial although its precise role is not known. The secretion also contains a number of proteins including acid phosphatase and canine prostate-specific esterase; unlike in men, these proteins are not accurate indicators of prostate disease. The gland has an abundant vascular supply via the prostatic vessels that branch from the internal pudendal arteries (Figure 16.2). The gland contains secretory epithelial tissue enclosed within a stromal capsule of fibrous, elastic and smooth muscle tissue. The vasa deferentia enter the gland bilaterally before reaching the urethra. The gland lies within the pelvic region until puberty but undergoes ordered glandular hyperplasia in the adolescent dog that causes it to adopt its adult posterior pelvic position. In some chondrodystrophoid dogs the gland is intra-abdominal from birth.

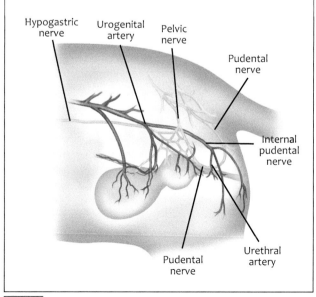

16.2 Vascular supply to the male urogenital tract.

Cytology and biopsy techniques

A variety of techniques are available for the recovery of prostatic samples for microbiological isolation or the identification of neoplastic disease.

Transurethral sampling

This technique has been described for microbiological isolation in cases of suspected prostatitis or prostatic abscessation; however, the increasing availability of ultrasound-guided aspirate sampling has rendered this method largely redundant.

Fine-needle aspiration

Both microbiological and cytological samples may be recovered using fine-needle aspiration. The procedure is most easily performed with the assistance of ultrasound guidance, which allows very accurate location of the biopsy sample.

Biopsy

The recovery of prostatic samples at surgery is very occasionally indicated for confirmation of neoplastic disease. The adult prostate gland is an entirely accessible abdominal organ and exposure for surgical procedures rarely gives rise to difficulty. In almost all cases of prostatic disease that require surgical intervention the gland will occupy a caudal abdominal position with minimal pelvic involvement. Wedge samples can be removed after pre-placement of several interrupted sutures that can be tightened once the sample has been removed to control parenchymal bleeding. Alternatively, core samples can be removed with the aid of a punch biopsy, in which case the urethra should be carefully identified.

Benign prostatic hyperplasia

Glandular hyperplasia occurs in the prostate gland under the influence of both testosterone and oestrogens secreted by the testicle. Testosterone itself is not the active hormone at the prostatic receptor sites but undergoes reduction by 5-alpha-reductase to dihydrotestosterone (DHT). This acts on receptor sites in the prostate gland to promote regulated glandular growth in the juvenile gland.

Juvenile forms

Glandular hyperplasia is a normal physiological process seen in the juvenile prostate gland and rarely gives rise to clinical signs. Occasionally, however, the glandular changes are associated with the development of discrete blood-filled areas or 'haematocysts' within the parenchyma. These can give rise to episodes of apparently spontaneous urethral bleeding that are not associated with urination. There is usually minimal prostatic enlargement in these cases and both palpation and radiography provide little clue as to the cause of the bleeding. Ultrasonography will highlight the discrete blood-filled lesions that can be confirmed by accurate fine-needle aspiration.

Adult forms

In the adult dog a complex form of hyperplasia begins to develop in the prostate gland. These changes also occur under the dominance of DHT, although the circulating levels remain normal. A disordered form of hyperplasia combining elements of both hyperplasia and atrophy begins to emerge. The hyperplastic regions have dilated cystic alveoli that contain eosinophilic material, while the atrophic regions contain an increasing amount of stromal material that interferes with epithelial differentiation and slows the rate of cell loss. The condition is found therefore only in intact dogs and often forms the basis of other prostatic diseases. BPH normally results in abdominal migration of the gland and, in advanced cases, obstruction of the movement of faecal boluses through the pelvic canal. The clinical signs therefore include defecatory tenesmus and constipation. Dysuria is rare, however.

A distinction has been drawn between the *glandular* and *complex* forms of hyperplasia. Glandular changes occur predominantly in young dogs (2–3 years onwards), while the complex form is more commonly associated with the development of cystic changes in the gland in dogs beyond 4 years of age. This histological distinction may not have direct relevance for the clinical syndromes and it may be more useful instead to classify the parenchymal changes seen on gross and ultrasound examination of the prostate gland as *non-cystic, cystic* or *haematocystic*.

Non-cystic BPH: Most cases of BPH are encountered in older dogs and appear to have non-cystic, or at least minimally cystic, changes on prostatic evaluation. They exhibit few complications once appropriate hormonal ablation is instigated.

Cystic BPH: Dogs that do have significant cystic changes in the parenchyma on both gross and ultrasound examination may be resistant to treatment with medical hormonal ablation and more prone to complications resulting from the establishment of ascending infections, resulting in cystic prostatitis. These cases are once again encountered in the older age group.

Haematocystic BPH: Haematocysts are encountered exclusively in young (<4 years) dogs that exhibit fresh urethral bleeding but minimal prostatomegaly. Ultrasonography of the prostate gland will identify small cystic lesions from which fine-needle aspirates will recover frank blood. The incidence of this condition in young dogs is very low but tends to suggest that it may be associated with the glandular, rather than the complex, form of BPH.

Management

The hyperplastic changes encountered in both juvenile and adult dogs can usually be successfully managed by ablation of testosterone. A number of medical options are theoretically available, although it should be emphasized that few are authorized for use in dogs.

- Antiandrogens: Delmadinone acetate (authorized in Europe) reduces testosterone production by supressing interstitial cell function. Osaterone acetate inhibits the effects of an excess of testosterone, competitively prevents the binding of androgens to their prostatic receptors and blocks the transport of testosterone into the prostate gland.
- Luteinizing hormone (LH) inhibitors: Megoestrol acetate inhibits LH release and suppresses 5 alpha reductase activity.
- Luteinizing hormone-releasing hormone (LHRH): Leuprolide reduces LHRH levels, causing a decrease in testosterone secretion.
- 5-Alpha-reductase inhibitor: Finasteride reduces the rate of conversion of testosterone to DHT.

- Oestrogens: These are rarely used for the management of prostatic disease. Because of their potential bone marrow toxicity and the risk of inducing metaplasia their use is NOT recommended.

Although medical management may seem an attractive alternative to surgery in the geriatric patient it should always be borne in mind that most medical options have potential side effects that may complicate the patient's long-term progress more than the perceived risks of a single anaesthestic episode.

Orchidectomy provides a surgical and permanent means of removing testosterone secretion. A rare but severe complication of BPH seen post-orchidectomy is cavitation of the periurethral parenchyma. This presumably represents sudden or severe parenchymal atrophy and leaves the still-enlarged capsule surrounding an unsupported prostatic urethra. Such dogs will be severely incontinent and, in some cases, the urethra itself may perforate and allow urine accumulation within the capsule of the gland.

Cystic hyperplasia, prostatitis and abscessation

Prostatitis

Infection of the prostate gland in dogs is thought to result from an ascending bacterial infection overcoming the normal urethral defence mechanisms and becoming established within the prostatic parenchyma. It seems likely that an underlying cystic parenchymal change must already be present to enable bacteria to become established in the presence of impoverished vascular access. Affected dogs are pyrexic, show caudal abdominal pain and pain on defecation and urination. Rectal examination usually reveals an enlarged and painful gland. Changes consistent with cystic BPH are commonly recognized on ultrasound examination of dogs with prostatitis. Infections may sometimes extend via the vas deferens to cause orchitis. Cytology and microbiological isolation is best performed on samples recovered by fine-needle aspiration of the prostate gland; samples recovered by transurethral washing are less specific but may nevertheless be helpful. Commonly isolated organisms include coliform species and other perineal contaminants.

Abscessation

Abscessation is thought to represent the extension of a pre-existing suppurative parenchymal infection that develops into microabscesses and then coalesces further into larger, loculated abscesses. The factors that are responsible for promoting the progression of a diffuse prostatitis into abscessation are unclear. The most commonly recovered organism is *E. coli*, with *Staphylococcus* spp. and *Proteus* spp. occasionally encountered. Dogs with prostatic abscesses are pyrexic and consistently have signs of caudal abdominal pain on rectal and transabdominal palpation of the prostate gland. The prostate gland is invariably enlarged and will have a 'doughy' feel when palpated. Many dogs will have aneutrophilia (>17 × 10^9 wbc/l) but this is not a consistent feature of the disease. Alkaline phosphatase concentrations may be elevated in some cases. Ultrasonographic imaging will demonstrate the characteristic loculations within the parenchyma that contain slightly echodense purulent fluid. Fine-needle aspiration may be used to recover purulent material but

should be performed with care to avoid the risk of peritonitis following this procedure.

Management

The removal of the underlying prostatic pathology that allows bacterial proliferation is a key step in the successful treatment of prostatic infections. Hormonal strategies to manage the cystic hyperplasia are likely to achieve only a temporary result and castration is undoubtedly the better option because it leads to involution of the glandular hyperplasia and any cystic changes and is an essential prerequisite for long-term resolution. Management of the prostatic change is combined with extended concurrent antibiotic therapy. Antibiotic selection is based, in the first instance, on the likely sensitivity of the organisms seen on smears of the exudate, and may then be modified in the light of the results of culture and sensitivity testing from prostatic aspirates. The selection of an appropriate antibiotic is somewhat controversial because penetration into normal prostatic tissue is impeded by a blood–lipid barrier that restricts the range of suitable antibiotics. In the diseased (i.e. inflamed) gland this barrier is no longer a consideration and selection of the antibiotic can be based primarily on the expected or proven bacterial presence. It is, however, wise to select antibiotics that are known to diffuse well into prostatic tissue, such as enrofloxacin, marbofloxacin and trimethoprim/sulphonamide. Uncastrated dogs may require extended courses (4 weeks) of antibiotic therapy to resolve the condition but the duration of therapy will be considerably shorter in castrated patients.

Chronic parenchymal lesions of the prostate gland, most notably abscesses, are remarkably difficult to resolve consistently by means of medical or surgical therapy. The use of antibiotic therapy, even in conjunction with castration, is notoriously ineffective in resolving prostatic abscessation because of the failure to achieve adequate therapeutic concentrations throughout the prostate gland. Moreover, it fails to provide effective ongoing drainage of the abscess cavity, and effective long-term management can therefore only be achieved through surgical drainage of the abscess cavities (see Operative Technique 16.2). The functions of the omentum that can be surgically exploited have been well documented and include:

- Promotion of angiogenesis that improves local vascularization
- Immune and phagocytic functions that confer an ability to remove bacterial contamination and resolve both acute and chronic infections
- Promotion of localized adhesions.

All of the above properties of the omentum have been shown to be valuable in the management of chronic prostatic parenchymal lesions.

Discrete prostatic cysts

Although separate aetiologies have been proposed for discrete cysts originating from the prostate gland it seems likely that these simply represent abnormal accumulations of prostatic secretions caused by obstruction of the parenchymal ducts. Cysts that tend to be intimately associated with the gland, often with evidence of communication with the prostatic urethra, are usually termed retention cysts; whereas, those that have only minimal structural communication with the prostate gland and do not communicate with the urethra have been classified as paraprostatic.

Both types of cyst are capable of attaining considerable size and are easily distinguished from the diffuse multiple cystic changes which occur within the parenchyma of dogs with BPH. Concurrent prostatic disease is always present and this includes BPH, squamous metaplasia, abscessation or neoplasia. Prostatic cysts are encountered primarily in medium/large-breed dogs, with Boxers being particularly at risk. Signs of urinary dysfunction, including stranguria, dysuria, haematuria and/or incontinence, and a caudal abdominal mass are invariably seen. Imaging will identify a posterior abdominal mass in the region of the bladder, and ultrasonography will confirm its fluid content.

Management

Simple aspiration of the cyst fluid will inevitably result in recurrence of the fluid accumulation. Complete resection of the cyst is feasible and is straightforward for paraprostatic lesions but more complex for the intimately attached retention cysts. Partial resection combined with omentalization is therefore a less extensive surgery with equally reliable results (see Operative Technique 16.3).

Prostatic neoplasia

Prostatic malignancy is an uncommon condition and, although there is no true breed predisposition, medium to large breeds of dog appear to be predisposed. There is some indication that orchidectomy may actually predispose to the disease. This tumour has great potential for secondary spread to the iliac lymph node chain, lumbar vertebrae, pelvic bones and more distant sites. Tumours commonly cause urinary signs (dysuria and haematuria). Metastatic spread to the bones of the pelvis and the lumbar vertebrae will cause lameness, pain and neurological deficits of the hindlimb. Per rectum, prostatic carcinoma will be felt as an irregular, immobile, asymmetrical enlargement of the prostate gland that is invariably painful. The pelvic lymph nodes may be similarly involved.

Management

Canine prostatic carcinoma continues to present serious therapeutic problems. Such tumours do not respond to the hormonal ablation strategies commonly used in humans. Similarly, they show little response to the commonly used cytotoxic drugs. Radiation therapy has been shown to improve survival times but outright cure has not been reported.

Total prostatectomy: Complete transurethral prostatectomy has been described for the management of early-stage lesions. However, this procedure is technically difficult to perform and requires careful dissection of the prostate gland so as to minimize damage to the neurovascular supply of the bladder and urethra. Following total prostatectomy the majority of dogs are incontinent to a varying degree, and this technique is no longer considered to be consistent with a good life quality. There are some reports of extended survival for dogs with transitional cell tumours but no study has yet shown any beneficial impact on survival following prostatectomy for malignant disease.

Subtotal prostatectomy: Removal of segments of the prostatic parenchyma with urethral preservation using a yttrium–aluminium–garnet (YAG) laser and an ultrasonic surgical aspirator (e.g. Cavitron instrument) have been described. These techniques have been put forward as a means of managing benign diseases such as abscesses, but their benefits are, as yet, unproven.

The penis and prepuce

Congenital anomalies

Intersexuality

A paediatric patient that has anatomical elements of both genders present is termed 'intersex'. The condition is mainly encountered in Yorkshire Terriers and Cocker Spaniels. These may be either ostensibly 'male' with penile and preputial remnants, or 'female' with a vulval structure and a clitoris that usually becomes exteriorized. Both forms of intersex have abdominal 'ovarotestes' that are hormonally active beyond puberty. 'Male' patients often present with severe post-voiding urinary incontinence due to the presence of a uterus masculinus attached to the dorsal urethra. This fills with urine during the voiding phase of micturition and then empties as the storage phase begins. The condition can be successfully managed by resection of this structure.

Hypospadias

Failure of fusion of the urogenital folds in the fetus results in the urethra remaining open ventrally. Possible sites for hypospadias include the penile, scrotal and perineal sections of the urethra. There is usually failure of concurrent preputial formation and a bipartite scrotum. The condition is especially associated with the English Bulldog. Depending on the site of the lesion, puppies may present with urine-soaked skin around the urethral orifice or have no clinical signs. Reconstruction may be practical for small lesions that permit dissection of the urethral mucosa and closure of the tubular structure. More extensive lesions may be better managed by urethrostomy, particularly if there is extensive preputial involvement.

Preputial anomalies

Preputial agenesis

Incomplete development of the prepuce leaves varying lengths of the distal penis unprotected. Reconstruction using skin flaps and extension of the mucosal lining is rarely successful because there is often a concurrent absence of the supporting preputial muscle that is necessary to prevent ingress of debris into the preputial orifice. Penile shortening or amputation with urethrostomy are therefore more feasible options.

Failure of urethropreputial separation

Fusion of the urethral mucosa with the preputial lining prevents normal extrusion of the penis, but otherwise causes few clinical signs. The condition may be managed by resection of the preputial mucosa from the prepuce, followed by reconstruction of the preputial orifice. Care should be taken to ensure that the repair creates an orifice of a diameter that prevents intrusion of foreign material, and that mucosa does not protrude from the orifice.

Failure of ventral closure

Failure of mucocutaneous fusion on the ventral aspect of the prepuce results in penile exposure with varying degrees of devitalization. Small deficits can be managed by primary closure of the preputial mucosa with recruitment of skin flaps. Larger deficits are often complicated by the absence of supporting preputial muscle and reconstruction may simply create a non-functional flaccid 'tube' that permits ingress of debris. Such cases are better managed by amputation and urethrostomy.

Penile trauma

Aetiology

Penile trauma is an unusual injury but may result from:

* Road traffic accidents
* Ballistic impacts
* Bite wounds
* Malicious intervention
* Self-inflicted injuries resulting from hypersexuality.

Clinical signs

Penile trauma and lacerations involving the cavernous tissue often result in severe haemorrhage. More chronic injuries may cause urethral obstruction and dysuria. Crush injuries may result in fracture of the os penis with further laceration of the cavernous tissue and leakage of urine into the periurethral tissues.

Management

Assessment of penile injuries is best undertaken following sedation of the patient and the placement of a tourniquet around the penis to control any bleeding. Superficial lacerations that involve only the mucosa can be managed by digital pressure or by the placement of fine sutures. More extensive wounds that lacerate the cavernous tissue may require closure of the cavernous spaces. Fractures of the os penis may be managed by orthopaedic intervention but with more serious injuries in which there is gross disruption of the cavernous tissue, amputation of the penis (with or without scrotal urethrostomy) is the most practical means of salvage (see Operative Technique 16.4).

Urethral prolapse

Aetiology

Prolapse of the penile urethral mucosa from the urethral orifice is encountered primarily in young brachycephalic dogs after periods of sexual excitement or hypersexuality. The prolapse results from chronic irritation and inflammation of the distal penile urethra that protrudes beyond the orifice as it becomes swollen.

Clinical signs

Affected patients will exhibit persistent attention to the prolapse and continually lick the prepuce and penis. The prolapsed tissue itself is seen as a small red pea-like lesion on the tip of the penis (Figure 16.3a). There may be associated bleeding and the patient may show urinary frequency.

Management

Many patients can be managed conservatively with a combination of sedation and anti-inflammatory drugs; additional management of the underlying hypersexuality is important for future prophylaxis. Where this approach is not successful or the prolapse has become chronic, the mucosa may be reduced under anaesthesia with a urethral catheter *in situ*. A purse-string suture of 0.7–1 metric (6/0–5/0 USP) monofilament material is used to prevent recurrence. In severe cases the protruding mucosa may become devitalized and this necessitates amputation of the prolapsed tissue. Sections of the mucosa are removed and the urethral mucosa repaired in quadrants with simple interrupted absorbable sutures (Figure 16.3b–d). In the English Bulldog, severe cases associated with ventral deviation of the penis and prepuce that predispose to trauma may exceptionally require penile shortening.

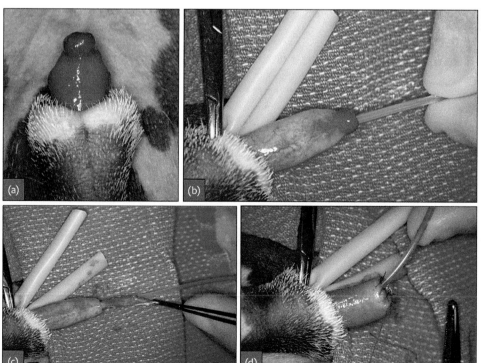

16.3 (a) Urethral prolapse in a young Bulldog. (b) A urethral catheter and Rummel tourniquet (Penrose drain) have been placed. (c) The prolapsed urethral mucosa is resected. (d) The urethral mucosa is sutured to the penile mucosa with simple interrupted absorbable sutures.

Penile tumours

Incidence

The penis is rarely affected by neoplasia. In the dog, the most common histological type is the squamous cell carcinoma, while papillomas are occasionally encountered. In areas of the world where transmissible venereal tumours are endemic, the tumour may occur with considerable frequency. Penile tumours are extremely rare in the cat.

Squamous cell carcinoma

Carcinoma is occasionally encountered affecting the glans of old dogs. It often presents as indurating ulceration of the glans and may be difficult to discern in the early stages. Lesions are usually slow growing and slow to metastasize to the inguinal nodes.

Clinical presentation: The clinical signs associated with penile carcinoma are frequently vague and have a chronic and insidious onset. Preputial discharge, preputial bleeding, licking around the prepuce, dysuria and blood associated with urination are often seen. Phimosis or paraphimosis are occasional complications. Dysuria or stranguria may be present in some dogs.

Diagnosis: The penis should be fully extruded from the sheath for adequate examination. Inspection of the penis may reveal irregular indurated areas of ulceration involving the glans. Cytological samples can be made from impression smears of the affected areas on microscope slides. The regional (superficial inguinal) nodes should be palpated and the abdomen radiographed for signs of metastatic disease.

Surgery and reconstruction: Penile amputation is the treatment of choice for early-stage carcinoma. The penis may be amputated cranially through its bulb, in which case the sheath is left intact. For more advanced lesions the penis is more radically removed at a point just cranial to the scrotum. For the latter procedure a scrotal urethrostomy is indicated together with castration, and scrotal and preputial ablation.

Prognosis: The outlook for early-stage lesions managed surgically is often favourable, although local recurrence and regional metastasis are possible complications.

Transmissible venereal tumour

In certain areas of the world, principally the tropics and subtropics including the Mediterranean countries, the Caribbean and the south-east USA, transmissible venereal tumour (TVT) is endemic, and it may be the most common canine tumour in those countries. In the UK it is seen occasionally in imported dogs. TVT is an unusual tumour transmitted from dog to dog by the transplantation of neoplastic cells, primarily during coitus. The chromosomal number in TVT cells is invariably 59 ± 5, giving rise to the theory that the tumour arose from a single cell transformation and that all present cases are clones of that original neoplasm. The possible aetiological role of a virus has also been examined but never substantiated.

Clinical presentation: TVT is readily transmitted at coitus and therefore commonly affects young adult dogs. The tumour presents as an erythematous vegetative lesion on the mucous membranes of the external genitalia. A serosanguineous or haemorrhagic discharge is usually present and this may be mistaken for oestrus, vaginitis, urethritis or prostatitis. The tumour may also affect the oral and nasal mucosae and a cutaneous form is also recognized. In most cases, the tumour undergoes spontaneous remission but, in a few, metastases develop in the local lymph nodes and more distant sites.

Diagnosis: The diagnosis is based upon clinical history and the appearance of the tumour, and may be confirmed histologically. Chromosomal counts can be helpful in difficult cases.

Treatment: The majority of cases regress spontaneously but some persist and metastasize. Electrosurgical excision may be used to resect the tumour but recurrence is common. This tumour is very radiosensitive and relatively low doses of radiation are curative. TVT is also extremely chemosensitive and this modality is the most practical treatment in most cases. Vincristine sulphate (0.5 mg/m^2) should be administered weekly for 4–6 weeks. Complete regression of the primary tumour and the secondary deposits can be expected.

Prognosis: Many cases of TVT regress spontaneously. The response to chemotherapy is usually excellent even for those that develop secondary deposits.

Penile prolapse

Prolapse of the penis from the prepuce is an unusual condition that should be distinguished from other causes of penile protrusion (i.e. paraphimosis and priapism; see the BSAVA Manual of Canine and Feline Reproduction and Neonatology). The condition occurs almost exclusively as a post-castration event and can be seen as soon as a few days after surgery. The underlying aetiology is not clear but may reflect failure of preputial muscle function. Exogenous testosterone replacement therapy is not effective.

Clinical signs

Affected dogs present with repeated protrusion of the penis beyond the preputial orifice. The prolapsed tissue rapidly dries and becomes devitalized, and paraphimosis due to 'in-rolling' of the preputial hairs is common. Although often initially intermittent, the frequency of prolapse usually increases as the preputial orifice is damaged by each episode.

Management

Reconstructive surgery for the preputial orifice and attempts to advance or elongate the prepuce are rarely successful. Although apparently drastic in the early stages of the condition, penile shortening (see Operative Technique 16.4) represents the most consistently effective means of dealing with prolapse.

Amputation of the penis

Penile resection (see Operative Technique 16.4) is indicated for the management of:

* Neoplasia
* Trauma
* Penile prolapse
* Severe urethral prolapse.

Urethrostomy procedures

The creation of a permanent stoma for urinary diversion through the urethral wall is occasionally indicated in the management of the following conditions:

- Stenosis of the urethra (resulting from iatrogenic intervention, recurrent urolithiasis or trauma)
- Prophylaxis of uroliths
- Neoplasia involving the urethra (e.g. carcinoma of penis)
- Severe penile trauma.

Urethrostomy sites in the dog

Although it is possible to create stomas in the urethra in several sites, most have potential complications.

Base of os penis

The 'low' site is unsuitable for a permanent stoma because there is a considerable risk of scarring and stenosis due to its narrow diameter; additionally the urine flow is less than ideal.

Scrotal

This is the optimal site because the urethra is superficial, the risk of stenosis is less here, the urethra is a reasonable diameter and urine does not flow over the surrounding tissues (see Operative Technique 16.5).

Perineal

This is undesirable because the urethra is deep at this point; hence there is a considerable risk of stenosis and urine flow over the perineum.

Prepubic

This should be regarded as a salvage site if all others have failed.

Urethrostomy sites in the cat

Perineal

See Operative Technique 16.6. The major site for urethrostomy in the cat is in the perineal urethra as it curves over the ischial brim. In the majority of cases, this site adequately addresses obstructive lesions in the distal (penile) urethra.

Prepubic

See Operative Technique 16.7. In a few rare cases, the obstructive lesion is found cranial to the perineal urethra and creating the stoma in a prepubic location is an option. The urethra at this point is in fact an extension of the bladder neck and patients can be expected to remain perfectly continent.

References and further reading

England G and von Heimendahl A (2010) *BSAVA Manual of Canine and Feline Reproduction and Neonatology, 2nd edn*. BSAVA Publications, Gloucester

Kirsch JA, Hauptman JG and Walshaw R (2002) A urethropexy technique for surgical treatment of urethral prolapse in the male dog. *Journal of the American Animal Hospital Association* **38**, 381–384

Newton JD and Smeak DD (1996) Simple continuous closure of canine scrotal urethrostomy. *Journal of the American Animal Hospital Association* **32**, 531–534

Shin SJ and Carmichael L (1999) Canine brucellosis caused by *Brucella canis*. In: *Recent Advances in Canine Infectious Diseases*, ed. L Carmichael. IVIS, Ithaca

Williams JM and Moores A (2009) *BSAVA Manual of Canine and Feline Wound Management and Reconstruction*. BSAVA Publications, Gloucester

---

OPERATIVE TECHNIQUE 16.1

Canine castration

PREPARATION AND POSITIONING

Castration in the dog can be performed with a variety of modifications but in all cases the scrotal and inguinal area is clipped and aseptically prepared. The patient is positioned in dorsal recumbency.

ASSISTANT

Optional but rarely required.

ANTIBIOTIC AND ANALGESIA REGIMES

Elective castration is considered to be a clean procedure and as such does not necessitate either peri- or postoperative antibiotic therapy. A combination of an opioid with non-steroidal anti-inflammatory drugs (NSAIDs) should be considered.

EQUIPMENT EXTRAS

Electrocautery is useful.

→ **OPERATIVE TECHNIQUE 16.1 CONTINUED**

Approach: prescrotal incision *versus* scrotal ablation

> **WARNING**
>
> Prescrotal incisions are undoubtedly quicker to perform and to close. However, they increase the possibility of complications such as haematoma and seroma development in the scrotal dead space. Although more time-consuming, ablation of the scrotum reduces dead space risks, particularly in dogs with a pendulous scrotum, larger dogs and patients with scrotal trauma

Prescrotal incision

Make a short skin incision in the midline immediately in front of the scrotum and push one testicle forward into the incision. The subcutaneous tissue and spermatic fascia are incised to expose the tunics. Closure is by repair of these layers.

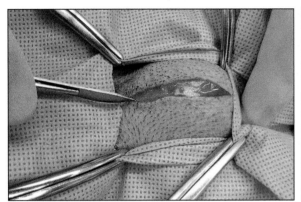
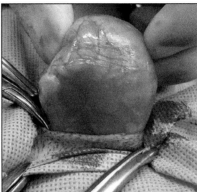

Scrotal ablation

Make two curvilinear incisions through the skin around the base of the scrotum. Haemostasis of scrotal vessels in the posterior midline is best achieved with electrocautery.

> **PRACTICAL TIP**
>
> The incisions should be positioned to ensure that once the scrotum is removed, sufficient skin remains to achieve closure without tension

The periscrotal fascia is repaired to reduce dead space prior to skin closure.

Surgical manipulations: 'closed' tunics

1 Once it has been exposed, grasp the parietal vaginal tunic and resect the spermatic fascia and scrotal ligament close to the testicle.

2 Withdraw the testicle from the scrotum and remove any adherent adipose tissue from the tunics by brushing with a surgical swab.

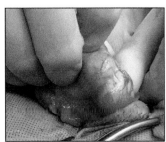
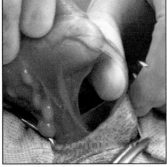
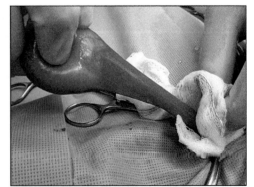

The testicle is exteriorized by incising the spermatic fascia but leaving the parietal vaginal tunic intact.

The testicle is further exteriorized by breaking the dense connective tissue between the tail of the epididymis and the scrotal wall (scrotal ligament).

Adherent adipose tissue is removed from the parietal tunic by brushing from the testicle downwards with a moist surgical swab.

→ **OPERATIVE TECHNIQUE 16.1 CONTINUED**

3 The point at which the spermatic cord is to be ligated may be crushed using artery forceps prior to the placement of a transfixing figure-of-eight ligature through the non-vascular component of the cord.

4 Sever the cord immediately above the ligature and lower the resected cord towards the inguinal canal, checking for any bleeding as the tension in the cord is released.

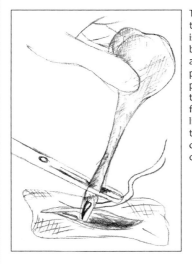
The point at which the spermatic cord is to be ligated may be crushed in artery forceps prior to the placement of a transfixing figure-of-eight ligature through the non-vascular component of the cord.

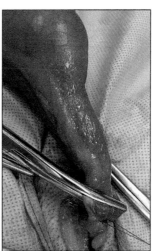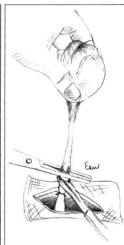
Sever the cord immediately above the ligature.

Surgical manipulations: 'open' tunics

1 Grasp and incise the parietal vaginal tunic to allow retraction of the testicle from within the tunics. Avoid incision of the tunica albuginea, to prevent bleeding from the testicular parenchyma itself.

2 Separate the spermatic cord from the tunics and cremaster muscle and ligate with a single transfixing ligature. Ligate the cremaster muscle and tunics separately alongside or over the cord.

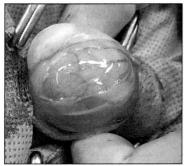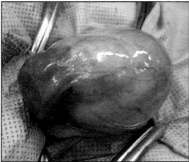
Grasp and incise the parietal vaginal tunic to allow retraction of the testicle from within the tunics.

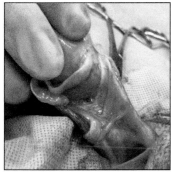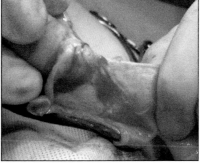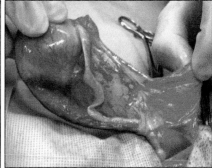
Separate the spermatic cord from the tunics and cremaster muscle.

→ **OPERATIVE TECHNIQUE 16.1 CONTINUED**

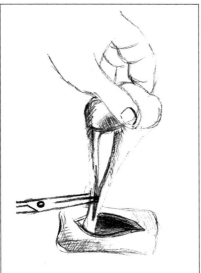

Ligate the cremaster muscle and tunics separately; transect immediately above the ligature.

Try not to resect the spermatic cord too far away from the testicle. In the event that the ligature slips off the cord it will retract through the inguinal canal towards the abdominal cavity. Leaving the cord long will increase the chances of being able to locate the bleeding end before it disappears into the abdomen. Do ensure, however, that all testicular tissue is removed!

Wound closure

Subcutaneous and skin closure is routine.

POSTOPERATIVE MANAGEMENT

Antibiotic therapy should not be regarded as a routine postoperative requirement, unless:

- Contamination occurs during surgery
- The procedure becomes prolonged for any reason
- The surgeon is inexperienced.

OPERATIVE TECHNIQUE 16.2

Prostatic abscess management (intracapsular prostatic omentalization)

POSITIONING

Dorsal recumbency.

ASSISTANT

Very helpful in all prostatic surgeries.

→ **OPERATIVE TECHNIQUE 16.2 CONTINUED**

- Dogs should receive perioperative broad-spectrum antibiotic therapy.
- In cases requiring omentalization this does not need to be extended into the postoperative period unless complications (e.g. major contamination of the abdominal cavity during/prior to surgery) are encountered.
- Appropriate analgesia should include an opioid for 24 hours. NSAIDs should be administered for a further 4–5 days.

EQUIPMENT EXTRAS

Electrocautery is useful. Gelpi and abdominal retractors; large artery forceps; umbilical tape.

SURGICAL TECHNIQUE

Approach

1 A caudal coeliotomy extending from the umbilicus to expose the pubic brim is normally adequate to permit access.

2 Pack off the gland from the remainder of the abdomen with moist laparotomy towels and gently elevate it from the abdomen by placing umbilical tape or a Penrose drain beneath it (i.e. around its dorsal aspect).

> **PRACTICAL TIP**
>
> Prior placement of a urethral catheter is always recommended to aid identification of the prostatic urethra during intracapsular procedures

The prostatic vascular supply, hypogastric and pelvic nerves are found on the dorsal aspect of the prostate gland and should be carefully preserved. Exceptions to the normal abdominal location of the prostate gland include cases of neoplastic disease, in which the gland may be fixed within the pelvic canal, and cystic disease, in which the affected portion of the gland may be found in the perineal region, necessitating a dorsolateral perineal approach.

Surgical manipulations

1 Make bilateral stab incisions into the lateral aspects of the prostate gland and remove pus from the abscess cavities by suction to minimize the potential for abdominal contamination.

2 Break down all abscess cavity walls and loculations within the parenchyma by digital exploration.

> **WARNING**
>
> It is important during this procedure to minimize any damage to the prostatic urethra, which should be identified by palpation of the pre-placed urethral catheter

Approximation of the omentum to the prostate gland can normally be achieved without the need for lengthening. In exceptional circumstances the prostatic lesion may be located within the perineal region and lengthening may be considered necessary.

3 Enlarge the stab incisions by resection of the lateral capsular tissue and control any haemorrhage from the capsular wall with electrocautery.

4 Position umbilical tape temporarily around the prostatic urethra within the parenchyma to help elevation of the gland.

5 Irrigate the common abscess cavity with warm saline to reduce the residual purulent debris.

6 Introduce artery or tissue forceps through one capsulectomy wound, under the urethra and exit through the contralateral wound.

7 Draw a leaf of omentum towards the caudal abdomen, grasp it with the forceps, and withdraw it into and through the dorsal abscess cavity.

8 After exiting, pass the omentum back through the ventral cavity and exit it through the original 'entry' capsulectomy wound, resulting in complete periurethral packing.

9 Anchor the tip of the omental leaf to its base with absorbable sutures outside the prostate gland.

→ **OPERATIVE TECHNIQUE 16.2 CONTINUED**

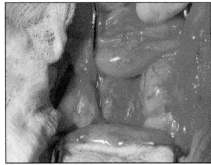

Exposure of the prostate gland via caudal laparotomy.

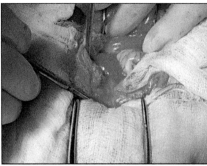

Pus draining from lateral stab incision in prostate gland.

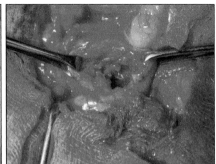

'Window' created in lateral aspect of the prostatic abscess.

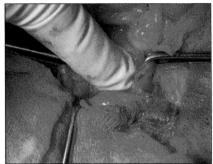

Digital exploration of the abscess cavities.

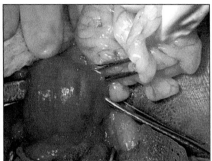

Forceps drawing omentum into ventral abscess cavity.

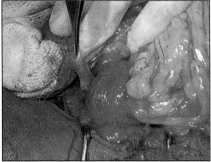

Omentum in ventral abscess cavity before packing into dorsal cavity.

Wound closure

Routine wound closure and castration are performed.

POSTOPERATIVE MANAGEMENT AND COMPLICATIONS

A significant advantage of omentalization drainage techniques for prostatic diseases is that patients can normally be discharged from the hospital within 24 hours of surgery.

- Omentalization is extremely successful in the management of prostatic abscesses. Compared with other drainage techniques, the level of surgical expertise required for successful omentalization is modest and postoperative complication rates are low.
- Abscess recurrence may be encountered if the abscess loculations are not broken down or if insufficient omentum is packed into the abscess cavity. To avoid this complication the surgeon should ensure that adequate lateral capsulectomy resections (normally sufficient to accommodate the easy entry of the forefinger into the abscess cavity) are performed.

OPERATIVE TECHNIQUE 16.3

Partial resection and omentalization for discrete prostatic cysts

POSITIONING

Dorsal recumbency.

ASSISTANT

Very helpful in all prostatic surgeries.

ANTIBIOTIC AND ANALGESIA REGIMES

- Dogs should receive perioperative broad-spectrum antibiotic therapy; this does not need to be extended into the postoperative period unless complications (e.g. major contamination of the abdominal cavity during/prior to surgery) are encountered.
- Appropriate analgesia should include an opioid for 24 hours and NSAIDs should be administered for a further 4–5 days.

EQUIPMENT EXTRAS

Electrocautery is useful. Gelpi and abdominal retractors; large artery forceps; umbilical tape.

SURGICAL TECHNIQUE

Approach

A caudal coeliotomy extending from the umbilicus to the pubic brim should be made initially; however, preparations should be made to extend this cranially should the cyst size dictate this. The cyst is normally easily identified.

Surgical manipulations

1 Exteriorize the cyst as far as possible and pack off from the remainder of the abdominal cavity with moist laparotomy towels.

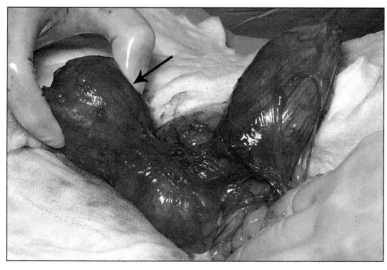

The paraprostatic cyst (arrowed) is exteriorized and the abdomen packed off with swabs.

2 Make a single stab incision through the cyst wall and use suction to remove its contents.

3 Resect the majority of the cyst wall, avoiding extensive dissection of the cyst in the region of the bladder neck and prostate gland so as to minimize the risk of damaging the neurovascular structures.

→ **OPERATIVE TECHNIQUE 16.3 CONTINUED**

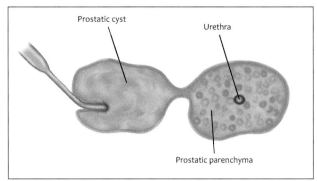

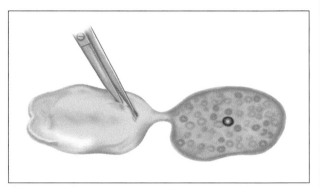

A single stab is made into the cyst and its contents are aspirated.

The majority of the cyst wall is resected.

4 Identify the prostatic urethra during this procedure by means of an indwelling catheter.

5 In some cases communication between the cyst and the urethra will be identified. Any such communication should not be dissected or oversewn.

6 Draw a leaf of omentum into the cyst remnant and secure it into its prostatic base with absorbable suture material, in a mattress pattern.

7 Carefully examine and palpate the prostate gland for any evidence of neoplastic disease that may underlie development of the cyst. Even in the absence of any gross evidence of neoplastic infiltration, an incisional or fine-needle aspirate biopsy should always be performed.

Wound closure

Routine abdominal closure and castration are performed.

POSTOPERATIVE MANAGEMENT AND COMPLICATIONS

Urinary incontinence seen in dogs with prostatic cysts may continue postoperatively owing to anatomical changes in the urethra. Omentalization is extremely successful in the management of discrete prostatic cysts.

OPERATIVE TECHNIQUE 16.4

Canine penile amputation

POSITIONING

Dorsal recumbency.

ASSISTANT

Useful but not essential.

ANTIBIOTIC AND ANALGESIA REGIMES

- Dogs should receive broad-spectrum antibiotic therapy perioperatively.
- Appropriate analgesia should include an opioid for 24 hours and NSAIDs should be administered for a further 4–5 days.

EQUIPMENT EXTRAS

Umbilical tape or Penrose tourniquet; bone cutters; fine needle holders.

→ **OPERATIVE TECHNIQUE 16.4 CONTINUED**

Approach

Extrude the penis and introduce a urethral catheter to permit later identification of the urethra.

Surgical manipulations: rostral amputation

1   Position a tape tourniquet or Penrose drain around the base of the penis, caudal to the bulb, to control bleeding.

2   Incise the mucosa and cavernous tissue circumferentially or, more frequently, in two V shapes to increase the circumference over which the repair can be made.

3   Dissect the cavernous tissue to expose the urethra and os penis.

4   Amputate the os penis with bone cutters and amputate the urethra further rostrally.

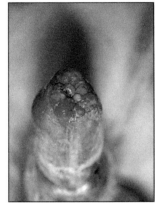 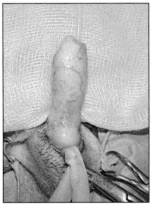 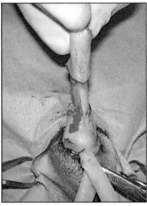 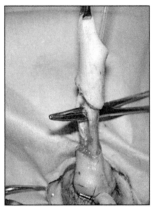

Carcinoma of penile glans.   Extrusion of the penis with tourniquet around the base.   Incision in penile mucosa.   Separation of the urethra from the os penis.

5   Close the cavernous openings with sutures at this point to limit subsequent bleeding.

6   Reflect the urethra back over the exposed cavernous tissue and suture to the incised edge of the mucosa with simple interrupted or continuous sutures.

7   Release the tourniquet and manage any major bleeding with additional sutures or digital pressure. Despite the shortened length of the penis the dog should be able to urinate without preputial pooling.

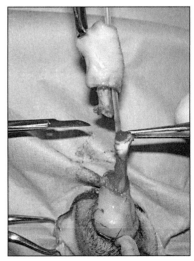 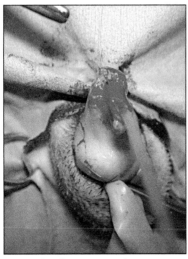 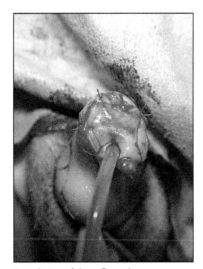

Amputation of the penis, leaving an extended section of urethra.   Oversewing the cavernous tissue to limit bleeding.   Spatulation of the reflected mucosa over the end of the amputated penis.

➜ **OPERATIVE TECHNIQUE 16.4 CONTINUED**

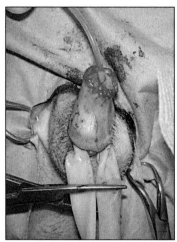

Completed urethral repair.

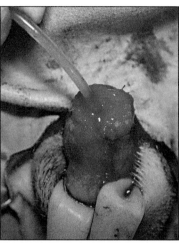

Bleeding following removal of tourniquet.

Surgical manipulations: total amputation

1 Make an approach over the base of the penis immediately cranial to the scrotum.

2 Dissect the penis caudal to the os free of the surrounding tissue. Cross-clamp the penis to limit bleeding and then amputate.

3 Oversew the tunics to close the cavernous tissues.

4 Perform castration, scrotal ablation and scrotal urethrostomy (see Operative Technique 16.5).

Wound closure

Routine closure is performed.

POSTOPERATIVE MANAGEMENT AND COMPLICATIONS

Patients should be monitored to ensure that urination occurs normally during the first 48 hours after surgery. Bleeding from the cavernous sinuses can continue for several days, especially at the end of urination, if the sinuses have not been adequately oversewn during the procedure.

OPERATIVE TECHNIQUE 16.5

Canine scrotal urethrostomy

POSITIONING

Dorsal recumbency. Right-handed surgeons will find it easier to operate from the right side of the patient.

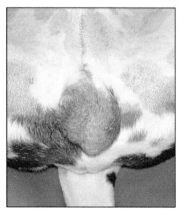

Patient positioned for scrotal urethrostomy.

→ **OPERATIVE TECHNIQUE 16.5 CONTINUED**

ASSISTANT

Unnecessary.

ANTIBIOTIC AND ANALGESIA REGIMES

- Dogs should receive broad-spectrum antibiotic therapy both peri- and postoperatively.
- Appropriate analgesia should include an opioid for 24 hours and NSAIDs should be administered for a further 4–5 days.

EQUIPMENT EXTRAS

Electrocautery is useful; urethral catheter; mini-Gelpi retractors; fine needle holders.

SURGICAL TECHNIQUE

Approach

Castration and scrotal ablation are prerequisites for urethrostomy at this site. Where possible, a urethral catheter should be used to allow the urethra to be located. In cases of urolithiasis, this may not be possible and identification of the urethra may be difficult. The skin is incised in the midline at the most convex point of the scrotal urethra.

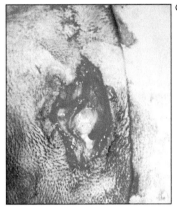

Castration with scrotal ablation.

PRACTICAL TIP

Enough skin should be left on the lateral aspects of the incision so that no tension is placed on the urethrostomy during closure

---

Surgical manipulations

1 Move the retractor penis muscle to one side and incise the urethra (this is usually accompanied by considerable bleeding, which is not easy to control). The urethral incision should be as long as reasonably possible, to increase the potential size of the stoma.

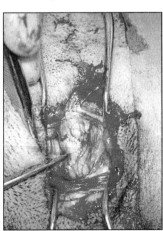

The retractor penis muscle is identified and displaced laterally to expose the urethra.

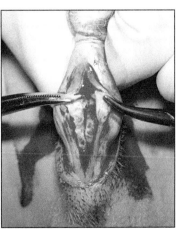

The urethra is incised longitudinally with a No. 11 scalpel blade; the urethral mucosa is identified.

→ **OPERATIVE TECHNIQUE 16.5 CONTINUED**

2   The urethral mucosa is often difficult to identify because of its vascular nature but should be sutured with 0.7–1.5 metric (6/0–4/0 USP) simple interrupted sutures directly to the skin.

WARNING

Failure to achieve accurate coaptation of the mucosa/skin repair may allow urine to leak into the periurethral space, leading to cellulitis and, ultimately, scarring around the stoma site

---

PRACTICAL TIP

Placement of a urethral catheter facilitates identification of the urethra. If a catheter cannot be placed, the incision should be made carefully to avoid damaging the dorsal surface of the urethra

---

WARNING

The urethral incision must be of sufficient length, because, once it has healed, the opening will decrease to approximately one-third to one-half of the original length

---

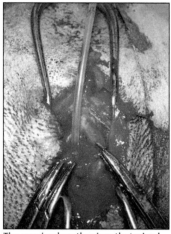

The proximal urethra is catheterized.

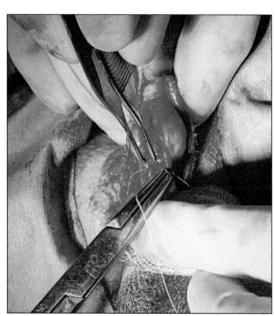

Monofilament, non-absorbable suture material (polypropylene) is used to suture the urethrostomy. A swaged-on taper cut needle should be used to minimize the size of the needle tract. The urethrostomy can be sutured using either a simple interrupted or a simple continuous pattern. A simple continuous pattern results in accurate apposition of the urethral mucosa to the skin and helps to achieve haemostasis. If the cranial aspect of the skin incision extends beyond the urethral incision, it should be closed with simple interrupted sutures. The needle should be driven from the urethral mucosa to the skin for best apposition. Each suture should comprise three tissue bites: the urethral mucosa; a 2–3 mm bite of the fibrous tunica albuginea; and a split-thickness bite of the skin.

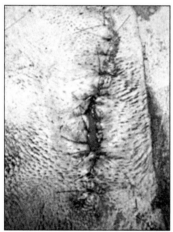

Completed scrotal urethrostomy.

POSTOPERATIVE MANAGEMENT AND COMPLICATIONS

- Micturition-related urethral haemorrhage is a common sequel to the surgery and may cause significant anaemia in a few cases.
- Periurethral haematoma can develop and may lead to urethral obstruction. Excessive scarring and stenosis at the site of surgery can lead to chronic urethral obstruction, necessitating revision of the stoma.
- Ascending infections are uncommon and urinary continence is not affected.

Owners should be made aware of these possible complications and, ideally, the dog should be hospitalized postoperatively to monitor the wound.

OPERATIVE TECHNIQUE 16.6

Feline perineal urethrostomy (PU)

DO

- Understand the anatomy of the procedure well before undertaking the surgery.
- Use meticulous dissection and haemostasis.
- Ensure that the urethral incision reaches the pelvic urethra, to produce a large urethrostomy opening, *but* disturb the pelvic structures as little as possible to avoid loss of urethral function.
- Place sutures as atraumatically as possible and ensure accurate urethral mucosa/skin coaptation.

DON'T

- Rush into perineal urethrostomy. Most feline lower urinary tract disorder (FLUTD)-related urethral obstructions can be managed medically and only rarely is surgery indicated.
- Perform a penile urethrostomy. Failure to create a stoma at the perineal site is the most common reason for subsequent stricture development.
- Use an indwelling catheter in the new stoma unless absolutely unavoidable because it may promote stricture formation.
- Attempt surgery without adequate guidance, practice and experience.

POSITIONING

Sternal recumbency and tilted downwards. The anus is closed with a purse-string suture and the urethra catheterized if possible.

ASSISTANT

Unnecessary, and may even hinder the procedure.

ANTIBIOTIC AND ANALGESIA REGIMES

- Cats should receive broad-spectrum antibiotic therapy both peri- and postoperatively.
- Appropriate analgesia should include an opioid (e.g. buprenorphine) for 24–48 hours and an NSAID may be used.

EQUIPMENT EXTRAS

Bipolar electrocautery is useful; urethral catheter; mini-Gelpi retractors; fine needle holders.

SURGICAL TECHNIQUE

Approach

Perform castration at this stage if necessary and make an elliptical skin incision around the penis and scrotum.

Surgical manipulations

1 The penis is dissected free of the underlying and surrounding fascial tissue.

2 Reflect the penis dorsally and to either side to enable the ischiocavernosus muscles to be isolated and sectioned. The muscles and their penile attachments are very vascular and can be resected with electrocautery or following ligation. Alternatively, periosteal dissection of the ischial attachment avoids the need for any haemostasis.

→ **OPERATIVE TECHNIQUE 16.6 CONTINUED**

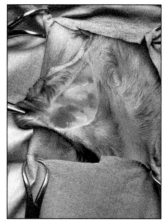
Incision surrounding the scrotum.

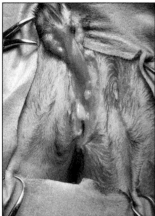
Dissection and dorsal reflection of the penis.

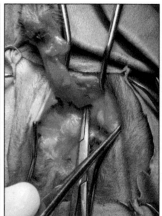
Incision of the ischiocavernosus muscle.

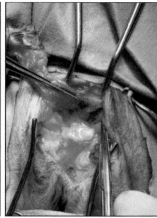
Resection of the ischiocavernosus muscle.

3 Again retract the penis dorsally to enable the penile ligament to be isolated in the midline and sectioned. The penis is now reflected ventrally. Trim the retractor penis muscle away from its dorsum.

4 Make a longitudinal incision into the dorsal penile urethra and amputate the distal penis.

5 Exposure of the urethra is facilitated considerably by the placement of a urethral catheter; where stenosis or unresolved obstruction prevents catheterization the urethra can be difficult to locate.

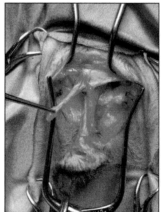
Resection of the retractor penis muscle.

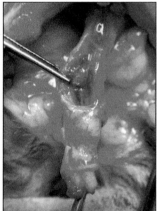
Exposure of penile urethra with urolith and localized cellulitis.

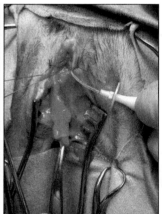
Spatulation of the urethral mucosa and cutaneous suturing.

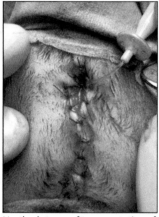
Urethral stoma after amputation of the penile stoma.

Wound closure

Suture the urethral mucosa using 0.7–1.5 metric (6/0–4/0 USP) suture material to the surrounding skin. Every care should be taken to ensure accurate coaptation, because periurethral leakage may have disastrous complications.

POSTOPERATIVE MANAGEMENT AND COMPLICATIONS

- Cats should be prevented from traumatizing the surgical site by use of a plastic collar and appropriate analgesia regimes.
- Urinary retention after surgery is common and may be caused by pain, ongoing FLUTD-related changes in the bladder or lack of familiarity with the environment. Try to avoid repeated catheterization of the stoma.

  Owners should be warned of possible complications, including the following:

- Rectal prolapse is usually only a temporary postoperative complication
- Periurethral cellulitis and perineal necrosis may follow failure to coapt the mucosa/skin junction adequately
- Stricture of the stoma site may be a possible sequel to cellulitis or, more commonly, failure to dissect the urethra adequately from its pelvic attachments
- Urinary incontinence may be encountered as the sequel to excessive dissection in the pelvic region with neurological damage.

OPERATIVE TECHNIQUE 16.7

Prepubic urethrostomy (PPU)

POSITIONING

Dorsal recumbency.

ASSISTANT

Unnecessary.

ANTIBIOTIC AND ANALGESIA REGIMES

* Cats should receive broad-spectrum antibiotic therapy both peri- and postoperatively.
* Appropriate analgesia should include an opioid (e.g. buprenorphine) for 24–48 hours and an NSAID may be used.

EQUIPMENT EXTRAS

Bipolar electrocautery is useful; urethral catheter; mini-Gelpi retractors; fine needle holders.

SURGICAL TECHNIQUE

Approach

Use a caudal laparotomy to expose the bladder neck and preprostatic urethra.

Surgical manipulations

1 Remove the periurethral adipose tissue by careful blunt dissection to expose the urethra.

2 Section the urethra as close to the pubis as possible.

3 Catheterize the proximal urethra to allow accurate identification of the mucosa.

4 Anchor the urethral mucosa to the skin through the laparotomy site. Alternatively, the urethra can be exteriorized through a separate paramedian stab incision.

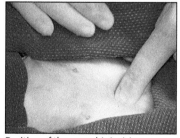
Position of the prepubic incision.

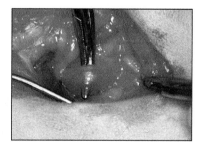
Dissection of the bladder neck and urethra.

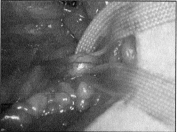
Elevation of the bladder neck and urethra.

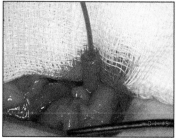
Exteriorization of the resected urethra.

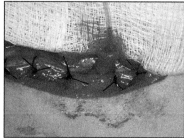
Resected urethra anchored in the laparotomy repair.

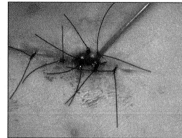
Complete urethral stoma.

→ **OPERATIVE TECHNIQUE 16.7 CONTINUED**

Wound closure

Routine abdominal closure is performed.

POSTOPERATIVE MANAGEMENT AND COMPLICATIONS

Following PPU, cats should be managed after surgery as for PU. Patients may take several days to accommodate to the new urinary stoma site but usually begin to adopt a modified posture for urination. Prepubic stomas will function well but this should be regarded as a 'salvage of a salvage procedure' because urine scalding of the inguinal region is a possible complication.

Chapter 17

The female reproductive system

Jane Ladlow

Elective neutering of female dogs and cats is one of the commonest surgeries performed in veterinary practice. Over the last decade, sterilization techniques in the bitch have advanced with the introduction of laparoscopic techniques and the acceptance of both ovariectomy and ovariohysterectomy for routine neutering. There is also debate over the best approach to be used in feline neutering with evidence supporting less discomfort associated with the midline *versus* a flank approach (Grint *et al.*, 2005). Led by the animal rehoming charities, prepubertal neutering is becoming an accepted procedure particularly in cats. Surgery may also be required to prevent, diagnose or treat various diseases. Indications for non-elective surgery include neoplasia, pyometra, dystocia, uterine torsion, uterine prolapse, metritis and intersexuality. Although the medical treatment of pyometra is now more commonplace, unless the bitch is a valuable breeding animal ovariohysterectomy is still regarded as the treatment of choice.

Anatomy

The female reproductive organs in dogs and cats include paired ovaries and uterine tubes (oviducts), a uterus (subdivided into horns, body and cervix), vagina and vulva (Figure 17.1).

- The ovaries are located adjacent to the caudal poles of the kidneys, concealed within a peritoneal pouch, the ovarian bursa. There is a narrow slit-like opening ventrally, which allows the egg to pass into the oviduct. The right ovary is cranial to the left. The ovarian pedicle is comprised of the suspensory ligament, ovarian vessels, and the ovary. The ovary itself is suspended within the mesovarium (cranial portion of the broad ligament) and attached caudally to the uterine tube by the proper ligament. The round ligament courses within the mesovarium from the ovary to the inguinal canal.
- The uterine horns are long, slender and flexible, extending from the ovaries to the uterine body. The uterine horns and body are supported within the mesometrium (caudal portion of the broad ligament).
- The cervix separates the relatively short uterine body from the vagina and acts as a sphincter to control access to the uterus. The lumen of the cervix is oriented in a dorsoventral direction, and the cranial orifice opens dorsally into the uterine body. Although the cervix may be difficult to locate visually, it can be

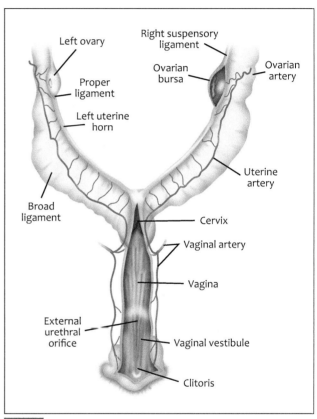

17.1 The anatomy of the female reproductive system in the bitch.

identified intraoperatively by palpation of a thickened segment of the caudal uterus.
- The vagina extends from the cervix to the external urethral orifice. In the canine, the cervical canal joins the vagina at a right angle, with ventral vaginal body ending in a blind-ending sac.
- The vestibule extends from the urethral orifice to the external opening of the reproductive tract at the vulva.

Ligamentous anatomy

The broad ligament attaches the uterus to the dorsolateral body wall. Cranially the broad ligament continues as the suspensory ligament, which attaches to the last rib. The ovaries are attached to the dorsolateral abdominal wall by the part of the broad ligament called the mesovarium, which contains the ovarian arteries. A lateral band of the broad ligament continues through the inguinal canal as the vaginal process and contains the round ligament of the uterus. The proper ligament is a continuation of the suspensory ligament and connects the ovary and the uterine horn.

The myometrium is smooth muscled and double layered with an outer longitudinal layer and an inner circular layer. These muscles hypertrophy during proestrus and oestrus allowing the cervical angle, which is at a right angle during anoestrus, to straighten prior to coitus. The tunica mucosa or endometrium is lined with columnar epithelium.

With regards to vascular supply, the reproductive tract is well supplied, with ovarian arteries which originate from the aorta caudal to the renal arteries and from the uterine arteries which branch from the vaginal artery. The right ovarian vein enters the vena cava, whilst the left ovarian vein usually drains into the left renal vein.

The lymphatic drainage is to the hypogastric and lumbar lymph nodes.

Surgical procedures

Ovariohysterectomy and ovariectomy

These procedures are used for the elective sterilization of the bitch and queen, as well as for treating ovarian and uterine diseases such as pyometra, mucometra and neoplasia. In addition, these techniques can be used to aid the management of endocrine abnormalities such as diabetes mellitus. Early neutering is also a preventative treatment for vaginal hyperplasia, pseudopregnancy, pyometra and mammary gland neoplasia.

Both ovariohysterectomy and ovariectomy (see Operative Techniques 17.1 to 17.3) are accepted techniques for elective sterilization. Ovariectomy has been traditionally performed in many European countries, whilst the UK and USA have historically advocated ovariohysterectomy. Proponents of ovariectomy suggest that it is less invasive as a smaller amount of tissue is removed, requiring a smaller skin incision and reducing manipulation of the abdominal organs (Peeters et al., 2011). As less tissue is removed, the incidence of complications such as ureteric entrapment, stump pyometra or ureterovaginal fistula is potentially reduced. Proponents of ovariohysterectomy are often concerned that leaving the uterus in place can lead to the development of pyometra in the future. If all the ovarian tissue is removed, then pyometra can only occur if exogenous progestagens are administered post-surgery.

Other forms of uterine disease, such as tumours, are possible following ovariectomy, but the incidence of uterine tumours in the bitch is very low (0.03%). These tumours are mostly benign and hormonally influenced and thus should not occur following ovariectomy. There is no published evidence that pyometra can occur following ovariectomy (Okkens et al., 1997). Ovariohysterectomy should be performed if the uterus has any obvious abnormalities.

Age at surgery

Traditionally, the age for neutering has been around 6–9 months in bitches and 4–6 months in cats. Interestingly, the recommended age for neutering has increased over the last century; bitches were routinely sterilized at 3–6 months in the early 1900s (Kustritz, 2007).

If a bitch is neutered prior to the first ovarian cycle, the incidence of mammary gland tumours has been reported to be reduced to <0.5% of that of an entire bitch, although this is an old study (Schneider et al., 1969). Providing the bitch is neutered after the second cycle, there is still a protective effect of 26% of the normal mammary gland tumour incidence in entire bitches. Tumour incidence is reported to be as high as 25% in entire bitches >10 years of age. There is also a protective effect of neutering on mammary gland tumours in cats, with intact queens having a seven-fold incidence of mammary gland neoplasia compared with neutered animals (Overly et al., 2005).

In the Rottweiler, a three-fold increased risk of osteosarcoma development has been reported in dogs that were neutered before 1 year of age (Cooley et al., 2002). Following this study, it is the author's view that it would seem sensible to delay neutering until after 1 year of age in the Rottweiler. However, it is also important to note that the risk of developing osteosarcoma is increased with gonadectomy at any age, and by a factor of 1.3–2 in at-risk breeds (Dobermann, Great Dane, Irish Setter, Irish Wolfhound, Rottweiler and St Bernard) (Root Kustritz, 2012). A recent study by Zink et al. (2014) suggests that neutered Vizslas have an increased risk of developing any form of cancer, particularly mast cell tumours and lymphoma. This study also demonstrated a higher risk of Vizslas developing haemangiosarcoma if they were neutered at <12 months of age compared with animals neutered after 12 months old.

Prepubertal neutering: Prepubertal neutering is advocated by many rescue shelters that have low compliance of owners returning rehomed animals for sterilization. Neutering is thus carried out at 6–14 weeks of age, prior to rehoming.

Advantages:

- Ease of surgery – younger animals have less abdominal fat and decreased vascularity of the reproductive tract, which means that identification of the uterus and ovaries and haemostasis of the ovarian pedicles is easier.
- Improved population control.
- Swifter recovery from surgery.
- Fewer perioperative complications.
- Decreased incidence of obesity, separation anxiety, inappropriate urination and roaming in dogs.
- In cats, gonadectomy prior to 5.5 months of age has been associated with a reduced incidence of feline asthma, gingivitis and hyperactivity.

Disadvantages:

- Paediatric animals are more vulnerable to hypothermia and hypoglycaemia under anaesthesia.
- There is an increased sensitivity to anaesthetic drugs with regard to effect and duration, which should be reflected in the drug dosages.
- The immature nervous system is less efficient at compensating for some of the side effects of commonly used anaesthetic drugs (e.g. alpha-2 agonists).
- Juvenile characteristics (small external genitalia) may be retained.
- An increased rate of cystitis and urinary incontinence has been reported in dogs neutered before 3 months of age, although the long-term significance has yet to be fully evaluated (Spain et al., 2004).

Several studies have shown radiographic delay in physeal closure amongst animals neutered before sexual maturity, but, ultimately, growth of neutered animals is essentially identical to that of intact littermates. Age at prepubertal gonadectomy has not been associated with the incidence of delayed physeal closure or the frequency of long-bone fractures in cats (Salmeri *et al.*, 1991; Stubbs *et al.*, 1996; Root *et al.*, 1997). Early neutering of cats does not result in an increased incidence of feline lower urinary tract disease or urinary obstruction, diabetes mellitus or physeal fracture.

For animal welfare charities concerned with rehoming, the benefits of prepubertal neutering outweigh any perceived disadvantages associated with the timing.

Oestrous cycle

In bitches that have had a season, timing of surgery should be related to the stage of the oestrous cycle. The cervix, uterine body and vagina undergo muscular hypertrophy in proestrus, which becomes most pronounced during oestrus and regresses through metoestrus. These changes are under the influence of oestrogens, which also increase the vascularity of the tract. Thus, during proestrus, oestrus and early metoestrus, the uterus and cervix are thickened, more friable and more vascular. In order to avoid operating when the tissues are more friable and vascular in animals which have undergone puberty, it is preferable to wait until anoestrus before performing elective sterilization (this is less of a problem when laparoscopic procedures are carried out). Along with changes to the uterus and cervix, the mammary glands develop during the luteal (dioestrus) phase of the cycle.

In pseudopregnancy, which is generally seen up to 12 weeks following oestrus, clinical signs and lactation can occur due to the high prolactin levels that arise as the progesterone levels decrease. Persistent signs of pseudopregnancy with lactation are a risk if the bitch is neutered whilst pseudopregnant or predisposed to pseudopregnancy and in the latter part of the luteal phase of the cycle (Allen, 1986). The work by Gobello *et al.* (2001) has shown that only in bitches predisposed to pseudopregnancy would an abrupt decrease in progesterone concentrations induce a substantial increase in prolactin concentrations, which would trigger the typical signs of pseudopregnancy.

Thus, to avoid congested tissue and minimize the risk of pseudopregnancy, surgery should be delayed until 8 weeks after oestrus. The mammary glands should be carefully palpated prior to surgery and if any discharge is noted, then the procedure should be postponed. In animals where lactation is not self-limiting, a prolactin inhibitor such as cabergoline can be used for 7–14 days to decrease prolactin levels.

Anaesthesia and analgesia

A number of suitable anaesthetic protocols have been described for routine ovariectomy or ovariohysterectomy in the bitch and queen (see *BSAVA Manual of Canine and Feline Anaesthesia and Analgesia*). Methods of analgesia for routine neutering have progressed with anaesthetic protocols incorporating drugs with an analgesic effect and local anaesthetics used as either a splash block on the pedicles and wound or as strips placed on either side of the wound at the end of the procedure. There is a wide selection of non-steroidal anti-inflammatory drugs (NSAIDs) available for postoperative analgesia. For patients that do not tolerate NSAIDs or require additional analgesia, the oral opioid tramadol or the gamma-aminobutyric acid (GABA) analogue gabapentin can be considered, but the latter two drugs are not authorized for veterinary use in the UK or USA (see the *BSAVA Small Animal Formulary*).

Open surgical techniques

Dogs: See Operative Techniques 17.1 and 17.2 for details on ovariohysterectomy and ovariectomy, respectively. Ligation of the ovarian pedicle is often the hardest part of the procedure, particularly for inexperienced surgeons. The types of ligature suitable for ligation of the ovarian pedicle (Figure 17.2) have been compared and the most secure knots were slip knots and single/double other side (SDOS) knots, narrowly followed by modified transfixing ligatures (Leitch *et al.*, 2012). With respect to suture material, there is a wide variety of absorbable monofilament and multifilament suture material that is suitable for pedicle ligation. Due to the potential risk of pedicle granulomas, non-absorbable suture material should never be used.

Cats: Ovariohysterectomy (see Operative Technique 17.3) and ovariectomy can be performed through a midline or left flank incision. In the UK, the flank route is the norm, whilst in the USA, Europe and Australasia, the midline approach is routine. The flank approach was introduced in the late 1920s and seems to have been advocated by two or three eminent surgeons of the time (May, 2012). It was considered safer when catgut was used routinely to close the abdominal wall, as any disruption to the sutures closing the body wall incision was less likely to result in herniation

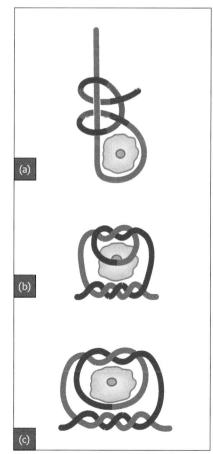

17.2 Different knots that are suitable for ovarian pedicle ligation. (a) Sliding knot. (b) Modified transfixing ligature. (c) Single/double other side knot.

of abdominal contents. However, with the advent of synthetic suture material, such failure is much less likely.

The midline approach incises through the linea alba rather than the muscle, so it is likely to cause less discomfort postoperatively; this is supported by prospective studies (Burrows *et al.*, 2006; Grint *et al.* 2006). The midline approach is preferable if there is doubt as to whether the cat has already been neutered; although the flank and midline of rescue cats should be carefully checked to identify a previous surgical scar. A coeliotomy is the approach of choice if the queen is pregnant, which is not always obvious on the pre-surgical check. The feline uterus can be very friable if pregnant or in oestrus, so clamps at the cervix should be placed with care, or ligatures applied directly to the uterine tissue instead of using forceps, in these cases.

> **WARNING**
>
> In oriental breeds, such as Siamese, fur is likely to darken after clipping due to the difference in temperature. In these cases, a midline approach is recommended

Prepubertal animals: Prepubertal ovariohysterectomy and ovariectomy is performed as in adult animals, but with some important considerations. When considering the surgical technique for non-laparoscopic procedures, the incision is made further caudally, approximately two-thirds the distance from the umbilicus to the pubic brim. Tissue handling needs to be minimal and gentle, and haemostasis exact, as the blood volumes are small.

The choice of anaesthetic needs to be carefully considered, especially in paediatric patients, as they are more vulnerable to hypothermia and hypoglycaemia. There is an increased sensitivity to anaesthetic drugs with regard to effect and duration, which should be reflected in the drug dosages. The immature nervous system is also less efficient at compensating for some of the side effects of commonly used anaesthetic agents (e.g. alpha-2 agonists), leaving the animal susceptible to hypotension. In addition, paediatric patients require oxygenation via an endotracheal (ET) tube to meet the increased tissue oxygen demand, as well as swift clipping and preparation for surgery (with warming devices in place) to avoid hypothermia.

Neonatal patients have minimal hepatic glycogen stores, therefore, food need only be withheld for 3–4 hours preoperatively and should be offered within 1–2 hours following extubation to avoid hypoglycaemia (Howe, 1997). Due to the smaller body mass of the patient, it is important to maintain body temperature before, during and after surgery. This can be achieved using a re-circulating warm water or air convection blanket or, preferably, a conductive polymer blanket. Great care should be taken with microwaveable heat pads and which are best avoided in such young patients due to the risk of thermal injury. As for adult animals, adequate sedation for anaesthetic induction must be provided. A balanced electrolyte solution should be administered intravenously with the addition of 5% dextrose. Paediatric animals have elevated respiratory and cardiac rates. Their oxygen consumption may be 2–3 times greater than that of an adult and they have a decreased ability for forced cardiac contraction, thus cardiac output depends primary on heart rate alone (Howe, 1997).

> **PRACTICAL TIP**
>
> When performing prepubertal ovariectomy or ovariohysterectomy, particular attention needs to be paid to gentle tissue handling because, although the surgical techniques used are similar, paediatric tissues are more delicate. Small gauge sutures should also be used (Aronsohn, 1993)

> **WARNING**
>
> If using a Snook ovariohysterectomy hook to locate the uterine body, be aware that the delicate structures around the uterus can be easily damaged, so the hook must be used with extreme care

> **Editors' note**
>
> Neither of the editors routinely use a Snook hook due to the risks associated with it

Laparoscopic techniques

Laparoscopic ovariectomy (Figures 17.3 and 17.4) and ovariohysterectomy have been shown to decrease the postoperative pain scores and surgical stress, and increase postoperative activity in bitches compared with open surgery (Davidson *et al.*, 2004; Hancock *et al.*, 2005; Culp *et al.*, 2009). Complication rates are not significantly different in the hands of an experienced surgeon, although surgical times are initially increased. These techniques are increasingly popular in general veterinary practice and owner awareness of 'keyhole' surgery is driving a willingness to pay a premium for the procedures. A variety of techniques have been described with one to three portal access and different methods of vessel ligation such electrocautery (monopolar and bipolar), ultrasonic devices, haemoclips, laser and extracorporeal sutures (see References and further reading).

Laparoscopic ovariectomy techniques have been described in the cat; although experienced surgeons will have a similar sized incision when using an open surgical approach. Laparoscopic ovariectomy is difficult to justify

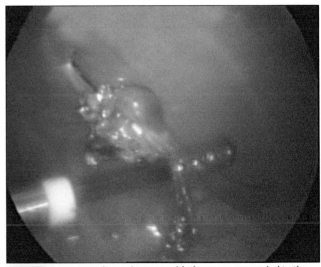

17.3 Laparoscopic ovariectomy with the ovary suspended to the body wall via an externally placed suture and a vessel-sealing device across the ovarian pedicle.

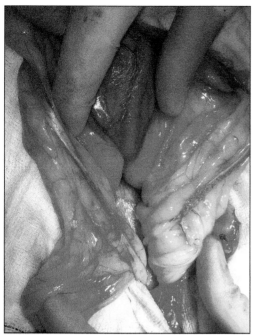

17.4 The appearance of the uterus in a 6-year-old Mastiff following bilateral laparoscopic ovariectomy 4 years previously.

in such small patients and would require smaller instrumentation than that routinely used in dogs. For a more detailed discussion on laparoscopic techniques, the reader is referred to Chapter 3.

Complications

Overall complication rates for ovariohysterectomy and ovariectomy range from 1% to 30%, although these are usually reports from veterinary teaching hospitals where the surgeons, though supervised, are usually inexperienced (Dorn and Swift, 1977; Burrows *et al.*, 2005). The type of complications can be divided into intraoperative and postoperative complications.

Intraoperative complications: These are reported to occur in 6–20% of cases and include haemorrhage and inadvertent damage to other abdominal organs such as the ureters or bladder. The most frequent intraoperative complication in the bitch is haemorrhage, usually from the right ovarian pedicle, presumably due to its more cranial position, and is more likely to occur if the incision is made slightly too caudal. This complication is more commonly reported in larger bitches (>22 kg). If haemorrhage occurs from the right ovarian pedicle once it has been replaced in the abdomen, picking up the duodenum and moving it over to the midline will trap most of the abdominal contents in the mesoduodenum, allowing visualization of the pedicle. On the left, the descending colon can be used to similar effect. In the queen, ligatures slipping off the ovarian pedicles is not an infrequent complication, although haemorrhage due to the trauma to the vessel is uncommonly seen. However, it is still preferable to relocate the pedicle, if possible, and replace the ligatures as even if haemorrhage is not present during surgery, increases in blood pressure during recovery may result in bleeding.

Postoperative complications: The complications following neutering can be divided into postoperative surgical complications and side effects from removing the hormonal influence of the gonads. Major postoperative complications include:

- Haemorrhage
- Wound dehiscence or infection
- Failure to remove all the ovarian tissue
- Ovarian pedicle granulomas
- Cervical granulomas or infection
- Damage to other abdominal organs (e.g. the ureters – ureteric ligation and ureterovaginal fistulae are rarely reported).

If a ureter is inadvertently ligated, the ligature should be removed as soon as is feasible. If the obstruction is removed within the first week, normal ureteric function is expected, whilst after 4 weeks permanent damage will have occurred resulting in hydronephrosis (Brunschwig *et al.*, 1964). This would then require a ureteronephrectomy to be performed (see Operative Technique 14.4).

The complication rate following surgery is usually related to surgical and anaesthetic time. Surgical time drops sharply with experience, so that most experienced veterinary surgeons (veterinarians) would expect a surgical time of <30 minutes. In procedures performed by inexperienced surgeons, complication rates range from 6–20%, but this decreases with experience, so in private practice major complication rates would be expected to be 1–4% (Pollari, 1996; Burrows *et al.*, 2005). Minor postoperative complications such as seroma formation, wound swelling and discharge, traumatization of the wound and granulomatous dermatitis at the site are reported at frequencies of between 1% and 24% in private practice (Pollari *et al.*, 1996).

Haemorrhage: When seen post-surgery, haemorrhage may occur from intra-abdominal structures such as the cervical vessels or from the skin and fascial wounds. If the animal is cardiovascularly stable, it is worth placing a body wrap prior to re-operating. If the bandage reduces the bleeding so that strikethrough does not occur and the heart rate and respiratory rate reduce to normal levels, the bitch can be left with the dressing in place for 24 hours with vital parameters being checked every 2 hours. If the animal is not cardiovascularly stable, it is unlikely to be bleeding from the superficial wound and, following stabilization, surgical exploration of the abdomen is advisable (Figure 17.5) with particular attention being paid to the cervical stump and ovarian pedicles.

Thromboelastography (TEG) can differentiate between postoperative coagulopathy and postoperative bleeding

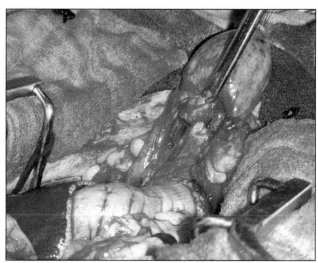

17.5 Postoperative haemorrhage following ovariohysterectomy. Exploratory surgery was required to stop the cervical bleeding.

(Kol, 2010), but is only currently available in some universities or larger referral practices. If no obvious source of bleeding is discovered in the abdomen, the midline should be closed, coagulation profiles run and the use of plasma considered. Rarely, haemorrhage from the cervical stump can be seen per vulva in the first couple of weeks following the procedure, which occurs due to erosion of the ligature through the cervical wall. This requires resection of the cervical stump if persistent.

Ovarian remnant syndrome: This occurs if ovarian tissue is left in the abdomen; the right pedicle is the most common location in dogs. Accessory ovaries are reported to occur in cats, but in all documented cases of feline ovarian remnant syndrome, ovarian remnants were found at surgery. Clinical signs consist of vulval swelling and preoestral bleeding, and behavioural changes with stump pyometra are also possible. Diagnosis is by a combination of history, surgical report, clinical signs, vaginal cytology and measurement of progesterone levels. On vaginal cytology, cornification is evidence of oestrogen secretion. In dogs, a functional corpus luteum is present if the progesterone level is >2 ng/ml, although this may only be detected in about 50% of cases (Ball *et al.*, 2010). Hormone stimulation tests provide a more reliable diagnosis (Ball *et al.*, 2010). In cats, human chorionic gonadotrophin is administered 1–3 days after signs of oestrus and progesterone levels measured 7 days later. Treatment consists of exploratory coeliotomy or laparoscopy and identification of the residual ovarian tissue, which is usually cystic and found at the pedicles or along the body wall.

PRACTICAL TIP

The resected tissue should be submitted for histopathology to confirm the presence of ovarian tissue and screen for neoplasia as there are a number of cases where ovarian tumours were diagnosed. These cases had a longer interval to diagnosis from initial ovariohysterectomy (Ball *et al.*, 2010). Prognosis is good following removal of the residual functional ovarian tissue

---

Inflammatory granulomas: Inflammatory granulomas or abscesses of the uterine stump can occur if non-absorbable sutures are used or an excessive amount of devitalized uterine stump is left in the abdomen following surgery. Granulomas of the ovarian pedicles are usually associated with non-absorbable suture material or traumatic surgical technique. Clinical signs of a cervical or uterine granuloma may include vaginal discharge or polyuria related to pressure on the bladder or signs of sepsis such as depression, lethargy, inappetence or vomiting. Ovarian granulomas usually involve the retroperitoneal space and often result in flank sinuses (Figures 17.6, 17.7 and 17.8). In all cases, surgical exploration and resection of the granuloma is required.

Side effects due to hormonal changes: Side effects due to hormonal changes following sterilization also occur. The most common side effects are weight gain and urinary incontinence. The most common risk factor for obesity is gonadectomy, with queens particularly affected (three-fold risk of obesity following neutering). In cats, neutering is associated with a decrease in basal metabolic rate; however, this has not been shown in the neutered bitch where increased appetite seems to be the more important factor

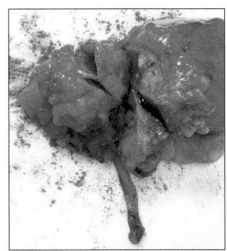

17.6 Ovarian granuloma that has resulted in ureteric entrapment, hydronephrosis and flank sinus. The granuloma was resected along with the left kidney and ureter.
(Courtesy of P Neath)

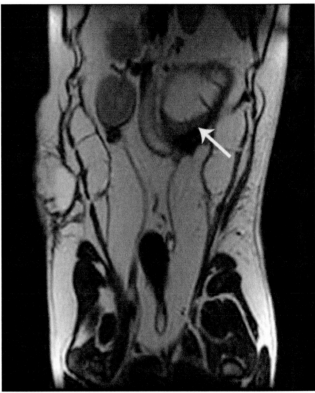

17.7 MR image showing ureteric entrapment by an ovarian granuloma (arrowed) with subsequent hydronephrosis.

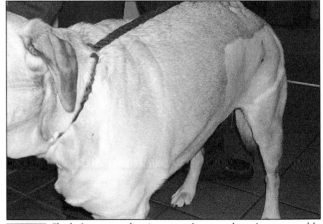

17.8 Flank sinus secondary to an ovarian granuloma in a 3-year-old bitch neutered 3 years previously.

(possibly related to oestrogen acting as a satiety factor). In a small (8 dog) study in Beagles, there was a small but significant weight gain following ovariectomy at 18 months of age; however, in a study of 44 working dogs there was no change in bodyweight over the year (Haupt *et al* .,1979; Le Roux *et al.*, 1984; Detilleux *et al.*, 2004). In both the bitch and queen, weight gain can be avoided by following a feeding regimen and this should be discussed with the owner at the time of neutering.

Urinary incontinence follows a decrease in the maximum urethral closure pressure, which is thought to be primarily due to withdrawal of oestrogen. The incidence of urinary incontinence following neutering varies from 5–20%, depending on the study, and is breed-dependent with large and giant breeds having a reportedly higher risk. Dogs neutered before 3 months of age are also reported to be at an increased risk according to one study (12.9% *versus* 5%; Spain *et al.*, 2004). Other reported consequences of neutering include an increased incidence of cruciate ligament rupture in neutered dogs, increased incidence of osteosarcoma in large breeds (Root Kustriz, 2012) and increased risk of haemangiosarcoma, particularly cardiac and splenic (Prymak *et al.*, 1988).

Caesarean section

Dystocia can occur for a variety of reasons, including uterine inertia, fetal oversize, developmental defects, faulty presentation and maternal deformity (narrowed pelvic inlet or vaginal hyperplasia). Maternal causes for dystocia are more common, with uterine inertia being seen most frequently in the bitch and queen. Primary uterine inertia can occur due to a small litter size, hypocalcaemia, large litter size with overstretching of the uterine wall, obesity, trauma, environmental disruption and septicaemia. Secondary uterine inertia results from exhaustion of the uterine muscle due to an oversized fetus, large litter size or dystocia. Malpositioning is the most common fetal cause of dystocia. In some brachycephalic breeds (particularly the Bulldog), there are some pedigree lines where all litters are delivered by Caesarean section due to cephalopelvic disproportion. The Kennel Club (UK) will only register puppies from the first two litters delivered by Caesarean section and, ethically, self-whelping lines are preferable.

Assessment of dystocia

The initial assessment of dystocia involves determining the expected date of labour (based on calculated due date, progesterone levels and temperature decrease) and a physical examination, particularly a careful vaginal examination. An abdominal examination should be carried out to assess uterine size and the number of fetuses present. If no fetus is present in the vaginal canal, ultrasonography can be used to confirm fetal number and assess viability, presentation and placental health. Radiography is also useful to assess the number, size and presentation of fetuses, along with maternal conformation. Blood calcium levels should be assessed and if there is any question as to the health of the bitch or queen full haematology and biochemistry profiles should be undertaken.

PRACTICAL TIP

A greenish vaginal discharge indicates placental separation and parturition should proceed within 2–3 hours

---

Medical management

In cases without obstruction of the birth canal, dystocia can be treated medically with ecbolics (oxytocin and calcium gluconate), lubrication and digital manipulation. In the bitch, if two or more injections of oxytocin plus calcium gluconate fail to cause fetal expulsion, surgical intervention is indicated. Only about a quarter of feline dystocia cases can be managed medically. A Caesarean section is also indicated if there is maternal deformity, if the fetus is malpositioned or oversized, or if the fetus or dam are showing signs of distress (fetal heart rate <170 bpm).

Anaesthesia and analgesia

The pregnant bitch or queen has a higher oxygen requirement and decreased functional lung residual capacity, as well as an increased sensitivity to anaesthetic drugs. The drugs suitable for sedation and anaesthesia or centrally-acting analgesia will pass into the placenta, allowing fetal exposure. In order to reduce fetal respiratory depression, anaesthetic drugs should be chosen with care; the use of agents where respiratory depression can be reversed, if necessary, are preferable. Short-acting opioids are a suitable choice and opioid epidural injections are a good method of decreasing anaesthetic requirements and providing postoperative analgesia. The use of local anaesthetic agents for epidural injection should be undertaken with care as they negatively affect ambulation of the bitch. Local anaesthetic agents can be used as a splash block on the wound to decrease postoperative discomfort. The time from induction to extraction of the fetuses should be kept to a minimum and a cuffed ET tube should be placed as soon as possible following induction as many animals will have eaten recently and aspiration is a risk.

Patient preparation

Patient preparation (including clipping) should be performed with the bitch conscious, if possible. The bitch should also be pre-oxygenated prior to the procedure.

Surgical techniques

A Caesarean section can be performed by incising into the uterine body or horns and extracting the fetuses or by *en bloc* ovariohysterectomy (see Operative Technique 17.4). The head and thorax of the animal should be elevated on the operating table to decrease abdominal pressure on the diaphragm. A midline coeliotomy is preferred. Speed of fetal extraction is imperative to increase survival rates.

Uterine body or horn incision: If the uterus is opened, the location of the incision should be made on a case-by-case basis. A puppy lodged in the vaginal canal is easier to extract via an incision in the uterine body; whereas, if there is a large litter, it is quicker to remove the fetuses by incising into each uterine horn. If the fetal membranes are firmly attached to the uterine wall, they should be left to pass naturally in cases with an open cervix to avoid excessive haemorrhage. The uterine incision may be closed with appositional simple continuous or interrupted sutures or with a double layer closure. Irrespective of how the uterine incision is closed, there are usually few complications with the wound and it is often difficult to locate the previous surgical incision if a second Caesarean section is performed.

> **PRACTICAL TIP**
>
> Oxytocin given after uterine closure helps involution of the uterus and facilitates fetal membrane detachment, as well as decreases haemorrhage

En bloc *ovariohysterectomy:* An *en bloc* Caesarean section is indicated where ovariohysterectomy is to be performed (see Operative Technique 17.4). This technique is also used in cases where infection is present or the litter is dead. In addition, this procedure may be preferable if the dam is in a critical condition, to decrease the surgical time. *En bloc* ovariohysterectomy can also aid speed of fetal extraction.

> **PRACTICAL TIP**
>
> If this technique is used when there is a large litter, it is ideal to have a number of assistants ready to deliver the puppies or kittens from the uterus and resuscitate them

Episiotomy: Very occasionally, an episiotomy is required to deliver a puppy or kitten that is lodged at the opening of the vulva (see Operative Technique 17.6). This procedure can often be performed under local anaesthesia.

Survival rates: The survival rate of puppies following traditional Caesarean section is in the range of 90%, with a slightly lower survival rate of 75% for *en bloc* ovariohysterectomy (although this may be a reflection that this procedure is used for more critical cases).

> **PRACTICAL TIP**
>
> As long as the puppies or kittens continue to suckle, milk production is not affected by these techniques, due to the neurohormonal reflex whereby suckling stimulates prolactin release from the pituitary gland

Uterus

A number of uterine disorders are seen, including:

- Cystic hyperplasia–pyometra complex (most common)
- Congenital abnormalities – unicornuate uterus (Figure 17.9), hypoplasia, agenesis, segmental aplasia, septate uterine body)
- Hydrometra/mucometra
- Metritis
- Torsion
- Neoplasia
- Prolapse
- Rupture.

Cystic hyperplasia–pyometra complex

Cystic endometrial hyperplasia (CEH) is often followed by pyometra, although the two conditions can occur independently. Cystic endometrial glandular hyperplasia is characterized by a thickened endometrium lined with thin-walled cysts. CEH progresses with diffuse plasma cell infiltration and an acute inflammatory reaction. In some cases, the

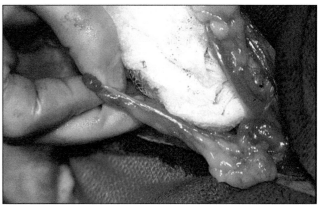

17.9 Unicornuate uterus as an incidental finding during a cat ovariohysterectomy. The ovary is in the correct position.

endometritis becomes chronic. It predisposes to infection with about 30% of CEH cases developing a bacterial infection during the luteal phase of the cycle, thus leading to pyometra (infection of the uterus). Hydrometra (accumulation of sterile watery fluid), mucometra (accumulation of sterile mucoid fluid) or haematometra (accumulation of sterile bloody fluid) may also follow from CEH and are difficult to differentiate from pyometra on diagnostic imaging; these conditions have no systemic effects but pyometra may be life-threatening. It has also been suggested that a low grade uterine infection introduced at proestrus or oestrus stimulates endometrial hyperplasia. The lymphoplasmacytic infiltrates that are seen in CEH may be an inflammatory reaction to the subclinical chronic bacterial infection. CEH also develops in response to a low grade mechanical irritation such as suture material or bacteria.

Aetiology

Pyometra commonly occurs in the luteal phase of the cycle (dioestrus), usually 5–90 days post-oestrus with some cases being reported in anoestrus. The dog is unusual in that the luteal phase of the cycle is a similar length to pregnancy. In cases that present in anoestrus, it is possible that the luteal phase was reduced due to the effect of prostaglandins stimulated by the uterine inflammation. Progesterone is the essential factor, suppressing the immune response, stimulating endometrial gland secretions, closing the cervix and decreasing myometrial activity, thus allowing secretions to accumulate within the lumen of the uterus. These effects are cumulative at subsequent oestrous cycles. The bacteria involved vary and are normal vaginal or perineal flora such as *Escherichia coli*, *Staphlococcus*, *Streptococcus*, *Pseudomonas* and *Proteus* species. *E. coli* is most commonly involved and adheres to specific binding sites in the endometrium through its uropathogenic virulence factor genes (*pap*, *sfa*, *hly A*, *cnF1* and *fim*). Pyometra can be reproduced experimentally by giving ovariectomized bitches cycles of stilboestrol and progesterone. A known risk factor for pyometra is the misalliance drug oestradiol benzoate, particularly in dogs <4 years of age. The oestrogen increases the effect of the progesterone on the endometrium and also relaxes the cervix, allowing infection to pass through.

Presentation

Pyometra has an incidence of about 2% per year in intact bitches <10 years of age seen at veterinary practices, but the risk increases with age with >20% of bitches developing pyometra by 10 years of age. Nulliparous bitches have an increased incidence and some breeds are more susceptible, noticeably Rough Collies, Rottweilers, St Bernards, Chow Chows, Cavalier King Charles Spaniels, Golden Retrievers, Bernese Mountain Dogs and Cocker Spaniels (Egenvall *et al.*, 2001). The incidence of pyometra in queens is lower than in bitches. It is more common in older cats and is uncommon during winter months when many queens are acyclic. It is seen in both mated and unmated queens due to the spontaneous ovulation that can occur and again is a disease of the luteal phase of the cycle, with most cases associated with retained corpora lutea. The use of exogenous progestagens in cats to delay oestrus or treat skin disorders increases the risk of CEH, which may progress to subsequent pyometra.

Pyometra is classified as closed or open, depending on the integrity of the cervix:

- Closed pyometra is usually associated with more severe systemic signs on presentation with an increased likelihood of systemic inflammatory response syndrome (SIRS) and death
- Open pyometra can still have a large accumulation of purulent discharge within the uterus, despite some drainage, and thus sepsis and rupture of the uterus are still possible.

Clinical signs

- ± Malodourous vaginal discharge.
- ± Abdominal distension.
- Polyuria/polydipsia.
- Depression.
- Anorexia.
- Vomiting and diarrhoea.

Cats generally have more subtle clinical signs, such as mild anorexia and depression.

Diagnosis

The history should include the stage of the oestrous cycle, possible matings and previous litters. A physical examination is indicated, including careful abdominal palpation as well as a rectal and vaginal examination. Cytology of the vaginal discharge helps differentiate pyometra from mucometra or haematometra, by the presence of large numbers of neutrophils, which are often degenerate in nature. Intracellular and extracellular bacteria may also be evident. Haematology profiles often reveal a leucocytosis with a left shift. Normocytic, normochromic anaemia is also common. Changes seen on biochemistry profiles include elevated alkaline phosphatase (ALP), hypoalbuminaemia, hyperglobulinaemia, elevated lactate, metabolic acidaemia and azotaemia.

The azotaemia has a prerenal component, but bitches with pyometra have decreased renal perfusion and decreased concentrating ability even when hydrated, with 20% of bitches having low urine specific gravity on presentation. This reduction in concentrating ability is usually reversible and is thought to be due to endotoxin-related tubulointerstitial inflammation. Over 50% of bitches have SIRS at presentation and this is associated with a poorer prognosis and longer hospitalization (Fransson *et al.*, 2007). Biochemical markers of SIRS include elevated C-reactive protein (CRP), serum amyloid A and haptoglobin. These markers can be monitored postoperatively to assess response to treatment, but it should be noted that these tests are not usually available in most general practices. In practice, haematology profiles can be monitored after treatment, with leucocytosis and neutrophilias typically resolving within 7 days (Bartoskova *et al.*, 2007).

Clinical findings are confirmed with ultrasonography, which reveals the uterus to be enlarged and convoluted. A thickened endometrium is diagnostic of CEH. The uterine fluid in cases of pyometra is usually anechoic to hypoechoic, although it may be echodense with a slow swirling pattern; thus a distended uterus with hyperechoic fluid should raise suspicion of mucometra or haematometra, especially if clinical signs are minimal. Radiographic examination is less sensitive for diagnosis because although an enlarged uterus is frequently visible, it is difficult to differentiate this from early pregnancy.

Treatment

In cases with systemic signs, stabilization prior to surgery or medical treatment includes intravenous fluid therapy and broad-spectrum antibiotics, pending culture results from the vaginal discharge or uterine contents. Good initial choices of antibiotics include amoxicillin, amoxicillin/clavulanate (co-amoxiclav), first- or second-generation cephalosporins and potentiated sulphonamides.

Surgical treatment: Surgical treatment in the form of an ovariohysterectomy usually results in a rapid resolution of the clinical signs and avoids recurrence. The uterus should be exteriorized (Figure 17.10), with care to avoid rupture, and packed off from the abdomen with laparotomy swabs. The suspensory ligaments are often stretched, making ligation of the ovarian pedicle easier. The cervical arteries should be ligated separately from the cervix, thus enabling an encircling ligature rather than a transfixing ligature to be used on the cervix. The cervical or uterine stump should be lavaged but not oversewn. Laparoscopic ovariohysterectomy for pyometra has been described and very careful handling is required to avoid uterine rupture.

In cases with generalized peritonitis or rupture of the uterus, abdominal drainage in the form of closed suction drains or open peritoneal drainage is indicated following copious abdominal lavage. If renal function is impaired following surgery, despite good hydration, furosemide may improve urine production; urine output and proteinuria should be monitored closely after surgery. Antibiotic therapy should be continued for 1–2 weeks following resolution of the clinical signs. Mortality rates after surgical

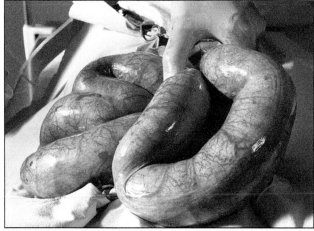

17.10 Closed pyometra in a 9-year-old Boxer. The uterine horns are engorged and friable and require delicate handling to prevent rupture.
(Courtesy of J Hall)

treatment of pyometra are in the range of 3–5% for dogs and 8% for cats, with death usually resulting from the progression of SIRS and myocardial injury (Kenney *et al.*, 1987; Egenvell *et al.*, 2001; Gibson *et al.*, 2013).

Medical treatment: A variety of medical treatments for pyometra have been successfully used in systemically healthy breeding bitches and queens, including:

* Drainage and lavage
* Prostaglandin F2α (PGF2α)
* Progesterone receptor antagonists (e.g. aglepristone)
* Dopamine agonists (e.g. bromocriptine or cabergoline)
* Antibiotics (2–3 week course).

Ideally, following resolution of the pyometra, the animal should be bred from at the next season to avoid recurrence. PGF2α and dopamine agonists cause luteolysis and a reduction in the plasma progesterone levels, which results in cervical relaxation, a decrease in endometrial secretions and expulsion of the uterine contents (Verstegen *et al.*, 2008). Prostaglandins relax the cervix and contract the myometrium, resulting in drainage of the uterus. When the cervix is closed, prostaglandins have been used (off license) with a dopamine agonist such as cabergoline or an antiprogestagen such as algepristone, although careful monitoring of such cases is warranted.

Editors' note:

Aglepristone and cabergoline are not authorized in the UK or USA for the treatment of pyometra. Expert advice should be sought for their use in pyometra

---

WARNING

Side effects of prostaglandins include abdominal pain, emesis, tachycardia, dyspnoea and hypersalivation. These side effects are less severe if a low dosage treatment of a natural prostaglandin (e.g. dinoprost tromethamine) is used

---

Intravaginal infusion of natural prostaglandins has also been reported to be effective with reduced side effects. Dopamine agonists work indirectly by decreasing prolactin and inducing functional arrest followed by luteolysis of the corpus luteum. Dopamine agonists result in a more rapid luteolysis than PGF and have few side effects. They are often used in combination with PGF (England *et al.*, 2007). Progesterone receptor agonists encourage opening of the cervix and aid expulsion of the uterine contents, although, as myometrial stimulation is poor they are usually used in combination with prostaglandins. In bitches with uterine CEH and degeneration, prolonging anoestrus with androgen receptor agonists such as mibolerone allows regeneration of the endometrium and improves subsequent fertility. For closed pyometra, additional drainage can be accomplished by placing a catheter into the uterine lumen via the vagina. The response to medical treatment is evaluated by the decreasing size of the uterus on ultrasound examination and by the resolution of leucogram changes.

The risks of medical treatment include uterine rupture, poor response to treatment and exacerbation of sepsis. Success rates are in the range of 75–90% depending on the therapy, with treatment being more likely to fail in bitches with ovarian cysts (Fieni *et al.*, 2006; Jurka *et al.*,

2010). Surgical treatment is reported to result in faster systemic recovery with normal haematology profiles by day 7 compared to day 10–15 with medical treatment.

WARNING

The recurrence rate following medical treatment in bitches that are not bred at the next season varies from 10–40%

Fertility following medical treatment of pyometra is reasonable in younger bitches (<5 years of age) with conception rates of 50–75% reported. Fertility results are higher in feline studies (Davidson *et al.*, 1990). Medical treatment can also be implemented prior to ovariohysterectomy to stabilize the animal and reduce the surgical risks associated with a pus-filled uterus. There is little information about the benefit of using medical treatment prior to definitive surgical treatment.

Hydrometra, mucometra and haematometra

* Hydrometra – the accumulation of sterile watery fluid.
* Mucometra – the accumulation of sterile mucoid fluid.
* Haematometra – the accumulation of sterile bloody fluid.

The incidence of these conditions is difficult to ascertain as many cases are misdiagnosed as pyometra, but in one study the incidence was reported as 6% (Fransson *et al.*, 2004). Unlike pyometra, these are local conditions and thus animals have fewer systemic clinical signs on presentation. The accumulation of sterile fluid results from endometrial gland secretion under progesterone stimulation and therefore occurs in the luteal phase of the cycle. Drainage may be impeded by a closed cervix or polypoid cyst as a result of CEH.

In addition to fewer clinical signs and being bright on presentation, with sterile fluid accumulations the changes on serum biochemistry and haematology profiles are mild with a low (if any) inflammatory response and a lower percentage of band neutrophils. CRP levels are lower in cases of mucometra/hydrometra compared with pyometra, but this assay is not widely available and also has a high individual variability. Plasma PGF2α is a more sensitive and specific method of differentiating mucometra/hydrometra from pyometra with levels of >4500 pmol/l having a 99% probability of pyometra (Hagman *et al.*, 2006). Vaginal cytology is also useful to differentiate these conditions from pyometra with minimal intracellular bacteria being noted and few degenerative neutrophils. On ultrasound examination, hydrometra usually contains hypoechoic fluid, whereas serous to viscous heterogeneous fluid is seen with mucometra and haematometra. The treatment for sterile fluid accumulations is ovariohysterectomy, as for pyometra, but the prognosis is improved.

Uterine cysts

Although CEH is the most common form of cystic disease affecting the uterus, a second type of endometrial hyperplasia – pseudo-placentational endometrial hyperplasia – is recognized to occur in the luteal phase of the cycle. In this condition, the endometrium responds to stimuli with highly organized proliferative remodelling, resembling placental sites. Other cysts that occur include:

- Congenital – cystic remnants of the mesonephric ducts
- Developmental adenomyosis – endometrial glandular tissue within the myometrium
- Acquired serosal inclusion cysts – develop from the peritoneal surface.

Uterine torsion and rupture

Uterine torsion (Figure 17.11) is reported rarely in both dogs and cats and usually occurs in gravid animals, in cases of pyometra or secondary to segmental aplasia of the uterine horn or vagina. Clinical signs consist of abdominal pain, but may progress to shock if the tissue becomes necrotic. Treatment consists of stabilization and emergency ovariohysterectomy.

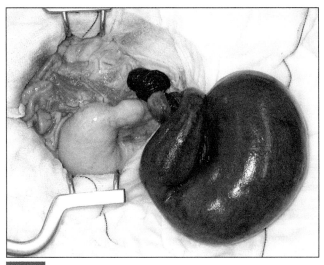

17.11 Uterine horn torsion in a cat.

Uterine rupture is also rare and usually occurs during parturition secondary to dystocia, although it may be traumatic in origin or follow segmental aplasia of the uterine horn, which is more common in the cat than the dog. Traumatic cases may be undiagnosed due to concurrent injuries. Uterine rupture is also reported after torsion. The fetus may be viable if placental circulation is intact and the animal may go into parturition before detection and develop signs of hypovolaemic shock. In these cases, obstructive dystocia will be noted and ovariohysterectomy is indicated.

Uterine prolapse

This condition is very rare and usually affects primiparous queens and bitches, occurring during or just after parturition when the cervix is dilated. If the uterus is healthy on presentation, the animal should be stabilized and the uterus can be reduced or ovariohysterectomy performed, depending on whether further litters are desired. Devitalized tissue requires ovariohysterectomy. In these cases, the cranial part of the uterine body is incised near the vulva to expose the uterine horns. Gentle traction may allow visualization of the ovarian arteries, which can then be ligated. If the ovarian arteries are not visible, the uterine horns should be ligated and transected and then a coeliotomy performed to remove the ovaries.

Uterine tumours

Uterine tumours are extremely rare, with a reported incidence of 0.03% in bitches, although they are reported more frequently in queens. Tumours usually occur in middle aged or older animals and a variety of neoplasms have been reported in both species with leiomyoma being by far the most commonly reported tumour (Schalfer, 2012). Other reported neoplasms include malignant endometrial adenocarcinoma, leiomyosarcoma, haemangiosarcoma and mixed Müllerian tumours (adenosarcoma). Clinical signs may be related to infertility, pyometra, abdominal masses or abdominal straining. The recommended treatment is ovariohysterectomy, although in the case of the most common malignant uterine tumour, endometrial adenocarcinoma, the prognosis is guarded. In one retrospective study, 50% of adenocarcinomas had metastasized at presentation and only two of the eight cats survived for longer than 5 months (Miller *et al.*, 2003).

Acute metritis

This is infection of the uterus, which occurs in the immediate postpartum period or following oestrus and mating. Clinical signs consist of a malodorous vaginal discharge and systemic signs of illness such as anorexia or inappetence, lethargy, pyrexia and vomiting. Post-oestrus metritis cases usually have less severe clinical signs compared with postpartum metritis or pyometra, and the uterine horns are less dilated (<1.5 cm in one study compared with >1.5 cm with pyometra; Gabor *et al.*, 1998). If the clinical signs are mild, medical treatment with PGF2α can be used (as described for pyometra), whilst in more severe cases ovariohysterectomy is indicated. The litter should be weaned and handfed.

Subinvolution of placental sites

Subinvolution is a disturbance in the normal postpartum placental degeneration and endometrial reconstruction, which is usually complete by 12 weeks postpartum. It typically occurs in younger females with only one or two whelpings or queenings. Following parturition, fetal myometrial attachments should degenerate and regress within 12 weeks. Clinical signs consist of a serosanguineous discharge 12–16 weeks after parturition, which is usually self-limiting. On abdominal palpation, enlargement of the uterine horns is evident. Treatment is usually unnecessary and the prognosis for dam health and fertility is excellent. If the discharge persists or results in severe anaemia, ovariohysterectomy is indicated.

Ovaries

Ovarian disorders include cysts, tumours, agenesis (often associated with uterine congenital abnormalities) and supernummary ovaries (Dow, 1960).

Ovarian cysts

Ovarian cysts (Figure 17.12) may be follicular, luteal or not of ovarian origin. Follicular cysts are those >8 mm in diameter that present in pro-oestrus or follicles of any size that present in late oestrus, dioestrus or anoestrus. They can result in prolonged oestrus, cystic mammary gland hyperplasia, CEH and pyometra, and fibroleiomyomas due to oestrogen secretion, although many are asymptomatic. Exogenous progestagens have been implicated in the development of follicular cysts in cats by inhibiting the luteinizing hormone surge required for ovulation. The diagnosis

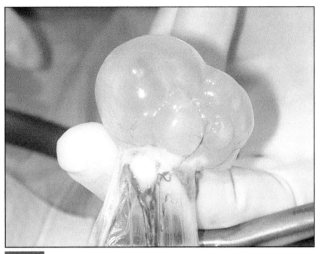

17.12 Ovarian cyst as an incidental finding during ovariectomy.

of ovarian follicular cysts is made by a combination of clinical signs, vaginal cytology where cornified cells are evident, and ultrasound examination of the ovaries. The diagnosis can be confirmed by measurement of plasma oestrogen concentration. In cats, human chorionic gonadotrophin (hCG) can be used to induce ovulation causing lysis of the cyst or progestagens can be used to suppress the clinical signs. Luteal cysts result from failure to ovulate due to inadequate or delayed LH release. Luteinized cysts are firm, thick-walled cysts that secrete progesterone. This may cause prolonged dioestrus and anoestrus, and contribute to CEH and pyometra in small animals. In both cats and dogs with ovarian cysts, ovariectomy or ovariohysterectomy is curative.

Ovarian tumours

Ovarian tumours (Figure 17.13) are found in about 6% of intact bitches. Four types of ovarian tumour are reported:

- Epithelial tumours – adenomas and adenocarcinomas constitute 40–50% of ovarian tumours in dogs
- Germ cell tumours – dysgerminomas, teratomas and teratocarcinomas
- Sex cord tumours – granulosa cell tumours (most common tumour reported in the cat)
- Mesenchymal tumours.

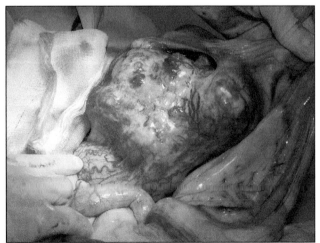

17.13 Ovarian tumour (carcinoma) in a 6-year-old Collie cross. (Courtesy of J Hall)

Epithelial tumours are often asymptomatic until they develop to such a size that space-occupying disease is noted, although they may also present with a malignant peritoneal or pleural effusion, or metastatic disease. The effusion may result from oedema within the ovarian tumour or from tumour cells exfoliating through the ovarian bursa. Of the germ cell tumours, dysgerminomas have a metastatic rate of 20–30%, whilst 50% of teratomas are malignant. Most granulosa cell tumours (80%) in dogs are benign, but may be functional with secretion of oestrogen and progestagens. However, in cats 50% of granulosa cell tumours are malignant. Clinical signs for these tumours include persistent oestrus, mammary gland hyperplasia, bone marrow hyperplasia, alopecia and CEH.

Diagnosis consists of serum haematology and biochemistry profiles, ultrasound assessment of the tumour, cytology of any pleural or peritoneal effusions, and staging of the tumour using inflated thoracic radiographs or thoracic computed tomography (CT) to screen for metastases. Differentiation between granulosa cell tumours and epithelial tumours on histopathology can be difficult, but can be aided by immunohistochemistry with cytokeratin 7 found in epithelial tumours and inhibin-α found in granulosa cell tumours (Riccardi *et al.*, 2007). Treatment is by ovariectomy or ovariohysterectomy. During surgery, tumours should be packed off from the abdomen, handled gently, and the abdomen lavaged post-surgery to decrease the risk of tumour seeding. The prognosis for ovarian tumours is good if there is no evidence of metastasis.

Vagina, vestibule and vulva

There are a number of conditions that affect the vagina, vestibule and vulva, including:

- Vaginal hyperplasia
- Vaginal or cervical prolapse
- Neoplasia
- Vulval hypoplasia or juvenile genital tract with associated vulval pyoderma
- Vaginal septum
- Persistent hymen
- Annular stenosis
- Segmental aplasia
- Rectovaginal fistula.

Vaginal oedema and vaginal fold prolapse

Vaginal oedema is excessive folding compounded by fibroplasia of the vaginal floor cranial to the urethral tubercle, which occurs in the follicular phase of the cycle or occasionally during pregnancy or parturition (Schaefers-Okkens, 2001). There is a reported increased incidence in brachycephalic and large-breed dogs. Clinical signs are excessive cleaning of the exposed vaginal wall and vulva, and in severe cases there can be trauma and infection of the exposed tissue or dysuria. The hyperplasia can be graded as:

- Type 1 where there is slight to moderate eversion of the vaginal floor with no tissue extruded through the vulva
- Type 2 where there is a complete prolapse of tissue through the vulva
- Type 3 where there is a circumferential prolapse, giving the appearance of a 'doughnut'.

In many type 1 cases treatment is not required; however, in more severely affected cases, the tissue requires moistening and lubrication with a view to removing it in dioestrus unless spontaneous regression occurs. Progestagen therapy may be used to decrease the size of the hyperplasia or gonadotropin-releasing hormone used to induce ovulation. The hyperplasia will regress following oestrus unless cystic ovaries, ovarian remnants or granulosa cell tumours are present, but is very likely to recur during the next oestrous cycle unless ovariectomy or ovariohysterectomy is performed. In cases where the tissue is unable to be reduced or is necrotic, surgical resection (Figure 17.14) and ovariectomy or ovariohysterectomy are required.

Mild cases should regress in dioestrus, whilst in moderate cases the tissue should be protected and reduced manually, with closure of the vulval lips until after oestrus to prevent recurrence. Severe cases where the tissue is completely prolapsed and oedematous require surgical resection and ovariohysterectomy. The urethral papilla should be identified and catheterized prior to surgery. Ice cold sterile saline is useful to control haemorrhage during surgery and the prolapse should be sectioned and sutured a quarter section at a time to decrease haemorrhage and aid orientation. Stay sutures should be placed after the first incision to avoid the cranial wall of the vagina slipping back into its normal position until the wall has been sutured.

True vaginal prolapse

Vaginal prolapse is rare (Tobias and Johnson, 2011). It is associated with parturition and may be partial or complete; the bladder and other organs may also be involved in the prolapsed tissue. It has the typical 'doughnut' appearance of a type 3 prolapse. True vaginal prolapse is distinguished from oedema by the inability to place a lubricated finger or probe between the vaginal wall and the prolapse. Such cases are usually managed by manual reduction of the prolapse and a standard abdominal ovariohysterectomy.

Vaginal tumours

Vaginal tumours constitute about 3% of the tumours that occur in dogs and tend to be seen in older bitches with a mean age at presentation of 10 years. They are rare in cats. The majority of vaginal tumours, such as leiomyomas, fibroleiomyomas, fibromas and lipomas, are benign and occur in intact females. About 20% of vaginal and vulval tumours are malignant with adenocarcinoma, squamous cell carcinoma (Figure 17.15), transmissible venereal tumour and leiomyosarcomas reported. Transmissible venereal tumours, which are found in many European countries, are now a real risk in the UK and there are unconfirmed reports in dogs that have travelled from continental Europe.

Clinical signs of vaginal tumours consist of perineal swelling, tissue protruding through the vulva, excessive vulval attention, vulval discharge, tenesmus, dysuria or urine leakage due to pooling of urine around larger vaginal tumours. Diagnosis consists of clinical examination, including a careful vaginal and rectal examination, vaginoscopy and fine-needle aspiration or an incisional or excisional biopsy. For larger tumours, ultrasonography, retrograde vaginourethrography, CT or magnetic resonance imaging (MRI) will delineate the tumour.

Treatment consists of surgical resection ± ovariohysterectomy, depending on the type of the tumour. Transmissible venereal tumours are easily treated with chemotherapy in the form of vincristine. Leiomyomas, which may be solitary or multiple, are often pedunculated and commonly seen affecting the dorsal wall of the vagina. They are hormonally dependent and thus do not recur if the animal is neutered at the time of resection. The surgical approach is usually via an episiotomy (see Operative Technique 17.6) and often even large tumours are resectable due to the redundancy of the vaginal wall. In the case of extensive malignant tumours, more radical procedures such as vulvovaginectomy with perineal urethrostomy (Bilbrey *et al.*, 1989) or subtotal vaginectomy through an episiotomy, ventral approach or combined

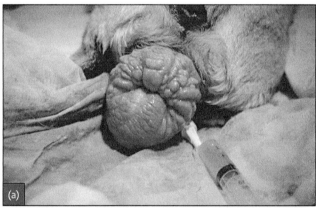
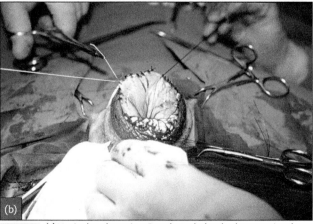

17.14 (a) Vaginal prolapse in a Pug that whelped 2 days previously. (b) Vaginal prolapse post-resection.

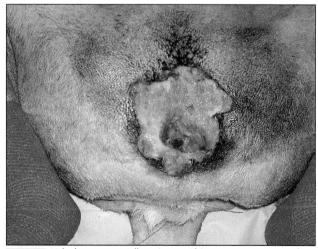

17.15 Vulval squamous cell carcinoma. This tumour was resected with 1 cm surgical margins, resulting in a perineal urethrostomy. Clean surgical margins were achieved.
(Courtesy of R Doust)

abdominal and vestibular approach (Nelissen and White, 2013) have been reported. These cases require thorough staging prior to surgery, but often have a good quality of life following radical resection.

Vulval fold pyoderma

This condition is most commonly seen in overweight or obese neutered dogs, often of large or giant breeds (Figure 17.16). These dogs usually have an infantile vulva or vulval hypoplasia, which retracts into the perineal skin folds. These redundant skin folds accumulate moisture, leading to skin fold pyoderma, vaginitis, perineal irritation and malodour. In addition, urine dribbling has been reported in these dogs due to the conformation of the vulva and overlying skin folds that act as a dam to retain urine within the vagina (Appledorn, 1990). These changes are often associated with chronic or recurrent urinary tract infection (UTI). In one study of 31 dogs with this condition, 50% had a chronic or recurrent UTI (Lightner et al., 2001).

Diagnosis is by careful examination of the vulval conformation with culture of the skin fold. Conservative medical treatment, such as weight reduction or regular cleansing of the affected perivulvar tissue, may be used as palliative therapy. However, this condition is most effectively treated by episioplasty (see Operative Technique 17.5), the aim of which is to remove the redundant skin folds dorsal and lateral to the vulva. The prognosis following surgery is good with resolution of the clinical signs and UTI occurring in >95% of reported cases.

Vaginal strictures

A variety of vaginal strictures or bands are reported in the literature, including:

- Longitudinal septa (most common)
- Annular strictures
- Persistent hymen.

Clinical signs associated with strictures include difficulty whelping or mating and, less commonly, dysuria, urinary incontinence and chronic vaginitis. Many strictures are likely to be asymptomatic and thus not reported. Diagnosis is by vaginal examination, endoscopy

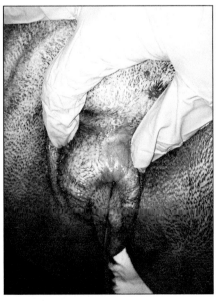

17.16 Vulval fold pyoderma in a 6-year-old neutered Newfoundland bitch.

or a retrograde vaginourethrogram. Treatment is by resection of the band or stricture, ovariohysterectomy or ovariectomy. Some bands can be broken down by digital manipulation, but more frequently episiotomy is required (Figure 17.17). Endoscopic laser ablation of the septae has also been reported with minimal complications (Burdick et al., 2014). This condition has not been shown to be hereditary in dogs, but prevalence is low. Vestibulovaginal stenosis has also been reported to cause chronic UTIs in dogs, although a study that looked at vestibulovaginal stenosis in dogs with and without lower urinary tract signs demonstrated no significant difference between the two groups as far as the vestibulovaginal ratio was concerned (Wang et al., 2006). There are reports of dogs showing improvement of urinary incontinence and infections and resolution of vaginitis after resection of the stenosis via a midline incision from the dorsal commissure of the labia to the ventral aspect of the anus.

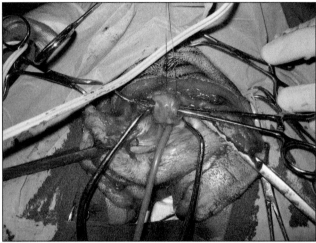

17.17 Vaginal septum (thick vertical band) approached by an episiotomy.

Rectovaginal fistulae

Rectovaginal fistulae are rare and usually congenital in origin, although traumatic rectovaginal fistulae have been reported. Clinical signs usually consist of recurrent or chronic UTIs, but vaginitis due to faecal contaminant can occur. Diagnosis is by retrograde positive contrast urethrography and endoscopy. Treatment consists of a linear midline incision ventral to the anal sphincter and identification of the fistula, which is then ligated, transected and oversewn. Identification of the fistula is aided by passing a small catheter or piece of suture material through the fistula or by injecting methylene blue through the fistula. Affected animals should not be used for breeding.

External genitalia

On occasion, the diagnosis of an intersexual condition can be made by examination of abnormal external genitalia. An os clitoris protruding from the vagina supports a tentative diagnosis of male pseudohermaphrodism. Female pseudohermaphrodites or hermaphrodites are very rare and occur less frequently than their male counterparts (Howard, 1986). These patients are often examined for evaluation of urinary incontinence or vaginal discharge; however, other presenting signs may include cryptorchism, pyometra and clitoral hypertrophy. A definitive diagnosis of intersexuality is based upon histological examination of the gonads. Objectives of management include removal of the internal genitalia and verification of a functional urinary tract. The os clitoris can be removed surgically and the external genitalia may be reconstructed for functional and cosmetic purposes. Differentiation of an os clitoris from an os penis is dependent upon identification of the urethra within the os penis, which does not occur with an os clitoris (Howard and Bjorling, 1989).

References and further reading

Adamovich-Rippe KN, Mayhew PD, Runge JJ et al. (2013) Evaluation of laparoscopic-assisted ovariohysterectomy for treatment of canine pyometra. Veterinary Surgery 42(5), 572–578

Allen WE (1986) Pseudopregnancy in the bitch: the current view of aetiology and treatment. Journal of Small Animal Practice 27, 419–424

Aronsohn MG and Faggella AM (1993) Surgical techniques for neutering 6–14 week-old kittens. Journal of the American Veterinary Medical Association 202, 53–57

Ball RL, Birchard SJ, May LR, Threlfall WR and Young GS (2010) Ovarian remnant syndrome in dogs and cats: 21 cases (2000–2007). Journal of the American Veterinary Medical Association 236, 548–553

Bartoshova A, Vitasek R, Leva L et al. (2007) Hysterectomy leads to fast improvement of haematological and immunological parameters in bitches with pyometra. Journal of Small Animal Practice 48, 564–568

Beal MW, Brown DC and Schofer FS (2000) The effects of perioperative hypothermia and the duration of anaesthesia on postoperative wound infection rate in clean wounds in a retrospective study. Veterinary Surgery 8, 89–91

Bertazzolo W, Bonfanti U, Mazzotti S et al. (2012) Cytologic features and diagnostic analysis of effusions for detection of ovarian carcinoma in dogs. Veterinary Clinical Pathology 41(1), 127–132

Bilbrey SA, Withrow SJ, Klein MK et al. (1989) Vulvovaginectomy and perineal urethrostomy for neoplasms of the vulva and vagina. Veterinary Surgery 18(6), 450–453

Breitkopf M, Hoffman B and Bostedt H (1997) Treatment of pyometra (cystic endometrial hyperplasia) in bitches with an antiprogestin. Journal of Reproduction and Fertility 51(Suppl.), 327–331

Brunschwig A, Barber HRK and Roberts S (1964) Return of renal function after varying periods of ureteral occlusion. Journal of the American Veterinary Medical Association 188, 5–8

Burdick S, Berent AC, Weisse C and Langston C (2014) Endoscopic-guided laser ablation of vestibulovaginal septal remnants in dogs: 36 cases (2007–2011) Journal of the American Veterinary Medical Association 244, 944–949

Burrows R, Batchelor D and Cripps P (2005) Complications observed during and after ovariohysterectomy of 142 bitches at a veterinary teaching hospital. Veterinary Record 157, 829–833

Burrows R, Wawra E, Pinchbeck G, Senior M and Dugdale A (2006) Prospective evaluation of postoperative pain in cats undergoing ovariohysterectomy by a midline or flank approach. Veterinary Record 158, 657–661

Coe R, Grint NJ, Tivers MS, Hotson Moore A and Holt P (2006) Comparison of flank and midline approaches to the ovariohysterectomy of cats. Veterinary Record 159, 309–313

Cooley DM, Beranek BC, Schittler DL et al. (2002) Endogenous gonadal hormone exposure and bone sarcoma risk. Cancer Epidemiology, Biomarkers and Prevalence 11, 1434–1440

Crawford JT and Adams WM (2002) Influence of vestibulovaginal stenosis, pelvic bladder and recessed vulva on response to treatment for clinical signs of lower urinary tract disease in dogs: 38 cases (1990–1999). Journal of the American Veterinary Medical Association 221, 995–999

Culp WTN, Mayhew PD and Brown DC (2009) The effect of laparoscopic versus open ovariectomy on postsurgical activity in small dogs. Veterinary Surgery 38, 811–817

Dabrowski R, Kostro K, Lisiecka U et al. (2009) Usefulness of C-reactive protein, serum amyloid A component and haptoglobin determinations in bitches with pyometra for monitoring early post-ovariohysterectomy complications. Theriogenology 72, 471–476

Davidson A, Feldman EC and Nelson RD (1992) Treatment of feline pyometra with prostaglandin F2α, 21 cases (1982–1990). Journal of the American Veterinary Medical Association 200(6), 825–828

Davidson EB, Moll HD and Payton ME (2004) Comparison of laparoscopic ovariohysterectomy and ovariohysterectomy in dogs. Veterinary Surgery 33, 62–69

Dow C (1958) The cystic hyperplasia–pyometra complex in the bitch. Veterinary Record 70, 1102–1108

Dow C (1960) Ovarian abnormalities in the bitch. Journal of Comparative Pathology 70, 59–69

Dupre G, Fiorbianco V, Skalicky M et al. (2009) Laparoscopic ovariectomy in dogs: comparison between single portal and two portal access. Veterinary Surgery 38, 818–824

Egenvall A, Hagman R, Bonnett BN et al. (2001) Breed risk of pyometra in insured dogs in Sweden. Journal of Veterinary Internal Medicine 15(6), 530–538

England GCW, Freeman SL and Russo M (2007) Treatment of spontaneous pyometra in 22 bitches with a combination of cabergoline and closprostenol. Veterinary Record 160, 293–296

Evans KM and Adams VJ (2010) Proportion of litters of purebred dogs born by Caesarean section. Journal of Small Animal Practice 51(2), 113–118

Fieni F (2006) Clinical evaluation of the use of aglepristone, with or without cloprostenol, to treat cystic endometrial hyperplasia–pyometra complex in bitches. Theriogenology 66, 1550–1556

Forsee KM, Davis GJ, Mouat EE, Salmeri KR and Bastian RP (2013) Evaluation of the prevalence of urinary incontinence in spayed female dogs: 566 cases (2003–2008). Journal of the American Veterinary Medical Association 242, 959–962

Fransson BA, Karlstam E, Bergstrom A et al. (2004) C-Reactive protein in the differentiation of pyometra from cystic endometrial hyperplasia/mucometra in dogs. Journal of the American Animal Hospital Association 40, 391–399

Gabor G, Siver L and Szenci O (1999) Intravaginal prostaglandin F2α for the treatment of metritis and pyometra in the bitch. Acta Veterinaria Hungarica 47(1), 103–108

Gelberg HB and McEntee K (1985) Feline ovarian neoplasms. Veterinary Pathology 22, 572–576

Gibson A, Dean R, Yates D and Stavisky J (2013) A retrospective study of pyometra at five RSPCA hospitals in the UK: 1728 cases from 2006 to 2011. Veterinary Record 173, doi: 10.1136/vr.101514

Gilbert RO, Nothling JO and Oettle EE (1989) A retrospective study of 40 cases of canine pyometra–metritis treated with prostaglandin F2 alpha and broad-spectrum antibacterial drugs. Journal of Reproduction and Fertility 39, 225–229

Gobello C, Baschar H, Castex G, de la Sota RL and Goya RG (2001) Dioestrous ovariectomy: a model to study the role of progesterone in the onset of canine pseudopregnancy. Journal of Reproduction and Fertility 57, 55–60

Gregory SP, Holt PE, Parkinson TJ et al. (1999) Vaginal position and length in the bitch: relationship to spaying and urinary incontinence. Journal of Small Animal Practice 40, 180–184

Grint NJ, Murison PJ, Coe R and Waterman-Pearson AE (2005) Assessment of the influence of surgical technique on postoperative pain and wound tenderness in cats following ovariohysterectomy. Journal of Feline Medicine and Surgery 8, 15–21

Gul A, Kotan C, Ugras S et al. (2000) Transverse uterine incision non-closure versus closure: an experimental study done in dogs. European Journal of Obstetrics, Gynaecology and Reproductive Biology 88, 95–99

Gunn-Moore DA and Thrusfield MV (1995) Feline dystocia: prevalence and association with cranial conformation and breed. Veterinary Record 136, 350–353

Hagman R (2012) Clinical and molecular characteristics of pyometra in female dogs. Reproduction in Domestic Animals 47, 323–325

Hagman R, Kindahl H, Fransson BA et al. (2006) Differentiation between pyometra and cystic endometrial hyperplasia/mucometra in bitches by prostaglandin F2 alpha metabolite analysis. Theriogenology 66(2), 198–206

Hammel SP and Bjorling DE (2002) Results of vulvoplasty for treatment of recessed vulva in dogs. Journal of the American Animal Hospital Association 38, 79–83

Hancock RB, Lanz O, Waldron DR et al. (2005) Comparison of postoperative pain after ovariohysterectomy by harmonic scalpel-assisted laparoscopy compared with median celiotomy and ligation in dogs. Veterinary Surgery 34, 273–282

Hayes G (2004) Asymptomatic uterine rupture in a bitch. Veterinary Record 154, 438–439

Heiene R, Kristiansen V, Teige J and Jansen JH (2007) Renal histomorphology in dogs with pyometra and control dogs, and long term clinical outcome with respect to signs of kidney disease. Acta Veterinaria Scandinavica 49(1), 13

Hosgood G (1992) Surgical and anaesthetic management of puppies and kittens. Compendium of Continuing Education for the Practicing Veterinarian 14, 345–357

Houpt KA, Coren B, Hintz HF et al. (1979) Effect of sex and reproductive status on sucrose preference, food intake and body weight of dogs. Journal of the American Veterinary Medical Association 174, 1083–1085

Joyce A and Yates D (2011) Help stop teenage pregnancy: early-age neutering in cats. Journal of Feline Medicine and Surgery 13, 3–10

Jurka P, Max A, Hawrynska K and Snochowski M (2010) Age-related pregnancy results and further examination of bitches after aglepristone treatment of pyometra. Reproduction in Domestic Animals 45, 525–529

Kenney KJ, Matthiesen DT, Brown NO and Bradley RL (1987) Pyometra in cats:183 cases (1979–1984). Journal of the American Veterinary Medical Association 191(9), 1130–1132

Kol A and Borjesson DL (2010) Application of thrombelastography/thromboelastometry to veterinary medicine. Veterinary Clinical Pathology 39(4), 405–416

Kooistra HS and Okkens AC (2001) Secretion of prolactin and growth hormone in relation to ovarian activity in the dog. Reproduction in Domestic Animals 36, 115–119

Kustritz MV (2007) Determining the optimal age for gonadectomy of dogs and cats. Journal of the American Veterinary Medical Association 231(11), 1665–1672

Kydd DM and Burnie AG (1986) Vaginal neoplasia in the bitch: a review of forty clinical cases. *Journal of Small Animal Practice* **27**, 255–263

Kyles AE, Vaden S, Hardie EM *et al.* (1996) Vestibulovaginal stenosis in dogs: 18 cases (1987–1995). *Journal of the American Veterinary Medical Association* **209**, 1889–1893

Leitch BJ, Bray JP, Kim NJG, Cann B and Lopez-Villalobos N (2012) Pedicle ligation in ovariohysterectomy: an *in vitro* study of ligation techniques. *Journal of Small Animal Practice* **53**, 592–598

LeRoux PH (1983) Thyroid status, oestradiol level, work performance and body mass of ovariectomised bitches and bitches bearing ovarian auto transplants in the stomach wall. *Journal of the South African Veterinary Association* **54**, 115–117

Lightner BA, McLoughlin MA, Chew DJ *et al.* (2001) Epsioplasty for the treatment of perivulvar dermatitis or recurrent urinary tract infections in dogs with excessive perivulvar skin folds: 31 cases (1983–2000). *Journal of the American Veterinary Medical Association* **219**, 1577–1581

Lucas X, Agit A, Ramis G *et al.* (2003) Uterine rupture in a cat. *Veterinary Record* **152**, 301–302

Luna SP, Cassu RN, Castro GB *et al.* (2004) Effects of four anaesthetic protocols on the neurological and cardiorespiratory variables of puppies born by Caesarean section. *Veterinary Record* **154(13)**, 387–389

Magne ML, Hoopes PJ, Kainer RA *et al.* (1985) Urinary tract carcinomas involving the canine vagina and vestibule. *Journal of the American Animal Hospital Association* **21**, 767–772

Manassero M, Leperlier D, Vallefuoco R and Viateau V (2012) Laparoscopic ovariectomy in dogs using a single-port multiple-access device. *Veterinary Record* doi: 10.1136/vr.100060

Manothaiudom K and Johnston K (1991) Clinical approach to vaginal/vestibular masses in the bitch. *Veterinary Clinics of North America: Small Animal Practice* **21(3)**, 509–521

Marcella KL, Ramirez M and Hammerslag ML (1985) Segmental aplasia of the uterine horn in a cat. *Journal of the American Veterinary Medical Association* **186**, 179–181

Matthews KA (2005) Analgesia for the pregnant, lactating and neonatal to pediatric cat and dog. *Journal of Veterinary Emergency and Critical Care* **15**, 273–284

May S (2012) The flank cat spay: eminence–driven fashions in veterinary surgery. *Veterinary Record* **170**, 450–461

McIntyre RL, Levy JK, Roberts JF *et al.* (2010) Developmental uterine anomalies in cats and dogs undergoing elective ovariohysterectomy. *Journal of the American Veterinary Medical Association* **237(5)**, 542–546

Meyers Wallen MH and Goldschmidt Flickinger GL (1986) Prostaglandin F2α treatment of canine pyometra. *Journal of the American Veterinary Medical Association* **189**, 1557–1561

Miller MA, Ramos-Vara JA, Dickerson MF *et al.* (2003) Uterine neoplasia in 13 cats. *Journal of Veterinary Diagnostic Investigation* **15**, 515–522

Moon PF, Erb HN and Ludders JW (2000) Perioperative risk factors for puppies delivered by Caesarean section in the United States and Canada. *Journal of the American Animal Hospital Association* **36**, 359–368

Moon PF, Erb HN, Ludders JW *et al.* (1998) Perioperative management and mortality rates of dogs undergoing Caesarean section in the United States and Canada. *Journal of the American Veterinary Medical Association* **213**, 365–369

Moon-Massat PF and Erb HN (2002) Perioperative factors associated with puppy vigour after delivery by Caesarean section. *Journal of the American Animal Hospital Association* **38**, 90–96

Nakamura K, Yamasaki M, Osaki T *et al.* (2012) Bilateral segmental aplasia with unilateral uterine horn torsion in a Pomeranian bitch. *Journal of the American Animal Hospital Association* **48**, 327–330

Nelissen P and White RAS (2012) Subtotal vaginectomy for management of extensive vaginal disease in 11 dogs. *Veterinary Surgery* **41**, 495–500

O'Farrell V and Peachey E (1990) Behavioural effects of ovariohysterectomy on bitches. *Journal of Small Animal Practice* **31**, 595–598

Öhlund M, Hoglund O, Olsson U and Lagerstedt AS (2011) Laparoscopic ovariectomy in dogs: a comparison of the LigaSure™ and the Sonosurg™ systems. *Journal of Small Animal Practice* **52**, 290–294

Okkens AC, Kooistra HS and Nickel RF (1997) Comparison of long-term effects of ovariectomy *versus* ovariohysterectomy in bitches. *Journal of Reproduction and Fertility* **51**, 227–231

Overly B, Shofer FS, Goldscmidt MH *et al.* (2005) Association between ovariohysterectomy and feline mammary carcinoma. *Journal of Veterinary Internal Medicine* **19**, 560–563

Peeters ME and Kirpensteijn J (2011) Comparison of surgical variables and short-term post-operative complications in healthy dogs undergoing ovariohysterectomy or ovariectomy. *Journal of the American Veterinary Medical Association* **238**, 189–194

Pollari FL and Bonnett BN (1996) Evaluation of postoperative complications following elective surgeries of dogs and cats at private practices using computer records. *Canadian Veterinary Journal* **37**, 672–678

Potter K, Hancock DH and Gallina AM (1991) Clinical and pathologic features of endometrial hyperplasia, pyometra, and endometritis in cats: 79 cases (1980–1985). *Journal of the American Veterinary Medical Association* **198**, 1427–1431

Prymak C, McKee LJ, Goldschmidt MH *et al.* (1988) Epidemiologic, clinical, pathological and prognostic characteristics of splenic haemangiosarcoma and splenic haematoma in dogs: 217 cases (1985). *Journal of the American Veterinary Medical Association* **193**, 706–712

Ramsey I (2014) *BSAVA Small Animal Formulary, 8th edn.* BSAVA Publications, Gloucester

Reichler IM (2009) Gonadectomy in cats and dogs: a review of risks and benefits. *Reproduction of Domestic Animals* **44(Suppl. 2)**, 29–35

Reichler IM, Pfeiffer E, Piche CA *et al.* (2005) Changes in plasma gonadotrophin concentrations and urethral closure pressure in the bitch during 12 months following ovariectomy. *Theriogenology* **63**, 1391–1402

Riccardi E, Greco V, Verganti S *et al.* (2007) Immunohistochemical diagnosis of canine ovarian epithelial and granulosa cell tumours. *Journal of Veterinary Diagnostic Investigation* **19**, 431–435

Robbins MA and Mullen HS (1994) En bloc ovariohysterectomy as a treatment for dystocia in dogs and cats. *Veterinary Surgery* **23**, 48–52

Rogers KS, Walker MA and Dillon HB (1998) Transmissible venereal tumor: a retrospective study of 29 cases. *Journal of the American Animal Hospital Association* **34**, 463–470

Root MV, Johnston SD and Johnstom GR (1995) Vaginal septa in dogs: 15 cases (1983–1992). *Journal of the American Veterinary Medical Association* **206**, 56–58

Root Kustritz MV (2012) Effects of surgical sterilization on canine and feline health and on society. *Reproduction in Domestic Animals* **47**, 214–222

Runge J, Curcillo PG, King SA *et al.* (2012) Initial application of reduced port surgery using the single port access technique for laparoscopic canine ovariectomy. *Veterinary Surgery* **41**, 803–806

Salomon JF, Gouriou M, Dutot E, Borenstein N and Combrisson H (2006) Experimental study of urodynamic changes after ovariectomy in 10 dogs. *Veterinary Record* **159**, 807–811

Schaefers-Okkens AC (2001) Vaginal edema and vaginal fold prolapse in the bitch, including surgical management. In: *Recent Advances in Small Animal Reproduction*, ed. PW Concannon *et al.* International Veterinary Information Service, New York

Schalfer DS (2012) Diseases of the canine uterus. *Reproduction in Domestic Animals* **47(Suppl. 6)**, 318–322

Schneider R, Dorn CR and Taylor DON (1969) Factors influencing canine mammary cancer development and postsurgical survival. *Journal of the National Cancer Institute* **43**, 1249–1261

Seymour C and Duke-Novakovski T (2007) *BSAVA Manual of Canine and Feline Anaesthesia and Analgesia, 2nd edn.* BSAVA Publications, Gloucester

Spain CV, Scarlett JM and Houpt KA (2004) Long term risks and benefits of early age gonadectomy in cats. *Journal of the American Veterinary Medical Association* **224**, 372–379

Spain CV, Scarlett JM and Houpt KA (2004) Long term risks and benefits of early age gonadectomy in dogs. *Journal of the American Veterinary Medical Association* **224**, 380–387

Taylor P (2002) Techniques for neutering kittens. *FAB Journal* **40**, 22–24

Thacher C and Bradley RL (1983) Vulvar and vaginal tumours in the bitch: a retrospective study. *Journal of the American Veterinary Medical Association* **183**, 690–692

Tobias K and Johnson S (2011) *Veterinary Surgery: Small Animal.* Saunders, Philadelphia

Traas AM (2008) Surgical management of canine and feline dystocia. *Theriogenology* **70**, 337–342

Van Goethem B, Schaefers-Okkens A and Kirpensteijn J (2006) Making a rational choice between ovariectomy and ovariohysterectomy in the dog: a discussion of the benefits of either technique. *Veterinary Surgery* **35**, 136–143

Van Haaften B and Taverne MAM (1989) Sonographic diagnosis of a mucometra in a cat. *Veterinary Record* **124**, 346–347

Van Nimwegen SA and Kirpensteijn J (2007) Comparison of Nd:YAG surgical laser and Remorgida bipolar electrosurgery forceps for canine laparoscopic ovariectomy. *Veterinary Surgery* **36**, 533–540

Verstegen J, Dhaliwal G and Verstegen-Onclin K (2008) Mucometra, cystic endometrial hyperplasia and pyometra in the bitch: advances in treatment and assessment of future reproductive success. *Theriogenology* **70**, 364–374

Volpato R, Rodello L, Abibe RB and Lopes MD (2012) Lactate in bitches with pyometra. *Reproduction in Domestic Animals* **47(6)**, 335–336

Wang KY, Samii VF, Chew DJ *et al.* (2006) Vestibular, vaginal and urethral relationships in spayed and intact normal dogs. *Theriogenology* **66**, 726–735

Wang KY, Samii VF, Chew DJ *et al.* (2006) Vestibular, vaginal and urethral relationships in spayed dogs with and without lower urinary tract signs. *Journal of Veterinary Internal Medicine* **20**, 1065–1073

Ware WA and Hopper DL (1999) Cardiac tumours in dogs: 1982–1995. *Journal of Veterinary Internal Medicine* **13**, 95–103

Whitehead ML (2008) Risk of pyometra in bitches treated for mismating with low doses of oestradiol benzoate. *Veterinary Record* **162**, 746–749

Yuri K, Nakata K, Katae H *et al.* (1999) Distribution of uropathogenic factors among Escherichia coli strains isolated from dogs and cats. *Journal of Veterinary Medical Science* **60**, 287–290

Zink CM, Farhoody P, Elser SE *et al.* (2014) Evaluation of the risk and age of onset of cancer and behavioral disorders in gonadectomized Vizslas. *Journal of the American Veterinary Medical Association* **244**, 309–319

OPERATIVE TECHNIQUE 17.1

Canine ovariohysterectomy

PREOPERATIVE PLANNING

Express the bladder prior to the procedure.

POSITIONING

Dorsal recumbency.

ASSISTANT

A scrubbed assistant can be useful in larger bitches to improve exposure.

EQUIPMENT EXTRAS

Self-retaining abdominal retractors (an ultrasonic or bipolar vessel-sealing device can be used for this procedure if available).

SURGICAL TECHNIQUE

Ovariohysterectomy, although a routine surgery, can be a difficult procedure, particularly in deep-chested or obese dogs. For inexperienced surgeons it is advisable to perform the surgery on several smaller breed dogs and young animals before tackling the more challenging breeds.

Approach

* Make a midline coeliotomy incision from 1–2 cm cranial to the umbilicus towards the pubis (this should extend to at least the proximal third (or longer) of the distance between the two points). The incision made with the scalpel will be approximately 4–8 cm, depending on the size and conformation of the bitch and the experience of the surgeon. Continue this through the subcutaneous tissue.
* Locate the linea alba and tent it outwards and make a stab incision into the abdominal cavity.
* Extend the incision in the linea alba with Mayo scissors.

Surgical manipulations

1 Locate the right uterine horn with a finger by following the body wall down into the gutter, distal to the kidney.

2 Place a clamp on the proper ligament of the ovary and break the suspensory ligament with a finger/thumb or dry swab as far cranially as possible to avoid traumatizing the ovarian pedicle.

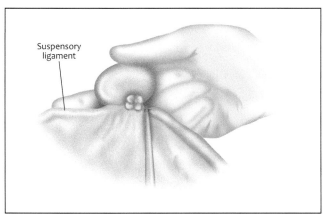

Ovary retracted whilst suspensory ligament is stretched/ruptured.

Suspensory ligament

3 Bluntly make a window in the mesovarium caudal to the ovarian vessels.

→ **OPERATIVE TECHNIQUE 17.1 CONTINUED**

4 Triple clamp the ovarian pedicle, if possible, with Rochester–Carmalt or Kelly forceps. If it is not possible to triple clamp the pedicle, two clamps can be placed on the pedicle and one on the proper ligament between the ovary and uterine horn.

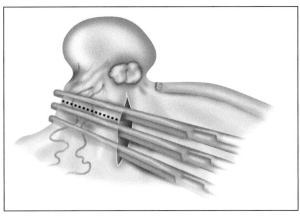

Ovarian pedicle (containing the ovarian artery and vein), with three clamps placed below the ovary. The dashed line shows the level of transection.

5 Remove the clamp most distant to the ovary and place a ligature of absorbable suture material in the groove of the clamp. A sliding knot or single/double other side knot is most secure; a transfixing ligature may also be used.

6 Place a second ligature proximal to the initial ligature.

7 Sever the pedicle between the two remaining clamps.

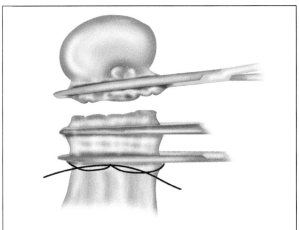
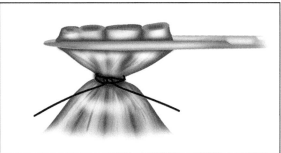

Ligature placed and tied in crush mark created by proximal clamp.

8 Remove the remaining clamp on the pedicle and gently holding the fat of the pedicle with a pair of forceps, allow the pedicle to return to the dorsal abdomen.

9 Check for bleeding, release the pedicle and check again for any bleeding.

10 Tear the broad ligament; in patients with a vascular broad ligament ligate the broad ligament before cutting it.

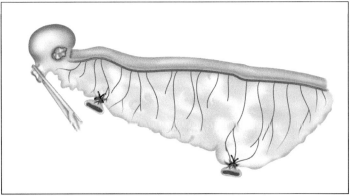

Broad ligament broken down and 'bunch' ligated if vascular.

→ **OPERATIVE TECHNIQUE 17.1 CONTINUED**

11 Repeat the procedure on the left ovarian pedicle and broad ligament.

12 Place three clamps on the uterine body, just cranial to the cervix.

13 Sever the uterine body between the proximal and middle clamps.

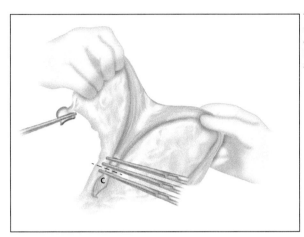

Three clamps applied to uterine body, immediately distal to the cervix (C). Dashed line indicates amputation site.

14 In older multiparous bitches or in cases of pyometra, ligate the uterine arteries separately just cranial to the most caudal clamp.

15 Remove the caudal clamp and ligate the uterine body in the groove that remains.

16 In younger animals, avascular clamps are not required and the uterine body and arteries can be ligated together with a transfixing ligature.

17 Grasp the uterine pedicle with forceps and remove the remaining clamp, replace the pedicle in the abdomen and observe for any haemorrhage.

18 Incise both ovarian bursas and check that the whole ovary has been removed.

19 Check both ovarian pedicles for haemorrhage prior to closure, using the mesocolon to check the left pedicle and the mesoduodenum to check the right pedicle.

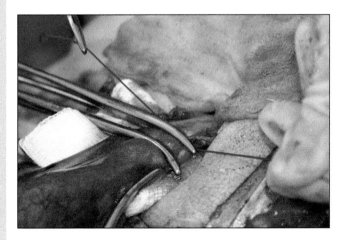

Wound closure

* Swab count prior to closure.
* Close the linea alba with absorbable sutures in a continuous pattern. The subcutaneous tissue should be closed with a continuous suture pattern and the skin can be closed with intradermal sutures, skin staples or skin sutures.

POSTOPERATIVE MANAGEMENT AND COMPLICATIONS

* Lead restriction for 10–14 days with a phased return to activity.
* Ligatures slipping, infection, stump pyometra, pedicle ligature rejection and wound dehiscence are the most common postoperative complications.

OPERATIVE TECHNIQUE 17.2

Canine ovariectomy

Express the bladder prior to the procedure.

Dorsal recumbency.

A scrubbed assistant can be useful in larger bitches to improve exposure.

Self-retaining abdominal retractors (an ultrasonic or bipolar vessel-sealing device can be used for this procedure if available).

Approach

Make the skin incision at the umbilicus.

Surgical manipulations

1   Follow the technique for canine ovariohysterectomy (see Operative Technique 17.1) to locate the ovaries.

2   Place a clamp on the proper ligament of the ovary to apply caudal traction and break the suspensory ligament with a finger/thumb or dry swab as cranially as possible to avoid traumatizing the ovarian pedicle.

3   Bluntly make a window in the mesovarium caudal to the ovarian vessels.

4   Triple clamp the ovarian pedicle, if possible, with Rochester–Carmalt or Kelly forceps. If it is not possible to triple clamp the pedicle, two clamps can be placed on the pedicle and one on the proper ligament between the ovary and uterine horn.

5   Remove the clamp most distant to the ovary and place a ligature of absorbable suture material in the groove of the clamp. A sliding knot or single/double other side knot is most secure; a transfixing ligature may also be used.

6   Place a second ligature proximal to the initial ligature.

7   Sever the pedicle between the two remaining clamps.

8   Remove the remaining clamp on the pedicle and gently holding the fat of the pedicle with a pair of forceps allow the pedicle to return to the dorsal abdomen.

9   Check for bleeding, release the pedicle and check again for any bleeding.

10 Place a clamp across the proper ligament, including the uterine artery and vein.

11 Move this clamp further cranially and tie a ligature around the artery and vein in the crush groove from the clamp.

12 Sever the uterine horn just cranial to the clamp.

13 Hold the uterine horn, remove the last clamp and check for haemorrhage.

14 Repeat the procedure on the left ovarian pedicle.

15 Incise both ovarian bursae and check the whole ovary has been removed.

→ **OPERATIVE TECHNIQUE 17.2 CONTINUED**

Wound closure

- Swab count prior to closure.
- Close the linea alba with absorbable sutures in a continuous pattern. The subcutaneous tissue should be closed with a continuous suture pattern and the skin can be closed with intradermal sutures, skin staples or skin sutures.

POSTOPERATIVE MANAGEMENT AND COMPLICATIONS

- Lead restriction for 10–14 days with a phased return to activity.
- Ligatures slipping, infection, stump pyometra, pedicle ligature rejection and wound dehiscence are the most common postoperative complications.

OPERATIVE TECHNIQUE 17.3

Feline ovariohysterectomy

POSITIONING

Feline ovariohysterectomy can be performed from either a ventral midline approach or a left flank incision. For the flank approach, the cat should be positioned in right lateral recumbency with the hindlimbs tied caudally.

ASSISTANT

Not usually required.

EQUIPMENT EXTRAS

None.

SURGICAL TECHNIQUE

Approach: flank

The cat is placed in right lateral recumbency with the legs gently extended and secured with ties.

Surgical manipulations

1   Make a 2 cm vertical incision (extended or shortened as necessary depending on surgeon experience) with a scalpel where an equilateral triangle would be bounded by a line dropped down from the cranial iliac wing, the greater trochanter and the centre point of the incision.

2   Incise the skin, subcutaneous fat, three layers of the abdominal wall and peritoneum.

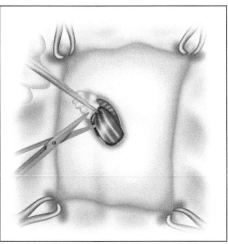

Subcutaneous fat is excised to expose the underlying muscles.

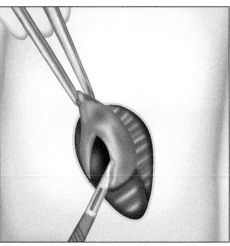

Incision through external abdominal oblique, internal abdominal oblique and rectus abdominis muscles, using a No. 15 scalpel blade.

→ **OPERATIVE TECHNIQUE 17.3 CONTINUED**

3   Identify the left uterine horn by feeling along the body wall with a finger. Avoid disrupting the fat pad dorsal to the bladder.

4   Ligate the ovarian pedicle in the manner described in Operative Technique 17.1 after disrupting the suspensory ligament.

5   Locate the right uterine horn by pulling the left uterine horn cranially and laterally and ligate the ovarian pedicle.

6   Ligate the uterine body with a transfixing suture (see Operative Technique 17.1).

7   Close the body wall in a single layer with absorbable suture material and close the subcutaneous tissue and skin routinely.

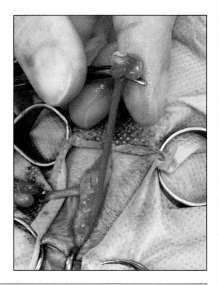

Editors' note:

An alternative to the flank approach described above is as follows:

1. Identify the wing of the ileum and make an incision 1-2 cm long through the skin and subcutaneous tissue approximately 2 cm below the wing of the ileum.
2. Excise the underlying subcutaneous fat.
3. Incise through the external abdominal oblique, internal abdominal oblique and rectus abdominis muscles, with either a No. 15 scalpel blade or Metzenbaum scissors.
4. Once in the peritoneum, differentiate between the white omental fat and the yellow sublumbar fat.
5. Grasp the yellow sublumbar fat with fine thumb forceps and gently lift it dorsally. This will exteriorize the left uterine horn.
6. Perforate the broad ligament and gently apply traction to exteriorize the left ovary.
7. Ligate the ovarian pedicle using absorbable suture material.
8. Pull the left uterine horn caudally to locate the bifurcation and the right uterine horn. Excise the right ovary in the same manner as the left ovary.
9. Ligate the uterine body as close to the cervix as possible. It may be necessary to transfix the uterus in mature cats or those in oestrus.
10. Close the laparotomy wounds routinely.

Approach: midline

Cats require a more cranial incision than dogs (see Operative Technique 17.1) for the midline approach to ovariohysterectomy.

Surgical manipulations

PRACTICAL TIP

Cats may only require two mosquito haemostats to be placed on the ovarian pedicle. The uterine body and cervix are often more friable in the cat, particularly at oestrus or in early pregnancy and haemostats should be placed with care. With particularly turgid uterine horns, it is safer and better practice to ligate the uterine body without prior placement of clamps

POSTOPERATIVE MANAGEMENT AND COMPLICATIONS

*   Keep the cat indoors and limit jumping activity for 10 days.
*   Infection, stump pyometra, pedicle ligature rejection (fistulous tract formation) and wound dehiscence are the most common postoperative complications.

OPERATIVE TECHNIQUE 17.4

Caesarean section

POSITIONING

Dorsal recumbency with the ventral abdomen clipped, prepared and draped from the xiphoid to the pubis. Tilting the surgical table so that the head is slightly higher than the feet helps relieve respiratory compromise due to the weight of the gravid uterus on the diaphragm.

ASSISTANT

Surgical assistants are optional. Non-sterile personnel are required to resuscitate and tend to the neonates.

EQUIPMENT EXTRAS

Electrocautery; laparotomy swabs; suction; incubator or warm towels and a hot water bottle in a box for the neonates.

SURGICAL TECHNIQUE

Approach

Ventral midline skin incision, extending from cranial to the umbilicus to just cranial to the pubis.

Surgical manipulations: hysterotomy

1 Make an incision from the umbilicus to the pubis, taking care only to incise the stretched linea alba and not damage the gravid uterus.

2 Exteriorize the uterine horns and pack off the remainder of the abdomen with laparotomy swabs.

3 Make an incision in the body of the uterus if a fetus is lodged in the vagina, or in one or both uterine horns depending on the location and number of fetuses.

4 Extend the incision with Metzenbaum scissors and gently 'milk' the fetuses out of the uterus.

5 Clamp the umbilical cord and pass the fetus to an assistant for revival and clearing of the airway.

6 If possible, use gentle traction to detach the placental membranes once the fetus has been removed. If the membranes are tightly adhered, leave them in place and administer oxytocin at the end of the procedure to encourage involution and membrane separation.

7 Inspect the uterus, cervix and proximal vagina carefully to identify and removed any further fetuses.

8 Close the uterine incision using a single or double layered closure (appositional suture patterns are suitable).

9 Lavage the abdomen.

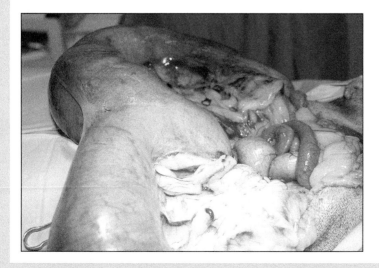

➜ **OPERATIVE TECHNIQUE 17.4 CONTINUED**

Surgical manipulations: *en bloc* ovariohysterectomy

An *en bloc* ovariohysterectomy can be used when further litters are not desired, where the fetuses are not in distress, if the bitch or queen is unstable, or the uterine contents are contaminated.

1 Make a coeliotomy incision from the umbilicus to the pubis.

2 Gently palpate the uterus and 'milk' any fetuses stuck in the vagina back into the uterus, if possible.

3 Double clamp the cervix and the ovarian pedicles.

4 Sever the tissue between the clamps and pass the uterus and ovaries to an assistant. The time from clamping the cervix and ovarian pedicles to removal of the uterus should be <30 seconds. The assistant should extract and revive the fetuses.

5 Ligate the ovarian pedicles and uterine arteries.

6 Ligate the cervix.

7 Lavage the abdomen.

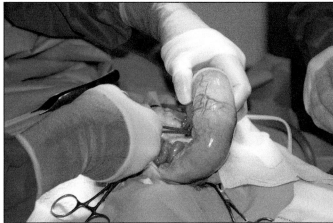

(Courtesy of J Hall)

Wound closure

Close the coeliotomy routinely using intradermal skin closure or tissue glue, if possible, to avoid the neonates disrupting skin sutures.

POSTOPERATIVE CARE OF THE NEONATES

- Clear the nasopharynx of the neonate by gently swinging its head in a downward direction or by suctioning the nares. Gentle rubbing and drying will stimulate respiration. If needed, a drop of doxapram may be placed sublingually to stimulate respiration.
- Keep the neonates warm while the dam is recovering from anaesthesia.
- The dam should be returned to the neonates as soon as she has recovered from the anaesthetic.
- The owner should monitor the dam closely for signs of uterine haemorrhage over the next 24–48 hours and ensure that all the litter are suckling.

OPERATIVE TECHNIQUE 17.5

Episioplasty

POSITIONING

Perineal stand (see Figure 8.11) with pelvic limbs positioned over the end of a well-padded table. Place a purse-string suture around the anus prior to surgery to avoid faecal contamination of the surgical field.

ASSISTANT

Not required.

EQUIPMENT EXTRAS

Electrocautery; skin marker; self-retaining retractor (Gelpi).

SURGICAL TECHNIQUE

Approach

Two concentric crescent-shaped incisions lateral and dorsal to the vulva are made to excise redundant skin and underlying subcutaneous tissues.

Surgical manipulations

1 Make two crescent-shaped incisions in the perivulvar skin, the first beginning lateral to the ventral commissure and extending in an arch dorsal to the vulva, ending at the contralateral commissure.

2 The second incision should be parallel to the first but in a wider arch. The depth of skin to be resected can be determined by making the first incision and then pulling the skin dorsally and laterally until the folds have been removed, marking the skin at this level, and then using this mark as a guide for the second incision.

3 Resect the crescent-shaped section of skin and subcutaneous tissue between the two incisions.

Wound closure

Close the subcutaneous tissue and skin in separate layers.

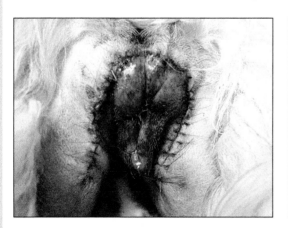 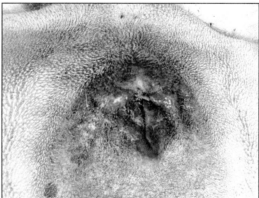

POSTOPERATIVE MANAGEMENT AND COMPLICATIONS

A buster/Elizabethan collar is advised.

OPERATIVE TECHNIQUE 17.6

Episiotomy

POSITIONING

Perineal stand (see Figure 8.11) with pelvic limbs positioned over the end of a well-padded table. Place a purse-string suture around the anus prior to surgery to avoid faecal contamination of the surgical field.

ASSISTANT

Not required.

EQUIPMENT EXTRAS

Electrocautery; skin marker; vaginal speculum; self-retaining retractors (Gelpi).

SURGICAL TECHNIQUE

Approach

Midline incision dorsal to the vulva extending from the vulvar opening through the vestibular wall. The dorsal margin of the incision should remain 1–2 cm ventral to the anus to avoid the external sphincter muscle.

Surgical manipulations

1 Make a midline skin incision from the dorsal commissure of the vulva to below the anus.

2 Place Doyen bowel clamps either side of the incision to decrease haemorrhage.

3 Extend the incision through the subcutaneous tissue, muscle layers and dorsal wall of the vagina.

4 Use ice cold saline to control any haemorrhage.

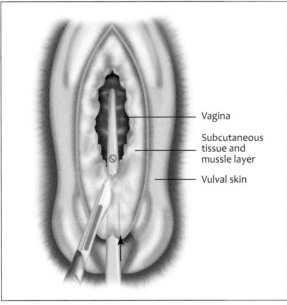

Vagina

Subcutaneous tissue and mussle layer

Vulval skin

Episiotomy incision. The dorsoventral incision begins 1–2 cm ventral to the anus and extends to include the dorsal vulvar commissure (arrowed). The incision is continued through the subcutaneous and muscle tissue layers, entering the vaginal wall.

Wound closure

Following resection of vaginal tumours or septae, close the episiotomy incision with absorbable sutures in a three-layer closure.

POSTOPERATIVE MANAGEMENT AND COMPLICATIONS

To avoid self-mutilation a buster/Elizabethan collar is advised until suture removal.

Chapter 18

Peritonitis

Lori Ludwig

Aetiology

Peritonitis is inflammation of the abdominal cavity that can occur spontaneously or as a result of pre-existing intra-abdominal pathology or penetration of the body wall. Peritonitis can be classified as primary or secondary, localized or generalized, and aseptic or septic. Primary peritonitis occurs without an obvious source of contamination and is thought to result from haematogenous spread of microorganisms. Feline infectious peritonitis is the most common example of primary peritonitis in small animals.

In most cases, peritonitis is secondary, resulting from disruption of the abdominal cavity or as a sequel to an intra-abdominal disease process. Sterile, mechanical or chemical irritation of the peritoneal surfaces results in aseptic peritonitis. The talcum powder from surgical gloves, barium sulphate, sterile foreign objects, urine, bile, pancreatic enzymes and gastric acid are all substances that can incite an inflammatory response when in contact with the peritoneal membranes. The degree of inflammation is dependent on the chemical and the length of time that it is in contact with the peritoneum. Bile, pancreatic enzymes and barium produce intense peritoneal irritation, whereas urine and blood cause minimal inflammation.

Septic peritonitis most commonly results from gastro-intestinal (GI) rupture, perforation or dehiscence. Penetrating trauma from bite wounds, stab wounds, gunshot wounds and foreign bodies can cause GI perforation. Blunt trauma can cause mesenteric avulsion with ischaemic injury to the GI tract and resulting necrosis. Ischaemic injury may also result from thromboembolism or mesenteric volvulus. Other causes of GI perforation include rupture of intestinal masses, gastric dilatation and volvulus with stomach rupture, and GI ulceration.

> **WARNING**
>
> GI ulceration is often secondary to the administration of corticosteroids or non-steroidal anti-inflammatory drugs (NSAIDs)

Intestinal dehiscence occurs in 7–15.7% of patients after GI surgery and may be more likely to occur when the procedure is associated with a traumatic injury or foreign body entrapment (Wylie and Hosgood, 1994). Additional factors that may be associated with dehiscence include the presence of preoperative peritonitis and hypoalbuminaemia (Ralphs et al., 2003). Septic peritonitis can also result from an abscessed abdominal organ (e.g. ruptured prostatic, hepatic, splenic, pancreatic or renal abscess) and leakage of infected urine or bile into the peritoneum. Rarely, fungal peritonitis caused by Candida spp. has been reported in dogs (Rogers et al., 2009; Bradford et al., 2013). Risk factors include peritoneal contamination with GI or biliary contents, inflamed intestinal mucosa, antimicrobial administration and immunosuppression. Chemical peritonitis may initially be sterile but become septic as a result of bacterial translocation. Patients with pyometra can develop septic peritonitis if the uterus ruptures due to over-distension, abdominal compression, or penetration with a needle during cystocentesis or abdominocentesis. Infected uterine contents can also leak out of the oviducts if the uterus is severely distended (see Chapter 17). Sclerosing encapsulating peritonitis is a rare form of peritonitis in which the abdominal organs become encased in a thick layer of collagenous connective tissue that resembles a cocoon; histology reveals marked peritoneal and serosal fibrosis. The aetiology is often unknown, but steatitis, ingestion of fibreglass, chylous and biliary effusions (Figure 18.1), leishmaniosis and bacterial contamination have been reported to be potential causes.

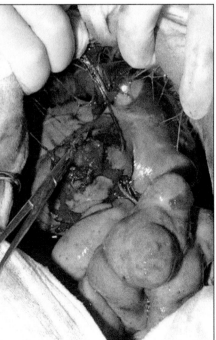

18.1 Sclerosing peritonitis resulting from a biliary effusion. It is difficult to identify any normal abdominal organs, owing to the thick fibrous covering.

Pathophysiology

In patients with peritonitis, vasodilatation and increased capillary permeability result in leakage of fluid and plasma proteins into the abdomen. Diaphragmatic lymphatics that normally function to return peritoneal fluid to the systemic circulation can no longer function as they become blocked by fibrin that is deposited in an effort to contain the contamination. If the patient is anorexic, vomiting or has diarrhoea, additional fluid and protein losses occur. The resulting hypovolaemia leads to decreased cardiac output, poor tissue perfusion, cellular hypoxia and cell death. Ischaemia and inflammation may result in compromise of the intestinal mucosa and allow bacterial translocation. Activation of macrophages and monocytes causes release of tumour necrosis factor-alpha (TNF-α), interleukins, platelet-activating factor, prostaglandins, thromboxanes, leucotrienes, free radicals and proteases. Neutrophils release proteases and endotoxins as they kill bacteria in the peritoneal fluid. The response of the body to this cascade of inflammatory mediators is peripheral vasodilatation, increased vascular permeability, decreased cardiac function and activation of the coagulation cascade. This systemic inflammatory response syndrome (SIRS) eventually leads to failure of the lungs, liver, kidneys and heart, resulting in death of the patient.

Diagnosis

A detailed and accurate history can provide many clues about the potential cause of peritonitis. The owner should be questioned about previous and current medical conditions, duration of clinical signs, whether or not the patient is neutered, if the patient is on medications (especially those that may cause GI ulceration) and whether there is a history of recent surgery. Additional information including the presence of GI signs and the possibility of trauma and foreign body ingestion should be obtained.

Clinical signs

Clinical signs in patients with peritonitis range from mild to severe and are often non-specific. They include:

- Anorexia/depression
- Vomiting
- Diarrhoea
- Dehydration
- Abdominal enlargement due to peritoneal effusion
- Tachypnoea and respiratory distress secondary to marked abdominal effusion
- Serosanguineous or purulent fluid dripping from a previous surgical wound
- Abdominal pain
- Lack of intestinal sounds on auscultation
- Progressive signs of shock (e.g. severe tachycardia, weak pulses, prolonged capillary refill time, pale mucous membranes).

A study of gastroduodenal perforation found that shock and acute collapse were uncommon signs at presentation (Hinton et al., 2002). Patients with bile peritonitis often have vague signs and presentation to the hospital may be delayed for several days or weeks, especially if the effusion is sterile.

> **WARNING**
>
> Patients with uroabdomen may still urinate and not show evidence of severe illness for 1–3 days

Physical examination

Physical examination often reveals abdominal tenderness that may be localized to the affected area in dogs. Cats with septic peritonitis rarely show signs of abdominal pain on palpation (Parsons et al., 2009). When pain is elicited in a dog or cat, careful distinction must be made between abdominal pain and pain from extra-abdominal sources, such as referred back pain. Animals with abdominal pain may splint on palpation or take a 'prayer position', with their sternum on the ground and hindquarters in the air. Abdominal palpation and ballottement can reveal free fluid or tympany associated with gas-distended bowel loops or pneumoperitoneum. Attention should be paid to the presence of organomegaly or palpable abdominal masses. An ocular examination may reveal signs of uveitis (aqueous flare, intraocular fibrin, miosis and low intraocular pressure) in septic patients and has been reported in cats with septic peritonitis (Pumphrey et al., 2011). An oral examination should include evaluation of mucous membrane colour, presence of ulcerations or petechiae, and examination under the tongue for a string foreign body. Rectal palpation may reveal ingested foreign material, melaena, haematochezia, prostatomegaly and masses or uroliths in the pelvic urethra. Females should be evaluated for vaginal discharge. Dogs with septic peritonitis are often tachycardic and tachypnoeic and may be hypo- or hyperthermic. In contrast, cats with septicaemia are often bradycardic. Figure 18.2 details the physical examination and laboratory findings in dogs and cats with septic peritonitis.

Parameter	Cats	Dogs
Abdominal palpation	No pain elicited	Usually painful
Heart rate	Tachycardia or bradycardia (>225 or <140 beats per minute)	Tachycardia (>80–120 beats per minute)
Serum glucose concentration	Low, normal or high	Normal or low
Red blood cell count	Often low	Low, normal or high
Blood to fluid lactate concentration difference	Not diagnostic	May be diagnostic

18.2 Differences in physical examination and laboratory findings between dogs and cats with septic peritonitis.

The history and physical examination determine the next step that should be taken for diagnosis. If patients have obvious free fluid on physical examination, abdominocentesis should be performed immediately. If the history suggests foreign body ingestion or trauma, or if the patient is tympanic on abdominal palpation, abdominal radiography is indicated. Life-threatening hypovolaemic shock should be treated prior to diagnostic imaging.

> **PRACTICAL TIP**
>
> Abdominocentesis is the most specific test for peritonitis

Haematology and biochemistry

In patients that are severely compromised, haematocrit, total protein, blood glucose and electrolyte concentrations will guide initial treatment and may aid in the diagnosis of peritonitis.

* An increased haematocrit and total protein suggest dehydration.
* In patients with acute haemorrhage, decreased total protein may be seen before a decrease in the haematocrit, due to splenic contraction and volume depletion.
* Patients with septic peritonitis are often hypoproteinaemic and hypoglycaemic.
* Hyperkalaemia in a patient with trauma should make the clinician suspicious of urine leakage.
* Most patients with biliary effusions will have icteric serum.

A complete blood cell count and serum chemistry panel should be performed in patients suspected of having peritonitis. An increase or decrease in the white blood cell count with an increase in the band neutrophil count suggests inflammation or sepsis.

> **WARNING**
>
> If an increasing band neutrophil count is found 4–6 days after intestinal surgery, dehiscence should be suspected

The serum chemistry panel may be helpful for determining the cause of peritonitis:

* Total bilirubin and liver enzyme concentrations are usually increased in cases of bile peritonitis
* Blood urea nitrogen, creatinine and potassium may be increased in cases of urinary obstruction, uroperitoneum, dehydration and renal failure
* Dogs with pancreatitis may have increased amylase and lipase, but these are not specific findings and are not helpful in cats. Serum canine and feline pancreatic lipase immunoreactivity (cPLI or fPLI) can be measured with a patient-side SNAP® test and a commercial Spec cPL® or fPL® test. These tests are currently the most sensitive tests for the diagnosis of pancreatitis. A positive SNAP® test should be followed by a cPL® or fPL® test to help confirm the diagnosis and aid in monitoring pancreatitis.

A coagulation panel should be performed in patients with unexplained haemorrhage or bruising and in patients with sepsis.

Abdominocentesis

A single needle (20–22 G) can be aseptically inserted 1–3 cm caudal to the umbilicus on the midline with the patient standing or in lateral recumbency (Figure 18.3).

> **PRACTICAL TIP**
>
> It is best to have the needle attached to a syringe if radiographs have not been taken prior to abdominocentesis, because free air can enter the abdomen through an open needle. This free air may be mistaken for free air introduced into the abdomen by rupture of a hollow viscus on radiographs taken later

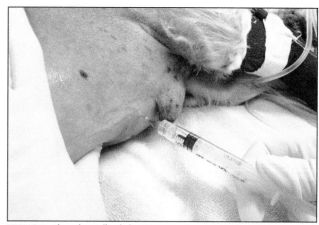

18.3 Closed-needle abdominocentesis prevents free air from entering the abdomen (which might make it difficult to interpret abdominal radiographs later).

Inserting a needle in each of the four quadrants of the ventral abdomen (right and left, cranial and caudal) may increase diagnostic yield. It has been reported that there must be at least 5–6 ml of fluid per kilogram bodyweight in the abdomen to obtain fluid via abdominocentesis. If a patient with peritonitis is dehydrated, rehydration will often result in an increased abdominal fluid volume and a positive abdominocentesis. Abdominal ultrasonography can be useful to guide aspiration of localized collections of fluid. If abdominocentesis is negative but there is still a high suspicion of peritonitis, diagnostic peritoneal lavage (DPL) is indicated.

Diagnostic peritoneal lavage

For DPL, a multi-fenestrated peritoneal lavage catheter can be used (Figure 18.4). The patient should be sedated and placed in dorsal or lateral recumbency. Local anaesthetic agents are injected 2 cm caudal to the umbilicus on the midline. The catheter is inserted into the abdomen in a caudal direction through a stab incision in the skin. The stylet is removed and, if no fluid is retrieved, warmed sterile 0.9% saline (15–20 ml/kg) is infused through the catheter. The animal is rolled from side to side and a collection system attached to the catheter is then placed ventral to the patient to collect fluid by gravity flow. Alternatively, a 16–20 G over-the-needle catheter with additional holes cut in it can be used to infuse the fluid. The fluid is allowed to dwell for a few minutes while the patient is gently rolled and then abdominocentesis is performed to collect the fluid for analysis.

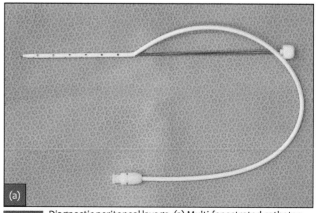

18.4 Diagnostic peritoneal lavage. (a) Multi-fenestrated catheter with trocar. (continues) ▶

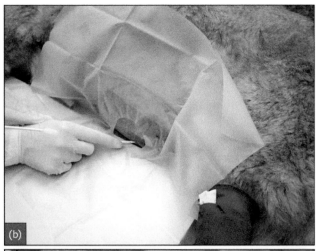

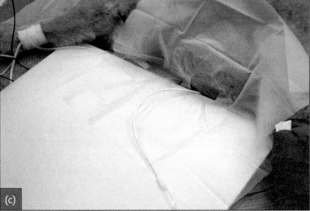

18.4 (continued) Diagnostic peritoneal lavage. (b) The catheter is placed aseptically into the abdomen after tranquillization and local anaesthesia. Fluid is infused via the catheter. (c) The catheter is connected to a collecting system after the patient has been rolled from side to side. This type of catheter can also be used to drain the abdomen of patients with uroperitoneum.

Abdominal fluid evaluation

Immediate cytological evaluation is performed on fluid that is retrieved by routine abdominocentesis or DPL (Figure 18.5). Fluid should also be submitted for analysis and bacterial culture and sensitivity testing. Additional fluid can be saved for chemical analysis. Samples that have been collected by DPL will be diluted, which may affect the results of fluid and chemical analysis.

> **WARNING**
>
> The presence of intracellular bacteria and degenerate neutrophils (Figure 18.6) in any fluid retrieved from the abdomen indicates septic peritonitis and immediate exploratory surgery is warranted

A large number of extracellular bacteria without neutrophils indicates that the needle may have penetrated the GI tract, and abdominocentesis should be repeated carefully. Patients with non-septic effusions usually have <13,000 nucleated cells/μl in the abdominal fluid. Green, yellow or brown pigment within macrophages or seen extracellularly is diagnostic for bile peritonitis.

In addition to abdominal fluid cytology, septic peritonitis can also be diagnosed by measuring the fluid glucose concentration. Patients with septic peritonitis would be expected to have a decrease in abdominal fluid glucose, because of glucose utilization by bacteria and phagocytic cells. One study demonstrated that all patients with septic peritonitis had an abdominal fluid glucose concentration that was less than the peripheral blood glucose concentration. This study showed a diagnostic accuracy of 100% in dogs and 92% in cats if the glucose concentration of the blood was 1.1 mmol/l greater than the glucose concentration of the fluid (Bonczynski *et al.*, 2003). In order for this test to be accurate, abdominal fluid and blood samples should be collected simultaneously and prior to intravenous glucose supplementation. This test is not reliable for patients with haemoperitoneum. A false negative may occur in patients with an acute onset of contamination, or a localized infection. This author has found that patients with gastric perforation due to ulceration may have a false-negative result, possibly due to the low number of bacteria present in the stomach or the containment of contamination by omentum.

Studies have also evaluated the accuracy of abdominal fluid lactate concentration for the diagnosis of septic peritonitis. The abdominal fluid lactate concentration would be expected to be higher in the fluid than in the blood, owing to neutrophilic glycolysis and bacterial metabolites. When a large number of patients with peritoneal effusions were evaluated, comparing the fluid lactate concentration to the blood lactate concentration was not found to be as accurate as the fluid glucose concentration for diagnosing septic peritonitis in dogs and cats (Levin *et al.*, 2004).

The cause of a chemical peritonitis can be determined by comparing abdominal fluid concentrations with blood concentrations.

- The bilirubin concentration of the effusion in patients with bile peritonitis is consistently higher than the serum concentration; however, the bilirubin concentration of the fluid may not be higher in cases of ruptured gallbladder mucocele, owing to localization of the congealed bile.
- In cases of uroabdomen, the fluid potassium and creatinine concentrations should be higher than serum concentrations.

Radiography

Abdominal radiographs should initially be evaluated for radiopaque foreign objects, organ enlargement, organ malposition, evidence of free or intraparenchymal air, or effusion.

- *Organ enlargement* may result from neoplasia, abscessation or torsion.
- *Organ malposition* may occur due to displacement by neoplastic masses, torsion, volvulus or herniation.
- *Free abdominal air* is associated with rupture of a hollow viscus or penetrating injury.
- *Intraparenchymal air* can be associated with organ necrosis, abscessation and gas-producing bacteria.

> **WARNING**
>
> Young or emaciated patients may have poor abdominal detail on radiographs, due to the lack of intra-abdominal fat, which can be mistaken for abdominal effusion

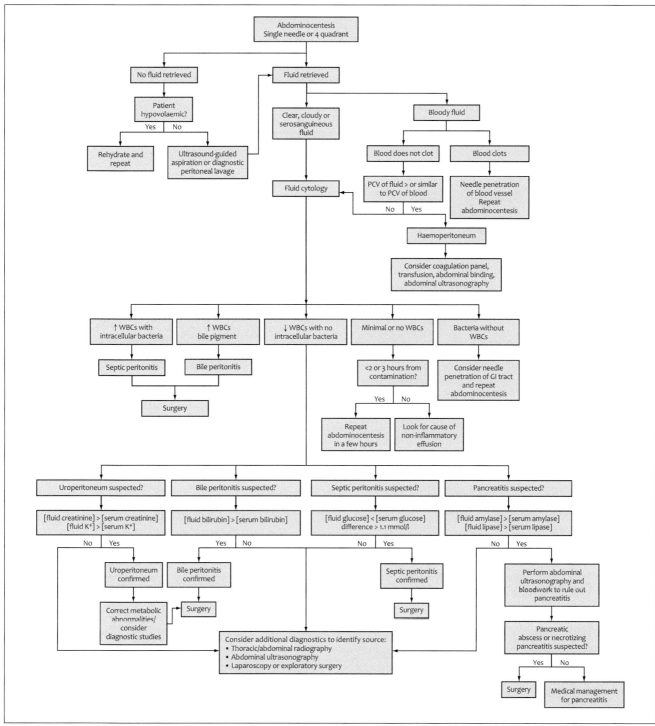

18.5 Diagnostic plan for fluid obtained by abdominocentesis. Peritonitis is present if lavage fluid contains >2 x 10⁹ nucleated cells/l in patients without prior abdominal surgery or >9 x 10⁹ nucleated cells/l in postsurgical patients. Diagnostic peritoneal lavage will dilute the sample, which may affect the results of fluid and chemical analysis. GI = gastrointestinal; PCV = packed cell volume, WBC = white blood cell.

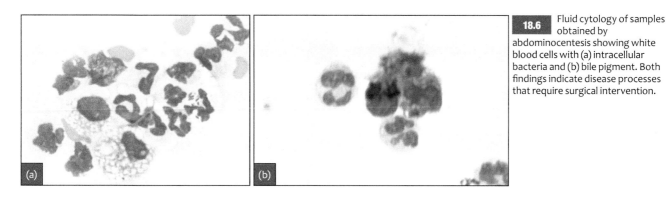

18.6 Fluid cytology of samples obtained by abdominocentesis showing white blood cells with (a) intracellular bacteria and (b) bile pigment. Both findings indicate disease processes that require surgical intervention.

Effusion is indicated by poor serosal detail. Loss of detail may be localized to the affected organ. For example, poor detail confined to the right cranial abdominal quadrant with lateral displacement of a gas-filled descending duodenum is indicative of pancreatitis. Poor detail or streaking of the retroperitoneum may be associated with haemorrhage (from a ruptured adrenal or kidney mass, or trauma) or urine leakage (from a damaged kidney or ureter). Free abdominal air and intraparenchymal air are important findings that indicate the need for exploratory surgery (Figure 18.7). It is important to determine whether abdominocentesis has been performed with an open needle prior to radiography, or if there is a history of surgery within 30 days of abdominal radiography, because these procedures will result in the appearance of free air within the abdomen that is not pathological.

The intestinal tract should be evaluated for evidence of bowel obstruction or plication. Diffuse intestinal distension is often associated with ileus and is not specific for peritonitis. Multiple severely dilated intestinal loops with abdominal effusion suggests an intestinal volvulus (Figure 18.8).

> **PRACTICAL TIP**
>
> Focal distension of an intestinal loop (intestinal diameter more than twice the width of the rib in dogs or >12 mm diameter in cats) is an indication of obstruction

Additional diagnostic imaging

After initial radiographic evaluation, the need for additional imaging may become apparent (see the *BSAVA Manual of Canine and Feline Abdominal Imaging*). GI contrast studies (preferably using water-soluble iodinated contrast medium), excretory urography, cystourethrography or ultrasonography are indicated, depending on the potential diagnosis. Thoracic radiographs are also often indicated in these patients to evaluate for the presence of traumatic injuries, pleural effusion or metastatic disease. Bicavitary effusion (pleural and peritoneal) can result from trauma, neoplasia, disseminated intravascular coagulopathy, heart failure, infection, pancreatitis, bile peritonitis and severe hypoproteinaemia.

Abdominal ultrasonography can be used to identify neoplastic masses and abscessed organs. Intestinal intussusception and obstruction related to foreign bodies may also be detected with ultrasonography. Small volumes of fluid (4 ml/kg) that may not have been detected on plain radiographs can be visualized and often aspirated by a skilled ultrasonographer. Localized fluid accumulation may be associated with the underlying disease (e.g. pancreatitis, biliary rupture). A distended gallbladder, immobile stellate or finely striated bile patterns, or gas in the gallbladder are signs of a gallbladder mucocele or necrotizing cholecystitis. Gallbladder wall discontinuity on ultrasound examination indicates rupture (Figure 18.9). Abdominal ultrasonography will, in skilled hands, aid in the diagnosis of pancreatitis without biopsy.

Computed tomography is a common imaging modality used in human patients for the diagnosis of intra-abdominal abscesses, but cost and availability have historically limited its usefulness in veterinary patients.

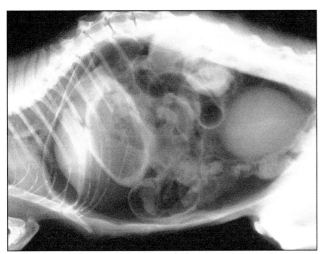

18.7 Lateral abdominal radiograph showing pneumoperitoneum. Note the free air. If this patient has not had recent surgery, penetrating trauma or open-needle abdominocentesis, exploratory surgery is indicated.

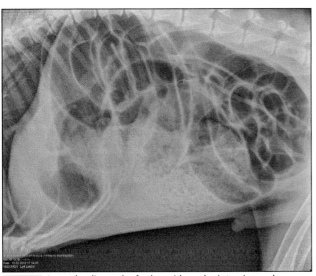

18.8 Lateral radiograph of a dog with a colonic torsion and peritonitis. All bowel loops are severely dilated and the extremely distended colon is seen ventrally. Poor serosal detail is related to abdominal effusion. This radiograph indicates the need for immediate surgical exploration.

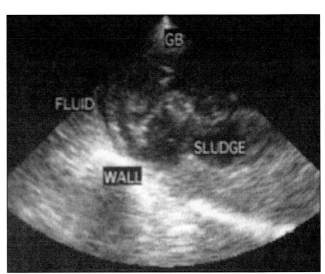

18.9 Abdominal ultrasonogram of the gallbladder (GB). The striated bile pattern and fluid outside the gallbladder wall are indicative of a ruptured gallbladder mucocele.

Preoperative treatment

Initial treatment of peritonitis involves providing haemodynamic support. Large volumes of fluid are lost into the abdominal cavity, and fluid replacement with crystalloids and/or colloids is essential (Figure 18.10). Fluid boluses are given and the patient is assessed after each bolus for response to therapy. Methods for monitoring fluid therapy range from basic parameters such as physical examination to more invasive parameters such as central venous pressure. There are several suggested resuscitation endpoint goals (Figure 18.11).

If hypotension is not corrected with adequate fluid replacement, vasopressors and/or inotropes should be used. Blood transfusions or blood substitutes may be required if the patient is anaemic. If coagulation abnormalities are present, fresh frozen plasma or whole blood should be given. Electrolytes should also be carefully monitored, because anorexic and vomiting animals may become severely hypokalaemic. Conversely, animals with acute renal failure or uroabdomen may have life-threatening hyperkalaemia that will require treatment.

Antibiotic therapy should be started as soon as there is a suspicion of septic peritonitis and should not be delayed

Fluid or drug	Indications for use	Dose
Isotonic crystalloids		
Plasma-Lyte®A, Normosol®-R, lactated Ringer's	Maintenance fluid therapy or to treat hypovolaemia	*Maintenance:* • Dogs: 60–90 ml/kg/day • Cats: 40–60 ml/kg/day *Dehydration:* % dehydration x weight (kg) = litres of fluid to add to maintenance rate* *Shock:* Give 10–30 ml/kg bolus for dogs or 5–15 ml/kg bolus for cats then reassess volume status. Repeat bolus administration up to the total daily maintenance dose (= one blood volume) given in 1 hour. Also combine with colloid bolus
Hypertonic crystalloids		
Hypertonic saline (7.5%)	Low volume resuscitation for shock	Bolus given over 10 min at dose of: • Dogs: 4–8 ml/kg • Cats: 1–4 ml/kg Follow with crystalloid or colloid
Colloid solutions		
Hetastarch, Dextran 70, Vetstarch™	For low volume resuscitation or hypoproteinaemia Total protein <35 g/l Albumin <25 g/l Colloid osmotic pressure <15 mmHg	*Maintenance:* • Dogs: 20 ml/kg/day • Cats: 15 ml/kg/day *Shock:* Give 5 ml bolus for dogs and cats and reassess volume status/perfusion parameters. Repeat bolus administration up to total daily maintenance dose in 1 hour
Haemoglobin glutamer-200	Packed cell volume (PCV) <25%	15 ml/kg at rate of 5 ml/kg/h
Albumin – canine (CSA) or human (HSA)	Albumin <20 g/l	• CSA: 800 mg/kg CSA as a 5% solution over 6 hours • HSA: 5% HSA at 2 ml/kg/h for 10 hours/day
Blood products		
Plasma	Coagulopathy	10 ml/kg i.v. given over 4–6 hours
Whole blood	Anaemia (PCV <25%) with coagulopathy; or >10% of blood volume loss	• Dogs: 20–25 ml/kg • Cats: 10 ml/kg Or: 2.2 ml of blood/kg bodyweight will increase PCV by 1%
Packed red blood cells	Anaemia (PCV <25%) with normal coagulation parameters	½ of dose calculated for whole blood
Inotropic and pressor agents		
	Systolic blood pressure <90 mmHg; or mean blood pressure <60 mmHg with normovolaemia and/or cardiac dysfunction	
Dopamine	Improves cardiac contractility and causes vasoconstriction Effects on alpha and beta receptors	5–20 µg/kg/min Vasoconstriction at rate >7 µg/kg/min
Dobutamine	Improves cardiac contractility Effects on beta receptors	5–20 µg/kg/min
Noradrenaline (norepinephrine)	Causes vasoconstriction Effects on alpha receptors	0.05–2 µg/kg/min
Fluid additives		
Potassium chloride	Potassium <3.5 mmol/l	0.125–0.25 mmol/kg/h i.v.
Glucose	Glucose <3.3 mmol/l	Bolus 0.5 g/kg diluted with crystalloid 2.5% or 5% constant infusion

18.10 Fluid therapy and drugs for dogs and cats with peritonitis. * Fluid boluses are usually given until the patient is stable and then the patient is maintained on 1.5 to 2 x maintenance fluids after surgery.

Parameter	Endpoint goal
Mucous membrane colour	Pink
Capillary refill time	1–2 seconds
Heart rate	Dogs: 80–120 beats/min Cats: 160–200 beats/min
Arterial blood pressure	Mean: >60 mmHg Systolic: ≥90 mmHg
Central venous pressure	5–10 cmH$_2$O
Packed cell volume	25–45%
Total protein	>35 g/l
Colloid osmotic pressure	15–20 mmHg
Lactate	<2.5 mmol/l
Core temperature	38–39.2°C
Urinary output	1–2 ml/kg/h
S$_a$O$_2$/P$_a$O$_2$	>95%/>80 mmHg

18.11 Resuscitation endpoint goals. P_aO_2 = partial pressure of oxygen; S_aO_2 = arterial oxygen saturation.

for collection of samples for culture. Ideally, a protocol is established to allow for antibiotic administration within 1–2 hours of the diagnosis of septic peritonitis (Abelson *et al.*, 2013). In humans with peritonitis, immediate adequate antibiotic therapy has been found to give the most profound decrease in mortality. The antibiotics chosen should be broad spectrum and based on the most likely types of organism involved (see Postoperative treatment below).

As soon as dehydration has been corrected and adequate perfusion has been restored, the patient with septic peritonitis should immediately be taken to surgery to correct the source of peritoneal contamination. Patients with uroabdomen should not be rushed to surgery until their metabolic derangements (hyperkalaemia and acidosis) have been corrected. A catheter (DPL catheter or large-gauge catheter with multiple fenestrations) can be placed into the peritoneal cavity, secured to the skin and attached to a collection system to provide evacuation of urine while the patient is given intravenous fluids. Abdominal lavage through the catheter is not necessary, because the intravenous fluids will dilute the urine that is leaking into the abdomen. Concurrent catheterization of the urinary bladder will keep the bladder decompressed to reduce urine flow into the abdomen. Hyperkalaemia (potassium >7–8 mmol/l) can result in abnormalities on electrocardiography, including peaked T waves, widening of the QRS complex, flattening and eventual loss of the P wave, atrial standstill, ventricular fibrillation and asystole. Recommended therapy to correct hyperkalaemia includes fluid diuresis and regular insulin (0.5–1 IU/kg i.v.) with concurrent administration of glucose (1–2 IU/g of insulin i.v. in addition to a continuous rate infusion of 2.5% dextrose). Intravenous calcium gluconate (0.5 ml/kg slow i.v. bolus) can be given for its cardioprotective effects if conduction disturbances are present. Sodium bicarbonate (0.5–1 mmol/kg) can be administered slowly as an intravenous bolus to correct severe metabolic acidosis (pH <7.2). As soon as the patient's hypovolaemia, metabolic acidosis and hyperkalaemia have been corrected, diagnostic tests (positive contrast cystourethrography or excretory urography) should be performed to determine the site of urine leakage, and the patient can be taken to surgery.

Surgical treatment

The main goal of surgery is to find and correct the source of contamination. In most patients, this can be accomplished in one procedure; however, some patients may benefit from planned repeat laparotomy (i.e. damage control surgery is performed initially). If the procedure required to provide definitive control of the source of peritonitis is time-consuming in an unstable patient, or in one that becomes destabilized during surgery, the abdomen is lavaged, perforations in leaking organs are rapidly closed and the patient is recovered and stabilized. Definitive corrective surgery is performed 1–5 days later, once the patient has been stabilized. A potential advantage of this technique is that it allows time for a clear demarcation to be established between healthy and devitalized tissue, which will facilitate surgical decision-making when determining how much tissue needs to be resected. Lavage has been recommended to help in the removal of foreign debris and to decrease the bacterial load and endotoxin concentration.

- Patients with a localized peritonitis may only need lavage of the affected area.
- Patients with generalized peritonitis will benefit from lavage of the entire abdomen with *large* volumes (from 500 ml to several litres, depending on the size of the animal) of sterile isotonic fluid.

Adding antiseptics and antibiotics to the lavage fluid is not currently recommended. All lavage fluid should be aspirated from the peritoneal cavity prior to closure, because fluid accumulation promotes bacterial proliferation and impairs bacterial phagocytosis. A sample of the abdominal fluid should be collected for bacterial culture and sensitivity testing. Although the goal of lavage is to decrease the number and concentration of bacteria present, one study was not able to demonstrate a significant difference between pre-lavage and post-lavage culture samples (Swayne *et al.*, 2012). Sample handling and timing of antimicrobial administration are likely to have an effect on culture results. Ideally, samples for culture should be obtained as soon as possible (i.e. fluid collected aseptically prior to surgery by abdominocentesis or upon entering the abdomen). If there is concern that contamination has occurred during surgery, post-lavage samples may be helpful. Regardless of when the samples are collected, antibiotic administration should not be delayed.

Abdominal drainage

Whether or not to provide postoperative abdominal drainage is controversial. The peritoneal membrane and omentum have the capacity to absorb large amounts of fluid and therefore the need for postoperative drainage is questionable.

PRACTICAL TIP

Preserve the omentum if possible. However, if the omentum is necrotic or heavily contaminated, omentectomy may be necessary

One retrospective study of dogs and cats with septic peritonitis failed to show a significant increase in survival rate for patients treated with open abdominal drainage *versus* those treated with primary closure (Staatz *et al.*, 2002). In human medicine, open abdominal drainage has been associated with higher morbidity and mortality rates and therefore it has been recommended to close the abdomen unless the source of contamination cannot be completely controlled, multiple surgeries are anticipated or it is not physically possible to close the abdomen. Criteria for deciding when to provide postoperative abdominal drainage in animals have not been defined, but indications may be similar to those for human patients.

If abdominal drainage is performed, open abdominal drainage (OAD) has been shown experimentally to be the most efficient method in small animals (see Operative Technique 18.1). It is more effective than Penrose drains or sump drains, which rely on gravity for drainage and rapidly become occluded with fibrin and omentum. However, the disadvantages of OAD include massive fluid and protein loss, increased nursing care and cost, enteric fistula formation, incisional hernia, evisceration, adhesion of abdominal viscera to the bandage and the need for a second surgery to close the abdomen.

Closed suction drains (most commonly Jackson–Pratt drains) have been reported to provide effective abdominal drainage (Mueller *et al.*, 2001). The drains in this report did not become occluded in any patient during the course of treatment (up to 8 days), which was probably related to drain number and placement (see Operative Technique 18.2). Advantages of this technique include ease of management and monitoring of abdominal fluid quantity and quality. A disadvantage is that the presence of the drain itself will result in some fluid production and it provides a route for ascending infection.

Vacuum-assisted drainage involves the application of pressure (50–150 mmHg) to the abdomen after the abdominal incision has been left partially open and covered (see Operative Technique 18.3). This technique has been reported to increase local blood flow and accelerate granulation tissue formation (Cioffi *et al.*, 2012). Potential advantages of this technique are that the pressure applied to the drainage tubing can be controlled and the abdominal incision is left open, which may result in more effective drainage of the peritoneal cavity than closed suction drains. In addition, it allows for collection of the drainage fluid and less frequent bandage changes than are required with OAD. However, like OAD, nosocomial infection and hypoproteinaemia are serious potential complications and a second procedure is required to close the abdomen.

> **WARNING**
>
> All patients with abdominal drainage, regardless of technique, are at risk of nosocomial contamination and hypoproteinaemia

Postoperative treatment

Fluids and electrolytes

Patients with peritonitis are usually critically ill and prone to many postoperative complications. Hypovolaemia and hypoproteinaemia result from loss of fluid and protein into the abdominal fluid, bandage or drain. Serial measurements of central venous pressure, blood pressure, bodyweight, urine specific gravity and urinary output can be used to determine the need for additional fluids. The goals of fluid therapy after surgery are the same as those prior to surgery.

Patients being treated with abdominal drainage should have the amount drained from the abdomen quantified daily and replaced intravenously. Usually patients will initially need a fluid rate that is ≥2 times maintenance requirements after surgery. Colloids should be provided at a maintenance rate if the total protein is <35 g/l or colloid osmotic pressure (COP) is <15 mmHg.

Hypoalbuminaemia should be treated with early nutritional support (see below). Plasma administration is often not a practical treatment for hypoalbuminaemia, because it takes 20 ml/kg of plasma to increase serum albumin by 0.5 g/dl and plasma transfusions are expensive. Canine-specific albumin may be available for transfusion, and when given at a dose of 800 mg/kg (reconstituted in 0.9% NaCl to yield a 5% solution) i.v. over 6 hours, it has been shown to increase albumin concentration and COP with minimal adverse reactions (Craft and Powell, 2012). Other colloid solutions should not be administered during albumin transfusion, and the patient should be monitored for transfusion reactions during administration (i.e. facial swelling, urticaria, pruritus, increased heart rate/respiratory rate or temperature and vomiting or diarrhea). The use of human serum albumin (HSA) has been reported, owing to a lack of available animal products; however, the infusion of a 25% solution has been associated with severe immediate and delayed anaphylactoid reactions (Trow *et al.*, 2008). Dilution of HSA to a 5 or 10% solution may be preferable. One study using 5% HSA at 2 ml/kg/h (total volume of 20 ml/kg/day) showed no severe adverse reactions (Vigano *et al.*, 2010).

Hypotension can be seen postoperatively and should initially be treated with volume loading. If a patient is normovolaemic but is still hypotensive, therapy should be directed towards myocardial depression and decreased systemic vascular resistance. Dobutamine and dopamine are the most commonly used inotropic agents (see Figure 18.10). Agents that have effects on alpha-adrenergic receptors cause vasoconstriction and should only be used at doses that will increase blood pressure enough to improve tissue blood flow. Excessive vasoconstriction will result in organ hypoxia. Hypotension that is *refractory* to fluid and vasopressor therapy may be related to relative adrenal insufficiency, characterized by a normal basal serum cortisol concentration but an inadequate response to adrenocorticotropic hormone (ACTH) administration. In one case report, the administration of dexamethasone (0.08 mg/kg i.v.) to a cat suffering from trauma and possible sepsis resulted in a rapid improvement in blood pressure that had been refractory to treatment with fluids and vasopressors (Durkan *et al.*, 2007). If glucocorticoids are to be given to patients with peritonitis, high doses should be avoided because of the risk of immunosuppression and GI complications.

Patients may become hypokalaemic and hypoglycaemic from decreased intake of nutrients and increased losses from vomiting or sepsis. Electrolytes and blood glucose should be monitored daily, and intravenous and oral supplementation can be used to correct any abnormalities. Excessive glucose supplementation should be avoided because of the potential negative effects of hyperglycaemia. Anaemia is commonly seen after surgery and may be related to blood loss at surgery or due to disseminated intravascular coagulation. Monitoring should include at least daily measurements of packed cell volume and total protein.

Ileus, gastric ulceration and bacterial translocation may be seen postoperatively in patients with peritonitis. Treatment with a combination of antiemetics, gastroprotectants (sucralfate) and antacids (histamine H2 receptor antagonists and proton pump inhibitors) is often indicated.

Antibiotics

Combination antibiotics are recommended in patients with septic peritonitis. Ampicillin (22 mg/kg i.v. q8h) or ampicillin/sulbactam (30 mg/kg i.v. q8h) may be used in conjunction with enrofloxacin (10 mg/kg i.v. q24h) or an aminoglycoside (amikacin at 15 mg/kg i.v. q24h or gentamicin at 6 mg/kg i.v. q24h) to provide the best spectrum of coverage. Aminoglycosides should only be used if there is no evidence of pre-existing renal disease and the patient is hydrated. Metronidazole (15 mg/kg i.v. q12h) or clindamycin (12 mg/kg i.v. q12h) should be used if additional anaerobic coverage is needed. Alternatively, a third-generation cephalosporin (cefotaxime 20–80 mg/kg i.v. q8h) can be used as a single agent. Antibiotic treatment should be modified once culture results are available.

> **Editors' note:**
>
> In the UK ampicillin/sulbactam is not available and the first-line use of enrofloxacin and third-generation cephalosporins is discouraged because of the risk of development of multi-drug resistance. Suitable alternatives would be clavulanic acid potentiated amoxicillin (co-amoxiclav) at 25 mg/kg i.v. q8h or cefuroximine at 30 mg/kg i.v. q8h

Additional postoperative monitoring

> **PRACTICAL TIP**
>
> Critically ill patients should have platelet counts and coagulation parameters evaluated daily, because of the risk of developing disseminated intravascular coagulation

Patients with septic peritonitis are at risk of developing acute respiratory distress syndrome (ARDS). In addition, patients with peritonitis are often depressed and vomiting, which puts them at risk of aspiration pneumonia. Careful lung auscultation should be performed at least twice daily in all patients. Hypoxaemia can be monitored by pulse oximetry or, ideally, arterial blood gas analysis when there is suspicion of respiratory compromise.

Cardiac arrhythmias may also be seen postoperatively due to hypovolaemia, electrolyte disturbances and hypoxia. Electrocardiography is indicated if an abnormal heart rhythm is auscultated or pulses are not synchronous with heart sounds. Initial treatment should involve controlling pain, hypoxia and electrolyte imbalances. Anti-arrhythmics are only used after extracardiac causes of arrhythmias have been eliminated and only if the arrhythmias are adversely affecting perfusion.

Analgesia

Analgesia is required to keep the patient comfortable and to avoid the negative effects of sympathetic stimulation on cardiovascular function. Tachycardia, tachypnoea, hypertension, restlessness, vocalization and depression can be indications of pain. Butorphanol (0.2–0.4 mg/kg i.m., i.v. q2–6h) or buprenorphine (0.005–0.04 mg/kg i.m., i.v. q4–8h) can be used to control pain in severely compromised patients, because these drugs do not result in as much bradycardia and respiratory depression as other narcotics. Morphine, methadone, oxymorphone, hydromorphone and

fentanyl can be used in stable patients for more potent pain relief. A combination of drugs can also be given as a continuous rate infusion: morphine (0.05–0.2 mg/kg/h), lidocaine (2–4 mg/kg/h) and ketamine (0.2–0.6 mg/kg/h) can be used in dogs, and fentanyl (2–4 μg/kg/h) and ketamine (0.05–0.2 mg/kg/h) in cats (see the *BSAVA Manual of Canine and Feline Anaesthesia and Analgesia*).

Nutrition

Nutritional support is a must for the postoperative care of patients with peritonitis (see the *BSAVA Manual of Canine and Feline Emergency and Critical Care*). A recent study reported that early nutritional support was associated with a decreased length of hospitalization in dogs with septic peritonitis (Lui *et al.*, 2012). Surgery produces a hypermetabolic state in these patients, who are often anorexic and malnourished. This contributes to delayed wound healing and impaired immune defences. Losses of fluid, electrolytes and proteins continue after surgery. In addition, hypoalbuminaemia is one of the factors that can be associated with intestinal dehiscence. Enteral nutrition is preferred to parenteral nutrition to decrease bacterial translocation and secondary sepsis. Animals that will not eat or accept syringe feeding should be tube fed.

> **PRACTICAL TIP**
>
> The need for a feeding tube should be anticipated during surgery and it should be placed so that the maximum amount of the GI tract is used

If the patient cannot tolerate anaesthesia, a naso-oesophageal tube should be placed. If anaesthesia is tolerated, an oesophageal tube or gastrostomy tube should be placed, because a larger-bore tube can be used (allowing for slurry diets and less clogging) and these tubes are better tolerated by the patient (see the *BSAVA Manual of Canine and Feline Emergency and Critical Care*). For comatose patients and for patients with pancreatitis, frequent vomiting or gastric outflow obstruction, the feeding tube should be placed distal to the pylorus. This can be achieved by surgical placement of a jejunostomy or gastro-jejunostomy tube (Figure 18.12).

Caloric requirements for patients >2 kg bodyweight (BW) can be calculated by the formula for resting energy requirement (RER):

$$RER\ (kcal/day) = 30 \times BW\ (kg) + 70$$

Feeding is started at one-third to one-quarter of the RER as a bolus, with the total volume divided over four to six feedings per day. The tube is flushed before and after each feeding. The volume fed is gradually increased over 3–4 days until the maintenance requirement is reached. Patients with a jejunostomy tube should be fed with a constant infusion of food to avoid the cramping and discomfort associated with bolus feeding.

Prognosis

Survival rates that have been reported for patients with peritonitis range from 32% to 80%. Development of respiratory disease, disseminated intravascular coagulation, cardiovascular collapse and refractory hypotension have been associated with a negative outcome in dogs and

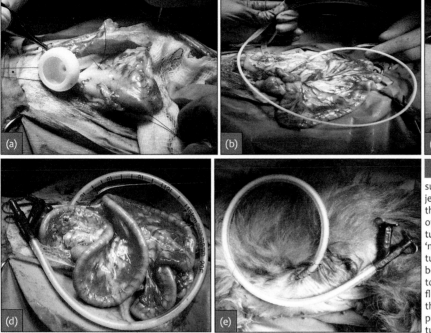

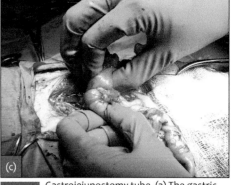

18.12 Gastrojejunostomy tube. (a) The gastric tube is placed through a purse-string suture in the body of the stomach. (b) The jejunostomy tube is measured so that 10–15 cm of the tube will be in the jejunum. (c) The external end of the stomach tube is cut off and the jejunostomy tube is placed through the stomach tube and 'milked' into the jejunum. (d) When the jejunostomy tube is in the jejunum, the stomach is sutured to the body wall around the gastric tube exit site. The port to the stomach tube can be used to evacuate air and fluid from the stomach while the patient is fed via the port to the jejunostomy tube. (e) When the patient can tolerate stomach feeding, the jejunal tube can be removed.

cats with septic peritonitis (King, 1994). A study of generalized peritonitis in patients treated by closed suction drainage found that postoperative hypotension was the only factor significantly different between patients that survived and patients that died (Mueller *et al.*, 2001). This study and another study of peritonitis resulting from gastroduodenal perforation showed a higher survival rate in dogs than in cats. A lower preoperative serum albumin concentration has been reported to be a poor prognostic indicator in dogs with peritonitis, whereas a high lactate concentration at the time of diagnosis may be an indication of a poor prognosis in cats (Parsons *et al.*, 2009; Craft and Powell, 2012).

The outcome may also be affected by the underlying cause of the peritonitis. Patients with intestinal dehiscence only have a 20–26% survival rate, with no difference in survival regardless of whether the peritonitis results from small intestinal or large intestinal leakage (Wylie and Hosgood, 1994). The prognosis for patients with bile peritonitis is affected by the presence of bacterial contamination. The survival rate for patients with a septic biliary effusion has been reported to be 27% to 45%, compared with 87% to 100% survival when the effusion is sterile (Ludwig *et al.*, 1997; Mehler *et al.*, 2004). Survival rates in patients with uroperitoneum range from 44% to 58% in dogs and up to 61.5% in cats (Stafford and Bartges, 2013). Mortality in these patients has been associated with concurrent injuries and a delay in diagnosis and treatment. The prognosis for cases of sclerosing encapsulating peritonitis (SEP) is generally poor. Major long-term management problems include chronic weight loss, progression of ascites and concurrent disease. Attempts to break down the fibrous membranes usually result in perforation of the intestinal wall, and treatment with antibiotics, corticosteroids and diuretics has been tried without success. Adjunctive therapy with tamoxifen is used in humans with SEP, and in a recent case report in the veterinary literature this showed some potential when used in combination with surgery (Etchepareborde *et al.*, 2010).

References and further reading

Abelson AL, Buckley GJ and Rozanski EA (2013) Positive impact of emergency department protocol on time to antimicrobial administration in dogs with septic peritonitis. *Journal of Veterinary Emergency and Critical Care* **23**, 551–556

Bonczynski JJ, Ludwig LL, Barton LJ, Loar A and Peterson ME (2003) Comparison of peritoneal fluid and peripheral blood pH, bicarbonate, glucose and lactate concentration as a diagnostic tool for septic peritonitis in dogs and cats. *Veterinary Surgery* **32**, 161–166

Bradford K, Meinkoth J, McKeirnen K and Love B (2013) Candida peritonitis in dogs: report of 5 cases. *Veterinary Clinical Pathology* **42**, 227–233

Cioffi KM, Schmiedt CW, Cornell KK *et al.* (2012) Retrospective evaluation of vacuum-assisted peritoneal drainage for the treatment of septic peritonitis in dogs and cats: 8 cases (2003–2010). *Journal of Veterinary Emergency and Critical Care* **22**, 601–609

Craft EM and Powell LL (2012) The use of canine-specific albumin in dogs with septic peritonitis. *Journal of Veterinary Emergency and Critical Care* **22**, 631–639

Durkan S, de Laforcade A, Rozanski E *et al.* (2007) Suspected relative adrenal insufficiency in a critically ill cat. *Journal of Veterinary Emergency and Critical Care* **17**, 197–201

Etchepareborde S, Heimann M, Cohen-Solal A and Hamaide A (2010) Use of tamoxifen in a German Shepherd Dog with sclerosing encapsulating peritonitis. *Journal of Small Animal Practice* **51**, 649–653

Hinton LE, McLoughlin MA, Johnson SE and Weisbrode SE (2002) Spontaneous gastroduodenal perforation in 16 dogs and seven cats (1982–1999). *Journal of the American Animal Hospital Association* **38**, 176–187

King LG (1994) Postoperative complications and prognostic indicators in dogs and cats with septic peritonitis: 23 cases (1989–1992). *Journal of the American Veterinary Medical Association* **204**, 407–414

King LG and Boag A (2007) *BSAVA Manual of Canine and Feline Emergency and Critical Care, 2nd edn.* BSAVA Publications, Gloucester

Levin GM, Bonczynski JJ, Ludwig LL *et al.* (2004) Lactate as a diagnostic test for septic peritoneal effusions in dogs and cats. *Journal of the American Animal Hospital Association* **40**, 364–371

Ludwig LL, McLoughlin MA, Graves TK and Crisp MS (1997) Surgical treatment of bile peritonitis in 24 dogs and 2 cats: a retrospective study (1987–1994). *Veterinary Surgery* **26**, 90–98

Lui DT, Brown DC and Silverstein DC (2012) Early nutritional support is associated with decreased length of hospitalization in dogs with septic peritonitis: a retrospective study of 45 cases (2000–2009). *Journal of Veterinary Emergency and Critical Care* **22**, 453–459

Mehler SJ, Mayhew PD, Drobatz KJ *et al.* (2004) Variables associated with outcome in dogs undergoing extrahepatic biliary surgery: 60 cases (1988–2002). *Veterinary Surgery* **33**, 644–649

Mueller MG, Ludwig LL and Barton LJ (2001) Use of closed-suction drains to treat generalized peritonitis in dogs and cats: 40 cases (1997–1999). *Journal of the American Veterinary Medical Association* **219**, 789–794

O'Brien R and Barr F (2009) *BSAVA Manual of Canine and Feline Abdominal Imaging*. BSAVA Publications, Gloucester

Parsons KJ, Owen LJ, Lee K *et al.* (2009) A retrospective study of surgically treated cases of septic peritonitis in the cat (2000–2007). *Journal of Small Animal Practice* **50**, 518–524

Pumphrey SA, Pirie CG and Rozanski EA (2011) Uveitis associated with septic peritonitis in a cat. *Journal of Veterinary and Emergency Critical Care* **21**, 279-284

Ralphs SC, Jesse CR and Lipowitz AJ (2003) Risk factors for leakage following intestinal anastomosis in dogs and cats: 115 cases (1991–2000). *Journal of the American Animal Hospital Association* **223**, 73–77

Rogers CL, Gibson C, Mitchell SI *et al.* (2009) Disseminated candidiasis secondary to fungal and bacterial peritonitis in a young dog. *Journal of Veterinary Emergency and Critical Care* **19**, 193–198

Seymour C and Duke-Novakovski T (2007) *BSAVA Manual of Canine and Feline Anaesthesia and Analgesia, 2nd edn.* BSAVA Publications, Gloucester

Staatz AJ, Monnet E and Seim HB (2002) Open peritoneal drainage versus primary closure for the treatment of septic peritonitis in dogs and cats: 42 cases (1993–1999). *Veterinary Surgery* **31**, 174–180

Stafford JR and Bartges JW (2013) A clinical review of pathophysiology, diagnosis, and treatment of uroabdomen in the dog and cat. *Journal of Veterinary Emergency and Critical Care* **23**, 216–219

Swayne SL, Brisson B, Weese JS *et al.* (2012) Evaluating the effect of intraoperative peritoneal lavage on bacterial culture in dogs with suspected septic peritonitis. *Canadian Veterinary Journal* **53**, 971–977

Trow AV, Rozanski EA, de Laforcade AM *et al.* (2008) Evaluation of use of human albumin in critically ill dogs: 73 cases (2003–2006). *Journal of the American Veterinary Medical Association* **233**, 607–612

Vigano F, Perissinotto L and Bosco VRF (2010) Administration of 5% human serum albumin in critically ill small animal patients with hypoalbuminemia: 418 dogs and 170 cats (1994–2008). *Journal of Veterinary Emergency and Critical Care* **20**, 237–243

Wylie KB and Hosgood G (1994) Mortality and morbidity of small and large intestinal surgery in dogs and cats: 74 cases (1980–1992). *Journal of the American Animal Hospital Association* **30**, 469–474

OPERATIVE TECHNIQUE 18.1

Open abdominal drainage

POSITIONING

Dorsal recumbency.

ASSISTANT

Not essential.

EQUIPMENT EXTRAS

Suction; large gauge (3 or 4 metric; 2/0 or 1/0 USP) monofilament non-absorbable suture material (polypropylene or nylon); sterile bandage material including:

- Petrolatum- or antibiotic-impregnated gauze (non-adherent contact layer)
- Laparotomy swabs (sponges) or gauze pads
- Roll cotton or cotton surgery towels
- Roll gauze
- Water-impermeable adhesive tape or additional gauze and co-adhesive tape.

SURGICAL TECHNIQUE

Approach

An abdominal incision is made on the ventral midline from the xiphoid process to the pubis to allow for complete abdominal exploration. The falciform fat is removed to improve exposure of the cranial abdomen and prevent obstruction of drainage.

Surgical manipulations

The source of the peritonitis is controlled by removal or closure of the source organ followed by copious lavage of the abdomen with warm sterile saline.

1   Remove as much fluid and necrotic debris as possible with suction. When the lavage solution appears clear on removal from the abdomen, flushing can be discontinued.

2   Preserve the omentum if possible and consider suturing it around the intestinal incisions with a few tacking sutures.

→ OPERATIVE TECHNIQUE 18.1 CONTINUED

3 Place a single layer of non-absorbable suture material in the external rectus fascia in a simple continuous pattern in the cranial two-thirds of the abdominal incision. The sutures should be placed loosely to create a gap of 3–6 cm in the body wall (depending on the size of the animal) that will allow for drainage. Each bite of the simple continuous pattern should be placed close to the next to prevent abdominal viscera or omentum from herniating through the open incision during the postoperative period.

4 Do not close the subcutaneous tissues or skin over the site of drainage, although some surgeons place a second loose suture layer in the skin, again leaving a 3–6 cm gap between the skin edges. The parapreputial incision in male dogs or the caudal one-third of the abdominal incision in females is closed routinely.

5 Place a sterile bandage over the open abdominal incision with bandage materials in the order listed above.

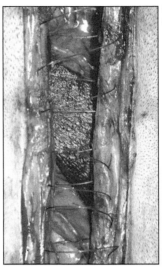

Open abdominal drainage incision.

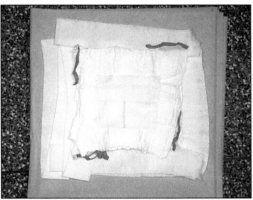

Preassembled sterile bandage that is placed over the open incision and secured to the patient with water-impermeable adhesive tape.

PRACTICAL TIP

In male dogs, a sterile urinary catheter should be placed and attached to a urine collection system to limit contamination of the bandage

---

POSTOPERATIVE MANAGEMENT

The bandage will initially need to be changed every 12 hours, or more frequently if it slips or becomes soaked with peritoneal fluid or soiled with urine or faeces. The patient may need to be sedated, but should be standing.

1 Preassemble the sterile bandage using sterile gloves, starting with the material that is farthest away from the patient's body and working towards the layer that will be in contact with the open incision.

2 Remove the old bandage and insert a sterile gloved finger into the open wound to break down adhesions blocking drainage.

3 Collect fluid aseptically for cytological examination and note the character of the draining fluid.

4 Place the preassembled sterile bandage over the open incision and secure it to the patient.

Editors' note:

There are several different ways to bandage an open abdomen. One of the editors [JN] prefers to place a sterile plastic sheet over the laparotomy swabs and sterile surgical towels (the plastic wrapping that comes around the laparotomy swabs is ideal) to help prevent strikethrough and ascending bacterial infection. The entire abdomen is then wrapped with padded bandage, conforming bandage and co-adhesive tape, rather than using water-impermeable tape

---

Drainage fluid quantity can be estimated from the appearance of the bandage or by weighing the bandage materials before application and after removal (1 g of weight gain = 1 ml of fluid). Daily bandage changes may be adequate after the first 24 hours.

→ **OPERATIVE TECHNIQUE 18.1 CONTINUED**

Wound closure

The patient is usually ready for abdominal closure within 3–5 days of the initial surgery. The decision to close the abdomen is based on an improvement in the patient's overall condition, a reduction in drainage fluid volume (bandage changes only needed once daily) and cytological evidence of resolution of the septic process (absence of bacteria, non-degenerative neutrophils).

1   With the patient under general anaesthesia, scrub the ventral abdomen for surgery, with a sterile sponge placed over the open incision to prevent soap from entering the peritoneal cavity.

2   Remove the sterile swab and continuous suture line from the open abdominal wound and submit a bacteriology swab from the abdominal cavity for culture.

3   Lavage the abdomen with warm sterile saline, which is completely aspirated after the final lavage.

The incision is closed routinely. If the patient is not improving clinically, the amount of peritoneal fluid is not decreasing after 3–5 days, or cytological examination of the abdominal fluid reveals continued (more than 3 days) or recurrent sepsis, full re-exploration of the abdominal cavity is indicated.

OPERATIVE TECHNIQUE 18.2

Closed suction drainage

POSITIONING

Dorsal recumbency.

ASSISTANT

Not essential.

EQUIPMENT EXTRAS

Jackson–Pratt drain (one for small dogs and cats, two for larger dogs); reservoir bulb(s); sterile bandage material.

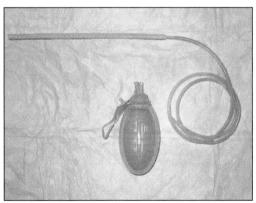

Closed suction drain (Jackson–Pratt drain with reservoir bulb).

SURGICAL TECHNIQUE

A thorough abdominal exploration is performed and the source of contamination is controlled. As much omentum as possible is preserved. The omentum is wrapped or sutured around any intestinal incisions. The abdominal cavity is copiously lavaged to remove gross contamination and all of the lavage fluid is aspirated from the abdominal cavity.

1   Make a paramedian stab incision near the cranial third of the incision and a second near the caudal third of the incision (cranial to the prepuce in male dogs).

→ **OPERATIVE TECHNIQUE 18.2 CONTINUED**

2   Insert two flat suction drains into the abdomen (one through each stab incision). Place the fenestrated portion of the cranial drain between the liver and diaphragm. Place the fenestrated portion of the caudal drain in the caudal abdomen along the ventral body wall. Placing the drains in this fashion decreases the likelihood that omentum will be able to occlude both drains. In patients weighing <5 kg, only the cranial drain between the liver and diaphragm is placed.

3   Secure the drain tubes to the skin with a purse-string suture and a Roman sandal suture.

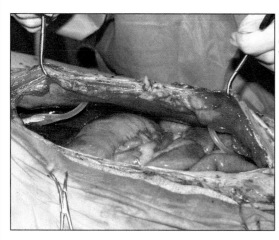

Placement of drains. The cranial drain is placed between the liver and diaphragm. The caudal drain is placed ventrally in the caudal abdomen.

Wound closure

The abdomen is closed routinely and the suction reservoir is attached to each flat suction drain. A vacuum is created by compressing the suction reservoir bulb. An abdominal bandage is placed with sterile bandage material in contact with the exit site of the drain tube.

POSTOPERATIVE MANAGEMENT

- The abdominal drain and suction reservoir are handled aseptically.
- The suction reservoir is emptied at 4–6 hour intervals and the volume of fluid is recorded.
- The abdominal bandage is changed daily to evaluate the abdominal incision and exit sites of the drains.
- Fluid is collected daily for cytological examination. The decision to remove the drains is based on a decrease in fluid production and cytological evidence that the fluid contains non-degenerative neutrophils without evidence of bacterial contamination.

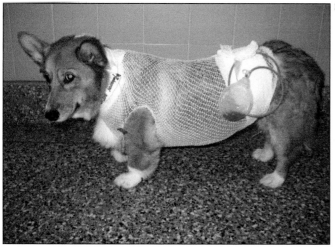

Postoperative bandage with drain.

Drains are usually removed between 3 and 5 days after the initial surgery. To remove the drains, the purse-string and Roman sandal sutures are removed, a sterile gauze swab (sponge) is placed over the exit site and traction is applied to the drain. There is no need to enlarge the exit site for removal, because the drains are soft and flexible. A sterile bandage is placed over the exit site for 12–24 hours after drain removal.

OPERATIVE TECHNIQUE 18.3

Vacuum-assisted peritoneal drainage

POSITIONING

Dorsal recumbency.

ASSISTANT

Not essential.

EQUIPMENT EXTRAS

Sterile open-cell reticulated polyurethane ether foam; sterile 14 Fr red rubber catheter; sterile suction tubing; sterile sealant drape; continuous suction unit; soft padded bandage material.

SURGICAL TECHNIQUE

A thorough abdominal exploration is performed and the source of contamination is controlled. As much omentum as possible is preserved. The omentum is wrapped or sutured around any intestinal incisions. The abdominal cavity is copiously lavaged to remove gross contamination and all of the lavage fluid is aspirated from the abdominal cavity.

1   Close the caudal half to two-thirds of the abdominal incision routinely in three layers.

2   Suture the cranial half to one-third of the linea alba in a loose, simple continuous pattern leaving a 1–5 cm wide gap between the edges. Place the sutures close together (approximately 1 cm apart) to prevent abdominal contents from herniating between the sutures. This closure is similar to that performed in Operative Technique 18.1.

3   Cut a piece of sterile polyethylene foam to fit over the partially open area of the incision and place a 14 Fr red rubber catheter into the foam. Place the foam with the catheter over the laparostomy.

4   Cover the ventral abdomen with a sterile sealant drape to completely cover the foam and red rubber catheter. An airtight seal should be formed.

5   Attach the red rubber catheter to sterile suction tubing and connect it to a suction unit. Turn on the vacuum to ensure an appropriate seal with no leaks. Maintain the suction at 125 mmHg.

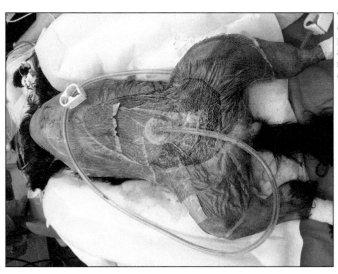

Vacuum-assisted peritoneal drainage. A catheter has been inserted into the foam and placed over the open portion of the abdominal incision. An adherent drape maintains an airtight seal. Sterile tubing connects the catheter to the suction unit.

POSTOPERATIVE MANAGEMENT

The bandage will need to be evaluated frequently (at least every 12 hours) for slippage, evidence of strikethrough or loss of the airtight seal. The bandage will need to be changed if this is seen. Drainage fluid should be monitored daily for volume collected. Fluid should also be submitted for cytological examination.

→ OPERATIVE TECHNIQUE 18.3 CONTINUED

Wound closure

The patient is usually ready for abdominal closure within 3–5 days of the initial surgery. The decision to close the abdomen is based on an improvement in the patient's overall condition, a reduction in drainage fluid volume and cytological evidence of resolution of the septic process (absence of bacteria, non-degenerative neutrophils).

1   With the patient under general anaesthesia, remove the soft padded bandage but leave the sterile sealant drape in place. Move the patient into the operating room and remove the sealant drape. Scrub the ventral abdomen for surgery, with a sterile sponge placed over the open incision to prevent soap from entering the peritoneal cavity. Use saline instead of alcohol during the surgical preparation.

2   Remove the sterile swab and continuous suture line from the open abdominal wound and submit a bacteriology swab from the abdominal cavity for culture.

3   Lavage the abdomen with warm sterile saline, which is completely aspirated after the final lavage. Perform an abdominal exploration to evaluate any intestinal incisions and drain any pockets of fluid.

The incision is closed routinely. If the patient is not improving clinically, the amount of peritoneal fluid is not decreasing after 3–5 days, or cytological examination of the abdominal fluid reveals continued (more than 3 days) or recurrent sepsis, full re-exploration of the abdominal cavity is indicated.

Index

Page numbers in *italics* indicate figures
Page numbers in **bold** indicate Operative Techniques

BSAVA Manual of Canine and Feline Abdominal Surgery, second edition. Edited by John M. Williams and Jacqui D. Niles. ©BSAVA 2015